Study Guide

CAMPBELL'S UROLOGY

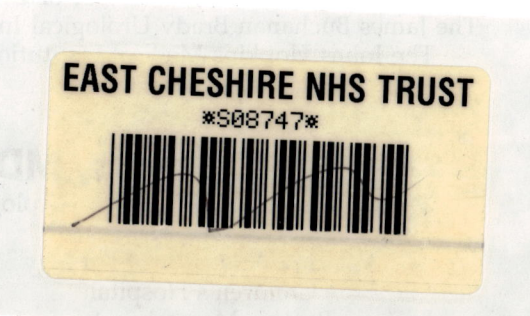

Editors

Alan B. Retik, MD
Professor of Surgery (Urology)
Harvard Medical School
Chief, Department of Urology
Children's Hospital
Boston, Massachusetts

E. Darracott Vaughan, Jr., MD
James J. Colt Professor of Urology
Weill Medical College of Cornell University
Chairman Emeritus
Department of Urology
The New York–Presbyterian Hospital
New York, New York

Alan J. Wein, MD
Professor and Chair, Division of Urology
University of Pennsylvania School of Medicine
Chief of Urology
University of Pennsylvania Health System
Philadelphia, Pennsylvania

Associate Editors

Louis R. Kavoussi, MD
Vice Chairman and Patrick C. Walsh Distinguished Professor of Urology
Director, Division of Endourology
The James Buchanan Brady Urological Institute
The Johns Hopkins Medical Institutions
Baltimore, Maryland

Andrew C. Novick, MD
Chairman, Urological Institute
The Cleveland Clinic Foundation
Professor of Surgery (Urology)
Ohio State University School of Medicine
Cleveland, Ohio

Alan W. Partin, MD, PhD
Bernard L. Schwartz Distinguished Professor of Urologic Oncology
The James Buchanan Brady Urological Institute
The Johns Hopkins Medical Institutions
Baltimore, Maryland

Craig A. Peters, MD
Associate Professor of Surgery (Urology)
Harvard Medical School
Associate Professor of Urology
Children's Hospital
Boston, Massachusetts

Study Guide

CAMPBELL'S UROLOGY

Second Edition

Editor-in-Chief

Patrick C. Walsh, MD

David Hall McConnell Professor
Director, Department of Urology
The Johns Hopkins University School of Medicine
Urologist-in-Chief
The James Buchanan Brady Urological Institute
The Johns Hopkins Medical Institutions
Baltimore, Maryland

W.B. SAUNDERS COMPANY
An Imprint of Elsevier Science
Philadelphia London Montreal New York St. Louis Sydney Tokyo Toronto

W.B. SAUNDERS COMPANY
An Imprint of Elsevier Science

The Curtis Center
Independence Square West
Philadelphia, Pennsylvania 19106

Copyright © 2002, 1998, Elsevier Science (USA)

All rights reserved. No part of this publication may be reproduced or transmitted in any form or by any means, electronic or mechanical, including photocopy, recording, or any information storage and retrieval system, without permission in writing from the publisher.

Notice

Medicine is an ever-changing field. Standard safety precautions must be followed, but as new research and clinical experience broaden our knowledge, changes in treatment and drug therapy may become necessary or appropriate. Readers are advised to check the most current product information provided by the manufacturer of each drug to be administered to verify the recommended dose, the method and duration of administration, and the contraindications. It is the responsibility of the treating physician, relying on experience and knowledge of the patient, to determine dosages and the best treatment for each individual patient. Neither the Publisher nor the editor assumes any liability for any injury and/or damage to persons or property arising from this publication.

The Publisher

Acquisitions Editor: Stephanie S. Donley
Developmental Editor: Hazel N. Hacker
Project Manager: Jennifer Ehlers
Designer: Karen O'Keefe-Owens

CAMPBELL'S UROLOGY STUDY GUIDE   ISBN 0-7216-9072-6

Printed in the United States of America

Last digit is the print number: 9 8 7 6 5 4 3 2 1

CONTRIBUTORS

MARK C. ADAMS, MD
Associate Professor of Urology and Pediatrics, Vanderbilt University School of Medicine, Nashville, Tennessee
Urinary Tract Reconstruction in Children

HAROLD J. ALFERT, MD
Department of Urology, The Johns Hopkins University School of Medicine; Assistant Professor, James Buchanan Brady Urological Institute, The Johns Hopkins Hospital, Baltimore, Maryland
Retropubic and Suprapubic Open Prostatectomy

RODNEY A. APPELL, MD
Professor of Urology, Baylor College of Medicine; F. Brantley Scott Chair, Department of Urology, St. Luke's Episcopal Hospital, Houston, Texas
Injection Therapy for Urinary Incontinence

ANTHONY ATALA, MD
Associate Professor of Surgery, Harvard Medical School; Director, Genitourinary Reconstruction Program, Associate in Surgery (Urology), Children's Hospital, Boston, Massachusetts
Vesicoureteral Reflux and Megaureter; Tissue Engineering Perspectives for Reconstructive Surgery

DAVID M. BARRETT, MD
Professor of Urology, Tufts University School of Medicine, Boston; CEO, Chairman, Board of Governors, and Senior Staff Consultant, Lahey Clinic, Burlington, Massachusetts
Implantation of the Artificial Genitourinary Sphincter

BRUCE J. BARRON, MD
Professor, University of Texas Medical School, Houston, Texas
Urinary Tract Imaging—Basic Principles

JOHN M. BARRY, MD
Head, Division of Urology and Division of Abdominal Organ Transplantation, Oregon Health and Science University; Staff Surgeon, University Hospital and Doernbecher Children's Hospital, Portland, Oregon
Renal Transplantation

STUART B. BAUER, MD
Professor of Surgery (Urology), Harvard Medical School; Senior Associate in Urology, Children's Hospital, Boston, Massachusetts
Anomalies of the Upper Urinary Tract; Voiding Dysfunction in Children: Neurogenic and Non-Neurogenic

CLAIR J. BEARD, MD
Assistant Professor of Radiation Oncology, Harvard Medical School; Co-Chair of Genitourinary Radiation Oncology, Brigham and Women's Hospital, Dana Farber Cancer Institute, Boston, Massachusetts
Radiation Therapy for Prostate Cancer

MARK F. BELLINGER, MD
Clinical Professor of Urology, University of Pittsburgh School of Medicine; Attending Physician, Children's Hospital of Pittsburgh, Pittsburgh, Pennsylvania
Abnormalities of the Testes and Scrotum and Their Surgical Management

MITCHELL C. BENSON, MD
George F. Cahill Professor of Urology, Columbia University College of Physicians and Surgeons; Director of Urologic Oncology, New York–Presbyterian Hospital—Columbia Campus, New York, New York
Cutaneous Continent Urinary Diversion

RICHARD E. BERGER, MD
Professor of Urology, University of Washington Medical School, Seattle, Washington
Sexually Transmitted Diseases: The Classic Diseases

JAY T. BISHOFF, MD
Assistant Clinical Professor of Surgery, University of Texas Health Science, San Antonio; Director, Endourology Section, Wilford Hall Medical Center, Lackland AFB, Texas
Laparoscopic Surgery of the Kidney

JERRY G. BLAIVAS, MD
Clinical Professor of Urology, Weill Medical College of Cornell University; Attending Surgeon, New York–Presbyterian Hospital and Lenox Hill Hospital, New York, New York
Urinary Incontinence: Pathophysiology, Evaluation, and Management Overview

JON D. BLUMENFELD, MD
Associate Professor of Medicine, Weill Medical College of Cornell University; Associate Attending in Medicine, The Rogosin Institute, New York–Presbyterian Hospital, New York, New York
Renal Physiology and Pathophysiology; The Adrenals

JOSEPH G. BORER, MD
Instructor in Surgery (Urology), Harvard Medical School; Assistant in Urology, Children's Hospital, Boston, Massachusetts
Hypospadias

CONTRIBUTORS

GEORGE J. BOSL, MD
Professor of Medicine, Weill Medical College of Cornell University; Chair, Department of Medicine, Memorial Sloan-Kettering Cancer Center, New York, New York
Surgery of Testicular Tumors

CHARLES B. BRENDLER, MD
Professor and Chairman, Section of Urology, Department of Surgery, University of Chicago School of Medicine, Chicago, Illinois
Examination of the Urologic Patient: History, Physical Examination, and Urinalysis

GREGORY A. BRODERICK, MD
Professor of Urology, Mayo Medical School, Mayo Clinic, Jacksonville, Florida
Evaluation and Nonsurgical Management of Erectile Dysfunction and Priapism

JAMES D. BROOKS, MD
Assistant Professor of Urology, Stanford University School of Medicine, Stanford, California
Anatomy of the Lower Urinary Tract and Male Genitalia

JEFFREY A. CADEDDU, MD
Assistant Professor, Department of Urology, and Director, Clinical Center for Minimally Invasive Urologic Cancer Treatment, University of Texas Southwestern Medical Center, Dallas, Texas
Other Applications of Laparoscopic Surgery

STEVEN C. CAMPBELL, MD, PhD
Associate Professor of Urology; Codirector of Urologic Oncology, Loyola University Medical Center, Maywood, Illinois
Renal Tumors

DOUGLAS A. CANNING, MD
Associate Professor in Surgery (Urology), The University of Pennsylvania School of Medicine; Director, Pediatric Urology, The Children's Hospital of Philadelphia, Philadelphia, Pennsylvania
Evaluation of the Pediatric Urologic Patient

MICHAEL A. CARDUCCI, MD
Associate Professor of Oncology and Urology, Johns Hopkins University School of Medicine; Head, Drug Development Program—Oncology Center, Johns Hopkins Hospital, Baltimore, Maryland
Chemotherapy for Hormone-Resistant Prostate Cancer

LESLEY K. CARR, MD, FRCSC
Lecturer, Division of Urology, University of Toronto Medical School; Director of Women's Pelvic Health Centre, Sunnybrook and Women's College Health Sciences Centre, Toronto, Ontario, Canada
Vaginal Reconstructive Surgery for Sphincteric Incontinence and Prolapse

MICHAEL C. CARR, MD, PhD
Assistant Professor of Urology, Department of Surgery, University of Pennsylvania School of Medicine; Attending Surgeon, Pediatric Urology, Children's Hospital of Philadelphia, Philadelphia, Pennsylvania
Anomalies and Surgery of the Ureteropelvic Junction in Children

PETER R. CARROLL, MD
Professor and Chair, Department of Urology, University of California–San Francisco, San Francisco, California
Cryotherapy for Prostate Cancer

H. BALLENTINE CARTER, MD
Professor of Urology and Oncology, Johns Hopkins University School of Medicine, Baltimore, Maryland
Basic Instrumentation and Cytoscopy; Diagnosis and Staging of Prostate Cancer

MICHAEL B. CHANCELLOR, MD
Professor of Urology; Director, Neuro-urology and Female Urology, University of Pittsburgh School of Medicine, Pittsburgh, Pennsylvania
Physiology and Pharmacology of the Bladder and Urethra

ROBERT CHEVALIER, MD
Benjamin Armistead Shepherd Professor and Chair, Department of Pediatrics, University of Virginia; Attending Pediatrician, Children's Medical Center, University of Virginia Health System, Charlottesville, Virginia
Renal Function in the Fetus, Neonate, and Child

RALPH V. CLAYMAN, MD
Professor and Chairman, Department of Urology, University of California–Irvine, Irvine, California
Basis of Laparoscopic Urologic Surgery

J. QUENTIN CLEMENS, BS, MD
Assistant Professor of Urology, Northwestern University College of Medicine, Chicago, Illinois
Pubovaginal Slings

JOHN M. CORMAN, MD
Assistant Clinical Professor, Department of Urology, University of Washington; Staff Urologist, Virginia Mason Medical Center, Seattle, Washington
AIDS and Related Conditions

PAUL J. COZZI, MD
University of New South Wales Department of Surgery, Pitney Clinical Sciences Building, St. George Hospital, Sydney, Australia
Surgery of Penile and Urethral Carcinoma

JUANITA CROOK, MD
Associate Professor of Radiation Oncology, University of Toronto; Radiation Oncologist, Princess Margaret Hospital, Toronto, Ontario
Radiation Therapy for Prostate Cancer

ANTHONY V. D'AMICO, MD, PhD
Associate Professor of Radiation Oncology, Harvard Medical School; Chief, Genitourinary Radiation Oncology, Brigham and Women's Hospital, Dana Farber Cancer Institute, Boston, Massachusetts
Radiation Therapy for Prostate Cancer

JEAN B. DEKERNION, MD
Professor and Chair, Department of Urology, University of California–Los Angeles, Los Angeles, California
Epidemiology, Etiology, and Prevention of Prostate Cancer

CONTRIBUTORS

JOSEPH DEL PIZZO, MD
Assistant Professor of Urology, Section of Laparoscopic and Minimally Invasive Surgery, and Director of Laparoscopic Surgery, Department of Urology, Weill Medical College of Cornell University, The New York–Presbyterian Hospital, New York, New York
The Adrenals

THEODORE L. DEWEESE, MD, PhD
Assistant Professor of Oncology, Johns Hopkins University School of Medicine, Baltimore, Maryland; Radiation Oncologist, Johns Hopkins Hospital, Baltimore, Maryland
Radiation Therapy for Prostate Cancer

DAVID A. DIAMOND, MD
Associate Professor of Surgery (Urology), Harvard Medical School; Associate in Urology, Children's Hospital, Boston, Massachusetts
Sexual Differentiation: Normal and Abnormal

CANER Z. DINLENC, MD
Assistant Professor of Urology, Albert Einstein College of Medicine; Physician-in-Charge of Endourology and Stone Disease, Beth Israel Medical Center, New York, New York
Percutaneous Approaches to the Upper Urinary Tract

ROGER DMOCHOWSKI, MD, FACS
Medical Director, North Texas Center for Urinary Control, Fort Worth, Texas
Surgery for Vesicovaginal Fistula, Urethrovaginal Fistula, and Urethral Diverticulum

STEVEN G. DOCIMO, MD
Professor of Urology, University of Pittsburgh School of Medicine; Pittsburgh's Children's Hospital, Pittsburgh, Pennsylvania
Pediatric Endourology and Laparoscopy

S. MACHELE DONAT, MD
Assistant Attending Physician in Urology, Cornell University Medical College; Assistant Attending Surgeon, Memorial Sloan-Kettering Cancer Center, New York Hospital–Cornell Medical Center, New York, New York
Surgery of Penile and Urethral Carcinoma

JAMES A. EASTHAM, MD
Associate Professor, Memorial Sloan-Kettering Cancer Center, New York, New York
Radical Prostatectomy

MARIO A. EISENBERGER, MD
Professor of Oncology and Urology, Johns Hopkins University; Active Full-Time Staff Physician, Johns Hopkins Hospital, Baltimore, Maryland
Chemotherapy for Hormone-Resistant Prostate Cancer

JACK S. ELDER, MD
Professor of Urology and Pediatrics, Case Western Reserve University School of Medicine, Cleveland, Ohio; Director of Pediatric Urology, Rainbow Babies and Children's Hospital, Cleveland, Ohio
Abnormalities of the Genitalia in Boys and Their Surgical Management

JONATHAN I. EPSTEIN, MD
Professor of Pathology, Urology, and Oncology, The Johns Hopkins Medical Institutions, Baltimore, Maryland
Pathology of Prostatic Neoplasia

ANDREW P. EVAN, PhD
Professor of Anatomy, Department of Anatomy and Cell Biology, Indiana University School of Medicine, Indianapolis, Indiana
Surgical Management of Urinary Lithiasis

ROBERT L. FAIRCHILD, PhD
Department of Immunology, Urological Institute, Cleveland Clinic Foundation, Cleveland, Ohio
Basic Principles of Immunology in Urology

DIANE FELSEN, PhD
Associate Research Professor of Pharmacology in Urology, Weill Medical College of Cornell University, New York, New York
Pathophysiology of Urinary Tract Obstruction

AMR FERGANY, MD
Fellow, Urological Institute, The Cleveland Clinic Foundation, Cleveland, Ohio
Renovascular Hypertension and Ischemic Nephropathy

JAMES H. FINKE, PhD
Department of Immunology, Urological Institute, Cleveland Clinic Foundation, Cleveland, Ohio
Basic Principles of Immunology in Urology

JOHN M. FITZPATRICK, MCh, FRCSI, FRCS
Professor and Chairman, Academic Department of Surgery, Mater Misericordiae Hospital and University College, Dublin, Ireland
Minimally Invasive and Endoscopic Management of Benign Prostatic Hyperplasia

STUART M. FLECHNER, MD
Section of Renal Transplantation, Urological Institute, The Cleveland Clinic Foundation, Cleveland, Ohio
Basic Principles of Immunology in Urology

JENNY J. FRANKE, MD
Assistant Professor, Department of Urology, Vanderbilt University School of Medicine, Nashville, Tennessee
Management of Upper Urinary Tract Obstruction

JOHN P. GEARHART, MD
Professor of Pediatric Urology and Professor of Pediatrics, Johns Hopkins University School of Medicine; Chief and Director of Pediatric Urology, Brady Urological Institute, Johns Hopkins Hospital, Baltimore, Maryland
Exstrophy, Epispadias, and Other Bladder Anomalies

GLENN S. GERBER, MD
Associate Professor, Department of Surgery (Urology), University of Chicago School of Medicine, Chicago, Illinois
Evaluation of the Urologic Patient: History, Physical Examination, and Urinalysis

ROBERT P. GIBBONS, MD
Clinical Professor of Urology, University of Washington, Seattle, Washington; Staff Urologist Emeritus, Section of Urology and Transplantation, Virginia Mason Medical Center, Seattle, Washington
Radical Perineal Prostatectomy

INDERBIR S. GILL, MD, MCh
Head, Section of Laparoscopic and Minimally Invasive Surgery, Urological Institute, and Director, The Minimally Invasive Surgery Center, The Cleveland Clinic Foundation, Cleveland, Ohio
Basis of Laparoscopic Urologic Surgery

KENNETH I. GLASSBERG, MD
Professor of Urology, Director of Division of Pediatric Urology, State University of New York, Downstate Medical Center, Brooklyn, New York
Renal Dysgenesis and Cystic Disease of the Kidney

DAVID A. GOLDFARB, MD
Head, Section of Renal Transplantation, Urological Institute, Cleveland Clinic Foundation, Cleveland, Ohio
Etiology, Pathogenesis, and Management of Renal Failure

STANFORD M. GOLDMAN, MD
Professor of Radiology and Urology, University of Texas–Houston Medical School; Chief, Genitourinary Radiology, Memorial Hermann Hospital, Houston, Texas
Urinary Tract Imaging—Basic Principles

MARC GOLDSTEIN, MD
Professor of Urology and Professor of Reproductive Medicine, Weill Medical College of Cornell University; Surgeon-in-Chief of Male Reproductive Medicine and Surgery and Coexecutive Director, Cornell Institute for Reproductive Medicine, New York Weill Cornell Medical Center, New York, New York
Surgical Management of Male Infertility and Other Scrotal Disorders

EDMOND T. GONZALES, JR., MD
Professor of Urology, Scott Department of Urology, Baylor College of Medicine; Chief, Urology Service, Texas Children's Hospital, Houston, Texas
Posterior Urethral Valves and Other Urethral Anomalies

RICHARD W. GRADY, MD
Assistant Professor, The University of Washington Medical School; Assistant Chief, Pediatric Urology, Children's Hospital and Regional Medical Center, Seattle, Washington
Surgical Technique for One-Stage Reconstruction of the Exstrophy-Epispadias Complex

ASNAT GROUTZ, MD
Lecturer, Sackler School of Medicine, Tel Aviv University; Urogynecology Unit, Lis Maternity Hospital, Tel Aviv Medical Center, Tel Aviv, Israel
Urinary Incontinence: Pathophysiology, Evaluation, and Management Overview

FREDERICK A. GULMI, MD
Assistant Professor of Urology, State University of New York Health Sciences Center at Brooklyn; Attending Urologist, Brookdale University Hospital and Medical Center, Brooklyn, New York
Pathophysiology of Urinary Tract Obstruction

MICHAEL L. GURALNICK, MD, FRCSC
Assistant Professor of Surgery (Urology), Medical College of Wisconsin, Milwaukee, Wisconsin
The Neurourologic Evaluation; Retropubic Suspension Surgery for Female Incontinence

MISOP HAN, MD
Chief Urology Resident, Department of Urology, The Johns Hopkins University School of Medicine; Chief Resident, James Buchanan Brady Urological Institute, The Johns Hopkins Hospital, Baltimore, Maryland
Retropubic and Suprapubic Open Prostatectomy

PHILIP M. HANNO, MD
Attending Urologist, Hospital of the University of Pennsylvania; Medical Director, Clinical Effectiveness and Quality Improvement Department, University of Pennsylvania Health System, Philadelphia, Pennsylvania
Interstitial Cystitis and Related Disorders

MATTHEW HARDY, PhD
The Population Council, Rockefeller University, New York, New York
Male Reproductive Physiology

HARRY W. HERR, MD
Professor of Urology, Cornell University Medical College; Attending Surgeon, Memorial Sloan-Kettering Cancer Center, New York Hospital–Cornell Medical Center, New York, New York
Surgery of Penile and Urethral Carcinoma

SENDER HERSCHORN, BSc, MDCM, FRCSC
Professor and Chairman, Division of Urology, University of Toronto; Director, Urodynamics Unit, Sunnybrook and Women's College Health Sciences Centre, Toronto, Ontario, Canada
Vaginal Reconstructive Surgery for Sphincteric Incontinence and Prolapse

STUART S. HOWARDS, MD
Professor of Urology, University of Virginia Medical School; Chief, Pediatric Urology, Children's Medical Center, University of Virginia Health System, Charlottesville, Virginia
Renal Function in the Fetus, Neonate, and Child

MARK HURWITZ, MD
Assistant Professor of Radiation Oncology, Harvard Medical School; Vice Chief of Genitourinary Radiation Oncology, Brigham and Women's Hospital, Dana Farber Cancer Institute, Boston, Massachusetts
Radiation Therapy for Prostate Cancer

JONATHAN P. JAROW, MD
Associate Professor of Urology, Johns Hopkins University School of Medicine, Baltimore, Maryland
Male Infertility

THOMAS W. JARRETT, MD
Associate Professor and Chief, Division of Endourology, Johns Hopkins University School of Medicine; Chief of Endourology, Johns Hopkins Hospital, Baltimore, Maryland
Management of Urothelial Tumors of the Renal Pelvis and Ureter

VENKATA R. JAYANTHI, MD
Clinical Assistant Professor, Section of Pediatric Urology, Children's Hospital, Division of Urology, Department of Surgery, The Ohio State University Medical Center; Director, Resident Education, Section of Pediatric Urology, Children's Hospital, Columbus, Ohio
Voiding Dysfunction in Children: Neurogenic and Non-Neurogenic

V. KEITH JIMINEZ, MD
Chief Resident, Department of Urology, Emory University School of Medicine, Atlanta, Georgia
Surgery of Bladder Cancer

CHRISTOPHER W. JOHNSON, MD
Resident, Department of Urology, College of Physicians and Surgeons of Columbia University, and New York–Presbyterian Hospital—Columbia Campus, New York, New York
Tuberculosis and Parasitic Diseases of the Genitourinary System

WARREN D. JOHNSON, JR., MD
B. H. Kean Professor of Tropical Medicine and Chief, Division of International Medicine and Infectious Diseases, Weill Medical College of Cornell University; Attending Physician, New York–Presbyterian Hospital—Cornell Campus, New York, New York
Tuberculosis and Parasitic Diseases of the Genitourinary System

GERALD H. JORDAN, MD
Professor and Chairman, Department of Urology, Eastern Virginia Medical School, Norfolk, Virginia
Surgery for Erectile Dysfunction; Surgery of the Penis and Urethra

DAVID B. JOSEPH, MD
Professor of Surgery, University of Alabama at Birmingham, Birmingham, Alabama; Chief of Pediatric Urology, Children's Hospital, Birmingham, Alabama
Urinary Tract Reconstruction in Children

JOHN N. KABALIN, MD
Adjunct Assistant Professor of Surgery, Section of Urologic Surgery, University of Nebraska College of Medicine, Omaha; Regional West Medical Center, Scottsbluff, Nebraska
Surgical Anatomy of the Retroperitoneum, Kidneys, and Ureters

MARTIN KAEFER, MD
Assistant Professor, Pediatric Urology, James Whitcomb Riley Hospital for Children, Indianapolis, Indiana
Surgical Management of Intersexuality, Cloacal Malformations, and Other Abnormalities of the Genitalia in Girls

IRVING KAPLAN, MD
Assistant Professor of Joint Center for Radiation Oncology, Harvard Medical School; Radiation Oncologist, Beth Israel Deaconess Medical Center, Boston, Massachusetts
Radiation Therapy for Prostate Cancer

LOUIS R. KAVOUSSI, MD
Patrick C. Walsh Distinguished Professor, Johns Hopkins University School of Medicine; Vice Chairman, The James Buchanan Brady Urological Institute, Johns Hopkins Medical Institutions, Baltimore, Maryland
Laparoscopic Surgery of the Kidney

AKIRA KAWASHIMA, MD, PhD
Associate Professor, Department of Radiology, Mayo Medical School; Senior Consultant, Department of Radiology, Mayo Clinic, Rochester, Minnesota
Urinary Tract Imaging—Basic Principles

MICHAEL A. KEATING, MD
Clinical Professor of Urology, University of South Florida, Tampa, Florida; Chairman, Department of Children's Surgery, Arnold Palmer Hospital for Children and Women, Orlando, Florida
Vesicoureteral Reflux and Megaureter

KURT KERBL, MD
Associate Professor of Urology, Alle Kassen, Kirchdorf, Austria
Basis of Laparoscopic Urologic Surgery

ADAM S. KIBEL, MD
Assistant Professor of Urologic Surgery, Washington University School of Medicine; Attending Physician, Barnes–Jewish Hospital, St. Louis, Missouri
Molecular Genetics and Cancer Biology

STEPHEN A. KOFF, MD
Professor of Surgery, Ohio State University Medical Center, Columbus, Ohio; Chief, Pediatric Urology, Children's Hospital, Columbus, Ohio
Voiding Dysfunction in Children: Neurogenic and Non-Neurogenic

JOHN N. KRIEGER, MD
Professor, University of Washington; Staff Urologist, Puget Sound VA Medical Center, Seattle, Washington
AIDS and Related Conditions

LAMK M. LAMKI, MD
Professor of Radiology and Chief of Nuclear Medicine, Department of Radiology, University of Texas Medical School at Houston, Houston, Texas
Urinary Tract Imaging—Basic Principles

JAY C. LEE, MD
University of Washington, Seattle, Washington
Sexually Transmitted Diseases: The Classic Diseases

HERBERT LEPOR, MD
Professor and Martin Spatz Chairman, Department of Urology, New York University School of Medicine; Chief of Urological Surgery, New York University Medical Center, New York, New York
Evaluation and Nonsurgical Management of Benign Prostatic Hyperplasia

RONALD W. LEWIS, MD
Witherington Chair in Urology, Professor of Surgery, Chief of Urology, Medical College of Georgia, Augusta, Georgia
Surgery for Erectile Dysfunction

EVANGELOS N. LIATSIKOS, MD
Instructor of Urology, University of Patras Medical School, University Hospital, Rio-Patras, Greece
Percutaneous Approaches to the Upper Urinary Tract

DAVID A. LIFSHITZ, MD
Lecturer, Sackler School of Medicine, Tel Aviv University, Tel Aviv; Head, Endourology Service, Rabin Medical Center, Petach Tikva, Israel
Surgical Management of Urinary Lithiasis

JAMES E. LINGEMAN, MD
Clinical Professor, Department of Urology, Indiana University School of Medicine; Director of Research, Methodist Hospital Institute for Kidney Stone Disease, Indianapolis, Indiana
Surgical Management of Urinary Lithiasis

FRANKLIN C. LOWE, MD, MPH
Associate Professor of Clinical Urology, Columbia University College of Physicians and Surgeons; Associate Director, Urology, St. Luke's/Roosevelt Hospital Center, New York, New York
Tuberculosis and Parasitic Diseases of the Genitourinary System; Evaluation and Nonsurgical Management of Benign Prostatic Hyperplasia

TOM F. LUE, MD
Professor and Vice Chairman, Department of Urology, University of California, San Francisco, San Francisco, California
Physiology of Penile Erection and Pathophysiology of Erectile Dysfunction and Priapism; Evaluation and Nonsurgical Management of Erectile Dysfunction and Priapism

DONALD F. LYNCH, JR., MD
Professor of Urology and Professor of Clinical Obstetrics and Gynecology, Eastern Virginia School of Medicine; Urologic Oncologist and Consultant Urologist, Sentara Hospitals, Southside Virginia, Norfolk, Virginia, and Virginia Beach, Virginia, and Howard and Georgianna Jones Institute for Reproductive Medicine, Norfolk, Virginia
Tumors of the Penis

STANLEY BRUCE MALKOWICZ, MD
Associate Professor of Urology, University of Pennsylvania School of Medicine; Chief of Urology, Philadelphia VA Medical Center, Philadelphia, Pennsylvania
Management of Superficial Bladder Cancer

DAVID J. MARGOLIS, MD, PhD
Associate Professor of Dermatology and Epidemiology, University of Pennsylvania School of Medicine, Philadelphia, Pennsylvania
Cutaneous Diseases of the Male External Genitalia

FRAY F. MARSHALL, MD
Professor of Urology, Emory University School of Medicine, Atlanta, Georgia
Surgery of Bladder Cancer

JACK W. MCANINCH, MS, MD
Professor of Urology, University of California–San Francisco; Chief of Urology, San Francisco General Hospital, San Francisco, California
Genitourinary Trauma

JOHN D. MCCONNELL, MD
Professor of Urology and Executive Vice President for Administration, The University of Texas Southwestern Medical Center, Dallas, Texas
Epidemiology, Etiology, and Pathophysiology of Benign Prostatic Hyperplasia

W. SCOTT MCDOUGAL, MD
Walter S. Kerr, Jr., Professor of Urology, Harvard Medical School; Chief of Urology, Massachusetts General Hospital, Boston, Massachusetts
Use of Intestinal Segments and Urinary Diversion

ELSPETH M. MCDOUGALL, MD
Professor of Urologic Surgery, Vanderbilt University Medical Center, Nashville, Tennessee
Percutaneous Approaches to the Upper Urinary Tract

EDWARD J. MCGUIRE, MD
Professor of Urology, The University of Michigan, Ann Arbor, Michigan
Pubovaginal Slings

JAMES MCKIERNAN, MD
Assistant Professor, Columbia University College of Physicians and Surgeons; Assistant Attending Physician, New York–Presbyterian Hospital, New York, New York
Surgery of Testicular Tumors

WINSTON K. MEBUST, MD
Emeritus Chair and Professor, Department of Urology, Kansas University Medical Center, Kansas City, Kansas
Minimally Invasive and Endoscopic Management of Benign Prostatic Hyperplasia

MANI MENON, MD
Professor of Urology, Case Western Reserve University, Cleveland, Ohio; The Raj and Padma Vattikuti Distinguished Chair/Director, Vattikuti Urology Institute, Henry Ford Health System, Detroit, Michigan
Urinary Lithiasis: Etiology, Diagnosis, and Medical Management

ANOOP M. MERANEY, MD
Fellow, Laparoscopic and Minimally Invasive Surgery, Cleveland Clinic Foundation Urological Institute, Cleveland, Ohio
Basis of Laparoscopic Urologic Surgery

EDWARD M. MESSING, MD
Chairman, Department of Urology, University of Rochester, Rochester, New York
Urothelial Tumors of the Urinary Tract

MICHAEL E. MITCHELL, MD
Professor, The University of Washington Medical School; Chief, Division of Pediatric Urology, Children's Hospital and Regional Medical Center, Seattle, Washington
Surgical Technique for One-Stage Reconstruction of the Exstrophy-Epispadias Complex

JOSEPH V. NALLY, JR., MD
Staff Nephrologist and Director of Fellowship Program, Department of Nephrology and Hypertension, Cleveland Clinic Foundation, Cleveland, Ohio
Etiology, Pathogenesis, and Management of Renal Failure

JOEL B. NELSON, MD
The Frederic N. Schwentker Professor and Chairman, Department of Urology, University of Pittsburgh School of Medicine; Attending Physician, UPMC Presbyterian Hospital, UPMC Shadyside Hospital, Pittsburgh, Pennsylvania
Molecular Genetics and Cancer Biology

J. CURTIS NICKEL, MD
Professor of Urology, Queen's University; Staff Urologist, Kingston General Hospital, Kingston, Ontario, Canada
Prostatitis and Related Conditions

VICTOR W. NITTI, MD
Associate Professor and Vice Chairman, Department of Urology, New York University School of Medicine, New York, New York
Postprostatectomy Incontinence

H. NORMAN NOE, MD
Chief of Pediatric Urology, University of Tennessee Health Science Center; Chief of Pediatric Urology, LeBonheur Children's Medical Center, Memphis, Tennessee
Renal Disease in Childhood

ANDREW C. NOVICK, MD
Professor of Surgery (Urology), Ohio State University School of Medicine; Chairman, Urological Institute, The Cleveland Clinic Foundation, Cleveland, Ohio
Renovascular Hypertension and Ischemic Nephropathy; Renal Tumors; Surgery of the Kidney

CARL A. OLSSON, MD
Professor and Chairman, Department of Urology, College of Physicians and Surgeons, Columbia University; Director of Squier Urological Clinic and Chief of Urology, New York–Presbyterian Hospital, Columbia Presbyterian Campus, New York, New York
Cutaneous Continent Urinary Diversion

JOHN M. PARK, MD
Assistant Professor of Urology and Director of Division of Pediatric Urology, University of Michigan Medical School, Ann Arbor, Michigan
Normal and Anomalous Development of the Urogenital System

ALAN W. PARTIN, MD, PhD
Professor of Urology, Oncology, and Pathology, Department of Urology, The Johns Hopkins University School of Medicine; Bernard L. Schwartz Distinguished Professor of Urologic Oncology, The James Buchanan Brady Urological Institute, The Johns Hopkins Medical Institutions, Baltimore, Maryland
The Molecular Biology, Endocrinology, and Physiology of the Prostate and Seminal Vesicles; Retropubic and Suprapubic Open Prostatectomy

CHRISTOPHER K. PAYNE, MD
Associate Professor of Urology, Stanford University Medical School; Director, Female Urology and Neuro-urology, Stanford Medical Center, Stanford, California
Urinary Incontinence: Nonsurgical Management

CRAIG A. PETERS, MD
Associate Professor of Surgery (Urology), Harvard Medical School; Associate Professor of Urology, Children's Hospital, Boston, Massachusetts
Perinatal Urology; Pediatric Endourology and Laparoscopy

CURTIS A. PETTAWAY, MD
Associate Professor of Urology and Urologic Oncologist, University of Texas, MD Anderson Cancer Center, Houston, Texas
Tumors of the Penis

ROBERT E. REITER, MD
Associate Professor, Department of Urology, University of California, Los Angeles; Codirector, Prostate Cancer Program, Jousson Comprehensive Cancer Center, Los Angeles, California
Epidemiology, Etiology, and Prevention of Prostate Cancer

MARTIN I. RESNICK, MD
Lester Persky Professor and Chair, Department of Urology, Case Western Reserve University School of Medicine; Director, Department of Urology, University Hospitals of Cleveland, Cleveland, Ohio
Urinary Lithiasis: Etiology, Diagnosis, and Medical Management

NEIL M. RESNICK, MD
Professor and Chief, Division of Gerontology and Geriatric Medicine, University of Pittsburgh Medical Center Health System, Pittsburgh, Pennsylvania
Geriatric Incontinence and Voiding Dysfunction

ALAN B. RETIK, MD
Professor of Surgery (Urology), Harvard Medical School; Chief, Department of Urology, Children's Hospital, Boston, Massachusetts
Ectopic Ureter, Ureterocele, and Other Anomalies of the Ureter; Hypospadias

JEROME P. RICHIE, MD
Elliott C. Cutler Professor of Surgery and Chairman of Harvard Program in Urology (Longwood Area), Harvard Medical School; Chief of Urology, Brigham and Women's Hospital, Boston, Massachusetts
Neoplasms of the Testis

RICHARD C. RINK, MD
James Whitcomb Riley Hospital for Children, Indianapolis, Indiana
Surgical Management of Intersexuality, Cloacal Malformations, and Other Abnormalities of the Genitalia in Girls

MICHAEL RITCHEY, MD
Professor of Surgery and Pediatrics, Director, Division of Urology, University of Texas–Houston Medical School, Houston, Texas
Pediatric Urologic Oncology

RONALD RODRIGUEZ, MD, PhD
Assistant Professor of Urology, Medical Oncology, Cellular and Molecular Medicine, Johns Hopkins University School of Medicine, The James Buchanan Brady Urological Institute, Baltimore, Maryland
The Molecular Biology, Endocrinology, and Physiology of the Prostate and Seminal Vesicles

CLAUS G. ROEHRBORN, MD
Professor and Chairman, Department of Urology, The University of Texas Southwestern Medical Center; Attending Chief, Zale Lipshy University Medical Center, Section of Urology, VA Medical Center, Dallas, Texas
Epidemiology, Etiology, and Pathophysiology of Benign Prostatic Hyperplasia

SHANE ROY, III, MD
Professor of Pediatrics, Section of Pediatric Nephrology, University of Tennessee Health Science Center, Memphis, Tennessee
Renal Disease in Childhood

ARTHUR I. SAGALOWSKY, MD
Professor of Urology, Chief of Urologic Oncology, University of Texas Southwestern Medical School, Dallas, Texas
Management of Urothelial Tumors of the Renal Pelvis and Ureter

CARL M. SANDLER, MD
Professor and Chairman of Surgery (Urology), The University of Texas Medical School–Houston; Adjunct Professor of Radiology, Baylor College of Medicine, Houston, Texas
Urinary Tract Imaging—Basic Principles

JAY I. SANDLOW, MD
Associate Professor, Director of Andrology and Male Infertility, University of Iowa Department of Urology, Iowa City, Iowa
Surgery of the Seminal Vesicles

RICHARD A. SANTUCCI, MD
Assistant Professor, Wayne State University School of Medicine; Chief of Urology, Detroit Receiving Hospital, Detroit, Michigan
Genitourinary Trauma

PETER T. SCARDINO, MD
Chairman, Department of Urology, Memorial Sloan-Kettering Cancer Center, New York, New York
Radical Prostatectomy

ANTHONY J. SCHAEFFER, MD
Herman L. Kretschmer Professor and Chairman, Department of Urology, Northwestern University Medical School, Chicago, Illinois
Infections of the Urinary Tract

STEVEN J. SCHICHMAN, MD
Assistant Clinical Professor of Urology, Division of Urology, Department of Surgery, University of Connecticut, Farmington, Connecticut
The Adrenals

PETER N. SCHLEGEL, MD
Acting Chairman and Associate Professor of Urology, Department of Urology, Weill Medical College of Cornell University; Acting Urologist-in-Chief, New York–Presbyterian Hospital–Weill Cornell Center, New York, New York
Male Reproductive Physiology

STEVEN M. SCHLOSSBERG, MD
Professor of Urology, Eastern Virginia Medical School, Norfolk, Virginia
Surgery of the Penis and Urethra

RICHARD N. SCHLUSSEL, MD
Department of Urology, Mount Sinai School of Medicine, New York, New York
Ectopic Ureter, Ureterocele, and Other Anomalies of the Ureter

FRANCIS X. SCHNECK, MD
Clinical Assistant Professor of Urology, University of Pittsburgh School of Medicine; Attending Physician, Children's Hospital of Pittsburgh, Pittsburgh, Pennsylvania
Abnormalities of the Testes and Scrotum and Their Surgical Management

MARK SCHOENBERG, MD
Associate Professor, The James Buchanan Brady Urological Institute, Director, Urologic Oncology, Johns Hopkins University School of Medicine, Baltimore, Maryland
Management of Invasive and Metastatic Bladder Cancer

MARTIN J. SCHREIBER, JR., MD
Staff Nephrologist, Department of Nephrology and Hypertension, Cleveland Clinic Foundation, Cleveland, Ohio
Etiology, Pathogenesis, and Management of Renal Failure

FRITZ H. SCHRÖDER, MD, PhD
Professor of Urology, Erasmus University, Rotterdam, The Netherlands
Hormonal Therapy of Prostate Cancer

PETER G. SCHULAM, MD, PhD
Associate Professor and Chief, Division of Endourology and Laparoscopy, University of California–Los Angeles Medical Center, Los Angeles, California
Urinary Tract Imaging—Basic Principles

RIDWAN SHABSIGH, MD
Associate Professor of Urology, College of Physicians and Surgeons of Columbia University; Director, New York Center for Human Sexuality, New York–Presbyterian Hospital, New York, New York
Female Sexual Function and Dysfunction

JOEL SHEINFELD, MD
Associate Professor, Weill Medical College of Cornell University; Vice Chairman, Department of Urology, Memorial Sloan-Kettering Cancer Center, New York, New York
Surgery of Testicular Tumors

KATSUTO SHINOHARA, MD
Department of Urology, University of California–San Francisco, San Francisco, California
Cryotherapy for Prostate Cancer

LINDA M. DAIRIKI SHORTLIFFE, MD
Professor and Chair of the Department of Urology, Stanford University School of Medicine; Chief of Urology, Stanford University Medical Center; Chief of Pediatric Urology, Lucile Salter Packard Children's Hospital, Stanford, California
Urinary Tract Infections in Infants and Children

MARK SIGMAN, BS, MD
Associate Professor of Urology, Division of Urology, Department of Surgery, Brown University School of Medicine; Staff Urologist, Rhode Island Hospital and VA Hospital, Providence, Rhode Island
Male Infertility

DONALD G. SKINNER, MD
Professor of Urology, University of Southern California, Norris Comprehensive Cancer Center, Los Angeles, California
Orthotopic Urinary Diversion

ARTHUR D. SMITH, MD
Professor of Urology, Albert Einstein College of Medicine, New York; Chairman, Long Island Jewish Medical Centre, New Hyde Park, New York
Percutaneous Approaches to the Upper Urinary Tract

EDWIN A. SMITH, MD
Assistant Clinical Professor of Urology and Director of Pediatric Urology, Emory University School of Medicine; Attending Pediatric Urologist, Children's Hospital of Atlanta, Atlanta, Georgia
Prune-Belly Syndrome

JOHN J. SMITH, III, MS, MD
Assistant Clinical Professor, Tufts University School of Medicine; Clinical Instructor of Surgery, Harvard Medical School, Boston; Senior Staff Consultant, Department of Urology, Lahey Clinic, Burlington, Massachusetts
Implantation of the Artificial Genitourinary Sphincter

JOSEPH A. SMITH, JR., MD
Professor and Chairman, Department of Urologic Oncology, Vanderbilt University, Nashville, Tennessee
Management of Upper Urinary Tract Obstruction

R. ERNEST SOSA, MD
Associate Professor of Urology, New York–Presbyterian Hospital, Weill Medical College, Cornell University, New York, New York
Ureteroscopy and Retrograde Ureteral Access; The Adrenals

GRAEME S. STEELE, MD
Assistant Professor, Harvard Medical School; Associate Surgeon, Brigham and Women's Hospital, Boston, Massachusetts
Neoplasms of the Testis

JOHN P. STEIN, MD
Assistant Professor of Urology, University of Southern California, Norris Comprehensive Cancer Center, Los Angeles, California
Orthotopic Urinary Diversion

STEVAN B. STREEM, MD
Head, Section of Stone Disease and Endourology, Urological Institute, Cleveland Clinic Foundation, Cleveland, Ohio
Management of Upper Urinary Tract Obstruction

LI-MING SU, MD
Assistant Professor of Urology and Director of Pelvic Laparoscopy and Stone Disease, Johns Hopkins Bayview Medical Center, The Brady Urological Institute, Johns Hopkins Medical Institutions, Baltimore, Maryland
Ureteroscopy and Retrograde Ureteral Access

MARTHA K. TERRIS, MD
Assistant Professor of Urology, Stanford University Medical Center, Stanford; Chief of Urology, Palo Alto Veterans Affairs Health Care System, Section of Urology, Palo Alto, California
Ultrasonography and Biopsy of the Prostate

E. DARRACOTT VAUGHAN, JR., MD
James J. Colt Professor of Urology, Weill Medical College of Cornell University; Chairman Emeritus, Department of Urology, New York–Presbyterian Hospital, New York, New York
Renal Physiology and Pathophysiology; Pathophysiology of Urinary Tract Obstruction; The Adrenals

PATRICK C. WALSH, MD
David Hall McConnell Professor and Director of Department of Urology, The Johns Hopkins University School of Medicine; Urologist-in-Chief, The James Buchanan Brady Urological Institute, The Johns Hopkins Medical Institutions, Baltimore, Maryland
Anatomic Radical Retropubic Prostatectomy

GEORGE D. WEBSTER, MB, FRCS
Professor of Surgery (Urology), Duke University, Durham, North Carolina
The Neurourologic Evaluation; Retropubic Suspension Surgery for Female Incontinence

ALAN J. WEIN, MD
Professor and Chair, Division of Urology, University of Pennsylvania School of Medicine; Chief of Urology, University of Pennsylvania Health System, Philadelphia, Pennsylvania
Pathophysiology and Categorization of Voiding Dysfunction; Neuromuscular Dysfunction of the Lower Urinary Tract and Its Management

ROBERT M. WEISS, MD
Donald Guthrie Professor of Surgery and Chief of Section of Urology, Yale University School of Medicine, New Haven, Connecticut
Physiology and Pharmacology of the Renal Pelvis and Ureter

RICHARD D. WILLIAMS, MD
Professor and Head, Rubin H. Flocks Chair, University of Iowa Department of Urology, Iowa City, Iowa
Surgery of the Seminal Vesicles

HOWARD N. WINFIELD, MD
Professor of Urology and Director of Laparoscopy and Minimally Invasive Surgery, Department of Urology, University of Iowa Hospitals and Clinics, Iowa City, Iowa
Other Applications of Laparoscopic Surgery

GILBERT J. WISE, AB, MD
Professor of Urology, State University of New York Health Science Center at Brooklyn; Director of Urology, Maimonides Medical Center, Brooklyn, New York
Fungal and Actinomycotic Infections of the Genitourinary System

JOHN R. WOODARD, MD
Clinical Professor of Urology, Emory University School of Medicine, Atlanta, Georgia
Prune-Belly Syndrome

SUBBARAO V. YALLA, MD
Professor of Surgery (Urology), Harvard Medical School; Chief, Urology Division, Boston Veterans Administration Medical Center, Boston, Massachusetts
Geriatric Incontinence and Voiding Dysfunction

NAOKI YOSHIMURA, MD, PhD
Associate Professor, Departments of Urology and Pharmacology, University of Pittsburgh School of Medicine, Pittsburgh, Pennsylvania
Physiology and Pharmacology of the Bladder and Urethra

CONTENTS

VOLUME I

I. Anatomy

Chapter 1
Surgical Anatomy of the Retroperitoneum, Kidneys, and Ureters 1
John N. Kabalin

Chapter 2
Anatomy of the Lower Urinary Tract and Male Genitalia 8
James D. Brooks

II. Urologic Examination and Diagnostic Techniques

Chapter 3
Evaluation of the Urologic Patient: History, Physical Examination, and Urinalysis 13
Glenn S. Gerber
Charles B. Brendler

Chapter 4
Basic Instrumentation and Cystoscopy 16
H. Ballentine Carter

Chapter 5
Urinary Tract Imaging—Basic Principles 17
Peter G. Schulam
Akira Kawashima
Carl M. Sandler
Bruce J. Barron
Lamk M. Lamki
Stanford M. Goldman

III. Physiology, Pathology, and Management of Upper Urinary Tract Diseases

Chapter 6
Renal Physiology and Pathophysiology 19
Jon D. Blumenfeld

Chapter 7
Renovascular Hypertension and Ischemic Nephropathy 30
Andrew C. Novick
Amr Fergany

Chapter 8
Etiology, Pathogenesis, and Management of Renal Failure 36
David A. Goldfarb
Joseph V. Nally, Jr.
Martin J. Schreiber, Jr.

Chapter 9
Basic Principles of Immunology in Urology 39
Stuart M. Flechner
James H. Finke
Robert L. Fairchild

Chapter 10
Renal Transplantation 42
John M. Barry

Chapter 11
Physiology and Pharmacology of the Renal Pelvis and Ureter 46
Robert M. Weiss

Chapter 12
Pathophysiology of Urinary Tract Obstruction 50
Frederick A. Gulmi
Diane Felsen
E. Darracott Vaughan, Jr.

Chapter 13
Management of Upper Urinary Tract Obstruction 56
Stevan B. Streem
Jenny J. Franke
Joseph A. Smith, Jr.

IV. Infections and Inflammations of the Genitourinary Tract

Chapter 14
Infections of the Urinary Tract 59
Anthony J. Schaeffer

Chapter 15
Prostatitis and Related Conditions 64
J. Curtis Nickel

Chapter 16
Interstitial Cystitis and Related Disorders 67
Philip M. Hanno

XV

Chapter 17
Sexually Transmitted Diseases: 71
    Richard E. Berger
    Jay Lee

Chapter 18
AIDS and Related Conditions 73
    John N. Krieger
    John M. Corman

Chapter 19
Cutaneous Diseases of the Male External Genitalia 74
    David J. Margolis

Chapter 21
Tuberculosis and Parasitic Diseases of the
Genitourinary System 76
    Warren D. Johnson, Jr.
    Christopher W. Johnson
    Franklin C. Lowe

Chapter 22
Fungal and Actinomycotic Infections of the
Genitourinary System 79
    Gilbert J. Wise

VOLUME II

V. Voiding Function and Dysfunction

Chapter 23
Physiology and Pharmacology of the Bladder and
Urethra 82
    Michael B. Chancellor
    Naoki Yoshimura

Chapter 24
Pathophysiology and Categorization of Voiding
Dysfunction 85
    Alan J. Wein

Chapter 25
The Neurourologic Evaluation 88
    George D. Webster
    Michael L. Guralnick

Chapter 26
Neuromuscular Dysfunction of the Lower Urinary
Tract and Its Management 94
    Alan J. Wein

Chapter 27
Urinary Incontinence: Pathophysiology, Evaluation,
and Management Overview 107
    Jerry G. Blaivas
    Asnat Groutz

Chapter 28
Post-prostatectomy Incontinence 110
    Victor W. Nitti

Chapter 29
Urinary Incontinence: Nonsurgical Management 112
    Christopher K. Payne

Chapter 30
Vaginal Reconstructive Surgery for Sphincteric
Incontinence and Prolapse 116
    Sender Herschorn
    Lesley K. Carr

Chapter 31
Retropubic Suspension Surgery for Female
Incontinence 121
    George D. Webster
    Michael L. Guralnick

Chapter 32
Pubovaginal Slings 123
    Edward J. McGuire
    J. Quentin Clemens

Chapter 33
Injection Therapy for Urinary Incontinence 126
    Rodney A. Appell

Chapter 34
Implantation of the Artificial Genitourinary
Sphincter 128
    John J. Smith, III
    David M. Barrett

Chapter 35
Surgery for Vesicovaginal Fistula, Urethrovaginal
Fistula, and Urethral Diverticulum 130
    Roger Dmochowski

Chapter 36
Geriatric Incontinence and Voiding Dysfunction 132
    Neil M. Resnick
    Subbarao V. Yalla

VI. Benign Prostatic Hyperplasia

Chapter 37
The Molecular Biology, Endocrinology, and
Physiology of the Prostate and Seminal Vesicles 135
    Alan W. Partin
    Ronald Rodriguez

Chapter 38
Etiology, Pathophysiology, Epidemiology, and
Natural History of Benign Prostatic Hyperplasia 138
    Claus G. Roehrborn
    John D. McConnell

Chapter 39
Natural History, Evaluation, and Nonsurgical
Management of Benign Prostatic Hyperplasia 143
    Herbert Lepor
    Franklin C. Lowe

Chapter 40
Minimally Invasive and Endoscopic Management of Benign Prostatic Hyperplasia 147
  John M. Fitzpatrick
  Winston K. Mebust

Chapter 41
Retropubic and Suprapubic Open Prostatectomy 149
  Misop Han
  Harold J. Alfert
  Alan W. Partin

VII. Reproductive Function and Dysfunction

Chapter 42
Male Reproductive Physiology 151
  Peter N. Schlegel
  Matthew Hardy

Chapter 43
Male Infertility 153
  Mark Sigman
  Jonathan P. Jarow

Chapter 44
Surgical Management of Male Infertility and Other Scrotal Disorders 159
  Marc Goldstein

VIII. Sexual Function and Dysfunction

Chapter 45
Physiology of Penile Erection and Pathophysiology of Erectile Dysfunction and Priapism 169
  Tom F. Lue

Chapter 46
Evaluation and Nonsurgical Management of Erectile Dysfunction and Priapism 174
  Gregory A. Broderick
  Tom F. Lue

Chapter 47
Surgery for Erectile Dysfunction 185
  Ronald W. Lewis
  Gerald H. Jordan

Chapter 48
Female Sexual Function and Dysfunction 190
  Ridwan Shabsigh

VOLUME III

IX. Pediatric Urology

Chapter 49
Normal and Anomalous Development of the Urogenital System 193
  John M. Park

Chapter 50
Renal Function in the Fetus, Neonate, and Child 196
  Robert Chevalier
  Stuart S. Howards

Chapter 51
Perinatal Urology 198
  Craig A. Peters

Chapter 52
Evaluation of the Pediatric Urologic Patient 200
  Douglas A. Canning

Chapter 53
Renal Disease in Childhood 202
  Shane Roy, III
  H. Norman Noe

Chapter 54
Urinary Tract Infections in Infants and Children 203
  Linda M. Dairiki Shortliffe

Chapter 55
Anomalies of the Upper Urinary Tract 206
  Stuart B. Bauer

Chapter 56
Renal Dysgenesis and Cystic Disease of the Kidney 208
  Kenneth I. Glassberg

Chapter 57
Anomalies and Surgery of the Ureteropelvic Junction in Children 213
  Michael C. Carr

Chapter 58
Ectopic Ureter, Ureterocele, and Other Anomalies of the Ureter 214
  Richard N. Schlussel
  Alan B. Retik

Chapter 59
Vesicoureteral Reflux and Megaureter 218
  Anthony Atala
  Michael A. Keating

Chapter 60
Prune-Belly Syndrome 225
  Edwin A. Smith
  John R. Woodard

Chapter 61
Exstrophy, Epispadias, and Other Bladder Anomalies 227
  John P. Gearhart

Chapter 62
Surgical Technique for One-Stage Reconstruction of the Exstrophy-Epispadias Complex 232
  Richard W. Grady
  Michael E. Mitchell

Chapter 63
Posterior Urethral Valves and Other Urethral Anomalies 233
Edmond T. Gonzales, Jr.

Chapter 64
Voiding Dysfunction in Children: Neurogenic and Non-Neurogenic 235
Stuart B. Bauer
Stephen A. Koff
Venkata R. Jayanthi

Non-Neurogenic Dysfunction 236
Stephen A. Koff
Venkata R. Jayanthi

Chapter 65
Hypospadias 238
Alan B. Retik
Joseph G. Borer

Chapter 66
Abnormalities of the Genitalia in Boys and Their Surgical Management 242
Jack S. Elder

Chapter 67
Abnormalities of the Testes and Scrotum and Their Surgical Management 244
Francis X. Schneck
Mark F. Bellinger

Chapter 68
Sexual Differentiation: Normal and Abnormal 246
David A. Diamond

Chapter 69
Surgical Management of Intersexuality, Cloacal Malformations, and Other Abnormalities of the Genitalia in Girls 249
Richard C. Rink
Martin Kaefer

Chapter 70
Pediatric Urologic Oncology 251
Michael Ritchey

Chapter 71
Urinary Tract Reconstruction in Children 286
Mark C. Adams
David B. Joseph

Chapter 72
Pediatric Endourology and Laparoscopy 263
Steven G. Docimo
Craig A. Peters

Chapter 73
Tissue Engineering Perspectives for Reconstructive Surgery 265
Anthony Atala

VOLUME IV

X. Oncology

Chapter 74
Molecular Genetics and Cancer Biology 268
Adam S. Kibel
Joel B. Nelson

Chapter 75
Renal Tumors 275
Andrew C. Novick
Steven C. Campbell

Chapter 76
Urothelial Tumors of the Urinary Tract 280
Edward M. Messing

Chapter 77
Management of Superficial Bladder Cancer 287
Stanley Bruce Malkowicz

Chapter 78
Management of Invasive and Metastatic Bladder Cancer 289
Mark Schoenberg

Chapter 79
Surgery of Bladder Cancer 291
V. Keith Jiminez
Fray F. Marshall

Chapter 80
Management of Urothelial Tumors of the Renal Pelvis and Ureter 293
Arthur I. Sagalowsky
Thomas W. Jarrett

Chapter 81
Neoplasms of the Testis 297
Jerome P. Richie
Graeme S. Steele

Chapter 82
Surgery of Testicular Tumors 303
Joel Sheinfeld
James McKiernan
George J. Bosl

Chapter 83
Tumors of the Penis 306
Donald F. Lynch, Jr.
Curtis A. Pettaway

Chapter 84
Surgery of Penile and Urethral Carcinoma 310
S. Machele Donat
Paul J. Cozzi
Harry W. Herr

XI. Carcinoma of the Prostate

Chapter 85
Epidemiology, Etiology, and Prevention of Prostate Cancer 313
    Robert E. Reiter
    Jean B. DeKernion

Chapter 86
Pathology of Prostatic Neoplasia 315
    Jonathan I. Epstein

Chapter 87
Ultrasonography and Biopsy of the Prostate 317
    Martha K. Terris

Chapter 88
Diagnosis and Staging of Prostate Cancer 318
    H. Ballentine Carter

Chapter 89
Radical Prostatectomy 320
    James A. Eastham
    Peter T. Scardino

Chapter 90
Anatomic Radical Retropubic Prostatectomy 323
    Patrick C. Walsh

Chapter 91
Radical Perineal Prostatectomy 326
    Robert P. Gibbons

Chapter 92
Radiation Therapy for Prostate Cancer 328
    Anthony V. D'Amico
    Juanita Crook
    Clair J. Beard
    Theodore L. DeWeese
    Mark Hurwitz
    Irving Kaplan

Chapter 93
Cryotherapy for Prostate Cancer 332
    Katsuto Shinohara
    Peter R. Carroll

Chapter 94
Hormonal Therapy of Prostate Cancer 334
    Fritz H. Schröder

Chapter 95
Chemotherapy for Hormone-Resistant Prostate Cancer 336
    Mario A. Eisenberger
    Michael A. Carducci

XII. Urinary Lithiasis and Endourology

Chapter 96
Urinary Lithiasis: Etiology, Diagnosis, and Medical Management 340
    Mani Menon
    Martin I. Resnick

Chapter 97
Ureteroscopy and Retrograde Ureteral Access 346
    Li-Ming Su
    R. Ernest Sosa

Chapter 98
Percutaneous Approaches to the Upper Urinary Tract 347
    Elspeth M. McDougall
    Evangelos N. Liatsikos
    Caner Z. Dinlenc
    Arthur D. Smith

Chapter 99
Surgical Management of Urinary Lithiasis 351
    James E. Lingeman
    David A. Lifshitz
    Andrew P. Evan

XIII. Urologic Surgery

Chapter 100
Basis of Laparoscopic Urologic Surgery 358
    Inderbir S. Gill
    Kurt Kerbl
    Anoop M. Meraney
    Ralph V. Clayman

Chapter 101
The Adrenals 361
    E. Darracott Vaughan, Jr.
    Jon D. Blumenfeld
    Joseph Del Pizzo
    Steven J. Schichman
    R. Ernest Sosa

Chapter 102
Surgery of the Kidney 365
    Andrew C. Novick

Chapter 103
Laparoscopic Surgery of the Kidney 369
    Jay T. Bishoff
    Louis R. Kavoussi

Chapter 104
Other Applications of Laparoscopic Surgery 373
    Howard N. Winfield
    Jeffrey A. Cadeddu

Chapter 105
Genitourinary Trauma 375
    Jack W. McAninch
    Richard A. Santucci

Chapter 106
Use of Intestinal Segments and Urinary Diversion 379
W. Scott McDougal

Chapter 107
Cutaneous Continent Urinary Diversion 382
Mitchell C. Benson
Carl A. Olsson

Chapter 108
Orthotopic Urinary Diversion 387
John P. Stein
Donald G. Skinner

Chapter 109
Surgery of the Seminal Vesicles 392
Jay I. Sandlow
Richard D. Williams

Chapter 110
Surgery of the Penis and Urethra 394
Gerald H. Jordan
Steven M. Schlossberg

SECTION I

ANATOMY

Chapter 1

Surgical Anatomy of the Retroperitoneum, Kidneys, and Ureters

John N. Kabalin

Questions

1. The lumbodorsal fascia originates from:

   a. the latissimus dorsi muscle.
   b. the lower rib cage posteriorly.
   c. the lumbar vertebrae.
   d. the iliac crest.
   e. the rectus sheath.

2. The lumbodorsal fascia consists of:

   a. a single layer.
   b. two distinct layers.
   c. three distinct layers.
   d. four distinct layers.
   e. five distinct layers.

3. The lumbodorsal fascia is contiguous anteriorly with:

   a. the transversalis fascia.
   b. the aponeurosis of the transversus abdominis muscle.
   c. the internal oblique fascia.
   d. the external oblique fascia.
   e. the rectus sheath.

4. The dorsal lumbotomy incision to expose the kidney:

   a. requires incision of the latissimus dorsi muscle.
   b. requires incision of the quadratus lumborum muscle.
   c. splits the lumbodorsal fascia horizontally from posterior to anterior.
   d. splits the lumbodorsal fascia vertically without incising muscle.
   e. requires excision of the 12th rib.

5. The psoas major muscle:

   a. flexes the thigh at the hip.
   b. extends the thigh at the hip.
   c. adducts the thigh at the hip.
   d. abducts the thigh at the hip.
   e. assists in full contraction of the diaphragm.

6. Which of the following muscles is NOT a boundary of the retroperitoneum?

   a. The psoas muscle
   b. The iliacus muscle
   c. The quadratus lumborum muscle
   d. The diaphragm
   e. The rectus muscle

7. In a subcostal flank approach to the kidney, which of the following may be incised to increase upward mobility of the 12th rib?

   a. The intercostal muscles between the 11th and 12th ribs
   b. The latissimus dorsi muscle
   c. The lumbodorsal fascia
   d. The quadratus lumborum muscle
   e. The costovertebral ligament

8. The first arterial branch(es) from the abdominal aorta is(are):

   a. the paired renal arteries.
   b. the right adrenal artery.
   c. the inferior phrenic arteries.
   d. the hepatic artery.
   e. the superior mesenteric artery.

9. Which of the following arteries branches from the celiac arterial trunk?

   a. The left gastric artery
   b. The right gastric artery
   c. The pancreaticoduodenal artery
   d. The superior mesenteric artery
   e. The inferior phrenic arteries

10. The renal arteries typically branch from the abdominal aorta at the level of the:

    a. 12th thoracic vertebral body.
    b. first lumbar vertebral body.
    c. second lumbar vertebral body.
    d. third lumbar vertebral body.
    e. fourth lumbar vertebral body.

11. The testicular arteries most commonly originate from:

    a. the renal arteries.
    b. the adrenal arteries.
    c. the abdominal aorta above the superior mesenteric artery.
    d. the abdominal aorta below the renal arteries.
    e. the common iliac arteries.

1

12. A 20-year-old man is undergoing retroperitoneal dissection for a testicular germ cell tumor. The inferior mesenteric artery is divided during reflection of the intestines to expose the retroperitoneum. This can be expected to result in:
    a. ischemia of the descending colon.
    b. ischemia of the sigmoid colon.
    c. ischemia of the rectum.
    d. ischemia of the transverse colon.
    e. none of the above.

13. Which of the following vessels drain(s) into the inferior vena cava?
    a. Renal veins
    b. Superior mesenteric vein
    c. Inferior mesenteric vein
    d. Splenic vein
    e. All of the above

14. The left gonadal vein typically drains into the:
    a. anterior aspect of the inferior vena cava.
    b. left lateral aspect of the inferior vena cava.
    c. inferior aspect of the left renal vein.
    d. left adrenal vein.
    e. inferior aspect of the common iliac vein.

15. The left renal vein crosses the abdominal aorta:
    a. anteriorly, just above the superior mesenteric artery.
    b. anteriorly, just below the superior mesenteric artery.
    c. posteriorly, at the level of the superior mesenteric artery.
    d. anteriorly, just below the inferior mesenteric artery.
    e. anteriorly, just above the inferior mesenteric artery.

16. Which of the following vessels commonly drains into the left renal vein?
    a. The left adrenal vein
    b. The second lumbar vein
    c. The left internal spermatic vein
    d. All of the above
    e. None of the above

17. On a CT scan, a male patient is found to have enlarged lymph nodes along the abdominal aorta between the left renal hilum and the inferior mesenteric artery. Sites of malignancy that would commonly drain directly to these lymph nodes would NOT include:
    a. the colon.
    b. the left kidney.
    c. the left testis.
    d. the left renal pelvis.
    e. the bladder.

18. Lymph flow in the lumbar lymphatic chains of the retroperitoneum proceeds:
    a. in a cephalad direction.
    b. in a cephalad direction and from right to left.
    c. in a cephalad direction and from left to right.
    d. caudally.
    e. caudally and from left to right.

19. The cisterna chyli is typically located at approximately the level of the first lumbar vertebral body:
    a. posterior to the inferior vena cava.
    b. posterior to the aorta.
    c. closely approximated to the posterior surface of the right adrenal gland.
    d. associated with the superior mesenteric artery.
    e. posterior to the right renal hilum.

20. The primary lymph node drainage site for the right testis is:
    a. the superficial right inguinal lymph nodes.
    b. the deep right inguinal lymph nodes.
    c. the right common iliac lymph nodes.
    d. lymph nodes at the right renal hilum.
    e. the interaortocaval lumbar lymph nodes.

21. The lumbar sympathetic chains:
    a. run vertically in the retroperitoneum, medial to the psoas muscles.
    b. contain numerous sympathetic ganglia.
    c. are closely associated with the lumbar blood vessels.
    d. contain postganglionic sympathetic neurons supplying the lower extremities.
    e. all of the above.

22. Disruption of which sympathetic nervous plexus on the anterior abdominal aorta during retroperitoneal dissection will probably cause loss of seminal emission in a male patient?
    a. Celiac plexus
    b. Renal plexus
    c. Superior mesenteric plexus
    d. Superior hypogastric plexus
    e. All of the above

23. In the lateral abdominal wall, the iliohypogastric nerve will be found coursing in the plane:
    a. deep to the transversalis fascia.
    b. between the transversalis fascia and the transversus abdominis muscle.
    c. between the transversus abdominis and internal oblique muscles.
    d. between the internal oblique and external oblique muscles.
    e. superficial to the external oblique muscle.

24. The cremaster muscle is innervated by:
    a. the ilioinguinal nerve.
    b. the iliohypogastric nerve.
    c. the obturator nerve.
    d. the genital branch of the genitofemoral nerve.
    e. the femoral branch of the genitofemoral nerve.

25. In the retroperitoneum, where can the genitofemoral nerve be found?
    a. Posterior to the psoas muscle
    b. On the anterior surface of the psoas muscle
    c. Lateral to the psoas muscle
    d. Medial to the psoas muscle
    e. The genitofemoral nerve is not typically found in the retroperitoneum.

26. The descending duodenum:
    a. lies within the retroperitoneum.
    b. receives the common bile duct.
    c. lies lateral to the head of the pancreas.
    d. lies anterior to the right renal hilum.
    e. all of the above.

27. The posterior surface of the tail of the pancreas is closely associated with the:
    a. splenic artery.
    b. splenic vein.
    c. upper pole of the left kidney.
    d. left adrenal gland.
    e. all of the above.

28. In cases of renal ectopia, the ipsilateral adrenal gland is typically:

a. absent.
b. found in its normal anatomic position in the upper retroperitoneum.
c. found in association with the contralateral adrenal gland.
d. found closely applied to the superior pole of the ectopic kidney.
e. found closely associated with the ipsilateral renal artery.

29. In cases of unilateral renal agenesis, the ipsilateral adrenal gland is commonly:

   a. absent.
   b. found in its normal anatomic position in the upper retroperitoneum.
   c. found in association with the contralateral adrenal gland.
   d. found just inside the ipsilateral internal inguinal ring.
   e. found in an ectopic, intrathoracic location.

30. Which of the following statements is NOT true?

   a. The right renal vein is much shorter than the left renal vein.
   b. The right adrenal vein is much shorter than the left adrenal vein.
   c. The right kidney is typically located lower in the retroperitoneum than the left kidney.
   d. The right adrenal gland is typically located lower in the retroperitoneum than the left adrenal gland.
   e. Both c and d.

31. As one proceeds outward from the adrenal medulla, the three separate functional layers of the adrenal cortex are, in correct order:

   a. the zona reticularis, zona fasciculata, then zona glomerulosa.
   b. the zona fasciculata, zona reticularis, then zona glomerulosa.
   c. the zona glomerulosa, zona fasciculata, then zona reticularis.
   d. the zona glomerulosa, zona reticularis, then zona fasciculata.
   e. the zona reticularis, zona glomerulosa, then zona fasciculata.

32. Which of the following statements is(are) NOT true?

   a. The adrenal medulla produces catecholamines in response to stimulation from the sympathetic nervous system.
   b. The zona glomerulosa produces aldosterone in response to angiotensin II.
   c. The zona reticularis of the adrenal cortex produces androgens in response to luteinizing hormone (LH).
   d. The zona fasciculata of the adrenal cortex produces glucocorticoids in response to adrenocorticotropic hormone (ACTH).
   e. Both b and c.

33. The adrenal arteries are branches from:

   a. the aorta.
   b. the inferior phrenic arteries.
   c. the renal arteries.
   d. the celiac arterial trunk.
   e. a, b, and c.

34. The kidney produces:

   a. renin.
   b. angiotensin.
   c. erythropoietin.
   d. both a and c.
   e. a, b, and c.

35. The normal kidney in an average-sized adult man weighs approximately:

   a. 1200 grams.
   b. 600 grams.
   c. 300 grams.
   d. 150 grams.
   e. 50 grams.

36. Persistent fetal lobation identified in the kidney of an adult patient:

   a. indicates the presence of a congenital renal disorder.
   b. indicates childhood renal injury due to infection.
   c. is observed only with long-standing obstructive uropathy.
   d. is a normal variant.
   e. is never seen.

37. The upper pole of the kidney lies anterior to:

   a. the 12th rib.
   b. the diaphragm.
   c. the pleura.
   d. all of the above.
   e. none of the above.

38. Which of the following statements regarding the typical anatomic positioning of the kidney is TRUE?

   a. The lower pole of the kidney lies more anterior than the upper pole.
   b. The lower pole of the kidney lies more lateral than the upper pole.
   c. The medial aspect of the kidney lies more anterior than its lateral aspect.
   d. The anterior renal calyces lie lateral to the posterior renal calyces.
   e. All of the above.

39. During left radical nephrectomy performed via a transabdominal approach, excessive traction on which of the following structures might be expected to produce a significant injury to the spleen?

   a. Left adrenal gland
   b. Splenorenal ligament
   c. Splenocolic ligament
   d. Both b and c
   e. a, b, and c

40. Gerota's fascia envelops and contains:

   a. the adrenal gland.
   b. the kidney.
   c. the ureter.
   d. the gonadal vessels.
   e. all of the above.

41. Following blunt trauma to the right kidney with a major laceration to the renal parenchyma and ongoing hemorrhage, the expanding hematoma contained within Gerota's fascia will tend to:

   a. extend across the midline into Gerota's fascia surrounding the left (contralateral) kidney.
   b. extend downward into the pelvis.
   c. extend upward into the thorax.
   d. extend anterolaterally, deep to the transversalis fascia.
   e. extend anterolaterally, between the peritoneum and transversalis fascia.

42. Proceeding from posterior to anterior, the structures encountered in the renal hilum are, in correct order:

   a. the renal artery, renal vein, and renal pelvis.
   b. the renal pelvis, renal artery, and renal vein.

c. the renal pelvis, renal vein, and renal artery.
d. the renal vein, renal artery, and renal pelvis.
e. the renal artery, renal pelvis, and renal vein.

43. The first branch segmental artery from the main renal artery is typically:

    a. the apical anterior segmental artery.
    b. the lower anterior segmental artery.
    c. the posterior segmental artery.
    d. the upper anterior segmental artery.
    e. the middle anterior segmental artery.

44. During pyeloplasty, the posterior segmental renal artery is inadvertently divided. This will produce:

    a. no effect on the kidney.
    b. ischemic loss of a large posterior segment of the renal parenchyma.
    c. ischemic loss of a small posterior segment of the renal parenchyma.
    d. ischemic loss of a segment of upper pole renal parenchyma.
    e. ischemic loss of a segment of lower pole renal parenchyma.

45. The sequential branches of the renal artery are, in order:

    a. the segmental, interlobar, arcuate, interlobular, and afferent arteriole.
    b. the segmental, interlobular, arcuate, interlobar, and afferent arteriole.
    c. the segmental, subsegmental, interlobar, interlobular, arcuate, and afferent arteriole.
    d. the segmental, arcuate, interlobar, interlobular, and afferent arteriole.
    e. the segmental, interlobar, interlobular, arcuate, and afferent arteriole.

46. During pyeloplasty, a large anterior segmental renal vein is inadvertently torn and subsequently ligated to control hemorrhage. This will produce:

    a. no effect on the kidney.
    b. segmental renal venous congestion and chronic pain.
    c. ischemic loss of a large anterior segment of the renal parenchyma.
    d. ischemic loss of a small anterior segment of the renal parenchyma.
    e. ischemic loss of a segment of lower pole renal parenchyma.

47. Which of the following vessels commonly drains into the right renal vein?

    a. The right adrenal vein
    b. The second lumbar vein
    c. The right gonadal vein
    d. All of the above
    e. None of the above

48. The most common renal vascular anomaly is:

    a. a supernumerary left renal artery.
    b. a supernumerary right renal artery.
    c. a supernumerary left renal vein coursing anterior to the aorta.
    d. a supernumerary left renal vein coursing posterior to the aorta.
    e. a supernumerary right renal vein.

49. After involvement of lymph nodes directly at the renal hilum, the primary lymph node drainage site for the left kidney is:

    a. the left lateral para-aortic lymph nodes.
    b. the interaortocaval lymph nodes.
    c. the right paracaval lymph nodes.
    d. left retrocrural lymph nodes.
    e. all of the above.

50. In a typical human kidney, there are approximately how many renal papillae and corresponding minor calyces?

    a. 3 to 5
    b. 7 to 9
    c. 11 to 12
    d. 14 to 15
    e. 17 to 18

51. A compound renal papilla and calyx:

    a. is protective against ascending infection.
    b. occurs least commonly at the upper pole of the kidney.
    c. is a rare finding.
    d. is commonly associated with formation of kidney stones.
    e. none of the above.

52. The ureteral smooth muscle consists of:

    a. a single layer of longitudinally oriented muscle bundles.
    b. a single layer of circular and obliquely oriented muscle bundles.
    c. a single layer of randomly oriented muscle bundles.
    d. two layers—an inner layer of longitudinal muscle and an outer layer of circular and oblique muscle.
    e. two layers—an inner layer of circular and oblique muscle and an outer layer of longitudinal muscle.

53. The ureter receives its blood supply from:

    a. the renal artery.
    b. the aorta.
    c. the common iliac artery.
    d. the gonadal artery.
    e. all of the above.

54. An invasive transitional cell carcinoma is diagnosed in the left proximal ureter, at the level of the third lumbar vertebral body. The primary site of potential nodal metastases from this lesion will be:

    a. the left para-aortic lymph nodes.
    b. the interaortocaval lymph nodes.
    c. the left common iliac lymph nodes.
    d. lymph nodes at the left renal hilum.
    e. the left external iliac lymph nodes.

55. During surgical dissection, the ureter can be identified as it enters the pelvis:

    a. at the aortic bifurcation.
    b. crossing the superior border of the sacrum.
    c. crossing the common iliac artery at the branching of the internal iliac artery.
    d. crossing the uterine artery.
    e. at the internal inguinal ring.

56. A young man with right-sided abdominal pain is diagnosed with right hydroureteronephrosis by renal ultrasonography. Which of the following inflammatory processes might impinge upon the right ureter and cause obstruction?

    a. Acute appendicitis
    b. Crohn's ileitis
    c. Perforated cecal carcinoma
    d. All of the above
    e. None of the above

57. Narrowing of the ureteral luminal caliber naturally occurs at:

    a. the ureteropelvic junction.
    b. the crossing of the iliac vessels.
    c. the ureterovesical junction.
    d. all of the above.
    e. none of the above.

58. Sympathetic nerve input to the kidney typically travels through the:
    a. celiac plexus.
    b. superior mesenteric plexus.
    c. superior hypogastric plexus.
    d. inferior hypogastric plexus.
    e. none of the above.

59. Ureteral peristalsis requires:
    a. intact sympathetic input.
    b. intact parasympathetic input.
    c. both sympathetic and parasympathetic input.
    d. intact spinal cord.
    e. intrinsic smooth muscle pacemakers in the renal collecting system.

60. The pain caused by an obstructing ureteral stone:
    a. is primarily related to distention of the collecting system above the stone.
    b. is transmitted via nerves from the eighth thoracic through the second lumbar spinal segments.
    c. may be referred over the somatic distribution of the subcostal, iliohypogastric, or ilioinguinal nerves.
    d. may be referred over the distribution of the genitofemoral nerve.
    e. all of the above.

Answers

1. **c. the lumbar vertebrae.** The lumbodorsal fascia originates from the lumbar vertebrae. [p 3]

2. **c. three distinct layers.** There are three distinct layers of the lumbodorsal fascia. [p 3]

3. **b. the aponeurosis of the transversus abdominis muscle.** All three layers of the lumbodorsal fascia join to form a single thick aponeurosis lateral to the quadratus lumborum muscle before extending further anterolaterally, where they are contiguous with the aponeurosis of the transversus abdominis muscle. [p 4]

4. **d. splits the lumbodorsal fascia vertically without incising muscle.** A vertical incision that parallels the lateral borders of the sacrospinalis and quadratus lumborum can be made through this lumbodorsal fascia, posteromedial to the first transverse muscle fibers of the transversus abdominis muscle, to gain surgical access to the retroperitoneum and kidney without cutting muscle (the so-called lumbodorsal approach, or dorsal lumbotomy) (see Fig. 1–6). [p 4]

5. **a. flexes the thigh at the hip.** The psoas major joins the iliacus muscle, which originates broadly over the inner aspect of the iliac wing of the pelvis, to become the iliopsoas and insert on the lesser trochanter of the femur and flex the thigh at the hip. [p 5]

6. **e. Rectus muscle.** The posterior surface of the retroperitoneum is formed by the lumbar vertebral bodies in the midline, which are covered by the shiny, longitudinal fibers of the anterior spinous ligament (see Fig. 1–7). These are flanked bilaterally by the psoas muscles. The psoas muscles are covered by a glistening white fibrous fascia, the so-called psoas sheath, which is contiguous with the transversalis fascia. As one moves laterally, the lateral portion of the quadratus lumborum extends from behind the lateral margin of the psoas. The anterior layer of the lumbodorsal fascia covers this muscle and continues as the aponeurosis of the transversus abdominis muscle. Farther laterally, the transversus abdominis muscle proper is encountered. Superiorly, the posterior wall of the retroperitoneum is formed by the posterior insertion of the diaphragm along the lower ribs (see Figs. 1–2 and 1–3). Inferiorly, below the level of the iliac crest, the iliopsoas muscle forms the posterior confine of the retroperitoneum. [p 5]

7. **e. The costovertebral ligament.** The costovertebral, or lumbodorsal, ligament is a strong fascial attachment between the inferior margin of the 12th rib and the transverse processes of the first and second lumbar vertebrae (see Fig. 1–5). It is encountered only in posterior approaches to the kidney and can be incised to produce greater mobility of the 12th rib and provide greater exposure and access to the structures of the upper retroperitoneum. [p 5]

8. **c. the inferior phrenic arteries.** The first abdominal branches of the aorta are the paired inferior phrenic arteries. [p 6]

9. **a. The left gastric artery.** The short celiac arterial trunk trifurcates into common hepatic, left gastric, and splenic branches. [p 6]

10. **c. second lumbar vertebral body.** Usually overlying the second lumbar vertebral body, but subject to considerable variation, the paired renal arteries emanate laterally from the aorta. [p 6]

11. **d. the abdominal aorta below the renal arteries.** The paired gonadal arteries arise from the anterolateral aorta—in atypical cases, from a single anterior trunk—at a level somewhat below the renal vessels. [p 6]

12. **e. none of the above.** The inferior mesenteric artery, especially in younger individuals without atherosclerotic occlusive arterial disease, can almost always be sacrificed without complication. [p 7]

13. **a. Renal veins.** Inferior mesenteric, superior mesenteric, and splenic veins join to form the portal vein and drain proximally into the liver rather than directly into the inferior vena cava. [p 8]

14. **c. inferior aspect of the left renal vein.** The left gonadal vein usually enters the inferior aspect of the left renal vein. [p 8]

15. **b. anteriorly, just below the superior mesenteric artery.** The left renal vein crosses the aorta anteriorly below the takeoff of the superior mesenteric artery. [p 8]

16. **d. All of the above.** The left renal vein commonly receives a lumbar vein (usually the second lumbar) on its posterior aspect. In addition, the left gonadal vein typically drains into its inferior margin and the left adrenal vein into its superior margin. [p 8]

17. **e. the bladder.** These lumbar nodal chains are extraregional or secondary drainage sites for any metastatic process arising from the lower pelvis. [p 9]

18. **b. in a cephalad direction and from right to left.** It is important that most of the lateral flow between ascending lymphatics moves from right to left ascending lumbar trunks. [p 9]

19. **b. posterior to the aorta.** The structure known as the cis-

terna chyli truly lies within the thorax, posterior to the aorta or slightly to the right, in a retrocrural position, usually anterior to the first or second lumbar vertebral body. [p 9]

20. **e. the interaortocaval lumbar lymph nodes.** The right testis drains primarily to the interaortocaval region. [p 10]

21. **e. all of the above.** The sympathetic trunks course vertically along the anterolateral aspect of the spinal column, in the retroperitoneum lying within the groove between the medial aspect of the ipsilateral psoas muscle and the spine, in some cases covered by the psoas (see Fig. 1–7). The lumbar arteries and veins, coursing posteriorly, are very closely associated with the sympathetic trunks, crossing them perpendicularly and at times proceeding directly through split portions of the sympathetic chain. The lumbar sympathetic trunks contain variable numbers of ganglia of variable size and position. Some of the preganglionic fibers of the sympathetic trunks synapse within these ganglia with postganglionic sympathetic neurons supplying the body wall and lower extremities. [pp 10 and 12]

22. **d. Superior hypogastric plexus.** At the lower extent of the abdominal aorta, much of the sympathetic input to the pelvic urinary organs and genital tract travels through the superior hypogastric plexus, which lies on the aorta anterior to its bifurcation and extends inferiorly on the anterior surface of the fifth lumbar vertebra. This plexus is contiguous bilaterally with inferior hypogastric plexuses, which extend into the pelvis. Disruption of the sympathetic nerve fibers that travel through these plexuses during retroperitoneal dissection can cause loss of seminal vesicle emission and/or failure of bladder neck closure, which results in retrograde ejaculation. [p 12]

23. **c. between the transversus abdominis and internal oblique muscles.** The iliohypogastric nerve and the ilioinguinal nerve originate together as a common extension from the first lumbar spinal nerve before splitting. These somatic nerves cross the anterior or inner surface of the quadratus lumborum muscle before piercing the transversus abdominis muscle and continuing their course between this and the internal oblique muscle. [p 14]

24. **d. the genital branch of the genitofemoral nerve.** The genital branch of the genitofemoral nerve supplies the cremaster and dartos muscles. [p 14]

25. **b. On the anterior surface of the psoas muscle.** The genitofemoral nerve lies directly atop and parallels the psoas muscle throughout most of its retroperitoneal course. [p 14]

26. **e. all of the above.** The second (descending) part of the duodenum descends vertically, directly anterior to the right renal hilum, and thus is intimately related on its posterior aspect to the medial margin of the right kidney, right renal vessels, renal pelvis, ureteropelvic junction, and often the upper right ureter. The common bile duct also lies posterior to and drains into this part of the duodenum. Directly medial and intimately related to the descending duodenum lies the head of the pancreas. [p 15]

27. **e. all of the above.** The tail of the pancreas on the left is related posteriorly to the left adrenal gland and upper portion of the left kidney. The splenic vein runs directly posterior to the pancreas, and the splenic artery runs just superior to the vein. [p 16]

28. **b. found in its normal anatomic position in the upper retroperitoneum.** In cases of renal ectopia, the adrenal gland is usually found in approximately its normal anatomic position. [pp 17–18]

29. **b. found in its normal anatomic position in the upper retroperitoneum.** In cases of renal agenesis, the adrenal gland on the involved side is typically present. [p 18]

30. **d. The right adrenal gland is typically located lower in the retroperitoneum than is the left adrenal gland.** The right adrenal tends to lie more superiorly in the retroperitoneum than does the left adrenal. [p 18]

31. **a. the zona reticularis, zona fasciculata, then zona glomerulosa.** Three cell layers can be identified in the adrenal cortex (see Fig. 1–19). The outermost layer is the zona glomerulosa, which produces aldosterone in response to stimulation by the renin-angiotensin system. Centripetally located are the zona fasciculata and zona reticularis, which produce glucocorticoids and sex steroids, respectively. [p 19]

32. **c. The zona reticularis of the adrenal cortex produces androgens in response to luteinizing hormone (LH).** The function of production of sex steroids by the zona reticularis is regulated by pituitary release of adrenocorticotropic hormone (ACTH). [p 19]

33. **e. a, b, and c.** Multiple small arteries supply each adrenal gland (see Fig. 1–15). These are branch vessels, which can be traced to three major arterial sources for each gland: (1) superior branches from the inferior phrenic artery, (2) middle branches directly from the aorta, and (3) inferior branches from the ipsilateral renal artery (see Fig. 1–9). [p 19]

34. **d. both a and c.** The kidneys play a central role in fluid, electrolyte, and acid-base balance in humans, but they also have important endocrine functions, known to include vitamin D metabolism and the production of both renin and erythropoietin. [p 19]

35. **d. 150 grams.** The normal kidney in the adult male weighs approximately 150 g. [p 20]

36. **d. is a normal variant.** It is neither unusual nor abnormal to see persistence of some degree of fetal lobation throughout adult life (see Fig. 1–20). [p 20]

37. **d. all of the above.** The diaphragm covers roughly the upper third or upper pole of each kidney. With the diaphragm travels the pleural reflection, and thus any direct approach to the upper portion of the kidney, whether percutaneous or open surgical, risks entering the pleural space. The 12th rib on either side crosses the kidney at approximately the lower extent of the diaphragm. [p 22]

38. **e. All of the above.** In part as a result of the contour of the psoas muscle, the lower pole of either kidney lies farther from the midline than does the upper pole, so that the upper poles tilt medially at a slight angle (see Fig. 1–27). Similarly, the kidneys do not lie in a simple coronal plane, but the lower pole of the kidney is pushed slightly more anterior than the upper pole. The medial aspect of each kidney is rotated anteriorly on a longitudinal axis at an angle of about 30 degrees from the true coronal plane, with the renal vessels and pelvis exiting the hilum medially in a relatively anterior direction (see Figs. 1–8 and 1–27). Typically, two longitudinal rows of renal pyramids and corresponding minor calyces, roughly perpendicular to one another, extend anteriorly and posteriorly. The anterior calyces extend laterally in a coronal plane, whereas the posterior calyces extend posteriorly in a sagittal plane. [pp 22 and 33]

39. **d. Both b and c.** There is typically a peritoneal extension between the perirenal fascia covering the upper pole of the left kidney and the inferior splenic capsule, called the splenorenal, or lienorenal, ligament. Just as with the adjacent and often contiguous splenocolic ligamentous attachment, care must be taken not to exert undue tension on the sple-

norenal ligament during operative procedures on the left kidney, to avoid inadvertent tearing of the spleen. [p 24]

40. **e. all of the above.** The kidneys and associated adrenal glands are surrounded by varying degrees of perirenal or perinephric fat, and these together are loosely enclosed by the perirenal fascia, commonly called "Gerota's fascia" (see Figs. 1–22C and D, 1–6, and 1–8). Inferiorly, Gerota's fascia remains an open potential space, containing the ureter and gonadal vessels on either side. [p 24]

41. **b. extend downward into the pelvis.** When very large, such collections can and do extend into the pelvis, following the potential space where Gerota's fascia does not fuse inferiorly. [p 25]

42. **b. the renal pelvis, renal artery, and renal vein.** The renal vein lies most anteriorly, and behind it lies the artery. Both normally lie anterior to the urinary collecting system, that is, the renal pelvis. [p 25]

43. **c. the posterior segmental artery.** The main renal artery typically divides into four or more segmental vessels, with five branches most commonly described (see Figs. 1–30 and 1–31). The first and most constant segmental division is a posterior branch. [p 25]

44. **b. ischemic loss of a large posterior segment of the renal parenchyma.** The posterior segmental artery usually exits the main renal artery before it enters the renal hilum and proceeds posteriorly to the renal pelvis to supply a large posterior segment of the kidney. The main renal artery and each segmental artery, as well as their multiple succeeding branch arteries, are all "end arteries," without anastomosis or collateral circulation, and occlusion of any of these vessels produces ischemia and infarction of the corresponding renal parenchyma that it supplies. [p 25]

45. **a. the segmental, interlobar, arcuate, interlobular, and afferent arteriole.** The segmental arteries course through the renal sinus and branch further into lobar arteries, which divide again and enter the renal parenchyma as interlobar arteries (see Fig. 1–32). The interlobar arteries branch into arcuate arteries, which arc parallel to the renal contour along the corticomedullary junction. The arcuate arteries, in turn, produce multiple radial arterial branches, the interlobular arteries. These have multiple side branches, which are the afferent arterioles to the glomeruli. [p 25]

46. **a. no effect on the kidney.** Unlike the renal arteries, none of which communicate, the renal parenchymal veins anastomose freely. [p 26]

47. **e. None of the above.** The right renal vein is short (2 to 4 cm) and enters the right lateral aspect of the inferior vena cava directly, usually without receiving other venous branches. [p 26]

48. **a. a supernumerary left renal artery.** The most common variation is the occurrence of supernumerary renal arteries. These supernumerary arteries usually arise from the lateral aorta, occur perhaps slightly more often on the left than on the right, and may enter the renal hilum or directly into the parenchyma of one of the poles of the kidney. [p 27]

49. **a. the left lateral para-aortic lymph nodes.** From the left kidney (see Fig. 1–36), the lymphatic trunks then drain primarily into the left lateral para-aortic lymph nodes, including nodes anterior and posterior to the aorta, from a level below the inferior mesenteric artery to the diaphragm. [p 30]

50. **b. 7 to 9.** The renal papillae may number as few as 4 or as many as 18, but 7 to 9 are present in the typical kidney. [p 33]

51. **e. none of the above.** A compound renal papilla and calyx often occurs at the renal poles. The compound papillae are of physiologic significance in that their configuration permits urinary reflux into the renal parenchyma with sufficient back pressure, also allowing bacterial reflux into the kidney in the presence of infected urine (see Fig. 1–42). Renal parenchymal scarring secondary to infection is typically most severe overlying such compound papillae. [pp 33–34]

52. **d. two layers—an inner layer of longitudinal muscle and an outer layer of circular and oblique muscle.** Smooth muscle covers the renal calyces, renal pelvis, and ureter. In the ureter, this muscle can usually be divided into an inner layer of longitudinally coursing muscle bundles and an outer layer of circular and oblique muscle (see Fig. 1–46). [pp 36–37]

53. **e. all of the above.** The ureter receives its blood supply from multiple feeding arterial branches along its course (see Fig. 1–47). In the retroperitoneum, the ureter may receive branches from the renal artery, gonadal artery, abdominal aorta, and common iliac artery. [p 37]

54. **a. the left para-aortic lymph nodes.** In the abdomen, the left para-aortic lymph nodes form the primary drainage sites for the left ureter. [pp 37–38]

55. **c. crossing the common iliac artery at the branching of the internal iliac artery.** The ureter is related posteriorly to the psoas muscle throughout its retroperitoneal course, crossing the iliac vessels to enter the pelvis at approximately the bifurcation of the common iliac artery into internal and external iliac arteries (see Fig. 1–1). [p 38]

56. **d. All of the above.** Anteriorly, the right ureter is related to the terminal ileum, cecum, appendix, and ascending colon and their mesenteries. [p 38]

57. **d. all of the above.** The ureter is not of uniform caliber, with three distinct narrowings normally present along its course (see Fig. 1–48). The first of these is the ureteropelvic junction, the second is the crossing of the iliac vessels, and the third is the ureterovesical junction in the pelvis. [pp 38–39]

58. **a. celiac plexus.** The kidneys receive preganglionic sympathetic input from the eighth thoracic through the first lumbar spinal segments. Postganglionic fibers arise primarily from the celiac and aorticorenal ganglia. [p 40]

59. **e. intrinsic smooth muscle pacemakers in the renal collecting system.** Normal ureteral peristalsis does not require outside autonomic input but rather originates and is propagated from intrinsic smooth muscle pacemaker sites located in the minor calyces of the renal collecting system. [p 40]

60. **e. all of the above.** Pain fibers leave the kidney, renal pelvis, and ureter, traveling with the sympathetic nerves. They are primarily stimulated by nociceptors sensitive to increased tension (distention) in the renal capsule, renal collecting system, or ureter. The resulting visceral pain is felt directly and is referred to somatic distributions that correspond to the spinal segments providing the sympathetic distribution to the kidney and ureter (eighth thoracic through second lumbar segments). Pain and reflex muscle spasm are typically produced over the distributions of the subcostal, iliohypogastric, ilioinguinal, and/or genitofemoral nerves. [p 40]

Chapter 2

Anatomy of the Lower Urinary Tract and Male Genitalia

James D. Brooks

Questions

1. The greater and lesser sciatic foramina are separated by:
   a. the sacrotuberous ligament.
   b. Cooper's (pectineal) ligament.
   c. the arcuate line.
   d. the sacrospinous ligament.
   e. the piriformis muscle.

2. During inguinal incisions, the vessels invariably encountered in Camper's fascia are:
   a. the superficial inferior epigastric artery and vein.
   b. the superficial circumflex iliac artery and vein.
   c. the external pudendal artery and vein.
   d. the gonadal artery and veins.
   e. the accessory obturator vein.

3. Rupture of the penile urethra at the junction of the penis and scrotum can result in urinary extravasation into all of the following structures except:
   a. the anterior abdominal wall up to the clavicles.
   b. the scrotum.
   c. the penis, deep to the dartos fascia.
   d. the perineum, in a "butterfly" pattern.
   e. the buttock.

4. During inguinal hernia repair in a male patient, the ilioinguinal nerve is injured in the canal, which will most likely produce:
   a. anesthesia over the dorsum of the penis.
   b. anesthesia over the pubis and scrotum, and loss of cremasteric contraction.
   c. anesthesia over the pubis and anterior scrotum only.
   d. anesthesia over the anterior and medial thigh.
   e. anesthesia over the pubis only.

5. A child has dense scarring after failed extravesical reimplantation. The landmark that can assist in locating the ureter in the pelvis is:
   a. the obturator nerve; the ureter will be medial to it.
   b. the obliterated umbilical artery; the ureter will be found lateral to it.
   c. the obliterated umbilical artery; the ureter will be found medial to it.
   d. the external iliac artery, as the ureter crosses it to enter the pelvis.
   e. the vas deferens; the ureter will pass anterior to it.

6. The levator ani attaches to all of the following except:
   a. the perineal body.
   b. the pubis.
   c. the coccyx.
   d. the vagina.
   e. the arcus tendineus fascia pelvis.

7. Accessory obturator veins (from the external iliac artery) and accessory obturator arteries (from the inferior epigastric artery) are encountered in:
   a. 50% and 25% of patients, respectively.
   b. 5% and 50% of patients, respectively.
   c. 50% and 75% of patients, respectively.
   d. 25% and 50% of patients, respectively.
   e. 25% and 5% of patients, respectively.

8. A retractor blade has rested on the psoas muscle during a prolonged procedure, resulting in a femoral nerve palsy. Postoperatively, the patient will experience:
   a. inability to flex the hip and numbness over the anterior thigh.
   b. inability to flex the knee and numbness over the thigh.
   c. numbness over the anterior thigh only.
   d. inability to extend the knee and numbness over the anterior thigh.
   e. inability to flex the knee only.

9. Autonomic nerves contributing to the pelvic plexus include:
   a. the superior hypogastric nerves from the para-aortic plexuses.
   b. the pelvic sympathetic trunks.
   c. pelvic parasympathetic neurons from the sacral spinal cord.
   d. a and c only.
   e. a, b, and c.

10. To preserve the vascular supply to the ureter, incisions in the peritoneum should be made:
    a. medially in the abdomen and laterally in the pelvis.
    b. laterally in the abdomen and medially in the pelvis.
    c. always medial to the ureter.
    d. always lateral to the ureter.
    e. directly over the ureter.

11. Relative to the ureter, the uterine vessels are found:
    a. laterally.
    b. posteriorly.
    c. anteriorly.
    d. medially.
    e. running together in a common sheath.

12. All of the following features of the ureterovesical junction cooperate to prevent vesicoureteral reflux except:
    a. fixation of the ureter to the superficial trigone.
    b. sphincteric closure of the ureteral orifice.
    c. detrusor backing.
    d. telescoping of the bladder outward over the ureter.
    e. passive closure of the intramural ureter caused by bladder filling.

13. In contrast to that of the male, the female bladder neck:
    a. has extensive adrenergic innervation.
    b. has a thickened middle smooth muscle layer.
    c. is largely responsible for urinary continence.
    d. is surrounded by type I (slow-twitch) fibers.
    e. has longitudinal smooth muscle fibers that extend to the external meatus.

14. Which of the following statements about the trigone is true:
    a. the epithelium is thicker than the rest of the bladder and densely adherent.
    b. the superficial smooth muscle is a continuation of Waldeyer's sheath.
    c. the smooth muscle enlarges to form thick fascicles.
    d. smooth muscle of the ureter forms the interureteric ridge (Mercier's bar).
    e. when the bladder empties, the trigone is thrown into thick folds.

15. During a perineal prostatectomy, the muscle that must be divided to gain access to the apex of the prostate is the:
    a. rectourethralis.
    b. internal anal sphincter.
    c. perineal body.
    d. external anal sphincter.
    e. puboanalis.

16. Arterial supply to the bladder includes:
    a. the superior vesical artery.
    b. the inferior vesical artery.
    c. the obturator artery.
    d. the uterine artery.
    e. all of the above.

17. The ducts of which of the following prostatic zones drain into the preprostatic urethra?
    a. The periurethral glands.
    b. The central zone.
    c. The transition zone.
    d. The peripheral zone.
    e. a and c.

18. Benign prostatic hyperplasia (BPH) may arise from:
    a. the periurethral glands.
    b. the central zone.
    c. the transition zone.
    d. the peripheral zone.
    e. a and c.

19. In BPH, blood supply to the adenoma arises from:
    a. the superior vesical artery.
    b. the urethral arteries extending down the urethra from the bladder neck.
    c. capsular arteries that arise laterally.
    d. the dorsal venous complex.
    e. the neurovascular bundle.

20. Which of the following statements concerning the striated urethral sphincter is true?
    a. It is composed of type I (slow-twitch) and type II (fast-twitch) fibers.
    b. It is bounded above by the superior fascia.
    c. It receives motor branches of the dorsal nerve of the penis.
    d. It is shaped like a signet ring and is 2 to 2.5 cm in length.
    e. It is densely supplied with proprioceptive muscle spindles.

21. The seminal vesicle:
    a. is normally palpable in a rectal examination.
    b. is a lateral outpouching of the prostate (central zone).
    c. contracts in response to excitatory efferents from the sacral parasympathetic nerves.
    d. is medial to the vas deferens.
    e. stores sperm.

22. From medial to lateral, the segments of the fallopian tube are:
    a. uterine, ampulla, infundibulum, isthmus, fimbriae.
    b. uterine, ampulla, isthmus, infundibulum, fimbriae.
    c. uterine, isthmus, ampulla, infundibulum, fimbriae.
    d. uterine, infundibulum, ampulla, isthmus, fimbriae.
    e. uterine, isthmus, infundibulum, ampulla, fimbriae.

23. The peritoneum may be accessed transvaginally through:
    a. the posterior fornix.
    b. the anterior fornix.
    c. the rectovaginal septum.
    d. the lateral fornices.
    e. the vesicovaginal space.

24. To avoid denervation of the striated urethral sphincter, incisions through the vaginal wall to enter the retropubic space should be made:
    a. perpendicular to the urethra.
    b. over the urethra.
    c. close to the lateral margins of the urethra.
    d. cephalad to the bladder neck.
    e. far lateral in the vaginal wall, parallel to the urethra.

25. When the endopelvic fascia lateral to the prostate and puboprostatic ligaments is opened, vessels are commonly encountered that pierce the levator ani to join the periprostatic plexus laterally. These vessels are communicating branches from:
    a. the pampiniform plexus of veins.
    b. the dorsal vein of the penis.
    c. the internal pudendal veins.
    d. the external pudendal veins.
    e. the accessory obturator veins.

26. Lymphatic drainage from the prostate flows to:
    a. the external iliac and common iliac nodes.
    b. the internal iliac and obturator nodes.
    c. the para-aortic nodes.
    d. the internal iliac and inguinal nodes.
    e. the perirectal and common iliac nodes.

27. The first branch of the pudendal nerve in the perineum is:
    a. the dorsal nerve of the penis.
    b. the inferior rectal nerve(s).
    c. the perineal nerve.
    d. the posterior femoral cutaneous branches.
    e. the posterior scrotal branches.

28. After fracture of the penis (disruption of the tunica albuginea), if Buck's fascia remains intact, the hematoma will be visible in:
    a. the perineum in a butterfly pattern.
    b. the penis and scrotum only.
    c. the penis, scrotum, and perineum, and tracking up the anterior abdominal wall.
    d. the shaft of the penis only.
    e. the shaft and glans of the penis.

29. The skin of the penile shaft and foreskin can be elevated as a rotational flap supplied by:

    a. the dorsal artery of the penis.
    b. the superficial inferior epigastric vessels.
    c. the gonadal vessels.
    d. the external pudendal vessels.
    e. several branches of the perineal vessels.

30. The dartos layer of smooth muscle and fascia in the scrotum is continuous with:

    a. the dartos layer of the penis.
    b. Colles' fascia.
    c. Scarpa's fascia.
    d. Buck's fascia.
    e. a, b, and c.

31. The cremaster muscle is supplied by:

    a. the ilioinguinal nerve.
    b. the genital branch of the genitofemoral nerve.
    c. the femoral branch of the genitofemoral nerve.
    d. terminal branches of the subcostal nerve (T12).
    e. the iliohypogastric nerve.

32. Lymphatic drainage from the bulbar urethra travels:

    a. through perianal nodes to reach the pelvis.
    b. directly to the deep pelvic lymph nodes.
    c. through the superficial and deep inguinal lymph nodes.
    d. to prepubic nodes.
    e. to para-aortic lymph nodes along with testicular drainage.

33. In their course from the seminiferous tubule to the epididymis, sperm pass through, in order:

    a. straight tubules, efferent ductules, rete testis.
    b. rete testis, straight tubules, efferent ductules.
    c. efferent ductules, rete testis, straight tubules.
    d. straight tubules, rete testis, efferent ductules.
    e. rete testis, efferent ductules, straight tubules.

34. The testicular artery may be ligated without sacrificing the testis because of collateral circulation from:

    a. the vasal and cremasteric arteries.
    b. the external pudendal and vasal arteries.
    c. the external pudendal, vasal, and cremasteric arteries.
    d. numerous anastomotic branches from scrotal arteries.
    e. the cremasteric and external pudendal arteries.

35. To avoid damage to subtunical testicular vessels, biopsy of the testis should be performed at:

    a. the lower pole of the testis.
    b. the anterior upper pole directly opposite the testicular mesentery.
    c. the medial surface of the lower pole.
    d. the lateral surface of the lower pole.
    e. the lateral or medial surface of the upper pole.

Answers

1. **d. the sacrospinous ligament.** The sacrospinous ligament separates the greater and lesser sciatic foramina. [p 42]

2. **a. superficial inferior epigastric artery and vein.** The superficial inferior epigastric vessels are encountered during inguinal incisions and can cause troublesome bleeding during placement of pelvic laparoscopic ports. [p 43]

3. **e. the buttock.** Blood and urine can accumulate in the scrotum and penis deep to the Dartos fascia after an anterior urethral injury. In the perineum, their spread is limited by the fusions of Colles' fascia to the ischiopubic rami laterally and to the posterior edge of the perineal membrane; the resulting hematoma is therefore butterfly-shaped. These processes will not extend down the leg or into the buttock, but they can freely travel up the anterior abdominal wall deep to Scarpa's fascia to the clavicles and around the flank to the back. [p 43]

4. **c. anesthesia over the pubis and anterior scrotum only.** The ilioinguinal nerve (L1) passes through the internal oblique muscle to enter the inguinal canal laterally. It travels anterior to the cord and exits the external ring to provide sensation to the mons pubis and anterior scrotum or labia majora. [p 54]

5. **c. the obliterated umbilical artery; the ureter will be found medial to it.** The obliterated umbilical artery in the medial umbilical fold serves as an important landmark for the surgeon. It can be traced to its origin from the internal iliac artery to locate the ureter, which lies on its medial side. [p 45]

6. **e. the arcus tendineus fascia pelvis.** The tendinous arc of the levator ani serves as the origin of the muscles of the pelvic diaphragm: pubococcygeus and iliococcygeus. The muscle bordering this hiatus has been referred to as "pubovisceral" because it provides a sling for (pubourethralis, puborectalis), inserts directly into (pubuvaginalis, puboanalis, levator prostatae), or inserts into a structure intimately associated with the pelvic viscera. The coccygeus muscle extends from the sacrospinous ligament to the lateral border of the sacrum and coccyx to complete the pelvic diaphragm. [p 46]

7. **a. 50% and 25% of patients, respectively.** In half of patients, one or more accessory obturator veins drain into the underside of the external iliac vein and can easily be torn during lymphadenectomy. In 25% of people, an accessory obturator artery arises from the inferior epigastric artery and runs medial to the femoral vein to reach the obturator canal. [pp 52 and 49]

8. **d. inability to extend the knee and numbness over the anterior thigh.** The femoral nerve (L2, L3, L4) supplies sensation to the anterior thigh and motor innervation to the extensors of the knee. [p 54]

9. **e. a, b, and c.** The presynaptic sympathetic cell bodies reach the pelvic plexus by two pathways: (1) the superior hypogastric plexus and (2) the pelvic continuation of the sympathetic trunks. Presynaptic parasympathetic innervation arises from the intermediolateral cell column of the sacral cord. [p 55]

10. **b. laterally in the abdomen and medially in the pelvis.** Blood supply to the pelvic ureter enters laterally; thus, the pelvic peritoneum should be incised only medial to the ureter. [p 58]

11. **c. anteriorly.** In women, the ureter first runs posterior to the ovary, then turns medially to run deep to the base of the

broad ligament before entering a loose connective tissue tunnel through the substance of the cardinal ligament. [p 58]

12. **b. sphincteric closure of the ureteral orifice.** The intravesical portion of the ureter lies immediately beneath the bladder urothelium and is therefore quite pliant; it is backed by a strong plate of detrusor muscle. With bladder filling, this arrangement is thought to result in passive occlusion of the ureter, like a flap valve. [p 61]

13. **e. has longitudinal smooth muscle fibers that extend to the external meatus.** At the female bladder neck, the inner longitudinal fibers converge radially to pass downward as the inner longitudinal layer of the urethra, as described earlier. The middle circular layer does not appear to be as robust as that of the male. The female bladder neck differs strikingly from the male in possessing little adrenergic innervation. [pp 60–61]

14. **d. smooth muscle of the ureter forms the interureteric ridge (Mercier's bar).** Fibers from each ureter meet to form a triangular sheet of muscle that extends from the two ureteral orifices to the internal urethra meatus. The edges of this muscular sheet are thickened between the ureteral orifices (the interureteric crest, or Mercier's bar) and between the ureters and the internal urethral meatus (Bell's muscle). [p 61]

15. **a. rectourethralis.** When approached from below, these fibers, the rectourethralis muscle, are 2 to 10 mm thick and must be divided to gain access to the prostate. [p 58]

16. **e. all of the above.** In addition to the vesical branches, the bladder may be supplied by any adjacent artery arising from the internal iliac artery. [p 62]

17. **a. The periurethral glands.** At its midpoint, the urethra turns approximately 35 degrees anteriorly, but this angulation can vary from 0 to 90 degrees (see Figs. 2–23, 2–25, and 2–28). This angle divides the prostatic urethra into proximal (preprostatic) and distal (prostatic) segments, which are functionally and anatomically discrete. Small periurethral glands, lacking periglandular smooth muscle, extend between the fibers of the longitudinal smooth muscle to be enclosed by the preprostatic sphincter. [p 63]

18. **e. a and c.** The periurethral glands can contribute significantly to prostatic volume in older men as one of the sites of origin of BPH. The transition zone commonly gives rise to BPH. [pp 63 and 64]

19. **b. the urethral arteries extending down the urethra from the bladder neck.** The urethral arteries penetrate the prostatovesical junction posterolaterally and travel inward, perpendicular to the urethra. They approach the bladder neck in the 1- to 5-o'clock and 7- to 11-o'clock positions, with the largest branches located posteriorly. They then turn caudally, parallel to the urethra, to supply it, the periurethral glands, and the transition zone. Thus, in BPH, these arteries provide the principal blood supply of the adenoma. [p 65]

20. **d. It is shaped like a signet ring and is 2 to 2.5 cm in length.** The membranous urethra spans on average 2.0 to 2.5 cm (range 1.2 to 5.0 cm). It is surrounded by the striated (external) urethral sphincter, which is often incorrectly depicted as a flat sheet of muscle sandwiched between two layers of fascia. The striated sphincter is actually shaped like a signet ring, broad at its base, and narrowing as it passes through the urogenital hiatus of the levator ani to meet the apex of the prostate. [p 65]

21. **c. contracts in response to excitatory efferents from the sacral parasympathetic nerves.** Innervation arises from the pelvic plexus, with major excitatory efferents contributed by the (sympathetic) hypogastric nerves. [p 67]

22. **c. uterine, isthmus, ampulla, infundibulum, fimbriae.** The tubes are divided into four segments: uterine, isthmus, ampulla, and infundibulum, which is crowned by the fimbriae. [p 67]

23. **a. the posterior fornix.** Because the apex of the vagina is covered with the peritoneum of the rectouterine pouch, the peritoneal cavity may be accessed through the posterior fornix. [p 68]

24. **e. far lateral in the vaginal wall, parallel to the urethra.** Somatic and autonomic nerves to the urethra travel on the lateral walls of the vagina near the urethra. During transvaginal incontinence surgery, the anterior vaginal wall should be incised laterally to avoid these nerves and prevent type III urinary incontinence. [pp 69–70]

25. **c. the internal pudendal veins.** The internal pudendal veins communicate freely with the dorsal vein complex by piercing the levator ani. These communicating vessels enter the pelvic venous plexus on the lateral surface of the prostate and are a common, often unexpected, source of bleeding during apical dissection of the prostate. [p 71]

26. **b. the internal iliac and obturator nodes.** Lymphatic drainage is primarily to the obturator and internal iliac nodes. [p 65]

27. **a. the dorsal nerve of the penis.** The pudendal nerve follows the vessels in their course through the perineum (see Fig. 2–37). Its first branch, the dorsal nerve of the penis, travels ventral to the main pudendal trunk in Alcock's canal. [p 71]

28. **d. the shaft of the penis only.** Bleeding from a tear in the corporal bodies (e.g., penile fracture) is usually contained within Buck's fascia, and ecchymosis is limited to the penile shaft. [p 72]

29. **d. the external pudendal vessels.** The blood supply of the skin of the penile shaft is independent of the erectile bodies and is derived from the external pudendal branches of the femoral vessels. [p 72]

30. **e. a, b, and c.** The dartos layer of smooth muscle is continuous with Colles' fascia, Scarpa's fascia, and the dartos fascia of the penis. [p 75]

31. **b. the genital branch of the genitofemoral nerve.** The genital branch of the genitofemoral nerve follows the cord through the inguinal canal, supplies the cremaster muscle, and supplies sensation to the anterior scrotum. [p 54]

32. **c. through the superficial and deep inguinal lymph nodes.** The penis, scrotum, and perineum drain into the inguinal lymph nodes. These nodes can be divided into a superficial groups and deep groups. [p 75]

33. **d. straight tubules, rete testis, efferent ductules.** Septa form 200 to 300 cone-shaped lobules, each containing one or more convoluted seminiferous tubules. Each tubule is U-shaped and has a stretched length of nearly 1 m. Interstitial (Leydig) cells lie in the loose tissue surrounding the tubules and are responsible for testosterone production. Toward the apices of the lobules, the seminiferous tubules become straight (tubuli recti) and enter the mediastinum testis to form an anastomosing network of tubules lined by flattened epithelium. This network, known as the rete testis, forms 12 to 20 efferent ductules and passes into the largest portion of epididymis, the caput. [p 76]

34. **a. the vasal and cremasteric arteries.** A rich arterial anastomosis occurs at the head of the epididymis, between the testicular and capital arteries, and at the tail between the testicular, epididymal, cremasteric, and vasal arteries. [p 77]

35. **e. the lateral or medial surface of the upper pole.** The testicular arteries enter the mediastinum and ramify in the tunica vasculosa, principally in the anterior, medial, and lateral portions of the lower pole and the anterior segment of the upper pole (see Fig. 2–45). Thus, placement of a traction suture through the lower pole tunica albuginea risks damaging these important superficial vessels and devascularizing the testis. Testicular biopsy should be carried out in the medial or lateral surface of the upper pole, where the risk of vascular injury is minimal. [p 77]

SECTION II

UROLOGIC EXAMINATION AND DIAGNOSTIC TECHNIQUES

Chapter 3

Evaluation of the Urologic Patient: History, Physical Examination, and Urinalysis

Glenn S. Gerber • Charles B. Brendler

Questions

1. What causes the pain associated with a stone in the ureter?
    a. Obstruction of urine flow with distention of the renal capsule
    b. Irritation of the ureteral mucosa by the stone
    c. Excessive ureteral peristalsis in response to the obstructing stone
    d. Irritation of the intramural ureter
    e. Urinary extravasation from a ruptured calyceal fornix

2. What is the most common cause of gross hematuria in a patient older than 50 years of age?
    a. Renal calculi
    b. Infection
    c. Bladder cancer
    d. Benign prostatic hyperplasia
    e. Trauma

3. What is the most common cause of pain associated with gross hematuria?
    a. Simultaneous passage of a kidney stone
    b. Ureteral obstruction due to blood clots
    c. Urinary tract malignancy
    d. Prostatic inflammation
    e. Prostatic enlargement

4. All of the following are typical lower urinary tract symptoms associated with benign prostatic hyperplasia except:
    a. urgency.
    b. frequency.
    c. nocturia.
    d. dysuria.
    e. weak urinary stream.

5. What is the most common cause of continuous incontinence (loss of urine at all times and in all positions)?
    a. Enterovesical fistula
    b. Noncompliant bladder
    c. Detrusor hyperreflexia
    d. Vesicovaginal fistula
    e. Sphincteric incompetence

6. All of the following are potential causes of anejaculation except:
    a. sympathetic denervation.
    b. pharmacologic agents.
    c. bladder neck and prostatic surgery.
    d. androgen deficiency.
    e. cerebrovascular accidents.

7. What percentage of patients with multiple sclerosis will present with urinary symptoms as the first manifestation of the disease?
    a. 1%
    b. 5%
    c. 10%
    d. 15%
    e. 20%

8. What important information is gained from pelvic bimanual examination that cannot be obtained from radiologic evaluation?
    a. Presence of bladder mass
    b. Invasion of bladder cancer into perivesical fat
    c. Presence of bladder calculi
    d. Associated pathologic lesion in female adnexal structures
    e. Mobility/fixation of pelvic organs

9. With what disease is priapism primarily associated?
    a. Peyronie's disease
    b. Sickle cell anemia
    c. Parkinson's disease
    d. Organic depression
    e. Leukemia

10. What is the most common cause of cloudy urine?
    a. Bacterial cystitis
    b. Urine overgrowth with yeast
    c. Phosphaturia
    d. Alkaline urine
    e. Significant proteinuria

11. Conditions that decrease urine specific gravity include all of the following except:

    a. increased fluid intake.
    b. use of diuretics.
    c. decreased renal concentrating ability.
    d. dehydration.
    e. diabetes insipidus.

12. Urine osmolality usually varies between:

    a. 10 and 200 mOsm/L.
    b. 50 and 500 mOsm/L.
    c. 50 and 1200 mOsm/L.
    d. 100 and 1000 mOsm/L.
    e. 100 and 1500 mOsm/L.

13. Elevated ascorbic acid levels in the urine may lead to false-negative results on a urine dipstick test for which of the following?

    a. Glucose
    b. Hemoglobin
    c. Myoglobin
    d. Red blood cells
    e. Leukocytes

14. Hematuria is distinguished from hemoglobinuria or myoglobinuria by:

    a. dipstick testing.
    b. the simultaneous presence of significant leukocytes.
    c. microscopic presence of erythrocytes.
    d. examination of serum.
    e. evaluation of hematocrit.

15. The presence of one positive dipstick reading for hematuria is associated with significant urologic pathologic findings on subsequent testing in what percentage of patients?

    a. 2%
    b. 10%
    c. 25%
    d. 50%
    e. 75%

16. The most common cause of glomerular hematuria is:

    a. transitional cell carcinoma.
    b. nephritic syndrome.
    c. Berger's disease (IgA nephropathy).
    d. poststreptococcal glomerulonephritis.
    e. Goodpasture's syndrome.

17. The most common cause of proteinuria is:

    a. Fanconi's syndrome.
    b. excessive glomerular permeability due to primary glomerular disease.
    c. failure of adequate tubular reabsorption.
    d. overflow proteinuria due to increased plasma concentration of immunoglobulins.
    e. diabetes.

18. Transient proteinuria may be due to all of the following except:

    a. exercise.
    b. fever.
    c. emotional stress.
    d. congestive heart failure.
    e. ureteroscopy.

19. Glucose will be detected in the urine when the serum level is above:

    a. 75 mg/dl.
    b. 100 mg/dl.
    c. 150 mg/dl.
    d. 180 mg/dl.
    e. 225 mg/dl.

20. The specificity of dipstick nitrite testing for bacteriuria is:

    a. 20%.
    b. 40%.
    c. 60%.
    d. 80%.
    e. >90%.

21. All of the following are microscopic features of squamous epithelial cells except:

    a. large size.
    b. small central nucleus.
    c. irregular cytoplasm.
    d. presence in clumps.
    e. fine granularity in the cytoplasm.

22. The number of bacteria per high-power microscopic field that correspond to colony counts of 100,000/ml is:

    a. 1.
    b. 3.
    c. 5.
    d. 10.
    e. 20.

23. Pain in the flaccid penis is usually due to:

    a. Peyronie's disease.
    b. bladder or urethral inflammation.
    c. priapism.
    d. calculi impacted in the distal ureter.
    e. hydrocele.

24. Chronic scrotal pain is most often due to:

    a. testicular torsion.
    b. trauma.
    c. cryptorchidism.
    d. hydrocele.
    e. orchitis.

25. Terminal hematuria (at the end of the urinary stream) is usually due to:

    a. bladder neck or prostatic inflammation.
    b. bladder cancer.
    c. kidney stones.
    d. bladder calculi.
    e. urethral stricture disease.

26. Enuresis is present in what percentage of children at age 5 years?

    a. 5%.
    b. 15%.
    c. 25%.
    d. 50%.
    e. 75%.

27. All of the following in the medical history suggest that erectile dysfunction is more likely due to organic rather than psychogenic causes except:

    a. sudden onset.
    b. peripheral vascular disease.
    c. absence of nocturnal erections.
    d. diabetes mellitus.
    e. inability to achieve adequate erections in a variety of circumstances.

28. All of the following should be routinely performed in men with hematospermia except:

    a. cystoscopy.
    b. digital rectal examination.
    c. serum prostate-specific antigen (PSA) level.
    d. genital examination.
    e. urinalysis.

29. Pneumaturia may be due to all of the following except:

    a. diverticulitis.
    b. colon cancer.
    c. recent urinary tract instrumentation.
    d. inflammatory bowel disease.
    e. ectopic ureter.

30. Which of the following disorders may commonly lead to irritative voiding symptoms?

    a. Parkinson's disease
    b. Renal cell carcinoma
    c. Bladder diverticula
    d. Prostate cancer
    e. Testicular torsion

Answers

1. **a. Obstruction of urine flow with distention of the renal capsule.** Pain is usually caused by acute distention of the renal capsule, usually from inflammation or obstruction. [p 84]

2. **c. Bladder cancer.** It should be remembered that the most common cause of gross hematuria in a patient older than 50 years is bladder cancer. [p 86]

3. **b. Ureteral obstruction due to blood clots.** Pain in association with hematuria usually results from upper urinary tract hematuria with obstruction of the ureters with clots. [p 86]

4. **d. dysuria.** Dysuria is painful urination that is usually caused by inflammation. [pp 86–87]

5. **d. Vesicovaginal fistula.** Continuous incontinence is most commonly due to a urinary tract fistula that bypasses the urethral sphincter. [p 87]

6. **e. cerebrovascular accidents.** Anejaculation may result from several causes: (1) androgen deficiency, (2) sympathetic denervation, (3) pharmacologic agents, and (4) bladder neck and prostatic surgery. [p 89]

7. **b. 5%.** In fact, 5% of patients with previously undiagnosed multiple sclerosis present with urinary symptoms as the first manifestation of the disease. [p 90]

8. **e. Mobility/fixation of pelvic organs.** In addition to defining areas of induration, the bimanual examination allows the examiner to assess the mobility of the bladder; such information cannot be obtained by radiologic techniques such as CT and MRI, which convey static images. [pp 93–94]

9. **b. Sickle cell anemia.** It occurs most commonly in patients with sickle cell disease but can also occur in those with advanced malignancy, coagulation disorders, and pulmonary disease, and in many patients without an obvious cause. [p 94]

10. **c. Phosphaturia.** Cloudy urine is most commonly caused by phosphaturia. [p 99]

11. **d. dehydration.** Conditions that decrease specific gravity include: (1) increased fluid intake, (2) diuretics, (3) decreased renal concentrating ability, and (4) diabetes insipidus. [p 99]

12. **c. 50 and 1200 mOsm/L.** Osmolality is a measure of the amount of material dissolved in the urine and usually varies between 50 and 1200 mOsm/L. [p 99]

13. **a. Glucose.** False-negative results for glucose and bilirubin may be seen in the presence of elevated ascorbic acid concentrations in the urine. [p 100]

14. **c. microscopic presence of erythrocytes.** Hematuria can be distinguished from hemoglobinuria and myoglobinuria by microscopic examination of the centrifuged urine; the presence of a large number of erythrocytes establishes the diagnosis of hematuria. [p 100]

15. **c. 25%.** Investigators at the University of Wisconsin found that 26% of adults who had at least one positive dipstick reading for hematuria were subsequently found to have significant urologic pathologic findings. [p 101]

16. **c. Berger's disease (IgA nephropathy).** IgA nephropathy, or Berger's disease, is the most common cause of glomerular hematuria, accounting for about 30% of cases. [p 101]

17. **b. excessive glomerular permeability due to primary glomerular disease.** Glomerular proteinuria is the most common type of proteinuria and results from increased glomerular capillary permeability to protein, especially albumin. Glomerular proteinuria occurs in any of the primary glomerular diseases such as IgA nephropathy or in glomerulopathy associated with systemic illness such as diabetes mellitus. [p 105]

18. **e. ureteroscopy.** Transient proteinuria occurs commonly, especially in the pediatric population, and usually resolves spontaneously within a few days. It may result from fever, exercise, or emotional stress. In older patients, transient proteinuria may be due to congestive heart failure. [p 105]

19. **d. 180 mg/dl.** This so-called renal threshold corresponds to a serum glucose level of about 180 mg/dl; above this level, glucose will be detected in the urine. [p 106]

20. **c. >90%.** The specificity of the nitrite dipstick test for detecting bacteriuria is over 90%. [p 107]

21. **d. presence in clumps.** Squamous epithelial cells are large, have a central small nucleus about the size of an erythrocyte, and have an irregular cytoplasm with fine granularity (see Fig. 4–5). [p 109]

22. **c. 5.** Therefore, 5 bacteria per high-power field reflects colony counts of about 100,000/ml. [p 109]

23. **b. bladder or urethral inflammation.** Pain in the flaccid penis is usually secondary to inflammation in the bladder or urethra, with referred pain that is experienced maximally at the urethral meatus. [p 85]

24. **d. hydrocele.** Chronic scrotal pain is usually related to noninflammatory conditions such as a hydrocele or varicocele, and the pain is usually characterized as a dull, heavy sensation that does not radiate. [p 85]

25. **a. bladder neck or prostatic inflammation.** Terminal hematuria occurs at the end of micturition and is usually secondary to inflammation in the area of the bladder neck or prostatic urethra. [p 86]

26. **b. 15%.** Enuresis refers to urinary incontinence that occurs during sleep. It occurs normally in children up to 3 years of age but persists in about 15% of children at age 5 and about 1% of children at age 15. [p 89]

27. **a. sudden onset.** A careful history will often determine whether the problem is primarily psychogenic or organic. In men with psychogenic impotence, the condition frequently develops rather quickly secondary to a precipitating event such as marital stress or change or loss of a sexual partner. [p 89]

28. **a. cystoscopy.** A genital and rectal examination should be done to exclude the presence of tuberculosis, a PSA assessment and digital rectal examination should be done to exclude prostatic carcinoma, and a urinary cytologic assessment should be done to exclude the possibility of transitional cell carcinoma of the prostate. [p 90]

29. **e. ectopic ureter.** Pneumaturia is the passage of gas in the urine. In patients who have not recently had urinary tract instrumentation or a urethral catheter placed, this is almost always due to a fistula between the intestine and bladder. Common causes include diverticulitis, carcinoma of the sigmoid colon, and regional enteritis (Crohn's disease). [p 90]

30. **a. Parkinson's disease.** The second important example of nonspecific lower urinary tract symptoms that may occur secondary to a variety of neurologic conditions is irritative symptoms resulting from neurologic disease, such as cerebrovascular accident, diabetes mellitus, and Parkinson's disease. [p 87]

Chapter 4

Basic Instrumentation and Cystoscopy

H. Ballentine Carter

Questions

1. The measurement system most often used when referring to catheter and instrument size is:

    a. English.
    b. French (Fr).
    c. metric.
    d. U.S.
    e. conventional.

2. A millimeter in diameter is approximately how many French?

    a. 1 French.
    b. 1.5 French.
    c. 3 French.
    d. 3.5 French.
    e. 5 French.

3. The size of a catheter or instrument refers to the:

    a. inside circumference.
    b. inside diameter.
    c. outside circumference.
    d. outside diameter.
    e. none of the above.

4. The catheter designed to help negotiate the male urethra when catheterization is difficult is the:

    a. Foley.
    b. Malecot.
    c. Pezzer.
    d. coudé.
    e. Council.

5. The catheter with the largest luminal size is the:

    a. No. 20 Fr Foley.
    b. No. 20 Fr three-way irrigation catheter.
    c. No. 20 Fr coudé Foley.
    d. No. 20 Fr Malecot.
    e. No. 18 Fr Malecot.

6. The catheter material best suited for long-term urethral catheterization is:

    a. latex.
    b. silicone.
    c. rubber.
    d. Dacron.
    e. polyurethane.

7. When multiple attempts to gently bypass a urethral obstruction are unsuccessful, the next best step is:

    a. a more vigorous attempt with stiffer catheters.
    b. balloon dilation of the obstruction under direct vision.
    c. incision of the obstruction under direct vision.
    d. placement of percutaneous cystostomy.
    e. perineal urethrostomy.

8. When cystoscopic electrocoagulation is planned, the irrigant solution that should be avoided is:

    a. sorbitol.
    b. normal saline.
    c. sterile water.
    d. glycine.
    e. mannitol.

Answers

1. **b. French (Fr).** Catheter size is usually referred to using the French (Fr) scale (circumference is in millimeters), in which 1 Fr = 0.33 mm in diameter. [p 112]

2. **c. 3 French.** For conversion from one scale to the other, it is easier to remember that each millimeter in diameter is approximately 3 Fr; thus, an 18 Fr catheter is about 6 mm in diameter. [p 112]

3. **c. outside circumference.** Catheter sizes refer to the outside circumference of the catheter, not the luminal diameter. [p 112]

4. **d. coudé.** Catheters with a curved tip (e.g., coudé catheters; see Fig. 4–1D) are specifically designed to help bypass areas of the male urethra that are difficult to negotiate with a straight catheter. [p 112]

5. **d. No. 20 Fr Malecot.** Catheters without a lumen for balloon inflation (e.g., Malecot) have a larger luminal size for bladder drainage than do Foley catheters of the same outer circumference. Likewise, for a given outer circumference, two-way catheters (with a balloon port) have a larger luminal size for urinary drainage than do three-way catheters (with a balloon port and fluid instillation port). [pp 112–113]

6. **b. silicone.** If long-term catheterization is anticipated (more than 1 week), it is advisable to use a Foley catheter made of the most biocompatible material. Catheters made of silicone in general are better tolerated over the long term than those made of materials such as latex and polyurethane. [p 113]

7. **d. placement of percutaneous cystostomy.** When it is not possible to gently bypass a bladder neck contracture by using other approaches (such as use of a guidewire to introduce a ureteral catheter or to guide passage of an Amplatz semirigid dilator), placement of a cystostomy tube is preferable to continued attempts at catheterization, to avoid urethral trauma. [p 114]

8. **b. normal saline.** If electrocoagulation is planned, it is necessary to avoid solutions containing electrolytes. [p 118]

Chapter 5

Urinary Tract Imaging: Basic Principles

Peter G. Schulam • Akira Kawashima • Carl Sandler • Bruce J. Barron • Lamk M. Lamki
Stanford M. Goldman

Questions

1. The primary physical characteristic of the high osmolar contrast agents that is responsible for their toxicity is:
   a. hypertonicity.
   b. ionicity.
   c. nonionicity.
   d. iodination.
   e. monomericity.

2. Risk factors associated with nephrotoxicity in patients receiving high osmolar contrast media include all of the following except:
   a. renal insufficiency.
   b. diabetic nephropathy.
   c. multiple administrations within a short interval.
   d. hyperuricemia.
   e. hypoalbuminemia.

3. Patients taking metformin (Glucophage) are at risk for lactic acidosis if renal failure occurs as a result of contrast agent–induced nephrotoxicity. The Food and Drug Administration (FDA) recommends that patients taking metformin who are administered contrast agents should: (select the one best answer)
   a. discontinue the medication 24 hours before injection.
   b. discontinue the medication 72 hours before and 24 hours after the injection.
   c. discontinue the medication for 48 hours after the injection.
   d. not discontinue the medication.
   e. discontinue the medication if lactic acidosis develops.

4. Contrast agent–induced reactions including urticaria, edema, and hypotension are thought to be:
   a. immunoglobulin G mediated.
   b. anaphylactoid.
   c. delayed-type hypersensitivity.
   d. immunoglobulin E mediated.
   e. a type 1 allergic reaction.

5. The filming sequence of an excretory urogram (EXU) can include various views not required in a routine study, with the exception of:
   a. nephrotomograms.
   b. delayed films.
   c. oblique films.
   d. prone films.
   e. erect films.

18 UROLOGIC EXAMINATION AND DIAGNOSTIC TECHNIQUES

6. The posterior urethra is best visualized by:
   a. static cystogram.
   b. retrograde urethrogram.
   c. voiding cystogram.
   d. postvoid film of an EXU.
   e. CT cystogram.

7. The most accurate method of detecting renal calculi is:
   a. unenhanced spiral CT.
   b. enhanced spiral CT.
   c. ultrasonography.
   d. EXU.
   e. KUB (kidneys, ureters, and bladder).

8. CT incidentally detects many adrenal lesions. No further work-up is necessary for small adrenal lesions with the following CT characteristics:
   a. less than 20 HU enhancement.
   b. equal to or less than 10 HU on an unenhanced CT scan.
   c. no enhancement.
   d. equal to or less than 20 HU on an unenhanced CT scan.
   e. less than 10 HU enhancement.

9. Pheochromocytomas of the adrenal gland have a very characteristic T_1/T_2 imaging profile. The profile is best described as:
   a. enhanced signal intensity on a T_2-weighted scan.
   b. reduced signal intensity on a T_2-weighted scan.
   c. enhanced signal intensity on a T_1-weighted scan.
   d. high signal intensity on T_1- and T_2-weighted scans.
   e. low signal intensity on a T_1-weighted scan.

10. All the following radiopharmaceuticals are cleared by glomerular filtration except:
    a. technetium Tc99m DTPA (pentetate).
    b. H-3 inulin.
    c. technetium Tc99m glucoheptonate.
    d. iothalamate sodium ^{125}I.
    e. technetium Tc99m mercaptoacetyl triglycine (MAG3).

11. The agent of choice for renal cortical imaging is:
    a. technetium Tc99m (dimercaptosuccinic acid) DMSA.
    b. technetium Tc99m MAG3.
    c. technetium Tc99m glucoheptonate.
    d. technetium Tc99m DTPA.
    e. technetium Tc99m pertechnetate.

12. Arteriography is least likely associated with:
    a. hematoma.
    b. pseudoaneurysm.
    c. allergic reactions.
    d. thrombosis.
    e. arterial dissection.

Answers

1. **a. hypertonicity.** A major disadvantage of these agents is their hypertonicity, with a mean osmotic load of 1400 to 2400 mOsm/kg water, which exceeds that of serum by a factor of 5 to 7. [p 124]

2. **e. hypoalbuminemia.** These risk factors include renal insufficiency, particularly when associated with small-vessel renal disease; diabetic nephropathy; congestive heart failure; hyperuricemia; proteinuria; and multiple administrations of contrast media within a short (i.e., 24-hour) interval. [p 124]

3. **c. discontinue the medication for 48 hours after the injection.** To minimize this risk, the FDA has recommended that patients taking metformin who receive contrast agents should have the drug withheld for 48 hours after receiving the contrast material. [p 125]

4. **b. anaphylactoid.** The mechanism of these reactions to contrast material most likely differs from that of type 1 allergic reactions and is therefore termed anaphylactoid. [p 125]

5. **a. nephrotomograms.** Nephrotomograms are essential for performance of an adequate study, especially when there is a history of hematuria or to exclude an unexpected mass. [p 126]

6. **c. voiding cystogram.** Voiding cystourethrography allows for evaluation of the bladder and urethra during the physiologic act of micturition and provides visualization of the posterior urethra. [p 130]

7. **a. unenhanced spiral CT.** Unenhanced spiral CT for the evaluation of patients with acute flank pain is more sensitive for detecting calculi than is excretory urography. [p 140]

8. **b. equal to or less than 10 HU on an unenhanced CT scan.** An adrenal adenoma can be differentiated from metastases when the lesion measures 10 HU or less on an unenhanced CT scan, and no further work-up is necessary. [p 140]

9. **a. enhanced signal intensity on a T_2-weighted scan.** The extremely high signal intensity of pheochromocytomas on T_2-weighted images is very helpful in diagnosing these lesions. [p 147]

10. **e. technetium Tc99m mercaptoacetyl triglycine (MAG3).** Because MAG3 is predominantly cleared by tubular secretion, it may be used to measure renal plasma flow. [p 157]

11. **a. technetium Tc99m (dimercaptosuccinic acid) DMSA.** Technetium Tc99m glucoheptonate is, however, not as accurate as technetium Tc99m DMSA and is therefore usually reserved for those times when technetium Tc99m DMSA may not be available. [p 160]

12. **c. allergic reactions.** Allergic reactions are uncommon during arterial injections. [p 163]

SECTION III

PHYSIOLOGY, PATHOPHYSIOLOGY, AND MANAGEMENT OF UPPER URINARY TRACT DISEASES

Chapter 6

Renal Physiology and Pathophysiology

Jon D. Blumenfeld

Questions

1. What proportion of the cardiac output is delivered to the kidney?

    a. 5%
    b. 20%
    c. 50%
    d. 85%
    e. 100%

2. Changes in preglomerular and postglomerular vascular resistances affect the glomerular filtration rate (GFR) in which of the following ways?

    a. Decrements in efferent arteriolar resistance increase the GFR.
    b. Increments in afferent arteriolar resistance increase the GFR.
    c. Afferent arteriolar dilatation and efferent arteriolar constriction enhance glomerular filtration pressure and, in turn, maintain glomerular filtration pressure.
    d. The GFR is unrelated to pre- and postglomerular resistances.
    e. The GFR is related to afferent but not efferent arteriolar resistance.

3. The filtration fraction is influenced by alterations in renal arteriolar tone in which of the following ways?

    a. The GFR and the renal plasma flow (RPF) change in parallel during afferent constriction, so no change occurs in the filtration fraction.
    b. The GFR and the RPF change reciprocally during afferent constriction, so no change occurs in the filtration fraction.
    c. The GFR and the RPF change in parallel during efferent constriction, so no change occurs in the filtration fraction.
    d. The filtration fraction is not related to changes in pre- and postglomerular resistances.
    e. The filtration fraction increases in parallel with increments in both afferent and efferent arteriolar resistances.

4. Which of the following is NOT true regarding nitric oxide synthase (NOS)?

    a. NOS I is predominantly active in neuronal and epithelial cells.
    b. NOS II is predominantly active in cytokine-induced cells and vascular smooth muscle.
    c. NOS III is predominantly active in endothelial cells.
    d. NOS III is constitutively expressed and is regulated by calcium and calmodulin.
    e. NOS II is dependent on calcium.

5. Inhibition of nitric oxide is characterized by each of the following except:

    a. marked increases in resistances in afferent and, predominantly, in efferent arterioles that result in elevated glomerular capillary pressure and reduced renal blood flow.
    b. a decline in the glomerular capillary ultrafiltration coefficient (K_f).
    c. a reduction in sodium reabsorption by the proximal tubule.
    d. development of systemic hypertension.
    e. development of systemic hypotension.

6. Creatinine is not an ideal marker for measuring GFR for each of the following reasons except which one?

    a. Creatinine is secreted by the organic cation transporter of the proximal tubule; therefore, creatinine clearance (Ccr) is not due solely to glomerular filtration.
    b. Creatinine is reabsorbed by the organic cation transporter of the proximal tubule; therefore, Ccr is not due solely to glomerular filtration.
    c. There is significant variability in the measurement of serum creatinine level.
    d. Creatinine generation may be affected by changes in muscle mass.
    e. The relationship between Ccr and GFR (Ccr/GFR) is not constant.

7. The proportion of the glomerular filtrate that is reabsorbed by the proximal tubule is:

    a. 5%.
    b. 25%.

c. 60% to 70%.
d. 80% to 90%.
e. 100%.

8. The main site of renal reabsorption of glucose is the:
   a. proximal tubule.
   b. medullary thick ascending limb (TAL) of Henle.
   c. cortical TAL of Henle.
   d. cortical collecting duct.
   e. medullary collecting duct.

9. Urea is not an ideal marker for determining the GFR because:
   a. the fractional excretion of urea varies according to the state of hydration.
   b. urea is secreted by the anionic transporter of the proximal tubule.
   c. urea is secreted by the cationic transporter of the proximal tubule.
   d. urea is a large molecule that is not freely filtered by the glomerulus.
   e. urea requires hepatic metabolism to creatinine before it is filtered.

10. In which nephron segment is the hypoosmotic filtrate initially formed?
    a. The proximal tubule
    b. The medullary TAL of Henle
    c. The cortical TAL of Henle
    d. The cortical collecting duct
    e. The medullary collecting duct.

11. Which of the following diuretics does not act at the loop of Henle?
    a. Bumetanide
    b. Furosemide
    c. Ethacrynic acid
    d. Spironolactone
    e. Torsemide

12. The distal nephron segments, which include the distal convoluted tubule, the connecting segment, and the collecting duct (cortical, inner, and outer medullary), have all of the following main functions except which one?
    a. Potassium secretion
    b. Urinary acidification
    c. Amino acid reabsorption
    d. Calcium reabsorption
    e. Maintaining maximal urine osmolality

13. The two major cell types that make up the collecting duct are:
    a. principal cell and intercalated cell.
    b. vasa recta and vasa vasorum.
    c. S_1 and S_2 segments.
    d. macula densa and juxtaglomerular cell.
    e. mesangial cell and Langerhans' cell.

14. Which of the following is NOT a major tubular action of arginine vasopressin (AVP)?
    a. To stimulate Na^+-K^+-$2Cl^-$ activity by the medullary TAL of Henle
    b. To increase inner medullary collecting duct permeability to water
    c. To increase inner medullary collecting duct permeability to urea
    d. To increase osmolarity of the renal medulla
    e. To increase glucose reabsorption by the inner medullary collecting duct

15. A major action of aldosterone is:
    a. to stimulate potassium secretion by the principal cells of the cortical and medullary collecting tubule.
    b. to decrease the number of apical sodium channels in the cortical collecting duct.
    c. to impair proton secretion by intercalated cells.
    d. to decrease sodium reabsorption by the epithelial sodium channel.
    e. to stimulate potassium secretion by the S_1 segment of the proximal tubule.

16. Which of the following statements is NOT true of renin?
    a. Renin is an aspartyl proteinase belonging to the same family as pepsin and cathepsin.
    b. Renin is synthesized predominantly in the kidney by specialized cells, referred to as juxtaglomerular cells.
    c. The substrate of renin is angiotensin I, which in turn forms angiotensin II, a potent vasoconstrictor that stimulates aldosterone production.
    d. The sole substrate of renin is angiotensinogen.
    e. Prorenin is the biosynthetic precursor.

17. Which of the following factors does NOT stimulate renin secretion?
    a. Renal ischemia
    b. Decreased NaCl delivery to the macula densa
    c. β-Adrenergic blockers
    d. β_1-Adrenergic stimulation
    e. Cyclic AMP

18. The main actions of angiotensin II include all of the following except:
    a. systemic vasoconstriction.
    b. stimulation of sodium reabsorption directly at the proximal tubule.
    c. promotion of aldosterone biosynthesis and secretion.
    d. inhibition of thirst and AVP secretion.
    e. stimulation of thirst and AVP secretion.

19. Each of the following governs potassium secretion by the cortical collecting duct except:
    a. aldosterone.
    b. serum potassium concentration.
    c. luminal flow rate.
    d. luminal Na^+ delivery.
    e. plasma calcitonin level.

20. After potassium is reabsorbed by the TAL of Henle and by the collecting duct, it re-enters the lumen of the TAL in a process referred to as "recycling." Which of the following is NOT a proposed consequence of potassium recycling?
    a. The TAL fluid potassium concentration is maintained.
    b. The TAL fluid potassium concentration is sufficient for reabsorption by the Na^+-K^+-$2Cl^-$ cotransporter of the large filtered load of Na^+ that enters the TAL.
    c. The TAL lumen-positive transepithelial voltage is maintained, which promotes a paracellular current.
    d. Potassium recycling promotes magnesium secretion by the TAL.
    e. The TAL lumen-positive transepithelial voltage promotes sodium, calcium, and magnesium reabsorption.

21. Which of the following diuretics is NOT referred to as potassium-sparing?
    a. Spironolactone
    b. Amiloride
    c. Torsemide

d. Furosemide
e. Triamterene.

22. The most abundant divalent cation in the body is:
    a. calcium.
    b. potassium.
    c. sodium.
    d. chloride.
    e. magnesium.

23. Which of the following is NOT a major nephron site of renal calcium reabsorption?
    a. Proximal convoluted tubule
    b. Medullary TAL of the loop of Henle
    c. Medullary thin ascending limb of Henle
    d. Distal convoluted tubule
    e. Medullary collecting duct

24. The effect of thiazide-type diuretics on calcium reabsorption is to:
    a. stimulate calcium reabsorption by the distal convoluted tubule.
    b. inhibit calcium reabsorption by the distal convoluted tubule.
    c. inhibit calcium reabsorption by the cortical collecting tubule.
    d. inhibit calcium reabsorption by the TAL.
    e. stimulate calcium secretion by the medullary collecting duct.

25. Which of the following is NOT a major renal action of parathyroid hormone (PTH)?
    a. Stimulation of calcium reabsorption at the distal tubule independently from Na^+ and water.
    b. Increased adenylate cyclase activity via a stimulatory G-protein that is coupled to the PTH receptor.
    c. Stimulation of adenylate cyclase activity via an inhibitory G-protein that is coupled to the PTH receptor.
    d. Stimulation of the production of 1,25-dihydroxyvitamin D_3.
    e. Inhibition of the Na^+-H^+ antiporter at the S_1 segment of the proximal nephron.

26. Which of the following does NOT increase renal calcium excretion?
    a. Extracellular fluid volume expansion
    b. Torsemide
    c. High dietary sodium intake
    d. Ethacrynic acid
    e. Hydrochlorothiazide

27. Which of the following statements is NOT true of the calcium-sensing receptor?
    a. It has been identified in the basolateral aspect of the cortical TAL.
    b. It is a G-protein–coupled receptor activated by high levels of extracellular calcium.
    c. It is isolated from the proximal tubule, cortical TAL and medullary TAL, and distal convoluted tubule.
    d. It is isolated from the parathyroid.
    e. It stimulates cAMP production.

28. All of the following are the major nephron sites of renal magnesium reabsorption except:
    a. proximal convoluted tubule.
    b. proximal straight tubule.
    c. TAL of Henle.
    d. distal tubule.
    e. inner medullary collecting duct.

29. Which of the following major factors influences renal magnesium reabsorption?
    a. Lumen-positive transepithelial potential of the TAL.
    b. Lumen-negative transepithelial potential of the TAL.
    c. Lumen-positive transepithelial potential of the cortical collecting duct.
    d. Binding to the Na^+-K^+-$2Cl^-$ cotransporter in the cortical collecting duct.
    e. Binding to the Na^+-Cl^- cotransporter in the distal tubule.

30. All of the following regulate phosphorus excretion except:
    a. phosphaturic effect of PTH.
    b. PTH stimulation of phosphorus reabsorption.
    c. GFR.
    d. vitamin D.
    e. dietary phosphorus intake.

31. Urate concentration in human plasma is saturated at which of the following concentrations?
    a. 6.5 to 7.0 mg/dl
    b. 1.5 to 3.0 mg/dl
    c. 10 to 12 mg/dl
    d. 15 to 20 mg/dl
    e. not saturable at physiologic pH

32. All of the following mechanisms of urate transport are active in the proximal tubule except:
    a. reabsorption of urate in the S_1 segment.
    b. entry into the cytoplasm in exchange for HCO_3^-.
    c. secretion of urate in the S_2 segment.
    d. metabolism of urea to urate in the cytoplasm.
    e. a and b.

33. Which of the following statements is NOT true regarding urate?
    a. Extracellular fluid volume expansion reduces excretion.
    b. Solubility decreases at low urinary pH.
    c. Radiocontrast agents inhibit reabsorption.
    d. Secreted diuretics (e.g., furosemide) inhibit tubular secretion of urate.
    e. Lead intoxication stimulates reabsorption.

34. Which of the following is NOT involved in vasopressin stimulation of water reabsorption by the collecting duct?
    a. Binding of vasopressin to the specific V_1 receptor (V_1R)
    b. Stimulation of a GDP-GTP exchange to occur on the GTP-binding protein G_s
    c. Aggregation of intramembranous particles in the membrane facing the lumen of principal cells of the collecting duct
    d. Insertion of water channels into the apical membrane in response to vasopressin stimulation, which increases water permeability by the collecting duct
    e. A link between acquired disorders of water balance to abnormalities in AQP-2, including nephrogenic diabetes insipidus caused by urinary tract obstruction, lithium, hypokalemia, and hypercalcemia

35. Each of the following is a major determinant used to calculate the total osmolality of body fluids except:
    a. plasma sodium concentration.
    b. plasma potassium concentration.
    c. plasma glucose concentration.
    d. blood urea nitrogen (BUN) value.
    e. plasma calcium concentration.

36. Which of the following is not an "effective osmole"?
    a. Urea
    b. Na$^+$
    c. K$^+$
    d. Glucose
    e. Betaine

37. Which of the following statements is NOT true?
    a. Na$^+$ concentration is proportional to total body osmolality because the body compartments are in osmotic equilibrium.
    b. K$^+$ concentration in cells is directly proportional to total body osmolality because K$^+$ is the predominant intracellular effective osmole.
    c. Alterations in total body osmolality, and thus serum Na$^+$ concentration, reflect changes in the *ratio* of the body content of K$^+$, Na$^+$, and total body water.
    d. Plasma Na$^+$ concentration correlates strongly with total body volume.
    e. Na$^+$ is the major determinant of normal plasma osmolality.

38. All of the following contribute to nonosmotic stimulation of thirst and vasopressin secretion except:
    a. acute blood loss.
    b. gastrointestinal losses.
    c. congestive heart failure.
    d. ascites.
    e. treatment with angiotensin-converting enzyme inhibitors.

39. Which of the following mechanisms does NOT contribute to the formation of a concentrated urine?
    a. Urine is initially concentrated in the descending limb of the loop of Henle by diffusion of water into the medulla.
    b. In the medullary TAL, NaCl is reabsorbed by active transport.
    c. The medullary TAL is relatively impermeable to water.
    d. The medullary TAL is highly permeable to water in the presence of vasopressin.
    e. During antidiuresis, when vasopressin levels are high, the collecting duct epithelium is highly permeable to water.

40. Which of the following statements is NOT true?
    a. Osmolar clearance (C_{Osm}) is the relative urinary excretion of isotonic fluid.
    b. Free water clearance (C_{H2O}) is the relative urinary excretion of solute free water.
    c. The total urine volume is the sum of $C_{Osm} + C_{H2O}$.
    d. Free water clearance is increased by diuretic treatment.
    e. Hyponatremia occurs when free water clearance is reduced excessively.

41. Which of the following conditions is not required to excrete solute-free water by the kidney?
    a. Adequate GFR
    b. Delivery of filtrate to the loop of Henle
    c. Adequate medullary solute content
    d. Normal loop of Henle function, whereby tubule fluid is diluted because NaCl is reabsorbed without water
    e. High levels of vasopressin together with collecting ducts that are permeable to water

42. Which of the following features does not characterize pseudohyponatremia?
    a. Life-threatening, characterized by low serum Na$^+$ concentration and neurologic abnormalities.
    b. Reduced aqueous phase of plasma, leading to reduction in the Na$^+$ concentration in total plasma.
    c. Occurring in disorders associated with hyperlipidemia
    d. Occurring in disorders associated with hyperproteinemia
    e. Normal Na$^+$ concentration in the aqueous phase of plasma

43. In regard to hypovolemic hyponatremia, which of the following statements is incorrect?
    a. Urinary Na$^+$ concentration identifies whether fluid losses are renal or extrarenal.
    b. Urinary Na$^+$ concentration less than 20 mEq/L reflects a normal renal response to volume depletion.
    c. Urinary Na$^+$ concentration greater than 20 mEq/L reflects an abnormal renal response to volume depletion.
    d. Syndrome of inappropriate antidiuretic hormone (SIADH) is the most common cause of hypovolemic hyponatremia.
    e. Physical examination is important in determining the pathophysiology of hyponatremia.

44. Which of the following is NOT a characteristic feature of SIADH?
    a. Hyponatremia with excretion of urine that is not maximally dilute (greater than 100 mOsm/kg).
    b. Maintained Na$^+$ balance, so that urine Na$^+$ concentration reflects intake and is usually high.
    c. Hypouricemia with plasma uric acid concentration less than 4 mg/dl, indicative of increased urate clearance.
    d. Associated with malignancies, pulmonary diseases, and central nervous system disorders.
    e. Low blood pressure because of volume depletion.

45. Which of the following electrolyte abnormalities is associated with nephrogenic diabetes insipidus?
    a. Hypercalcemia
    b. Hypokalemia
    c. Hyperkalemia
    d. Hypocalcemia
    e. Both a and b

46. Which of the following is NOT true in the assessment of the polyuric patient?
    a. U_{Osm} below 250 mOsm/kg usually indicates a water diuresis.
    b. U_{Osm} greater than 300 mOsm/kg most commonly reflects a solute diuresis.
    c. High-protein feeding is associated with U_{Osm} less than 250 and diabetes insipidus.
    d. Intravenous contrast material is an osmotic diuretic.
    e. Some psychiatric disorders may be manifested by hyponatremia.

47. The predominant buffering system in humans is:
    a. bicarbonate.
    b. titratable acids.
    c. ammonium (NH$_4^+$).
    d. urea.
    e. phosphate.

48. Which of the following is NOT characteristic of the buffering response to an acid load?
    a. Hydrogen ions are initially buffered primarily by HCO$_3^-$.
    b. Hydrogen ions are initially buffered intracellularly by proteins.
    c. Approximately 50% of the acid load occurs intracellularly within a few hours.
    d. The relative amount of intracellular to extracellular buffering can increase so that more than twice as much buffering occurs intracellularly.

e. About 40% to 45% of an acid load can be buffered extracellularly within 30 minutes.

49. Which of the following is not an effect of organic and inorganic acidosis on serum potassium concentration?

   a. Plasma potassium concentration increases to a greater extent during an acute load with an inorganic acid than during an organic acid load.
   b. During organic acidosis, transcellular potassium shifts are minor because the proton is accompanied into the cell by the organic anion rather than in exchange for potassium.
   c. Hyperkalemia does not usually occur during organic acidosis despite reductions in pH, which are comparable to those in mineral acidosis.
   d. Intracellular buffering during an inorganic acid load requires transcellular ion transport, including sodium/proton, potassium/proton, and chloride/bicarbonate exchanges.
   e. In ketoacidosis, profound hyperkalemia is characteristic because intracellular buffering by sodium/proton exchange is maximized.

50. Which of the following does NOT occur during respiratory compensation to metabolic acidosis?

   a. Stimulation of chemoreceptors that control respiration.
   b. Compensation, which is fully operational within about 14 hours.
   c. An increase in alveolar ventilation and a decline in P_{CO_2}.
   d. A decrease in alveolar ventilation and an increase in P_{CO_2}.
   e. Hyperventilation, characterized by a predominant increase in tidal volume (Kussmaul respiration).

51. The main site of renal HCO_3^- reabsorption is the:

   a. proximal convoluted tubule.
   b. medullary TAL of Henle.
   c. distal convoluted tubule.
   d. cortical collecting duct.
   e. medullary collecting duct.

52. Which of the following statements is NOT true?

   a. 80% of filtered HCO_3^- is reabsorbed in the proximal convoluted tubule.
   b. 80% of filtered HCO_3^- is reabsorbed in the medullary TAL.
   c. H^+ secretion in the proximal tubule is driven by the Na^+-H^+ exchanger.
   d. Carbonic anhydrase minimizes H^+ concentration in the proximal tubule lumen.
   e. Acetazolamide inhibits carbonic anhydrase activity.

53. Which of the following statements is NOT true?

   a. Very steep gradients for H^+ can be maintained in the medullary collecting duct.
   b. Urinary pH cannot decrease below 4.5, which is equivalent to an $[H^+]$ of less than 0.1 mEq/L.
   c. Urine is buffered by titratable acid.
   d. Urine is buffered by ammonium.
   e. Under normal circumstances, urinary pH cannot decrease below 7.0 despite buffering by ammonium and titratable acid.

54. Which of the following statements is NOT true?

   a. Titratable acidity refers to the quantity of NaOH required to titrate urine back to a pH 7.40.
   b. Filtered phosphates are ideal urinary buffers because 80% are present in dibasic form (HPO_4^{2-}), with a pK_a of 6.8.
   c. Filtered phosphates are ideal urinary buffers because their rate of excretion is approximately 40 to 60 mmol/day, leading to the excretion of about 30 to 40 mEq/L of titratable acid daily.
   d. Titratable acid excretion increases two- to threefold during metabolic acidosis.
   e. Filtered phosphates are ideal urinary buffers because 80% are present in dibasic form (HPO_4^{2-}) with a pK_a of 7.4.

55. Which of the following statements is NOT true?

   a. In the proximal tubule, NH_4^+ is secreted into the lumen by replacing H^+ on the Na^+-H^+ exchanger.
   b. After entering the medullary TAL of Henle, approximately 50% to 80% of the NH_4^+ present in the lumen is then reabsorbed by replacing K^+ on the Na^+-K^+-$2Cl^-$ cotransporter.
   c. With the "single effect" of the countercurrent mechanism, very large amounts of NH_3 accumulate in the medulla.
   d. The low pH of urine in the cortical collecting duct, together with the high pK_a (9.3) of NH_3, leads to the formation of NH_4^+ and its accumulation in the tubule lumen.
   e. Renal NH_4^+ production is stimulated during acute and chronic respiratory acidosis, but not by metabolic acidosis.

56. Which of the following does NOT have a major effect on net acid excretion?

   a. Luminal HCO_3^- concentration.
   b. Extracellular volume and body contents of K^+ and Cl^-.
   c. Peritubular HCO_3^-.
   d. Serum K^+ concentration.
   e. Hydroxymethylglutaryl coenzyme A reductase activity.

57. Which of the following statements regarding metabolic alkalosis is NOT true?

   a. As with an acid load, a bicarbonate load is distributed throughout the extracellular compartment within 30 minutes.
   b. Only about 30% of a bicarbonate load is buffered in the intracellular compartment.
   c. The respiratory response occurs over several hours.
   d. Renal excretion of the excess base is required to restore base stores to normal.
   e. This process occurs very slowly, compared with the renal response to an acid load.

58. Laboratory information on all of the following is essential for the diagnosis of an acid-base disorder except:

   a. bicarbonate.
   b. ammonium.
   c. pH.
   d. chloride.
   e. P_{CO_2}.

59. Which of the following factors is NOT included in the calculation of the anion gap?

   a. pH
   b. K^+
   c. Cl^-
   d. HCO_3^-
   e. Both a and b

60. Which of the following does NOT characterize hyperchloremic metabolic acidosis?

   a. Excess HCO_3^- is lost from the gastrointestinal tract (e.g., in diarrhea).
   b. Excess HCO_3^- is lost from the kidney (e.g., in renal tubular acidosis).
   c. Dilution of HCO_3^- occurs during saline infusion.

d. It occurs during exogenous acid load.
e. It occurs during generation of excess lactic acid.

61. Which of the following is NOT a characteristic of the urinary anion gap?

   a. The NH_4^+ excretion rate can be estimated by the urinary anion gap, assuming that the major urinary cations are NH_4^+, Na^+, and K^+ and that Cl^- is the predominant anion.
   b. The urinary anion gap value is normally approximately zero.
   c. It is markedly negative during gastrointestinal losses of HCO_3^-, when the NH_4^+ excretion rate can exceed 200 mEq/day.
   d. It is inappropriately near zero in the renal tubular acidoses.
   e. It is markedly positive during gastrointestinal losses of HCO_3^-, when the NH_4^+ excretion rate can exceed 200 mEq/day.

62. Which of the following is NOT a characteristic of proximal renal tubular acidosis?

   a. Impaired proximal tubular reabsorption of HCO_3^- with increased fractional excretion of HCO_3^- ($FE_{HCO3} \geq 10\%$ to 30%)
   b. Bicarbonaturia with a reduction in net acid excretion
   c. Extracellular fluid volume contraction
   d. Low plasma renin activity level
   e. Hypokalemia caused by secondary hyperaldosteronism and increased delivery of an impermeable anion (HCO_3^-) to the collecting duct

63. Which of the following is NOT a characteristic of distal renal tubular acidosis?

   a. The ability of the collecting duct to secrete H^+ against this gradient is impaired and urine pH cannot be reduced below 5.3 despite the low blood pH.
   b. Net acid excretion is reduced because a defect in H^+ secretion impairs excretion of titratable acids and ammonia even though ammonia production is normal.
   c. The relatively small fraction of filtered HCO_3^- that is delivered to the distal nephron is not reabsorbed.
   d. In distal renal tubular acidosis, the acidosis is progressive and may be severe because the urine cannot be maximally acidified.
   e. In distal renal tubular acidosis, the acidosis is self-limited and is usually mild.

64. Which of the following factors does NOT generate metabolic alkalosis?

   a. Gastrointestinal proton loss
   b. Renal proton loss
   c. Proton translocation into cells
   d. Activation of the renin-angiotensin-aldosterone system
   e. Inhibition of the renin-angiotensin-aldosterone system.

65. Which of the following factors does NOT contribute to the persistence of metabolic alkalosis?

   a. Reduced extracellular fluid volume
   b. Chloride depletion
   c. Hypokalemia
   d. Hyperaldosteronism
   e. Hypoaldosteronism

Answers

1. **b. 20%.** Under resting conditions, the blood flow to the kidney is about 20% of the cardiac output. Approximately 20% of the plasma reaching the glomeruli is filtered into renal tubules; the plasma that is not filtered exits the glomerulus through the efferent arteriole into the postglomerular capillaries. [p 169]

2. **c. Afferent arteriolar dilatation and efferent arteriolar constriction enhance glomerular filtration pressure and, in turn, maintain glomerular filtration pressure.** The glomerular circulation promotes ultrafiltration of large volumes of fluid because of the excess transcapillary hydraulic pressure relative to oncotic pressure. Because the glomerulus is located between the afferent and the efferent arterioles, selective changes in the arteriolar resistances that are caused by vasoactive substances will have a significant impact on glomerular hemodynamics. When the afferent arteriole dilates, more arterial perfusion pressure is transmitted to the glomerulus and both capillary flow and GFR increase. Conversely, afferent arteriolar vasoconstriction decreases both the GFR and the glomerular plasma flow. In contrast, a selective increase in efferent arteriolar constriction reduces glomerular plasma flow but increases glomerular pressure and, thus, GFR increases. [p 170]

3. **a. The GFR and the renal plasma flow (RPF) change in parallel during afferent constriction, so no change occurs in the filtration fraction.** The relationship between the RPF and the GFR depends on whether the predominant change in tone occurs at the afferent or the efferent arteriole. The GFR and the RPF change in parallel during afferent constriction and so no change occurs in the filtration fraction, defined as the ratio GFR:RPF. In contrast, during efferent constriction, reciprocal changes in the GFR and the RPF occur. This change in the ratio of GFR to RPF signifies that, in general, a change in the filtration fraction accompanies constriction of the efferent but not the afferent arteriole. [pp 170–171]

4. **e. NOS II is dependent on calcium.** NOS is the enzyme that catalyzes the production of nitric oxide and citrulline from arginine. There are three isoforms of this enzyme: NOS I (in neuronal and epithelial cells), NOS II (in cytokine-induced cells and vascular smooth muscle), and NOS III (in endothelial cells). Isoform II is not dependent on calcium and is inducible by cytokines (i.e., interleukin-1) and lipopolysaccharide and participates in the vasodilatation associated with septic shock. In contrast, NOS isoform III is constitutively expressed in endothelial cells, where it is regulated by calcium and calmodulin. Eplerenone is a mineralocorticoid receptor antagonist and is not a direct vasodilator. [pp 175–176]

5. **e. development of systemic hypotension.** After nitric oxide is formed in endothelial cells, it diffuses to adjacent vascular smooth muscle, where it stimulates soluble guanylyl cyclase, increases cGMP, and consequently dilates blood vessels. Characteristic changes that occur during NOS inhibition include (1) marked increases in resistances in afferent and, predominantly, in efferent arterioles that result in elevated glomerular capillary pressure and reduced renal blood flow; (2) a decline in the glomerular capillary ultrafiltration coefficient K_f; (3) a reduction in sodium reabsorption by the proximal tubule; and (4) the development of systemic hyper-

tension that occurs in concert with these changes in renal hemodynamic and excretory function. [p 176]

6. **b. Creatinine is reabsorbed by the organic cation transporter of the proximal tubule, and therefore Ccr is not due solely to glomerular filtration.** Creatinine is generated by the nonenzymatic conversions from creatine and phosphocreatine that are present in muscle. It is a small molecule that is freely filtered by the glomerulus and is not metabolized by the kidney. However, creatinine is secreted by the organic cation transporter of the proximal tubule. Therefore, Ccr is not due solely to glomerular filtration but also reflects tubular secretion. There is also significant variability in the measurement of serum creatinine level. The absolute difference between Ccr and GFR is greatest within the range of GFR 40 to 80 ml/min/1.73 m^2, for which the Ccr/GFR ratio is 1.5 to 2.0. [p 178]

7. **c. 60% to 70%.** The proximal tubule reabsorbs approximately 60% to 70% of the glomerular filtrate. Although most of the glomerular filtrate is reabsorbed by the proximal tubule, there are substantial differences in the amounts of individual solutes that are reabsorbed by this segment; almost all of the filtered glucose and amino acids are reabsorbed, but only about 70% of filtered sodium is reclaimed there. [p 179]

8. **a. the proximal tubule.** Glucose reabsorption by the proximal tubule occurs in two steps: (1) carrier-mediated, sodium-glucose cotransport across the apical membrane, followed by (2) facilitated glucose transport and active sodium extrusion across the basolateral membrane. Two sodium-glucose cotransporters have been identified in the apical membrane: SLGT-1 and SLGT-2. The driving force for the apical translocation of sodium and glucose is secondary active transport, whereby sodium moves down its electrochemical gradient from the lumen to the intracellular space. Transport of glucose across the basolateral membrane does not consume energy but is mediated by specific carriers belonging to the GLUT gene family. In the outer cortex, a high-capacity, low-affinity glucose transport system is present, with a sodium/glucose ratio of 1:1, identified as SLGT-2. Glucose exits the basolateral membrane via a high-capacity transporter, GLUT-2. In the outer medullae, a high-affinity system carries two Na$^+$ per glucose, identified as SLGT-1. [p 186]

9. **a. the fractional excretion of urea varies according to the state of hydration.** The fractional excretion of urea varies according to the state of hydration. Approximately 40% to 50% of filtered urea is reabsorbed by the proximal tubule, regardless of the state of hydration. During antidiuresis, urea is secreted into the loop of Henle, so that the amount of urea delivered to the early distal nephron may exceed the filtered load. A significant fraction of urea is reabsorbed by the medullary collecting duct, and consequently only 30% to 40% of the filtered load is excreted during antidiuresis. In contrast, during diuresis, neither secretion nor reabsorption occurs beyond the proximal nephron, so that urea clearance is 55% to 60% of the GFR. [pp 178–179]

10. **b. Medullary TAL of Henle.** The medullary TAL reabsorbs solute but is impermeable to water. Filtrate entering the loop of Henle from the proximal tubule is isoosmotic with plasma, decreasing to about 50 mOsm/kg as it exits the loop and enters the distal tubule. Solute reabsorbed by the loop of Henle of juxtamedullary nephrons accumulates in the medulla, thereby increasing the tonicity of the medullary interstitium. Tubular fluid becomes progressively more dilute as it flows from the thin ascending limb through the thick ascending limb of Henle and is hypoosmotic to plasma when it enters the distal tubule, regardless of whether vasopressin is present. [pp 180, 201–202]

11. **d. Spironolactone.** Bumetanide, furosemide, torsemide, and ethacrynic acid are loop diuretics. They inhibit the Na$^+$-K$^+$-2Cl$^-$ cotransporter and thus promote diuresis as well as increased excretion of Na$^+$, K$^+$, Cl$^-$, Ca^{2+}, and Mg^{2+}. Loop diuretics reduce medullary solute content and impair urinary concentrating and diluting capacity. Spironolactone is a mineralocorticoid receptor antagonist. [pp 180–181]

12. **c. Amino acid reabsorption.** Approximately 10% to 15% of the filtered load of NaCl exits the loop of Henle and enters the distal nephron. It is at this point that the characteristics of the final urine are established, including the magnitude of potassium secretion, calcium excretion, urinary acidification, and maximal osmolality. [pp 181, 182–183]

13. **a. principal cell and intercalated cell.** The principal cell has receptors for vasopressin and aldosterone that promote reabsorption of water and NaCl and also stimulate K$^+$ secretion. The intercalated cell contains an H$^+$,K$^+$-ATPase pump at the luminal membrane that actively absorbs K$^+$ in exchange for H$^+$ and thus participates in K$^+$ and acid-base homeostasis. [pp 181–182, 187, 188]

14. **e. To increase glucose reabsorption by the inner medullary collecting duct.** AVP stimulates Na$^+$-K$^+$-2Cl$^-$ activity by the medullary TAL of Henle and thus increases electrolyte, but not water, reabsorption by that segment. At the cortical and outer medullary collecting ducts, AVP stimulates reabsorption of NaCl and water but does not increase urea permeability. The main action of AVP in the inner medullary collecting duct is to increase water and urea permeability. [pp 201–202]

15. **a. to stimulate potassium secretion by the principal cells of the cortical and medullary collecting tubule.** Potassium secretion by the principal cells of the cortical and medullary collecting tubule is directly stimulated by aldosterone. Aldosterone binds to a cytoplasmic receptor, forming an aldosterone-receptor complex that subsequently activates gene transcription and synthesis of aldosterone-induced proteins. During the early phase of mineralocorticoid action, a greater number of apical sodium channels are in the open state so that sodium entry into principal cells increases. During this phase, Na$^+$,K$^+$-ATPase activity increases with Na$^+$ entry into these cells, although the maximum activity of the enzyme is not increased initially. This electrogenic reabsorption of Na$^+$ increases the lumen-negative transepithelial potential. During the late phase of aldosterone action, more Na$^+$,K$^+$-ATPase units are added to the basolateral membrane. Together these aldosterone responses augment the electrochemical gradient for potassium secretion. [pp 181–182, 188]

16. **c. Renin's substrate is angiotensin I, which in turn forms angiotensin II, a potent vasoconstrictor that stimulates aldosterone production.** Renin is an aspartyl proteinase belonging to the same family as pepsin and cathepsin. It is synthesized predominantly in the kidney by specialized cells, referred to as juxtaglomerular cells, that are located at the afferent arteriole of each nephron. The juxtaglomerular cells are specialized myoendocrine cells that are close to both the macula densa cells of the ascending limb of Henle and the extraglomerular mesangium at the hilum of the glomerulus. Together they form the juxtaglomerular apparatus. [p 183]

17. **c. β-Adrenergic blockers.** The major factors that control renin secretion include the following: (1) The baroreceptor mechanism: increased renal perfusion pressure sensed by the juxtaglomerular cells inhibits renin secretion, and decreased perfusion pressure stimulates secretion. (2) The neural mech-

anism: low levels of renal sympathetic nerve activity, mediated through β_1-adrenoceptors, stimulate renin secretion. (3) The macula densa mechanism: increases in Cl^- delivery to this specialized cell in the thick ascending limb suppress renin secretion, and decreases in Cl^- delivery stimulate renin secretion. [pp 183, 184]

18. **d. inhibit thirst and AVP secretion.** Angiotensin II is the first effector of the renin system, and its actions, mediated through the AT_1 receptor subtype, include systemic vasoconstriction, stimulation of sodium reabsorption directly at the proximal tubule, promotion of aldosterone biosynthesis and secretion and thus increased Na^+ reabsorption at the cortical collecting tubule, and stimulation of thirst and AVP secretion. Thus, the renin-angiotensin-aldosterone system plays a central role in maintaining blood pressure, body volume, and potassium homeostasis. [pp 172, 183–184, 213]

19. **e. plasma calcitonin level.** The cell model for K^+ transport by the principal cell of the cortical collecting duct is illustrated in Figure 6–12. The basolateral Na^+,K^+-ATPase pump maintains a high intracellular K^+ concentration and promotes the coupling of Na^+ reabsorption and K^+ secretion. Na^+ diffusion from lumen to cell through apical Na^+ channels occurs down a concentration gradient. The resulting lumen-negative transepithelial potential difference promotes K^+ secretion down the electrochemical gradient. Maneuvers that increase the electrochemical potential, such as high urinary flow (by decreasing luminal K^+ concentration) and high serum K^+ levels, enhance K^+ secretion. K^+ secretion by the principal cells of the cortical and medullary collecting tubule is also directly stimulated by aldosterone. Accordingly, at any level of serum K^+, urinary K^+ levels will increase as aldosterone levels rise. [pp 181–182]

20. **d. Potassium recycling promotes magnesium secretion by the TAL.** There are two consequences of this recycling: (1) the TAL fluid potassium is replenished and remains sufficient for reabsorption by Na^+-K^+-$2Cl^-$ of the large filtered load of Na^+ that enters the TAL, and (2) potassium recycling into the lumen produces a lumen-positive transepithelial voltage that promotes a paracellular current, carrying 50% of the total amount of Na^+ reabsorbed by the TAL. [p 180]

21. **c. Torsemide.** Potassium-sparing diuretics include spironolactone, amiloride, and triamterene. Aldactone competitively inhibits the binding of aldosterone to the aldosterone receptor located in the cytoplasm of principal cells. Amiloride directly blocks the Na^+ channel located on the luminal surface of the collecting duct. By inhibiting the Na^+ conductance, these diuretics attenuate the electrochemical driving force for K^+ secretion. The precise tubular action of triamterene is not completely defined. [p 189]

22. **a. calcium.** Calcium is the most abundant divalent cation in the body, accounting for about 2% of the body weight, and is present in extracellular fluid at a concentration of 10 mg/dl (equal to 5 mEq/L and 2.5 mmol/L). This level is tightly regulated despite the wide range of dietary calcium intakes (500 to 1200 mg/day). [p 191]

23. **c. Medullary thin ascending limb of Henle.** Approximately 65% of filtered calcium is reabsorbed in the proximal convoluted tubule, 25% in the medullary TAL of the loop of Henle, and 8% in the distal convoluted tubule. Micropuncture studies have demonstrated that calcium reabsorption by this segment, and in the kidney as a whole, parallels that of Na^+ and water. [p 192]

24. **a. stimulate calcium reabsorption by the distal convoluted tubule.** Thiazide diuretics stimulate calcium reabsorption by the distal convoluted tubule. One proposed mechanism for this phenomenon is that thiazides hyperpolarize the cell, thereby activating apical calcium channels and stimulating calcium entry. Alternatively, the reduced intracellular sodium increases the electrochemical gradient, thereby promoting calcium reabsorption by the basolateral Na^+-Ca^{2+} exchanger. In contrast, loop diuretics reduce the magnitude of the lumen-positive potential and thus reduce the driving force for calcium reabsorption by the TAL. [p 181]

25. **c. Stimulation of adenylate cyclase activity via an inhibitory G-protein that is coupled to the PTH receptor.** PTH stimulates calcium reabsorption at the distal tubule independently from Na^+ and water. This action is mediated by increased adenylate cyclase activity via a stimulatory G-protein that is coupled to the PTH receptor on the basolateral membrane. PTH also stimulates the production of 1,25-dihydroxyvitamin D_3 by inducing production of the cytochrome P450 monooxygenase, 25-hydroxyvitamin D-1α-hydroxylase, in the proximal tubule. Vitamin D increases renal calcium reabsorption at distal nephron segments. [pp 194–195]

26. **e. Hydrochlorothiazide.** Extracellular fluid volume expansion and loop diuretics increase renal calcium excretion. In contrast, thiazide diuretics and potassium-sparing diuretics decrease calcium excretion. [p 195]

27. **e. It stimulates cAMP production.** A calcium-sensing receptor has been identified in the basolateral aspect of the cortical TAL, where receptors for PTH reside (see Fig. 6–27). It has also been isolated from parathyroid, thyroid, brain, and intestine and has been found in the apical membrane of the proximal tubule, cortical TAL and medullary TAL, and distal convoluted tubule. This G-protein–coupled receptor is activated by high levels of extracellular calcium, thereby attenuating cAMP production and consequently reducing renal tubular reabsorption. The receptor also binds Mg^{2+} and other polyvalent ions. [p 195]

28. **e. inner medullary collecting duct.** Of the 2100 mg of Mg^{2+} filtered daily by the glomerulus, 97% is reabsorbed along the nephron: 20% to 30% by the proximal convoluted tubule, 15% by the proximal straight tubule, 65% in the TAL of Henle, and 2% to 5% in the distal tubule. [p 195]

29. **a. Lumen-positive transepithelial potential of the TAL.** As with Ca^{2+}, Mg^{2+} reabsorption in the TAL occurs in parallel with reabsorption of Na^+ and Cl^-. A major driving force for Mg^{2+} reabsorption by this segment is the lumen-positive transepithelial potential. [pp 195–196]

30. **b. PTH stimulation of phosphorus reabsorption.** PTH is the predominant hormonal regulator of urinary phosphate excretion—PTH infusion is phosphaturic, and parathyroidectomy decreases phosphate excretion by the kidney. The major site of PTH-sensitive P_i transport is the proximal tubule, with activity also present in the distal nephron. Other factors include GFR, vitamin D, and dietary intake. [p 197]

31. **a. 6.5 to 7.0 mg/dl.** Saturation of human plasma occurs at a urate concentration of approximately 6.5 to 7.0 mg/dl, with lower solubility at lower temperatures and higher sodium concentrations. [p 197]

32. **d. metabolism of urea to urate in the cytoplasm.** Reabsorption of urate by the proximal tubule occurs predominantly in the S_1 segment, where it enters the cytoplasm in exchange for hydroxyl anions, HCO_3^-, Cl^-, hippurate, and

lactate. Urate secretion also occurs in the proximal tubule, with the secretory rate exceeding reabsorption in the S_2 segment of the proximal tubule. [p 197]

33. **a. Extracellular fluid volume expansion reduces excretion.** Urate clearance is increased by volume expansion. Secretion is inhibited by certain secreted diuretics (such as furosemide); reabsorption is stimulated by chronic lead intoxication and is inhibited by radiocontrast agents. Uric acid is relatively insoluble in its nonionized form in acidified urine (pH 4.5). [pp 197–198]

34. **a. Binding of vasopressin to the specific V_1 receptor (V_1R).** Binding of vasopressin to the specific V_2 receptor (V_2R) stimulates a GDP-GTP exchange to occur on the GTP-binding protein G_s, located on the basolateral plasma membrane of the TAL and of the principal cells of the collecting duct. Stimulation of adenylate cyclase, in turn, promotes cAMP generation. Within minutes, aggregates of intramembranous particles appear in the membrane facing the lumen of principal cells of the collecting duct. These particles contain water channels that are inserted into the apical membrane in response to vasopressin stimulation and that increase water permeability by the collecting duct. When vasopressin is withdrawn, endocytosis of the membrane-containing water channels breaks their contact with the aqueous luminal surface, and water permeability decreases markedly. The link between aqueporin-2 (AQP-2), a water channel, and vasopressin-mediated water transport by the kidney was established with the discovery that the aqueporin-2 gene is mutated in patients with congenital nephrogenic diabetes insipidus. Subsequent studies have linked acquired disorders of water balance to abnormalities in AQP-2, including nephrogenic diabetes insipidus caused by urinary tract obstruction, lithium, hypokalemia, and hypercalcemia. [p 202]

35. **b. plasma potassium concentration.** $P_{Osm} = (2 \times$ plasma $[Na^+]) + ([glucose]/18) + (BUN/2.8)$, where plasma sodium concentration is multiplied by 2 to account for the accompanying anion (predominantly Cl^- and HCO_3^-), and glucose and BUN are expressed as millimoles per liter. [p 198]

36. **a. Urea.** Urea is unlike Na^+ and K^+ because it diffuses freely across cell membranes and is present in equal concentrations in the extracellular and intracellular spaces. Urea is referred to as an ineffective osmole because it does not generate an osmotic gradient and therefore does not affect the distribution of water. [p 198]

37. **d. Plasma Na^+ concentration correlates strongly with total body volume.** Serum Na^+ concentration is proportional to total body osmolality because the body compartments are in osmotic equilibrium. Similarly, the concentration of K^+ in cells is also directly proportional to total body osmolality because K^+ is the predominant intracellular effective osmole. Therefore, alterations in total body osmolality, and thus serum Na^+ concentration, reflect changes in the *ratio* of the body content of K^+, Na^+, and total body water. This linear relationship is expressed as plasma $[Na^+] = (Na^+_e + K^+_e)/TBW$, where $(Na^+_e + K^+_e)$ refers to exchangeable Na^+ and K^+ ions that are not sequestered in body tissues and TBW is total body water. Plasma Na^+ concentration does *not* correlate with body volume, and so the plasma Na^+ concentration does not provide information for predicting a patient's volume status: hyponatremia can occur when total body volume is increased (e.g., congestive heart failure) or decreased (e.g., gastrointestinal losses). [p 199]

38. **e. treatment with angiotensin-converting enzyme inhibitors.** Examples of nonosmotic stimuli of thirst associated with decreased extracellular fluid volume include acute blood loss, gastrointestinal losses, congestive heart failure, ascites, and unilateral renovascular hypertension. The renin-angiotensin-aldosterone system is intensely activated in each of these conditions, and angiotensin II has been demonstrated to be one of the mediators of this potent dipsogenic response and is a direct stimulus of vasopressin secretion through its actions at central nervous system structures located near the third ventricle. Other nonosmotic stimuli include nausea, pain, and several pharmacologic agents, including general anesthetics. [pp 199–200]

39. **d. The medullary TAL is highly permeable to water in the presence of vasopressin.** Urine is initially concentrated in the descending limb of the loop of Henle by the diffusion of water into the medulla. In the medullary TAL, NaCl is reabsorbed by active transport. However, this nephron segment is relatively impermeable to water, so that the osmolality of the tubule lumen is reduced to a level below that of the surrounding medullary tissue and the interstitial solute gradient is not dissipated by water fluxes. During water diuresis, when vasopressin secretion is reduced, tubule fluid hypotonicity is maintained in the distal tubule and collecting ducts because water permeability in these segments is low. During antidiuresis, when vasopressin levels are high, the collecting duct epithelium is highly permeable to water, and diffusion of water occurs from the collecting duct lumen into the hyperosmotic medulla. [pp 200–201]

40. **d. Free water clearance is increased by diuretic treatment.** To calculate the amount of water excreted or retained by the kidney, it is useful to consider that urine has two components, one that contains all of the solute in an isotonic solution (termed C_{Osm}, or osmolar clearance) and another that contains only solute-free water (termed C_{H2O}, or free water clearance). The total urine volume (e.g., liters per day) is the sum of C_{Osm} and C_{H2O}. Hyponatremia occurs when one or more of these requirements are not fulfilled, such as when GFR is impaired, when diuretics impair NaCl reabsorption, or when vasopressin is in excess (e.g., syndrome of inappropriate antidiuretic hormone). Urine that is hyperosmotic to plasma consists of an isoosmotic solution and also a volume of free water that was reabsorbed by the kidney to raise the urine osmolality. The term T^c_{H2O} refers to this volume of water removed from the urine. [p 203]

41. **e. High levels of vasopressin together with collecting ducts that are permeable to water.** To excrete dilute urine, vasopressin levels should be low and collecting ducts should be relatively impermeable to water. [p 203]

42. **a. Life-threatening, characterized by low serum Na^+ concentration and neurologic abnormalities.** Plasma consists of 93% water, and the remaining nonaqueous phase is composed primarily of proteins and lipids. The Na^+ concentration in the aqueous phase is normally about 151 mEq/L; however, the value reported by the clinical laboratory is lower (i.e., 140 mEq/L) because it is expressed as the ratio of Na^+ in total plasma volume. Pseudohyponatremia occurs when the proportion of the nonaqueous phase increases, such as in disorders associated with hyperlipidemia or hyperproteinemia, because the Na^+ concentration in the total plasma volume is decreased even though both the Na^+ concentration in plasma water and the total body osmolality are normal. [p 203]

43. **d. Syndrome of inappropriate antidiuretic hormone**

(SIADH) is the most common cause of hypovolemic hyponatremia.** Measurement of urinary Na^+ concentration can provide important diagnostic information about whether the fluid losses are renal or extrarenal in patients with hypovolemic hyponatremia. A urinary Na^+ concentration less than 20 mEq/L reflects a normal renal response to volume depletion and indicates that extrarenal fluid loss has occurred. In contrast, when urine Na^+ concentration is greater than 20 mEq/L in the patient with hypovolemic hyponatremia, volume loss by the kidney has occurred. Physical evidence of volume depletion includes postural changes in blood pressure and pulse, decreased jugular venous pressure, and dry mucous membranes. These findings, together with a relevant clinical history and physical examination, provide the basis for the hyponatremia. [pp 204–205]

44. **e. Low blood pressure because of volume depletion.** SIADH occurs most commonly with bronchogenic tumors and is found in 8% of patients with small cell carcinoma of the oat cell type. It is associated with volume expansion. [p 206]

45. **e. Both a and b.** Hypercalcemia causes impaired urine concentration. The mechanisms that contribute to this include decreased GFR with increased solute load per nephron, reduced medullary solute as a result of impaired NaCl reabsorption, decreased vasopressin sensitivity by the collecting duct caused by increased prostaglandin E_2 production, and attenuated vasopressin-sensitive adenylate cyclase activity. Hypokalemia also leads to a vasopressin-resistant concentrating defect. [p 208]

46. **c. High-protein feeding is associated with U_{Osm} less than 250 and diabetes insipidus.** In the polyuric patient, U_{Osm} below 250 mOsm/kg usually indicates water diuresis, and an evaluation for diabetes insipidus is needed. Conversely, U_{Osm} greater than 300 mOsm/kg most commonly reflects solute diuresis (e.g., high-protein feedings, glucose). [pp 209–210]

47. **a. bicarbonate.** The bicarbonate buffer is predominant in humans; in this system, bicarbonate (HCO_3^-) is the proton acceptor (base) and carbonic acid (H_2CO_3) is the proton donor (acid). One important feature of the bicarbonate system that makes it ideally suited as a body buffer is that the components of this system are regulated independently: the HCO_3^- concentration is maintained at 24 mmol/dl by the kidneys, and PCO_2 is fixed at 40 mm Hg by the lungs. The ability to regulate alveolar ventilation over a wide range enhances the buffering capacity of the bicarbonate system. [pp 210–211]

48. **b. Hydrogen ions are initially buffered intracellularly by proteins.** The initial response to an acid load is the distribution of hydrogen ions in the extracellular fluid, where these ions are buffered primarily by HCO_3^-. This process can buffer approximately 45% of the acid load and is completed within 30 minutes. However, extracellular buffering is insufficient, and additional buffering of approximately 50% of the acid load occurs intracellularly within a few hours. As the duration of the acid loading increases, the relative amount of intracellular to extracellular buffering can increase so that more than twice as much buffering occurs intracellularly. [p 211]

49. **e. In ketoacidosis, profound hyperkalemia is characteristic because intracellular buffering by sodium/proton exchange is maximized.** Intracellular buffering requires transcellular ion transport, including sodium/proton, potassium/proton, and chloride/bicarbonate exchanges. During an acute load with an inorganic acid, plasma potassium concentration increases by approximately 0.6 mEq/L for each 0.1 unit decrease in pH. In contrast, during organic acidosis (e.g., ketoacidosis), transcellular potassium shifts are minor because the proton is accompanied into the cell by the organic anion rather than in exchange for potassium. Therefore, hyperkalemia does not usually occur during organic acidosis despite reductions in pH, which are comparable to those in mineral acidosis. [p 211]

50. **d. A decrease in alveolar ventilation and an increase in PCO_2.** When the blood pH decreases (e.g., as in acidemia) during an acid load, chemoreceptors that control respiration are stimulated. During this compensatory process, which is fully operational within about 14 hours, alveolar ventilation increases and PCO_2 declines. [p 211]

51. **a. proximal convoluted tubule.** The bulk of the filtered HCO_3^- is reclaimed in the proximal nephron, with approximately 80% of the filtered HCO_3^- reabsorbed within the proximal convoluted tubule. [p 211]

52. **b. 80% of filtered HCO_3^- is reabsorbed in the medullary TAL.** Carbonic anhydrase minimizes the H^+ concentration in the tubule lumen, thereby providing a favorable gradient for H^+ secretion by the proximal tubule cell. Inhibition of carbonic anhydrase (e.g., by acetazolamide) reduces the H^+ secretion rate by approximately 80%. [p 212]

53. **e. Under normal circumstances, urinary pH cannot decrease below 7.0 despite buffering by ammonium and titratable acid.** Although very steep gradients for H^+ can be maintained in the medullary collecting duct, the urinary pH cannot decrease to below 4.5, which is equivalent to an $[H^+]$ of less than 0.1 mEq/L. Therefore, urine buffering by titratable acid and ammonium is required. [p 212]

54. **c. Filtered phosphates are ideal urinary buffers because 80% are present in dibasic form (HPO_4^{2-}) with a pK_a of 7.4.** The term *titratable acidity* refers to the quantity of NaOH required to titrate urine back to a pH of 7.40, which is similar to that of blood. Other buffers, such as uric acid (pK_a, 5.75) and creatinine (pK_a, 4.97) contribute to the titratable acidity, but only to a minor extent. Filtered phosphates are ideal urinary buffers for two reasons: (1) 80% is present in dibasic form (HPO_4^{2-}) with a pK_a of 6.8, and (2) the rate of phosphate excretion is approximately 40 to 60 mmol/day, leading to the excretion of about 30 to 40 mEq/L of titratable acid daily. Titratable acid excretion increases two- to threefold during metabolic acidosis. [p 212]

55. **e. Renal NH_4^+ production is stimulated during acute and chronic respiratory acidosis, but not by metabolic acidosis.** The urinary excretion of NH_4^+ is a complex process. In the proximal tubule, NH_4^+ is secreted into the lumen by replacing H^+ on the Na^+-H^+ exchanger. After entering the medullary TAL of Henle, 50% to 80% of the NH_4^+ present in the lumen is reabsorbed by replacing K^+ on the Na^+-K^+-$2Cl^-$ cotransporter. This accounts for the "single effect" of the countercurrent mechanism, whereby very large amounts of NH_3 accumulate in the medulla. NH_3 then diffuses into the cortical collecting duct. The low pH of urine in the cortical collecting duct, together with the high pK_a (9.3) of NH_3, leads to the formation of NH_4^+ and its accumulation in the tubule lumen. [p 212]

56. **e. Hydroxymethylglutaryl coenzyme A reductase activity.** Factors affecting acid excretion include luminal HCO_3^- concentration; extracellular volume and body contents of K^+ and Cl^-; peritubular HCO_3^-, PCO_2, and pH; aldosterone; angiotensin II; PTH; neural and adrenergic effects; and atrial natriuretic peptide. Net acid excretion = titratable acidity + urinary NH_4^+-urinary HCO_3^-. [pp 212–213]

57. **e. This process occurs very slowly, compared with the renal response to an acid load.** When confronted with an alkaline load, the strategies used by the body to eliminate the excess base include distribution and buffering in the extracellular and intracellular compartments and respiratory and renal responses. As with an acid load, a bicarbonate load is distributed throughout the extracellular compartment within 30 minutes. However, a greater proportion of the base load remains in the extracellular fluid; only about 30% is buffered in the intracellular compartment. When a bicarbonate load is buffered, additional CO_2 is produced and alveolar ventilation increases. This is often followed by hypoventilation, during which PCO_2 increases, thereby compensating for the persistently elevated bicarbonate concentration. This respiratory response occurs over several hours. Renal excretion of the excess base is necessary for restoring base stores to normal. This process occurs rapidly in comparison with the renal response to an acid load. [pp 211, 213]

58. **b. ammonium.** Essential information provided by the clinical laboratory includes blood levels of bicarbonate, potassium, and chloride in addition to the arterial blood PCO_2, pH, and oxygen partial pressure (PO_2). [p 214]

59. **e. Both a and b.** Anion gap = $C' = Na^+ - (Cl^- + HCO_3^-)$. In an anion gap acidosis, the anion gap increases when non-Cl^-–containing acids (e.g., lactic acid) are added to the blood. In this case, HCO_3^- is buffered and the unmeasured anion is retained to maintain electroneutrality. The plasma Cl^- concentration is unchanged so that the anion gap is increased. This type of acidosis is often acute and severe, with rapid generation of large amounts of acid. [p 215]

60. **e. It occurs during generation of excess lactic acid.** In this type of acidosis, extracellular HCO_3^- is consumed and replaced by an equivalent amount of Cl^-; thus, the anion gap remains within the normal range. It occurs in the following settings (see Table 6–16): (1) excess HCO_3^- is lost from the gastrointestinal tract (e.g., as in diarrhea) or kidney (e.g., as in renal tubular acidosis), (2) HCO_3^- is diluted during saline infusion, and (3) there is an exogenous acid load. In contrast to the non-anion gap acidosis, cases of hyperchloremic acidosis are often less severe and tend to be more chronic processes. [p 216]

61. **e. It is markedly positive during gastrointestinal losses of HCO_3^- when the NH_4^+ excretion rate can exceed 200 mEq/day.** The NH_4^+ excretion rate can be estimated by the urinary anion gap, under the assumptions that the major urinary cations are NH_4^+, Na^+, and K^+ and that Cl^- is the predominant anion. The anion gap is defined as $Na^+ + K^+ - Cl^- = NH_4^+$, so if $[Cl^-] > [Na^+] + [K^+]$, then $[NH_4^+]$ is high, and if $[Cl^-] < [Na^+] + [K^+]$, then $[NH_4^+]$ is low or NH_4^+ excretion is with anions other than Cl^-. The urinary anion gap value is (1) normally approximately zero because other unmeasured electrolytes are present, (2) markedly negative during gastrointestinal losses of HCO_3^- when the NH_4^+ excretion rate can exceed 200 mEq/day, and (3) inappropriately near zero in the renal tubular acidoses. [p 216]

62. **d. Low plasma renin activity level.** Approximately 80% of filtered HCO_3^- is reabsorbed in the proximal convoluted tubule. In proximal renal tubular acidosis, this process is impaired, and the augmented delivery of HCO_3^- to more distal nephron segments exceeds their capacity to reabsorb the HCO_3^- load. This leads to increased fractional excretion of HCO_3^- (about 10% to 30%), bicarbonaturia with a reduction in net acid excretion, and extracellular fluid contraction (see Fig. 6–39). Stimulation of the renin-angiotensin-aldosterone system promotes NaCl reabsorption and hyperchloremic metabolic acidosis. Ultimately, a new steady state is reached in which serum HCO_3^- is decreased and hence the filtered load, distal delivery, and urinary excretion of HCO_3^- are all reduced. [p 216]

63. **e. In distal renal tubular acidosis, the acidosis is self-limited and is usually mild.** In distal renal tubular acidosis, the ability of the collecting duct to secrete H^+ against this gradient is impaired and urine pH cannot be reduced below 5.3 despite the low blood pH. Net acid excretion is reduced because this defect in H^+ secretion impairs excretion of titratable acids and ammonia even though ammonia production is normal. The buffering capacity of ammonia is decreased at the higher urinary pH. In addition, the relatively small fraction of filtered HCO_3^- that is delivered to the distal nephron is not reabsorbed. As a consequence, metabolic acidosis develops because the kidney is unable to excrete the entire daily load of acid generated by the diet (50 to 100 mEq/day) and additional acid is retained daily. In distal renal tubular acidosis, the acidosis is progressive and may be severe because the urine cannot be maximally acidified. Other features of distal renal tubular acidosis include abnormal calcium metabolism with hypercalciuria, nephrocalcinosis, and nephrolithiasis. [p 217]

64. **e. Inhibition of the renin-angiotensin-aldosterone system.** Factors that generate metabolic alkalosis include excess acid loss, both nonrenal (gastric fluid loss; intestinal acid loss; translocation of acid into cells, as in potassium deficiency) and renal (persistent mineralocorticoid activity with potassium deficiency and distal delivery of sodium); excess HCO_3^- gain (ingestion or infusion of HCO_3^-; metabolism of lactate, ketones, or other organic ions to HCO_3^-); and contraction alkalosis. [p 218]

65. **e. Hypoaldosteronism.** Metabolic alkalosis is maintained by factors that impair renal HCO_3^- excretion. These factors include reduced effective circulating volume and potassium depletion. [p 218]

Chapter 7

Renovascular Hypertension and Ischemic Nephropathy

Andrew C. Novick • Amr Fergany

Questions

1. The rate-limiting step in the renin-angiotensin-aldosterone cascade is:
   a. secretion of angiotensinogen by the liver.
   b. conversion of angiotensinogen to angiotensin I.
   c. conversion of angiotensin I to angiotensin II.
   d. secretion of aldosterone from the adrenal cortex.
   e. secretion of adrenocorticotropic hormone from the anterior pituitary.

2. The major site of synthesis of systemic renin is the:
   a. liver.
   b. lung.
   c. brain.
   d. kidney.
   e. adrenal gland.

3. Renin secretion is mediated by all the following except:
   a. decreased potassium delivery to the distal tubule.
   b. decreased chloride delivery to the distal tubule.
   c. diminished stretch of the afferent arteriole.
   d. β-adrenergic stimulation of the kidney.
   e. exogenous prostaglandins.

4. Angiotensin-converting enzyme (ACE):
   a. is a specific enzyme that converts angiotensin I to angiotensin II.
   b. is a nonspecific enzyme that has several functions in vivo.
   c. forms angiotensin I from angiotensinogen.
   d. is the only enzyme in the formation of angiotensin II that cannot be pharmacologically modulated.
   e. is the major enzyme for degradation of angiotensin II.

5. Angiotensin II stimulates all the following actions except:
   a. cardiac muscle hypertrophy.
   b. thirst.
   c. vasoconstriction.
   d. secretion of aldosterone.
   e. secretion of epinephrine.

6. Under conditions of decreased renal perfusion, angiotensin II regulates glomerular filtration through:
   a. afferent arteriolar vasodilatation.
   b. afferent arteriolar vasoconstriction.
   c. efferent arteriolar vasodilatation.
   d. efferent arteriolar vasoconstriction.
   e. main renal artery vasoconstriction.

7. Experimental models of renovascular hypertension are characterized by:
   a. close resemblance to human clinical renovascular hypertension.
   b. the early volume-dependent phase of hypertension.
   c. the late renin-dependent phase of hypertension.
   d. constant sensitivity to ACE inhibition.
   e. dynamic change through different pathophysiologic phases.

8. Atheroembolism (cholesterol embolism):
   a. frequently contributes to renal function deterioration in patients with atherosclerotic renal artery stenosis.
   b. occurs mainly in younger patients with fibromuscular renal artery stenosis.
   c. is usually managed by exploration and immediate surgical repair.
   d. is usually managed by percutaneous transluminal angioplasty.
   e. is a benign phenomenon, usually limited to the lower extremities, that rarely involves the kidney.

9. The presence of anatomic renal artery stenosis:
   a. confirms the diagnosis of renovascular hypertension.
   b. predicts cure of hypertension after correction of the stenosis.
   c. predicts improvement of renal function, especially in unilateral cases.
   d. is not clinically significant if stenosis is less than 70%.
   e. is always a clinically significant finding.

10. The diagnosis of renal artery stenosis:
    a. is usually confirmed through laboratory testing.
    b. is based on wide-scale radiologic screening of asymptomatic patients.
    c. is based on radiologic confirmation of clinically suspicious cases.
    d. is generally not pursued in azotemic patients.
    e. can be confirmed by clinical examination alone.

11. Definitive diagnosis of renal artery stenosis is currently provided through:
    a. duplex ultrasonography.
    b. rapid-sequence intravenous urography.
    c. intraoperative digital subtraction angiography.
    d. magnetic resonance angiography.
    e. intra-arterial angiography.

12. Duplex ultrasonography:
    a. provides accurate three-dimensional imaging of renal arterial lesions.
    b. estimates renal artery stenosis through measurement of blood flow velocity.
    c. is a dependable technique for diagnosing branch renal artery disease.
    d. loses its diagnostic utility in patients with compromised renal function.
    e. can provide all the necessary information for treatment of patients with ischemic nephropathy.

13. Carbon dioxide digital subtraction angiography:
    a. is an invasive diagnostic modality that is especially useful in patients with renal insufficiency.
    b. is a noninvasive diagnostic technique that minimizes the risk associated with iodinated contrast angiography.
    c. is associated with a higher incidence of arterial wall trauma than is standard angiography.
    d. cannot be used if angioplasty is contemplated.
    e. is associated with a high incidence of allergic complications and gas embolism.

14. Medical management for patients with renal artery stenosis:
    a. rarely succeeds in controlling hypertension.
    b. presents the best chance for maintaining renal function.
    c. is appropriate therapy for young patients with ischemic nephropathy.
    d. is generally preferred for children.
    e. is appropriate therapy for older patients with mild hypertension.

15. Nephrectomy as a treatment option for renal artery stenosis:
    a. is indicated for hypertension caused by a unilateral, small, poorly functioning kidney.
    b. is indicated for bilateral renal artery stenosis provided that total renal function is normal.
    c. is usually indicated in cases of ischemic nephropathy rather than renovascular hypertension.
    d. should be performed only by using an open surgical technique as opposed to laparoscopy.
    e. rarely provides long-term therapeutic benefit even in properly selected cases.

16. Revascularization of ischemic kidneys:
    a. should be performed only in patients with ischemic nephropathy.
    b. should be performed only in patients with renovascular hypertension.
    c. provides inferior long-term therapeutic benefit compared with medical therapy.
    d. leads to stabilization, but not improvement, of renal function.
    e. may be performed surgically or percutaneously.

17. Percutaneous transluminal angioplasty of the renal arteries:
    a. can be performed under ultrasonographic guidance.
    b. is currently performed by using coaxial dilators placed through the femoral artery.
    c. currently employs a dilatation balloon passed through the femoral or axillary artery.
    d. is useful only for cases of atherosclerotic renal artery disease.
    e. is the preferred modality for treating branch renal artery disease.

18. The best therapeutic results after percutaneous angioplasty can be expected with the following arterial lesions:
    a. renal artery aneurysm.
    b. ostial renal artery atherosclerotic stenosis.
    c. branch renal artery atherosclerotic stenosis.
    d. main renal artery fibrous stenosis.
    e. branch renal artery fibrous stenosis.

19. Complications of percutaneous angioplasty:
    a. should never be managed surgically.
    b. include contrast allergy as well as femoral and renal artery trauma.
    c. occur in 30% to 50% of cases.
    d. are not related to operator experience.
    e. should always be managed by immediate surgery.

20. Technical success for percutaneous angioplasty in cases of fibrous dysplasia can be expected to be:
    a. less than 50%.
    b. 50% to 60%.
    c. 65% to 75%.
    d. 75% to 85%.
    e. 90% or more.

21. Results of percutaneous angioplasty in cases of atherosclerotic renal artery stenosis are worse than in cases of fibrous disease because:
    a. atherosclerotic plaque is more difficult to dilate using angiographic balloons.
    b. atherosclerotic lesions are tighter and do not allow passage of the guide wire.
    c. the presence of femoral artery atherosclerosis usually prevents arterial access.
    d. renal artery atherosclerotic lesions are usually ostial and part of aortic wall plaque.
    e. renal artery atherosclerosis usually involves arterial branches and responds poorly to dilatation.

22. The use of endovascular stents as treatment for renal artery stenosis:
    a. has increased the rate of emergency surgery because of complications of angioplasty.
    b. has increased the rate of immediate postangioplasty success.
    c. is reserved mainly for cases of fibrous renal artery stenosis.
    d. is the preferred technique for angioplasty in children.
    e. necessitates arterial access through the axillary artery.

23. Continued deterioration of renal function after renal artery stent placement may be due to all of the following except:
    a. acute thrombosis of the renal artery.
    b. cholesterol embolism.
    c. use of a slightly larger stent than the renal artery diameter.
    d. restenosis of the renal artery.
    e. progressive glomerulosclerosis.

24. Which of the following statements regarding atherosclerotic renal artery disease is incorrect?
    a. It is the most common type of renal artery disease.
    b. It is more common in men than in women.
    c. It is usually not associated with manifestations of generalized atherosclerosis.
    d. It is more commonly observed in patients older than 50 years of age.
    e. It usually involves the proximal 2 cm of the main renal artery.

25. The most useful clinical marker or markers of progressive atherosclerotic renal artery obstruction are:
    a. poorly controlled hypertension.
    b. poorly controlled hypertension and a decrease in kidney size.
    c. poorly controlled hypertension and an increase in the serum creatinine level.
    d. a decrease in kidney size and an increase in the serum creatinine level.
    e. all of the above.

26. All of the following represent clinical clues to the presence of atherosclerotic renal artery disease except:

a. evidence of generalized atherosclerosis.
b. patient age younger than 50 years.
c. unilateral small kidney.
d. mild azotemia.
e. severe hypertension.

27. The most common cause of unilateral renal atrophy in patients older than 50 years of age is:

    a. congenital hypoplasia.
    b. chronic pyelonephritis.
    c. atherosclerotic renal artery disease.
    d. fibrous renal artery disease.
    e. chronic glomerulonephritis.

28. Clinical clues suggesting renal salvageability with complete arterial occlusion include all of the following except:

    a. kidney size greater than 9 cm.
    b. angiographic evidence of collateral vascular supply.
    c. nondiseased glomeruli as seen on a renal biopsy specimen.
    d. function of the involved kidney as revealed by isotope renography.
    e. absence of contralateral compensatory renal hypertrophy.

29. The percentage of end-stage renal disease cases that are currently thought to be caused by ischemic nephropathy is:

    a. 0% to 5%.
    b. 6% to 10%.
    c. 15% to 20%.
    d. 50% to 60%.
    e. 80% to 90%.

30. The natural history of renal artery atherosclerosis is best characterized as being:

    a. unpredictable and varying in each case.
    b. gradually improving.
    c. progressive and unremitting.
    d. not a threat to renal function.
    e. associated with remissions and exacerbation.

31. The usual cause of renal artery stenosis causing ischemic nephropathy is:

    a. atherosclerosis of the renal arteries.
    b. bilateral renal artery aneurysms.
    c. fibroplasia of the renal arteries.
    d. inflammatory vasculitis of the intrarenal arteries.
    e. abdominal or thoracic aortic aneurysm.

32. The class of antihypertensive drugs having a specific deleterious effect on renal function in cases of renal artery stenosis is:

    a. vasodilators.
    b. calcium channel blockers.
    c. ACE inhibitors.
    d. β blockers.
    e. ganglion blockers.

33. Which of the following investigations is best suited as an initial screening test for renal artery stenosis in a 65-year-old woman with generalized atherosclerosis, diabetes mellitus, and a serum creatinine value of 2.5 mg/dl?

    a. CT angiography
    b. Intra-arterial digital subtraction angiography
    c. Captopril test
    d. Duplex ultrasonography of the renal arteries
    e. Determination of differential renal vein renin

34. Which of the following best describes the outcome of patients with ischemic nephropathy who undergo dialysis?

    a. They have the poorest survival of all patients.
    b. They have the best survival of all patients.
    c. Infection is a major cause of mortality.
    d. Long-term survival is a realistic goal.
    e. Complications with vascular access make peritoneal dialysis attractive.

35. Patients with end-stage renal failure from ischemic nephropathy:

    a. are always beyond the point of regaining renal function with revascularization.
    b. are the best candidates for revascularization.
    c. may be suitable candidates for revascularization if renal salvage criteria are met.
    d. tolerate permanent dialysis exceptionally well.
    e. should undergo only angioplasty for revascularization.

36. Which of the following is the most common type of renal arterial aneurysm?

    a. Fusiform
    b. Saccular
    c. Dissecting
    d. Post-traumatic
    e. Intrarenal

37. Factors that predispose to rupture of a renal arterial aneurysm include all of the following except:

    a. noncalcification.
    b. aneurysmal size greater than 2.0 cm.
    c. hematuria.
    d. hypertension.
    e. pregnancy.

38. Arteriovenous fistulas resulting from needle biopsy of the kidney:

    a. generally heal spontaneously within 2 weeks.
    b. are not amenable to transcatheter angiographic occlusion.
    c. usually require total or partial nephrectomy for treatment.
    d. generally heal spontaneously within 18 months.
    e. are an uncommon cause of acquired renal arteriovenous fistulas.

39. In which of the following clinical settings is surgical excision of a renal arterial aneurysm clearly NOT indicated?

    a. Dissecting aneurysm
    b. Calcified aneurysm 1.5 cm in diameter
    c. Aneurysm causing hypertension
    d. Noncalcified aneurysm 3.0 cm in diameter
    e. Aneurysm increasing in size on sequential angiograms

40. Renal arterial aneurysms may cause hypertension through all of the following mechanisms except:

    a. extrinsic compression of renal arterial branches.
    b. turbulent blood flow within an aneurysm.
    c. associated arteriolar nephrosclerosis.
    d. associated renal artery stenosis.
    e. peripheral renal embolism.

41. The most common cause of an acquired renal arteriovenous fistula is:

    a. blunt renal trauma.
    b. renal carcinoma.
    c. renal surgery.
    d. penetrating renal trauma.
    e. closed renal biopsy.

42. The most common method of surgical treatment of symptomatic congenital arteriovenous fistulas has been:

a. aortorenal bypass with saphenous vein.
b. total or partial nephrectomy.
c. bench surgery and autotransplantation.
d. individual ligation of interconnecting arteriovenous vessels.
e. aortorenal bypass with hypogastric artery.

43. The most appropriate method of management for a patient with unilateral renal arterial embolism secondary to a myocardial ventricular aneurysm is:

a. systemic anticoagulation.
b. observation.
c. aortorenal bypass.
d. surgical renal arterial embolectomy.
e. segmental renal arterial resection and reanastomosis.

44. Which of the following statements regarding acute renal arterial thrombosis is NOT correct?

a. It commonly occurs in the proximal two thirds of the main renal artery.
b. It may be due to trauma.
c. It more commonly involves the right renal artery.
d. It may be due to atherosclerosis.
e. It may be managed with percutaneous intra-arterial infusion of streptokinase.

Answers

1. **b. conversion of angiotensinogen to angiotensin I.** The basic cascade of the renin-angiotensin-aldosterone system (RAAS) involves conversion of angiotensinogen to angiotensin I through the action of renin. This is the rate-limiting step for the entire system, and, accordingly, control of renin release regulates the activity of the whole system. [p 235]

2. **d. kidney.** Renin is a single polypeptide chain aspartyl protease that is secreted from the juxtaglomerular cells of the afferent arteriole. The kidney is the major site of renin production, although renin mRNA is found in several other tissues where the local renin-angiotensin system functions. [p 235]

3. **a. decreased potassium delivery to the distal tubule.** Reduction of distal tubule salt delivery stimulates renin secretion and vice versa. Although sodium was initially thought to be responsible for this action, it now appears that the signal for macula densa–controlled renin release is the alteration of tubular chloride concentration. [p 235]

4. **b. is a nonspecific enzyme that has several functions in vivo.** ACE is expressed in several tissues where the local RAAS functions. Renal ACE is localized to the glomerular endothelial cells and the proximal tubule brush border, where it might play a role in cleaving filtered protein for reabsorption. Within the central nervous system (CNS), ACE is found in several locations, where it functions in the local RAAS. This local CNS RAAS is thought to have dipsogenic and hypertensive effects as well as to stimulate vasopressin secretion. Adrenal ACE is found predominantly in the medulla, where it is thought to stimulate catecholamine secretion. ACE is found abundantly in the testes and prostate, in the Leydig cells, and in cytoplasmic droplets in sperm. In the female reproductive tract, ACE is found in follicular and fallopian tube oocytes. The precise role of ACE in the reproductive system has not been elucidated. [p 236]

5. **e. secretion of epinephrine.** Angiotensin II acts directly on the adrenal glomerulosa cells to stimulate aldosterone secretion, which is accomplished through increased desmolase activity and increased conversion of corticosterone to aldosterone. This serves to augment the salt reabsorptive actions of angiotensin II to conserve sodium. Vasoconstriction and release of aldosterone occur immediately and are of short duration, supporting the role of angiotensin II in maintaining tissue perfusion in hypovolemia. Other actions such as vascular growth and ventricular hypertrophy are slower in onset and longer in duration, lasting for several days or weeks. [pp 236–237]

6. **d. efferent arteriolar vasoconstriction.** One of the most important actions of angiotensin II is the autoregulation of glomerular filtration rate (GFR) in response to changes in renal perfusion. This action is effected through changes in vascular resistance as well as mesangial cell tone. Angiotensin II causes a marked increase in efferent arteriolar resistance in cases of renal hypoperfusion but does not affect afferent arteriolar resistance unless there is an increase in renal perfusion pressure. The result of this disproportionate increase in efferent over afferent resistance is an increase in capillary hydraulic pressure, and subsequently in filtration pressure, maintaining GFR in the face of decreased renal perfusion. [p 236]

7. **e. dynamic change through different pathophysiologic phases.** Renovascular hypertension has been demonstrated in two models of experimental Goldblatt hypertension: the two-kidney, one-clip model (2K,1C), in which one renal artery is clipped and the contralateral kidney is in place and normal; and the one-kidney, one-clip model (1K,1C), in which one renal artery is clipped and the contralateral kidney is removed. Both models do not remain static but rather pass through an acute phase, a transition phase, and then a final chronic phase. In cases of 2K,1C hypertension, a chronic phase is eventually reached after several days or weeks when unclipping of the stenotic kidney fails to normalize blood pressure. In this chronic phase, the elevated perfusion pressure as well as high levels of angiotensin II have resulted in widespread arteriolar damage to the contralateral kidney. Excretory function (natriuresis) of the contralateral kidney declines, resulting in extracellular volume expansion, decrease of circulating angiotensin II levels, and gradual development of a "volume-dependent" type of hypertension. [p 238]

8. **a. frequently contributes to deterioration of renal function in patients with atherosclerotic renal artery stenosis.** The organs most commonly affected by atheroembolism are the kidney, spleen, pancreas, and gastrointestinal tract. Renal effects take the form of deteriorating renal function, usually after a precipitating event. The decline in renal function can vary in severity from slowly progressive to rapid acute renal failure. Gradual improvement of renal function occurs after the event, but recurrent episodes lead to progressive loss of renal function with time. [p 240]

9. **d. is not clinically significant if stenosis is less than 70%.** For ischemic injury to occur, the reduction in renal blood flow needs to exceed the compensatory ability of the kidneys. Renal autoregulation fails to maintain the GFR when renal perfusion decreases below 70 to 80 mm Hg. This occurs when the luminal diameter of the renal artery is ste-

nosed by more than 70% of the original size. At this point, the stenosis becomes hemodynamically significant, resulting in a gradual deterioration of the GFR with an accompanying rise in serum creatinine level. [p 239]

10. **c. is based on radiologic confirmation of clinically suspicious cases.** The clinical clues serve in the selection of patients who should be studied for the possible presence of renal artery stenosis. For patients with suspected renovascular hypertension, a number of tests are available for functional diagnosis of renovascular hypertension. These tests (plasma renin activity, captopril test, captopril renography, and renal vein renin assays) diagnose hyperactivity of the RAAS but provide no anatomic information regarding the offending arterial lesion. Anatomic delineation of the arterial lesion guides the treatment decisions and is obtained by intra-arterial angiography, which remains the most definitive study and the "gold standard" against which other diagnostic techniques are compared. [pp 242–243]

11. **e. intra-arterial angiography.** Intra-arterial angiography remains the gold standard for diagnosing renal artery disease, and it is the test against which other tests are compared. However, angiography is not suitable for use as a preliminary screening tool for all patients suspected of having renal artery stenosis. [p 246]

12. **b. estimates renal artery stenosis through measurement of blood flow velocity.** Duplex ultrasonography of the renal arteries is a noninvasive anatomic study that has shown excellent ability for diagnosis of renal artery stenosis. It combines the use of real-time B-mode renal ultrasonography with color-coded pulsed Doppler imaging to obtain blood flow velocities within the major abdominal vessels. The basis for diagnosing renal artery stenosis is the altered flow pattern distal to the stenosis, with a turbulent jet during systole and a decrease in diastolic flow. [p 244]

13. **a. is an invasive diagnostic modality that is especially useful in patients with renal insufficiency.** Carbon dioxide has been introduced as a contrast agent for intra-arterial injection in an effort to reduce contrast nephrotoxicity from iodinated contrast material. Carbon dioxide has no effect on renal function, making it an ideal agent for use in patients with renal insufficiency. [p 247]

14. **e. is appropriate therapy for older patients with mild hypertension.** In patients with atherosclerotic renal vascular hypertension, more vigorous attempts at medical management are warranted, because these patients are older and often have extrarenal vascular disease. Therefore, multiple-drug regimens that control blood pressure are often the preferred approach. [p 248]

15. **a. is indicated for hypertension caused by a unilateral, small, poorly functioning kidney.** Advances in both surgical renal vascular reconstruction and medical antihypertensive therapy have limited the role of total or partial nephrectomy in the management of patients with renal artery disease. These operations are only occasionally indicated in patients with severe arteriolar nephrosclerosis, severe renal atrophy, noncorrectable renal vascular lesions, and renal infarction. [p 252]

16. **e. may be performed surgically or percutaneously.** Intervention with surgery or endovascular therapy is best reserved for patients whose hypertension cannot be adequately controlled or when renal function is threatened by advanced vascular disease. [p 248]

17. **c. currently employs a dilatation balloon passed through the femoral or axillary artery.** The original Gruntzig coaxial technique utilizes an 8 or 9 Fr renal guiding catheter through which a 4.3 or 4.5 Fr balloon catheter is passed over a guide wire traversing the stenotic segment through a femoral arterial puncture. Modification of the original technique and balloon catheters have allowed the use of a 5 Fr femoral artery puncture through which a 5 Fr diagnostic catheter is passed to the renal artery using the Seldinger technique. An axillary approach may be used to perform renal percutaneous transluminal angioplasty when the renal arteries originate at an acute angle from the abdominal aorta as well as in cases with severe pelvic atherosclerosis, occlusion, or the presence of bypass grafts in the pelvic or abdominal areas. [p 255]

18. **d. main renal artery fibrous stenosis.** The results of angioplasty for fibrous dysplasia of the main renal artery have been excellent and equal to those obtained with surgical revascularization; therefore, angioplasty is the initial treatment of choice in such cases. [p 248]

19. **b. include contrast allergy as well as femoral and renal artery trauma.** The complications of percutaneous transluminal angioplasty include those of standard angiography (complications related to arterial puncture and to the use of iodinated contrast material), as well as specific complications related to manipulation of the renal arteries. Transient deterioration of renal function is the most frequent complication and is related to the contrast load delivered during the procedure. Technical mishaps during percutaneous transluminal angioplasty may lead to an intimal dissection or even thrombosis of the renal artery. [p 255]

20. **e. 90% or more.** Percutaneous transluminal angioplasty is usually performed in cases of fibrous dysplasia without stent placement and has become the primary modality of treatment for these lesions. With the use of modern equipment and increasing experience with the technique, technical success has been more than 90%. A beneficial blood pressure response—that is, cure of hypertension or improvement in blood pressure control—can be expected in more than 80% and up to 100% of cases. [p 256]

21. **d. renal artery atherosclerotic lesions are usually ostial and part of aortic wall plaque.** Renal artery stenosis in cases of arteriosclerosis obliterans is usually bilateral and ostial or very proximal in the main renal artery. In most ostial cases, this represents encroachment of the atherosclerotic plaque in the abdominal aorta upon the origin of the renal artery rather than primary renal artery disease. The patients affected by atherosclerotic renal artery stenosis are also different from patients with fibrous dysplasia of the renal arteries in that they are generally older and have a number of comorbid medical conditions as well as generalized atherosclerosis affecting the coronary and carotid arteries or the peripheral vascular tree. Associated essential hypertension and nephrosclerosis are usually present. All of the previously mentioned factors, as well as the propensity for atheroembolism in patients with generalized arteriosclerosis obliterans, make percutaneous transluminal angioplasty in cases of arteriosclerosis obliterans renal artery stenosis less successful and associated with higher morbidity (and some mortality) than in cases of fibrous dysplasia. [p 257]

22. **b. has increased the rate of immediate postangioplasty success.** In the only prospective study comparing percutaneous transluminal angioplasty alone versus the procedure with stenting in ostial atherosclerosis, 85 patients were randomized to receive either treatment. Technical success was higher in the group receiving stents (88% versus 57%), and patency at 6 months was 75% for patients in the group receiving stents versus 29% for the patients undergoing the procedure alone. In patients with successful primary proce-

dures, restenosis occurred in 14% of the patients with stents and in 48% of patients undergoing percutaneous transluminal angioplasty alone. Stenting for immediate or late failure of the procedure was required in 12 (of 42) patients in the group undergoing percutaneous transluminal angioplasty alone. This study reflects the overall higher success of percutaneous transluminal angioplasty with stenting in treating ostial atherosclerosis when compared with the procedure alone and probably also justifies the increasing trend to perform primary stenting in these cases to avoid exposing patients to a secondary procedure. [p 261]

23. **c. use of a slightly larger stent than the renal artery diameter.** Complications of percutaneous transluminal angioplasty with stenting were not found to be significantly different from those of percutaneous transluminal angioplasty alone in a prospective study comparing both procedures. Specifically, rates in both groups for bleeding-related complications were 19% and for cholesterol embolism were 10%; the rate for access site pseudoaneurysm and renal artery injury was slightly higher with stent placement (7% versus 5%). Transient deterioration of renal function secondary to contrast nephrotoxicity was noted in 24% of patients undergoing the procedure alone and in 21% of patients undergoing the procedure with stent placement. [p 261]

24. **c. It is usually not associated with manifestations of generalized atherosclerosis.** Recent epidemiologic studies indicate that atherosclerotic renal artery disease is quite common in patients with generalized atherosclerosis obliterans, regardless of whether renovascular hypertension is present. [p 241]

25. **d. a decrease in kidney size and an increase in the serum creatinine level.** Clinical follow-up of patients in our study also revealed that significantly more patients with progressive disease developed deterioration of overall renal function (a decrease in kidney size or an increase in the serum creatinine level) compared with patients with stable disease. Interestingly, serial blood pressure control was equivalent in these two groups, indicating that it is not a useful clinical marker for progressive atherosclerotic renal artery stenosis. [p 232]

26. **b. patient age younger than 50 years.** Studies indicate that clinical screening for atherosclerotic renal artery disease is appropriate in older patients with most or all of the following features: (1) evidence of generalized atherosclerosis; (2) a decrease in the size of one or both kidneys; (3) renal insufficiency, even of a mild extent, particularly in patients with no obvious underlying cause; (4) the development of progressive azotemia after restoration of normotension with medical antihypertensive therapy; (5) coronary artery disease; (6) a history of congestive heart failure; and (7) peripheral vascular disease. [p 242]

27. **c. atherosclerotic renal artery disease.** The screening of patients for atherosclerotic renal artery disease is based in part on an early (1965) study by Gifford and colleagues. These investigators found that in 53 of 75 older patients (71%) with unilateral renal atrophy, the renal atrophy was caused by stenosing atherosclerotic renal artery disease. Of equal importance was the finding that 22 of these 53 patients (42%) also had unsuspected atherosclerotic renal artery disease involving the opposite normal-sized kidney. Subsequently, Lawrie and colleagues reviewed 40 patients with renal atrophy caused by total arterial occlusion and noted contralateral atherosclerotic renal artery stenosis in 31 patients (78%). These observations underscore the high incidence of renal artery disease, often bilateral, in patients with generalized atherosclerosis and diminished renal size. [p 242]

28. **e. absence of contralateral compensatory renal hypertro-** phy. Complete occlusion of the renal artery most often ends in irreversible ischemic damage of the involved kidney. In some patients with gradual arterial occlusion, however, the viability of the kidney can be maintained through the development of collateral arterial supply. Helpful clinical clues suggesting renal salvageability in such cases include the following: (1) angiographic demonstration of retrograde filling of the distal renal arterial tree, by collateral vessels on the side of the total arterial occlusion; (2) a renal biopsy showing well-preserved glomeruli; (3) kidney size greater than 9 cm; and (4) function of the involved kidney as revealed by isotope renography or intravenous pyelography. When such criteria are present, restoration of normal renal arterial flow can lead to recovery of renal function. [p 249]

29. **b. 6% to 10%.** The exact incidence of end-stage renal disease caused by atherosclerotic renal artery disease in the United States is not known. In a report from England, Scoble and colleagues prospectively performed renal arteriography in all new patients with end-stage renal disease during an 18-month period. Atherosclerotic renal artery disease was the cause of end-stage renal disease in 6% of all patients and in 14% of patients older than 50 years of age. Approximately 300,000 patients in the United States are currently being maintained by chronic dialysis. Their median age is greater than 60 years, and a majority of patients have evidence of generalized atherosclerosis obliterans. Although the exact number of patients with end-stage renal disease caused by atherosclerotic renal artery disease is not known, these data suggest that there are several thousand patients in this category. [p 232]

30. **c. progressive and unremitting.** Natural history data clearly show that atherosclerotic renal artery disease progresses in many patients and that loss of functioning renal parenchyma is a common sequela of such progression. [p 232]

31. **a. atherosclerosis of the renal arteries.** Following angiographic diagnosis of atherosclerotic renal artery stenosis, and with knowledge of the natural history of this disease, one can identify those patients in whom such disease poses a significant threat to overall renal function. This designation applies to patients with high-grade (>75%) arterial stenosis affecting their entire renal mass, namely, when such stenosis is present bilaterally or involves a solitary kidney. [p 248]

32. **c. ACE inhibitors.** Another important clinical clue to the presence of significant atherosclerotic renal artery stenosis is the development of progressive azotemia after medical control of blood pressure in patients with significant hypertension. ACE inhibitor agents can lead to deterioration of renal function through loss of efferent arteriolar vasoconstrictor tone in the kidney. [p 242]

33. **d. Duplex ultrasonography of the renal arteries.** Duplex ultrasonography offers significant advantages as a diagnostic tool for renal artery stenosis. It is noninvasive, uses portable equipment that is relatively inexpensive and widely available, does not utilize iodinated contrast material, and has no effect on renal function. Azotemia does not affect the results of the study, and no discontinuation of antihypertensive medications is required. [p 245]

34. **a. They have the poorest survival of all patients.** Patients with renal vascular disease as the cause of end-stage renal disease had the poorest survival of all patients who have had dialysis, with a 27-month median survival time and a 12% 5-year survival rate. [p 232]

35. **c. may be suitable candidates for revascularization if renal salvage criteria are met.** Occasional patients with end-stage renal disease from ischemic nephropathy have been en-

countered in whom renal function has been salvageable with revascularization. The basis for this has been the presence of chronic bilateral total renal arterial occlusion when, fortuitously, the viability of one or both kidneys has been maintained through collateral vascular supply. In such cases, revascularization can yield dramatic recovery of renal function. [p 250]

36. **b. Saccular.** Saccular aneurysms are the most common type and account for about 75% of renal artery aneurysms. They generally occur at the bifurcation of the renal artery, perhaps because of an inherent weakness in the wall of the artery at this point. [p 262]

37. **c. hematuria.** Factors that appear to predispose to aneurysmal rupture include absent or incomplete calcification, aneurysmal diameter greater than 2.0 cm, coexisting hypertension, and pregnancy. [p 262]

38. **d. generally heal spontaneously within 18 months.** Approximately 70% of fistulas occurring after needle biopsy of the kidney close spontaneously within 18 months. [p 264]

39. **b. Calcified aneurysm 1.5 cm in diameter.** A small (<2.0 cm) well-calcified renal arterial aneurysm in an asymptomatic normotensive patient does not require operative intervention. These aneurysms can be followed with serial plain abdominal radiographs to detect any change in size. [p 262]

40. **c. associated arteriolar nephrosclerosis.** The majority of renal arterial aneurysms are small and asymptomatic. Renovascular hypertension is reported to occur in 15% to 75% of patients and may be due to turbulent flow within an aneurysm, associated arterial stenosis, dissection, arteriovenous fistula formation, thromboembolism, or compression of adjacent arterial branches by a large aneurysm. [p 262]

41. **e. closed renal biopsy.** Acquired fistulas are the most common type of fistula, accounting for 70% to 75% of all renal arteriovenous fistulas. On angiography, they appear as solitary communications between an artery and a vein. By far the most common cause is iatrogenic trauma resulting from needle biopsy of the kidney. [p 264]

42. **b. total or partial nephrectomy.** Various operations have been used in the surgical treatment of renal arteriovenous fistulas. Most congenital or cirsoid fistulas have been managed with total or partial nephrectomy because of the difficulty of completely excising the many small communicating vessels. [p 264]

43. **a. systemic anticoagulation.** Patients with unilateral renal arterial embolic occlusion generally have serious underlying extrarenal disease and are best managed nonoperatively with systemic anticoagulation. [p 265]

44. **c. It more commonly involves the right renal artery.** Renal arterial thrombosis commonly involves the proximal or middle third of the main renal artery, whereas renal arterial embolization generally involves peripheral arterial branches. Acute arterial occlusion is more common on the left side because of the more acute angle between the left renal artery and the aorta. [pp 264–265]

Chapter 8

Etiology, Pathogenesis, and Management of Renal Failure

David A. Goldfarb • Joseph V. Nally, Jr. • Martin J. Schreiber, Jr.

Questions

1. Creatinine clearance overestimates glomerular filtration rate (GFR) in renal insufficiency because:

    a. tubular creatinine reabsorption is increased.
    b. creatinine production is decreased.
    c. the proportion of tubular creatinine secretion is increased.
    d. total body creatinine is increased.
    e. glomerular creatinine selectivity is increased.

2. In patients with occult renal artery stenosis, angiotensin-converting enzyme (ACE) inhibitors cause acute renal failure (ARF) because of:

    a. sodium retention.
    b. increased antidiuretic hormone.
    c. afferent arteriolar vasoconstriction.
    d. efferent arteriolar vasodilatation.
    e. decreased sympathetic nervous system activity.

3. Six days after partial nephrectomy in a solitary kidney, a patient becomes oliguric. Large amounts of fluid are coming from the flank drain. The serum creatinine level increases from 1.7 to 3.2 mg/dl. What is the next step in management?

    a. Renal angiography
    b. Computed tomography
    c. Renal scan
    d. Immediate surgical exploration
    e. Duplex ultrasonography

4. After a 7-hour-long, complex urethral reconstruction performed in the extended lithotomy position, the patient has severe thigh and buttock pain. The creatine phosphokinase levels are dramatically elevated. To prevent ARF, the next step should be:

    a. dopamine infusion.
    b. plasmapheresis.
    c. dobutamine infusion.
    d. forced alkaline diuresis.
    e. percutaneous nephrostomy.

5. The sentinel cellular change in renal ischemic injury is:
   a. loss of cell polarity.
   b. depletion of ATP.
   c. alteration of Na$^+$ metabolism.
   d. increased intracellular Ca^{2+}.
   e. increased oxidant stress.

6. The renal structure at greatest risk for ischemic injury is the:
   a. vasa recta.
   b. cortical collecting duct.
   c. juxtaglomerular apparatus.
   d. medullary thick ascending loop of Henle.
   e. distal convoluted tubule.

7. A patient with ARF has a urinary sodium concentration of 10 mEq/L, urinary osmolality of 650, and a renal failure index of less than 1. Urinalysis shows 10 to 20 red blood cells (RBCs) per high-power field (HPF), 3 to 5 white blood cells per HPF, 2+ proteinuria, and RBC casts. What is the most likely diagnosis?
   a. Acute tubular necrosis (ATN)
   b. Prerenal azotemia
   c. Acute glomerulonephritis
   d. Acute interstitial nephritis
   e. Obstruction

8. When renal impairment is demonstrated in a patient, the first therapeutic intervention should be to:
   a. begin low-dose dopamine.
   b. administer a cardiac inotropic agent.
   c. restore adequate circulating blood volume.
   d. administer a loop diuretic.
   e. begin a mannitol infusion.

9. Loop diuretics are of benefit in the management of ATN because of:
   a. improved patient survival.
   b. decreasing metabolic demand.
   c. decreasing hypoxic cell swelling.
   d. free radical scavenging.
   e. increased renal vascular resistance.

10. Which statement is true with regard to the pharmacologic management of ARF?
    a. Mannitol has a demonstrated beneficial effect.
    b. Improved outcome results in patients who respond to loop diuretics.
    c. Atrial natriuretic peptide is associated with hypertension.
    d. Calcium channel blockers adversely affect renal outcomes.
    e. Growth factors prevent renal ischemic injury.

11. Dopamine therapy in ARF:
    a. causes efferent arteriolar vasodilatation.
    b. is recommended for routine use after renal transplantation.
    c. is effective because of improved cardiac function.
    d. is an unproven treatment.
    e. improves patient survival.

12. A patient with ATN after partial nephrectomy has a serum potassium level of 6.9 mEq/L and widening of the QRS complex on an electrocardiogram. The initial step in management should be:
    a. intravenous calcium.
    b. intravenous insulin and glucose.
    c. sodium polystyrene sulfonate resin.
    d. intravenous furosemide.
    e. dialysis.

13. A patient with a serum creatinine level of 2.7 mg/dl requires renal angiography. The best way to protect renal function is with:
    a. saline diuresis.
    b. mannitol infusion.
    c. furosemide before the study.
    d. dopamine throughout the study.
    e. atrial natriuretic factor before the study.

14. In response to a reduction in renal mass, a number of events occur within the kidney that include all of the following except:
    a. activation of the sympathetic nervous system.
    b. hyperfiltration.
    c. glomerular hypertrophy.
    d. intrarenal vascular occlusion.
    e. interstitial fibrosis.

15. The ACE genotype *DD* is associated with:
    a. renal artery stenosis.
    b. low serum ACE levels.
    c. progressive renal disease.
    d. hyperaldosteronism.
    e. decreased need for dialysis.

16. The most rapidly progressing chronic renal disease is associated with:
    a. hypertensive nephrosclerosis.
    b. autosomal dominant polycystic kidney disease (PKD).
    c. chronic interstitial nephritis.
    d. diabetes mellitus.
    e. minimal change disease.

17. The most common cause for end-stage renal disease (ESRD) in the United States is:
    a. focal segmental glomerular sclerosis (FSGS).
    b. membranoproliferative glomerulonephritis (type 2).
    c. membranous glomerulonephritis.
    d. autosomal dominant polycystic kidney disease.
    e. diabetes mellitus.

18. The most accurate monitoring tool for assessment of progression of renal failure is:
    a. urinary creatinine clearance.
    b. Cockcroft-Gault formula.
    c. serum creatinine level.
    d. Modification of Diet and Renal Disease study equation.
    e. iothalamate GFR measurement.

19. A hypertensive 38-year-old man has a serum creatinine level of 2.4 mg/dl. The urinalysis shows 10 to 20 RBCs/HPF, 3+ protein, and RBC casts. Ultrasonography shows echogenic kidneys without hydronephrosis. What is the best method to achieve a diagnosis?
    a. Renal angiography
    b. Renal biopsy
    c. Retrograde pyelography
    d. Magnetic resonance imaging
    e. Spiral CT

20. The most effective agents for preserving residual renal function in chronic renal insufficiency are:
    a. α blockers.
    b. dihydropyridine calcium channel blockers.
    c. ACE inhibitors.
    d. β blockers.
    e. nitrates.

21. Chronic renal failure patients treated with an ACE inhibitor may experience a decrease in residual renal function in the setting of:

    a. unilateral renal artery stenosis.
    b. concomitant treatment with an α blocker.
    c. acquired renal cystic disease.
    d. left ventricular hypertrophy.
    e. autosomal dominant PKD with cysts larger than 10 cm.

22. What is the best renal replacement therapy for an otherwise healthy 37-year-old woman with chronic interstitial nephritis?

    a. Performing pre-emptive transplantation
    b. Stabilizing with hemodialysis for 1 year, then performing transplantation
    c. Stabilizing with peritoneal dialysis for 1 year, then performing transplantation
    d. Providing home hemodialysis
    e. Using peritoneal dialysis with an automated cycler

23. Based on the National Kidney Foundation Kidney Disease Outcome Quality Initiative (K/DOQI) Clinical Guidelines, dialysis should be initiated in chronic renal failure patients except under which condition?

    a. The weekly K_rT/V_{urea} is less than 2.
    b. The patient has a greater than 6% involuntary reduction of edema-free water.
    c. Body weight is less than 90% of standardized body weight according to the National Health and Nutrition Examination Survey II.
    d. The albumin level is reduced by more than 0.3 g/dl.
    e. The hematocrit is higher than 25%.

24. Late referral for dialysis is associated with:

    a. a hematocrit less than 20%.
    b. K_t/V higher than 2.
    c. an increased mortality rate.
    d. vascular access problems.
    e. increased edema-free body weight.

25. The strongest predictor of hospitalization in chronic dialysis patients is:

    a. African-American race.
    b. hematocrit less than 30%.
    c. glomerulonephritis.
    d. poor nutritional status.
    e. age younger than 30 years.

Answers

1. **c. the proportion of tubular creatinine secretion is increased.** Serum creatinine is produced at a constant rate by muscle and more accurately reflects the GFR. When renal function deteriorates, tubular secretion represents an increasing proportion of creatinine excretion. Therefore, creatinine clearance may overestimate the GFR as renal function slowly declines when measured in the steady state. [p 273]

2. **d. efferent arteriolar vasodilatation.** Angiotensin II has selectively greater vasoconstrictor effects on the efferent than on the afferent arteriole, whereas vasodilatory prostaglandins cause afferent arteriolar vasodilatation. Drugs that block angiotensin II synthesis (ACE inhibitors), block angiotensin II receptor binding (angiotensin II receptor antagonists), or inhibit vasodilatory prostaglandin synthesis (nonsteroidal anti-inflammatory drugs) may cause ARF in selected clinical settings. [p 273]

3. **c. Renal scan.** Ways to confirm urinary extravasation include intravenous administration of a vital dye excreted by the kidneys (such as indigo carmine or methylene blue) and radiographic demonstration of a fistula (isotope renography, retrograde pyelography, cystography, computed tomography). [p 275]

4. **d. forced alkaline diuresis.** The combination of renal hypoperfusion and the nephrotoxic insult of myoglobin or hemoglobin within the proximal tubule may result in acute tubular necrosis (ATN). Early recognition of this disorder is crucial, because a forced alkaline diuresis is indicated to minimize nephrotoxicity. [p 276]

5. **b. depletion of ATP.** The sentinel biochemical event in renal ischemia is the depletion of ATP, which is the major energy currency for cellular work. [p 277]

6. **d. medullary thick ascending loop of Henle.** Structures that sustain injury in this region include the medullary thick ascending limb, which is metabolically active and rich in the energy-requiring Na^+,K^+-ATPase. [p 279]

7. **c. Acute glomerulonephritis.** A low fractional excretion of sodium (or renal failure index) may be associated with either prerenal azotemia or acute glomerulonephritis. These entities could be separated clinically by examination of the urinalysis results. Conditions associated with prerenal azotemia would have a bland urinalysis, whereas proteinuria, RBCs, and RBC casts would be seen with acute glomerulonephritis. [p 281]

8. **c. restore adequate circulating blood volume.** During the initial stages, a trial of parenteral hydration with isotonic fluids may correct ARF secondary to prerenal causes. [p 282]

9. **b. decreasing metabolic demand.** They decrease active NaCl transport in the thick ascending limb of Henle and thereby limit energy requirements in the metabolically active segment, which often bears the greatest ischemic insult. [p 283]

10. **a. Mannitol has a demonstrated beneficial effect.** Mannitol has shown some benefit in the clinical setting of ARF, particularly when administered prophylactically or within a short time after an ischemic or nephrotoxic insult. [p 283]

11. **d. is an unproven treatment.** Results of clinical studies have not conclusively proved that dopamine infusion improves ARF. [p 284]

12. **a. intravenous calcium.** Priorities for treatment of acute hyperkalemia with electrocardiographic changes include stabilizing the electrical membrane of the cardiac conduction system, which may be accomplished with the use of intravenous calcium salts, which have an immediate effect and a rather short duration of action. [p 285]

13. **a. saline diuresis.** A study by Solomon and coworkers confirmed that prestudy intravenous hydration with saline was crucial in limiting the nephrotoxic effect of radiocontrast agents in patients with pre-existing azotemia. The addition of either a loop diuretic or mannitol did not improve outcome. [p 286]

14. **d. intrarenal vascular occlusion.** In response to reduced nephron mass, a mosaic of events occurs linking sympathetic nervous system activation, renal structural remodeling, altered gene expression and regulation, and several regulatory mechanisms for progression. [p 288]

15. **c. progressive renal disease.** The *DD* genotype imparts an increased risk for disease progression, and this genotype is also associated with an earlier need for dialysis. [p 290]

16. **b. autosomal dominant polycystic kidney disease (PKD).** Among a group of 866 patients, patients with PKD and chronic glomerulonephritis experienced a faster mean rate of progression of renal failure in comparison with patients with hypertensive nephrosclerosis or chronic interstitial nephritis. [p 290]

17. **e. diabetes mellitus.** Diabetes mellitus and hypertension account for the greatest percentage of cases (70.4%), followed by glomerular diseases (24.1%) (e.g., FSGS, membranous glomerulonephritis) and then secondary glomerulonephritis (2.5%) associated with systemic diseases (e.g., systemic lupus erythematosus, Wegener's granulomatosis). [p 291]

18. **e. iothalamate GFR measurement.** The iothalamate GFR assay is the "gold standard" for measuring renal function, but it requires a dedicated staff and laboratory to carry out the tests. [p 293]

19. **b. Renal biopsy.** For definitive diagnosis, a renal biopsy is required to aid prognosis and therapy decisions, especially in the setting of abnormal renal function. [p 293]

20. **c. ACE inhibitors.** ACE inhibitors and nondihydropyridine calcium antagonists are effective in decreasing proteinuria and renal scarring. At this time, it would appear that ACE inhibitors and angiotensin receptor blockers are preferential drugs for achieving these therapeutic goals. [p 295]

21. **e. autosomal dominant PKD with cysts larger than 10 cm.** Individuals with bilateral renal artery stenosis and autosomal dominant PKD patients with cyst size greater than 10 cm may also experience a decrease in residual renal function while being given ACE inhibitor therapy. [p 295]

22. **a. Performing pre-emptive transplantation.** A comparison of outcomes suggests that renal transplantation is the best overall treatment for ESRD patients. [p 297]

23. **e. The hematocrit is higher than 25%.** The K/DOQI guidelines recommend that dialysis be initiated when the weekly renal $K_r t/V_{urea}$ decreases to less than 2, unless all three of the following criteria are met: (1) stable or increased edema-free body weight, (2) randomized protein equivalent of total nitrogen appearance greater than 0.8, and (3) absence of clinical symptoms and signs attributable to uremia. The patient should begin some sort of renal replacement therapy if $K_r t/V_{urea}$ is less then 2 and more than 6% involuntary reduction of edema-free weight exists or the patient weighs less than 90% of standard body weight from the National Health and Nutrition Examination Survey III standard, or there is a reduction in albumin by ≥ 0.3 g/dl. [p 298]

24. **c. increased mortality rate.** Historically, mortality among late referrals for dialysis is consistently higher than among those with more timely initiated renal replacement therapy patterns. [p 298]

25. **d. poor nutritional status.** The strongest predictors of the number of hospitalizations per year of patients at risk include low serum albumin, decreased activity level, diabetes mellitus as a primary cause of ESRD, peripheral vascular disease, white race, increasing age, and congestive heart failure. Both nutritional status (levels of serum albumin, creatinine, transferrin, and prealbumin, and lean body mass) and inflammatory response (e.g., C-reactive protein) are independent predictors of hospitalization in chronic hemodialysis patients. [p 299]

Chapter 9

Basic Immunology in Urology

Stuart M. Flechner • James H. Finke • Robert L. Fairchild

Questions

1. Antigen presentation involves both uptake of foreign proteins and processing to form complexes between peptides and major histocompatibility complex (MHC) molecules. Each of the following immune responsive cell types can carry out this function except:

    a. granulocytes.
    b. vascular endothelial cells.
    c. monocytes.
    d. macrophages.
    e. dendritic cells.

2. Transplants between two siblings who are HLA identical (a perfect class I and class II match) can be rejected. This is primarily a consequence of:

    a. direct antigen presentation.
    b. differences in complement proteins.
    c. indirect antigen presentation.
    d. differences in childhood antimicrobial vaccination.
    e. differences in numbers of circulating platelets.

3. Lymphocyte activation depends on complex interactions among many intracellular enzymes, transcription factors, and electrolytes. The influx of which electrolyte is most important for T cell activation?

    a. Sodium
    b. Magnesium
    c. Potassium
    d. Phosphorus
    e. Calcium

4. Anergy describes a state of immune nonresponsiveness to antigenic stimulation. The most effective way to induce a state of anergy is by:

   a. splenic irradiation.
   b. delivery of signal 1 and signal 2.
   c. depletion of complement proteins.
   d. delivery of signal 1 without signal 2.
   e. depletion of helper CD4+ T cells.

5. Each of the following characteristics describes the utility and adaptability of the immune system except:

   a. memory.
   b. rapid amplification.
   c. identification of self.
   d. antigen restriction.
   e. specificity.

6. Innate immune responses are nonspecific and include all of the following except:

   a. natural killer cells.
   b. antibody-dependent cell-mediated cellular cytotoxicity.
   c. complement.
   d. acute phase proteins.
   e. physical and mucosal barriers.

7. Which cell surface glycoprotein is commonly referred to as the pan–T cell marker because of its presence on all T lymphocytes?

   a. CD3
   b. CD4
   c. CD8
   d. CD28
   e. CD45

8. Which part of an IgG antibody molecule interacts with cell surface receptors on other immune reactive cells such as natural killer cells?

   a. Hypervariable region
   b. Disulfide bonds
   c. Amino-terminal end of the antibody
   d. Fc fragment
   e. Fab fragment

9. The family of transcription factors termed NFAT is essential for T cell activation and clonal expansion through the expression of the gene for:

   a. interferon-γ.
   b. transferrin.
   c. tumor necrosis factor.
   d. interleukin-2.
   e. interleukin-10.

10. The receptor on B cells that recognizes antigen and transmits signals to the nucleus for gene expression is:

    a. the T cell receptor.
    b. the surface IgD molecule.
    c. the surface IgM molecule.
    d. CD40.
    e. CD28.

11. The Jak (Janus family of kinases)/STAT (signal transducers and activators of transcription) signaling pathways are crucial in regulating cytokine expression. Inborn deficiencies in these pathways may lead to diseases such as:

    a. Burkitt's lymphoma.
    b. Wilms' tumor.
    c. neuroblastoma.
    d. retinoblastoma.
    e. severe combined immunodeficiency.

12. The initial contact of host immunoresponsive cells with foreign antigen or transplanted donor tissue takes place in:

    a. peripheral lymph nodes.
    b. the thymus gland.
    c. the spleen.
    d. the bursa of Fabricius.
    e. the bone marrow.

13. Programmed cell death, apoptosis, is a mechanism responsible for the elimination of aged, damaged, autoimmune, or redundant cells. Caspase proteins are responsible for executing the suicide program by:

    a. release of granzyme B.
    b. activating the alternative complement pathway.
    c. activating natural killer cells.
    d. mediating DNA fragmentation and condensation.
    e. release of perforin.

14. Tolerance describes the absence of lymphocyte reactivity to specific antigens that have been previously encountered by the immune system. Known mechanisms of tolerance include each of the following except:

    a. deletion of reactive T cells.
    b. deletion of reactive B cells.
    c. blocking by antigen-antibody complexes.
    d. clonal anergy by delivery of signal 1 without costimulation.
    e. suppression of immune responses by regulatory cells.

15. Chemokines are chemoattractant cytokines that localize various cell populations to tissue sites of inflammation. Each of the following cell types responds to chemokines except:

    a. erythrocytes.
    b. granulocytes.
    c. natural killer cells.
    d. dendritic cells.
    e. monocytes.

16. Although most human tumors are antigenic, the immune system is often not a significant barrier to tumor growth and metastasis. A major reason for the relative weakness of the immune system in eradicating tumors is:

    a. the absence of costimulation by tumors, leading to anergy.
    b. tumor-induced alterations of immune function.
    c. impaired function of tumor neovasculature.
    d. rapid tumor cell proliferation.
    e. lack of tumor cell Fc receptors.

17. Tumor cell destruction by the immune system is often weak because of tumor cell escape mechanisms, which include all of the following except:

    a. tumor cell release of interleukin-2.
    b. a reduced expression of MHC class I and class II molecules on tumor cells.
    c. tumor cell and local release of interleukin-10.
    d. the ligation of tumor cell Fas by Fas ligand to induce apoptosis of host T cells.
    e. tumor cell and local release of transforming growth factor-β.

18. Immunotherapy for metastatic renal cell carcinoma in humans has included the use of cytokines such as interferon-γ and interleukin-2. The objective response rate (both complete and partial responses) has been demonstrated in what percentage of patients?

a. 95%
b. 75%
c. 55%
d. 35%
e. 15%

19. Extracellular bacteria are susceptible to killing by phagocytosis and complement, but some have developed capsules to block these mechanisms. What is the most effective immune countermeasure against bacterial encapsulation?

    a. The classic complement pathway
    b. The alternative complement pathway
    c. Opsonization of bacteria by circulating antibodies
    d. Increased secretion of transforming growth factor-β in tears
    e. Increased beating of bronchial cilia

20. Clearance of intracellular bacteria is most dependent on which of the following immune cell populations?

    a. Macrophages
    b. Plasma cells
    c. Natural killer cells
    d. Dendritic cells
    e. Primed T lymphocytes

21. Passive immune therapy may be particularly useful for patients with immunodeficiency. Passive therapy is delivered via:

    a. attenuated viral organisms.
    b. lyophilized vaccines.
    c. heterologous serum.
    d. live viral organisms.
    e. cow's milk.

22. The anatomic blood-testis barrier has few regions where gaps have been identified. These include:

    a. the rete testis.
    b. the vas deferens.
    c. the proximal urethra.
    d. the epididymis.
    e. the seminiferous tubules.

23. Which of the following statements is true of human anti-sperm antibodies?

    a. They are found at a titer of less than 1:16 in the serum of more than 50% of adult men.
    b. Those of the IgM class are often found in the semen.
    c. Those identified are most often of the IgA class.
    d. They impair fertilization most effectively when they bind to the tail of the spermatozoa.
    e. They are found in all men after vasectomy.

Answers

1. **a. granulocytes.** Macrophages, monocytes, some B cells, Langerhans cells of the skin, dendritic reticulum cells, and vascular endothelial cells can process and present antigen. [p 312]

2. **c. indirect antigen presentation.** The evidence for an indirect recognition pathway for alloantigens comes from observations that rejection can take place even if donor and recipient share most, if not all, MHC antigens. [p 317]

3. **e. Calcium.** This event also leads to the opening of the calcium channels in the plasma membrane, which further increases Ca^{2+} levels. Elevated intracellular Ca^{2+} results in the activation of the enzyme calcineurin, which is a cytosolic serine/threonine protein phosphatase that regulates the activation of a family of transcription factors termed NFAT (nuclear factor of activated T cells). [p 319]

4. **d. delivery of signal 1 without signal 2.** In fact, stimulation by signal 1 alone leads to a state of anergy, whereby the T cell becomes unresponsive to further stimulation by antigen. [p 315]

5. **d. antigen restriction.** Unique characteristics that help explain the utility and adaptability of the immune system against many different foreign invaders. These include (1) the ability to identify self from non-self; (2) specificity; (3) memory; and (4) rapid amplification. [p 308]

6. **b. antibody-dependent cell-mediated cellular cytotoxicity.** Innate defense mechanisms represent nonspecific barriers to invaders, which rely primarily on physical barriers, phagocytic cells, natural killer cells, complement, acute phase proteins, lysozyme, and the interferons. [p 308]

7. **a. CD3.** Each T cell precursor retains the pan–T cell CD3 marker, which is the signal-transducing complex closely linked to the T cell receptor. [p 311]

8. **d. Fc fragment.** The Fc fragment does not bind antibody but is responsible for fixation to complement and attachment of the molecule to the cell surface. [p 313]

9. **d. interleukin-2.** NFAT along with other transcription factors plays a critical role in T cell activation and clonal expansion through activation of the interleukin-2 gene. [p 319]

10. **b. surface IgD molecule.** The receptor on B cells that recognizes antigen and transmits signals to the nucleus for gene expression is composed of a cell surface immunoglobulin containing heavy and light chains with variable regions. [p 320]

11. **e. severe combined immunodeficiency.** The biologic importance of different Jaks and STATs has been revealed by deficiencies of these proteins both in humans and in animal models. Mutations in Jak3 have resulted in patients' having severe combined immunodeficiency (SCID) that is similar to X-linked SCID, which occurs because of a mutation in the common cytokine receptor γ chain. [p 320]

12. **a. peripheral lymph nodes.** Activation of specific T cells and the generation of an immune response require transport of antigenic components to the lymphoid tissue. For the induction of most T cell–mediated immune responses, the crucial antigen-presenting cell is the dendritic cell, which is interspersed throughout peripheral tissues. [p 320]

13. **d. mediating DNA fragmentation and chromatin condensation.** The proteins responsible for executing the suicide program, the caspases, are essentially common to all the stimuli and pathways and mediate the nuclear and cytoplasmic alterations characteristic of apoptotic cell death. The specific roles of each member of the caspase cascade are gradually becoming defined, whereby caspases 3, 6, and 7 have been identified as the terminal effectors mediating DNA fragmentation and chromatin condensation. [p 325]

14. **c. blocking by antigen-antibody complexes.** An important

mechanism mediating tolerance to self-proteins is the deletion of self-reactive T cells and B cells during maturation. Clonal anergy of T cells is induced by T cell receptor engagement of peptide-MHC complexes in the absence of costimulatory signals. An active mechanism of tolerance mediated by T cells with suppressive or down-regulatory activities may also be induced to inhibit immune responses to self and exogenous antigens. [pp 327–329]

15. **a. erythrocytes.** Cytokines with chemoattractant properties, chemokines, are also crucial in mediating localization and trafficking of leukocytes to tissue sites during physiologic processes, including inflammation and homeostasis. [p 331]

16. **b. tumor-induced alterations of immune function.** Tumor-induced alterations in the functional status of immune cells may be responsible for the poor development of antitumor immunity in many cancer patients. [p 332]

17. **a. tumor cell release of interleukin-2.** Natural killer cells can recognize and destroy some tumors, particularly those of lymphoid origin, without any exogenous activation. Reduction in or loss of MHC class I and class II expression by tumors, including renal cell carcinoma, has been well documented. In some tumors, there is also decreased expression of transporter proteins associated with antigen processing (TAP proteins). Among the best studied immunosuppressive molecules overexpressed in the tumor microenvironment is the TH2 cytokine interleukin-10. Transforming growth factor-β is also thought to contribute to the suppression of tumor immunity. Evidence suggests that the down-regulation of antitumor immunity may be due in part to the induction of the Fas apoptotic pathway in T cells. [pp 334–336]

18. **e. 15%.** It is clear from these and other studies that a subset of individuals with metastatic renal cancer does respond favorably to cytokine therapy; however, they represent a minority of patients (<15% response rate). [p 337]

19. **c. Opsonization of bacteria by circulating antibodies.** Many of these bacterial mechanisms can be overridden by host antibodies, which are soluble or secreted on external mucosal surfaces. Circulating antibodies can directly bind to bacterial exotoxins and "neutralize" them. They can also bind to the encapsulated bacteria, which will permit ingestion by polymorphs and macrophages. [p 338]

20. **e. Primed T lymphocytes.** Clearance of these intracellular microbes depends directly on T cells, which in turn must activate the infected macrophages. Specifically primed T cells react with processed antigen derived from the intracellular bacteria in association with MHC class II molecules on the macrophage surface. [p 339]

21. **c. heterologous serum.** Protection against a specific infection can be passively transferred from one individual to another via serum containing preformed antibodies. This type of passive immunity is generally short-lived, because the half-life of immunoglobulins is generally 1 to 2 weeks. Patients with immunodeficiency diseases may actually be sustained by regular treatments with pooled nonspecific human immune globulin treatments. [p 339]

22. **a. the rete testis.** Although the anatomic blood-testis barrier appears to continue along the epididymis, vas deferens, and proximal urethra, gaps have been identified. The rete testis and efferent ductules are two locations where a weaker morphologic barrier exists. [p 340]

23. **a. They are found at a titer of less than 1:16 in the serum of more than 50% of adult men.** Low titers of less than 1:16 of serum-only antibodies that bind sperm can be found in up to 60% of normal males and likely arise from bacterial cross-reactivity. Serum antibodies can be found in 50% to 80% of men after vasectomy. The IgG class represents the most frequently encountered antibody, which is derived from both local genital tract production and transudation from the blood. [p 340]

Chapter 10

Renal Transplantation

John M. Barry

Questions

1. The number of patients starting renal replacement therapy for end-stage renal disease (ESRD) in the United States is about how many per million population per year?

    a. 100
    b. 150
    c. 200
    d. 250
    e. 300

2. Permanent renal failure in adults is defined as an irreversible glomerular filtration rate (GFR) of less than how many milliliters per minute or a serum creatinine level of greater than how many milligrams per decaliter?

    a. 5 ml/min, 10 mg/dl
    b. 10 ml/min, 8 mg/dl
    c. 15 ml/min, 10 mg/dl
    d. 5 ml/min, 8 mg/dl
    e. 10 ml/min, 10 mg/dl

3. The most common form of treatment for adults with end-stage renal disease is:

    a. kidney transplantation.
    b. home hemodialysis.
    c. in-center hemodialysis.
    d. chronic ambulatory peritoneal dialysis.
    e. combination hemodialysis and chronic ambulatory peritoneal dialysis.

4. When was the first human kidney transplantation performed?

    a. 1926
    b. 1933

c. 1939
d. 1945
e. 1951

5. Which of the following renal diseases has a high probability of recurrence in patients with a kidney transplant, resulting in failure of the kidney graft?

    a. Chronic glomerulonephritis
    b. Chronic pyelonephritis
    c. Membranoproliferative glomerulonephritis
    d. Focal segmental glomerulosclerosis
    e. Alport's syndrome

6. Lymphoproliferative disorders are most commonly associated with which of the following viruses?

    a. Herpes simplex virus type 1
    b. Herpes simplex virus type 2
    c. Human papillomavirus
    d. Epstein-Barr virus (EBV)
    e. Varicella-zoster virus

7. To reduce the risk of cancer recurrence, a minimum waiting time of how many cancer-free years from the time of last cancer treatment is recommended for patients who have had invasive malignancies?

    a. 1
    b. 2
    c. 3
    d. 4
    e. 5

8. A disadvantage of intestinal augmentation cystoplasty in an anephric hemodialysis patient is:

    a. hyperkalemia.
    b. hypernatremia.
    c. metabolic alkalosis.
    d. metabolic acidosis.
    e. mucus.

9. Pretransplant nephrectomy is indicated for:

    a. hypertension controlled with medication.
    b. prior renal infection.
    c. renal calculi unsuitable for minimally invasive procedures.
    d. 100 mg/dl proteinuria.
    e. most polycystic kidneys.

10. The best renal imaging of a living renal donor to define renal anatomy and renal vasculature and to rule out renal stones is:

    a. kidney, ureter, bladder (KUB) radiography and selective renal arteriography.
    b. magnetic resonance (MR) nephrotomography and MR angiography.
    c. helical CT with and without intravenous contrast.
    d. KUB radiograph and helical CT with intravenous contrast.
    e. renal ultrasonography and selective renal arteriography.

11. After living donor nephrectomy, the renal donor is expected to have what level of total renal function?

    a. 50%
    b. 65%
    c. 80%
    d. 90%
    e. 95%

12. Kidney transplant survival rates are poorer for cadaver kidneys from donors younger than and older than how many years of age?

    a. 6, 45
    b. 6, 40
    c. 10, 45
    d. 10, 40
    e. 12, 45

13. The initial goals of resuscitation of the brain-dead cadaver donor are systolic blood pressure of what level and urinary output exceeding how many milliliters per kilogram per hour?

    a. 100 mm Hg, 0.25 ml/kg/hour
    b. 60 mm Hg, 0.5 ml/kg/hour
    c. 90 mm Hg, 0.5 ml/kg/hour
    d. 90 mm Hg, 0.3 ml/kg/hour
    e. 80 mm Hg, 0.4 ml/kg/hour

14. Which of the following is required for the cellular sodium-potassium pump to maintain a high intracellular concentration of potassium and a low intracellular concentration of sodium?

    a. ADP
    b. ATP
    c. CMP
    d. CTP
    e. Nitric oxide

15. The best solution for preservation of all abdominal organs is:

    a. EuroCollins.
    b. Collins 2.
    c. Sach's solution.
    d. University of Wisconsin (UW) solution.
    e. Ringer's lactated solution with heparin.

16. A cadaver kidney transplant recipient receives points on the national waiting list for all of the following except:

    a. time on the waiting list.
    b. age younger than 17 years.
    c. full-time employment.
    d. histocompatibility with donor.
    e. panel reactive antibody greater than 80%.

17. In the absence of significant recipient arteriosclerosis, the renal artery is usually anastomosed to the:

    a. aorta.
    b. common iliac artery.
    c. native renal artery.
    d. internal iliac artery.
    e. internal pudendal artery.

18. The renal vein is usually anastomosed to the recipient's:

    a. inferior vena cava.
    b. common iliac vein.
    c. external iliac vein.
    d. internal iliac vein.
    e. posterior gluteal vein.

19. The standard method of urinary tract reconstruction during renal transplantation is:

    a. ureteropyelostomy.
    b. ureteroureterostomy.
    c. transureteroureterostomy.
    d. ureteroneocystostomy.
    e. cutaneous ureterostomy.

20. The usual solution for intravenous fluid replacement after renal transplantation is:

    a. 0.25% saline.
    b. 0.45% saline.

c. 0.67% saline.
d. 0.85% saline.
e. 0.90% saline.

21. The risk of a hyperacute rejection after kidney transplantation is high when which of the following cross-matches is positive?

    a. B cell flow cross-match
    b. T cell flow cross-match
    c. Mixed lymphocyte culture
    d. Warm B cell cross-match
    e. Complement-dependent microlymphocytotoxicity cross-match

22. Which of the following immunosuppressants inhibits cell cycle progression?

    a. Azathioprine
    b. Mycophenolate mofetil
    c. Cyclosporine
    d. Tacrolimus
    e. Sirolimus

23. Which of the following paired immunosuppressants have similar mechanisms of action and toxicity?

    a. Azathioprine and cyclosporine
    b. Azathioprine and tacrolimus
    c. Cyclosporine and tacrolimus
    d. OKT3 and azathioprine.
    e. OKT3 and mycophenolate mofetil

24. Which of the following two drugs have been used to reduce cyclosporine dosing and cost while maintaining blood levels and immunosuppressive effect?

    a. Diltiazem and ketoconazole
    b. OKT3 and Atgam
    c. Phenytoin and phenobarbital
    d. Rifampin and trimethoprim-sulfamethoxazole
    e. Prednisone and azathioprine

25. Steroid-resistant rejection is often treated with:

    a. sirolimus.
    b. mycophenolate mofetil.
    c. antilymphocyte antibody.
    d. tacrolimus.
    e. higher doses of glucocorticoids.

26. Prophylaxis against *Pneumocystis* infection is best achieved with:

    a. trimethoprim-sulfamethoxazole.
    b. metronidazole.
    c. cytomegalovirus immune globulin.
    d. second-generation cephalosporin.
    e. erythromycin.

27. Prophylaxis against cytomegalovirus infection is best done with:

    a. trimethoprim-sulfamethoxazole.
    b. metronidazole.
    c. valacyclovir.
    d. second-generation cephalosporin.
    e. erythromycin.

28. A cadaver kidney transplant recipient has a serum creatinine level of 1.9 mg/dl. A large, asymptomatic perigraft fluid collection is aspirated, and the creatinine level is 2.0 mg/dl. What is the most likely diagnosis?

    a. Hydrocele
    b. Lymphocele
    c. Urinary leak
    d. Resolving hematoma
    e. Perinephric abscess

29. Which of the following interferes with the tubular secretion of creatinine and can cause an increase in serum creatinine levels?

    a. Azathioprine
    b. Cyclosporine
    c. Trimethoprim
    d. Sulfamethoxazole
    e. Mycophenolate mofetil

30. Fluconazole is prescribed to treat cystitis caused by yeast. Which of the following medications will need to have the dose reduced?

    a. OKT3
    b. Tacrolimus
    c. Daclizumab
    d. Azathioprine
    e. Prednisone

31. Hemorrhagic cystitis in an immunosuppressed patient has been associated with which of the following viruses?

    a. Cytomegalovirus
    b. Adenovirus
    c. Coxsackievirus
    d. Varicella-zoster virus
    e. Herpes simplex virus type 2

32. Which of the following antihypertensive agents is least likely to cause erectile dysfunction?

    a. Propranolol
    b. Clonidine
    c. Methyldopa
    d. Terazosin
    e. Labetolol

33. A successful kidney transplant recipient and his wife desire to have a child. What is the recommended length of time between transplantation and impregnation?

    a. 3 months
    b. 6 months
    c. 12 months
    d. 24 months
    e. 36 months

34. At what frequency would preterm delivery be expected in a pregnant kidney transplant recipient?

    a. 10%
    b. 20%
    c. 30%
    d. 40%
    e. 50%

35. The most common cancer after kidney transplantation is:

    a. skin.
    b. lymphoma.
    c. Kaposi's sarcoma.
    d. renal cell carcinoma.
    e. carcinoma of the cervix.

36. A kidney transplant recipient has recurrent superficial transitional cell carcinoma of the urinary bladder. Each of the following treatments is acceptable except:

    a. fulguration.
    b. laser ablation.
    c. intravesical bacille Calmette-Guérin (BCG).

d. intravesical thiotepa.
e. transurethral resection.

37. Hyperlipidemia is most associated with which of the following three-drug combinations?

a. Prednisone, cyclosporine, sirolimus
b. Prednisone, tacrolimus, azathioprine
c. Cyclosporine, mycophenolate mofetil, OKT3
d. Azathioprine, cyclosporine, propranolol
e. Atgam, tacrolimus, mycophenolate mofetil

Answers

1. **e. 300.** The estimated number of patients starting renal replacement therapy each year for ESRD in the United States is about 300 per million population. [p 346]

2. **b. 10 ml/min, 8 mg/dl.** Permanent renal failure in adults is commonly defined as an irreversible GFR of less than 10 ml/min or a serum creatinine level of greater than 8.0 mg/dl. [p 346]

3. **c. in-center hemodialysis.** In-center hemodialysis is the predominant form of therapy for adults with ESRD. In the United States, it accounts for about 60% of all treated ESRD patients. [p 346]

4. **b. 1933.** In 1933, the first human renal allograft was performed by Voronoy in the Ukraine. The recipient was a 26-year-old woman who had attempted suicide by ingesting mercuric chloride. The donor was a 66-year-old man whose kidney had been removed 6 hours after death. [p 347]

5. **d. Focal segmental glomerulosclerosis.** Patients with focal segmental glomerulosclerosis, hemolytic-uremic syndrome, or primary oxalosis should be counseled about the significant probability of disease recurrence and the risk of secondary graft failure. [p 348]

6. **d. Epstein-Barr virus (EBV).** EBV titers are determined in children, and, for the EBV-seronegative child, a kidney from an EBV-seronegative donor is preferred to reduce the risk of a post-transplant lymphoproliferative disorder, the most common de novo malignancy in pediatric organ transplant recipients. [p 349]

7. **b. 2.** To reduce the risk of cancer recurrence, a waiting time of 2 to 5 cancer-free years from the time of last cancer treatment is recommended for patients who have had invasive malignancies. [p 349]

8. **e. mucus.** A urothelial-lined augmentation is best because mucus does not have to be rinsed from the bladder on a regular basis. Advantages of gastrocystoplasty over enterocystoplasty are the lack of both metabolic acidosis and significant mucus. [p 351]

9. **c. renal calculi unsuitable for minimally invasive procedures.** The generally accepted indications for pretransplant nephrectomy, as outlined in Table 10–6, include the following: renal stones not cleared by minimally invasive techniques or lithotripsy; solid renal tumors with or without acquired renal cystic disease; polycystic kidneys that are symptomatic, extend below the iliac crest, have been infected, or have solid tumors; persistent antiglomerular basement membrane antibody levels; significant proteinuria not controlled with medical nephrectomy or angioablation; recurrent pyelonephritis; and grade 4 or 5 hydronephrosis. [p 351]

10. **c. helical CT with and without intravenous contrast.** Three-dimensional CT angiography without and with intravenous contrast followed by a radiograph of the abdomen has been widely accepted for use with living renal donors because it satisfactorily excludes stone disease, demonstrates renal and vascular anatomy, and defines the urinary collecting system, all with minimal donor morbidity and at reasonable expense. [p 352]

11. **c. 80%.** Hyperfiltration injury has not been a problem for living renal donors. Endogenous creatinine clearance rapidly approaches 70% to 80% of the preoperative level, and this has been shown to be sustained for more than 10 years. The development of late hypertension is nearly the same as that for the general population, and the development of proteinuria is negligible. [p 352]

12. **a. 6, 45.** Kidney transplant survival rates are poorer for cadaver kidneys from donors younger than the age of 6 years and older than the age of 45 years. [p 352]

13. **c. 90 mm Hg, 0.5 ml/kg/hour.** The initial goals of resuscitation of the brain-dead cadaver donor are a systolic blood pressure of 90 mm Hg and a urinary output exceeding 0.5 ml/kg/hour. [p 354]

14. **b. ATP.** ATP is required for the cellular sodium-potassium pump to maintain a high intracellular concentration of potassium and a low intracellular concentration of sodium. [pp 354–355]

15. **d. University of Wisconsin (UW) solution.** The UW solution minimizes cellular swelling with the impermeable solutes lactobionate, raffinose, and hydroxyethyl starch. Phosphate is used for its hydrogen ion buffering qualities, adenosine is for ATP synthesis during reperfusion, glutathione is a free radical scavenger, allopurinol inhibits xanthine oxidase and the generation of free radicals, and magnesium and dexamethasone are membrane-stabilizing agents. A major advantage of this preservation solution has been its utility as a universal preservation solution for all intra-abdominal organs. [p 357]

16. **c. full-time employment.** A point system that has evolved in the United States for the selection of cadaver kidney transplant recipients, presented in Table 10–9, includes the following variables: waiting time; human leukocyte antigen panel reactive antibody greater than 80%; age of 17 years or younger; donor of kidney, liver segment, lung segment, partial pancreas, or small bowel segment; and histocompatibility points. [p 357]

17. **d. internal iliac artery.** The renal artery is usually anastomosed to the end of the internal iliac artery or to the side of the external iliac artery. [pp 358–359]

18. **c. external iliac vein.** The renal vein, with or without an extension, is usually anastomosed end-to-side to the external iliac vein. [p 359]

19. **d. ureteroneocystostomy.** Urinary tract reconstruction is usually by antireflux ureteroneocystostomy, of which there are several techniques. [p 359]

20. **b. 0.45% saline.** Intravenous fluid of 0.45% saline in 5%

dextrose is given to replace estimated insensible losses, and 0.45% saline in 0% dextrose is given at a rate equal to the previous hour's urinary output. [p 362]

21. **e. Complement-dependent microlymphocytotoxicity cross-match.** Hyperacute rejection is very rare when the microlymphocytotoxicity cross-match between recipient serum and donor lymphocytes is negative. [p 364]

22. **e. Sirolimus.** Sirolimus (formerly called rapamycin) inhibits cell cycle progression. [p 364]

23. **c. Cyclosporine and tacrolimus.** Cyclosporine and tacrolimus have similar mechanisms of action, effectiveness, and cost, but slightly different side effect profiles, and they are not used together. [p 365]

24. **a. Diltiazem and ketoconazole.** Diltiazem and ketoconazole have been used to reduce cyclosporine dosing and cost while maintaining blood levels and immunosuppressive effect. [p 365]

25. **c. antilymphocyte antibody.** Conventional treatment for acute renal allograft rejection is high-dose pulses of glucocorticoids. Treatment of steroid-resistant rejection is with antilymphocyte antibody preparations such as OKT3, Atgam, and Thymoglobulin. [p 365]

26. **a. trimethoprim-sulfamethoxazole.** Commonly used regimens to prevent infections and peptic ulcer disease, as listed in Table 10–16, include trimethoprim-sulfamethoxazole for 3 months for prophylaxis against *Pneumocystis* pneumonia. [pp 365 and 368]

27. **c. valacyclovir.** Prophylaxis against cytomegalovirus disease is possible with ganciclovir, acyclovir, valacyclovir, or cytomegalovirus immune globulin. [p 365]

28. **b. Lymphocele.** Lymph, urine, and blood can be differentiated from each other by creatinine and hematocrit determinations. Lymph has a creatinine concentration that is the same as serum, urine has a creatinine concentration higher than that of serum and approaching that of bladder urine, and blood has a high hematocrit level when compared with the other two fluids. [p 368]

29. **c. Trimethoprim.** Trimethoprim interferes with the tubular secretion of creatinine, and this can cause an increase in serum creatinine levels. [p 370]

30. **b. Tacrolimus.** Cyclosporine and tacrolimus doses usually have to be reduced when ketoconazole or fluconazole is given because these drugs interfere with the metabolism of both of those immunosuppressants. [p 370]

31. **b. Adenovirus.** Hemorrhagic cystitis can be caused by adenovirus. The disease is usually self-limited and resolves within a week or two. [p 370]

32. **d. Terazosin.** Erectile dysfunction can be due to any one or a combination of factors. Included are the antihypertensives clonidine, methyldopa, propranolol, and labetalol. [pp 370 and 371]

33. **c. 12 months.** Among male recipients who have fathered children, there has been no increase in congenital abnormalities in the offspring. However, it is recommended that impregnation be delayed for at least 1 year after transplantation. [p 371]

34. **e. 50%.** Successful renal transplantation usually restores female fertility. In a report based on thousands of pregnancies in renal transplant recipients, Davison and Milne noted, among other findings, that 50% of the deliveries were preterm. [pp 371–372]

35. **a. skin.** Immunosuppressed patients are more likely to develop cancer than age-matched control subjects in the general population. Among several thousand tumors that occurred in renal transplant recipients, the common cancers, in order, were skin, lymphoma, Kaposi's sarcoma, carcinomas of the cervix, renal tumors, and carcinomas of the vulva and perineum. [p 372]

36. **c. intravesical bacille Calmette-Guérin.** BCG vaccine should be avoided for the treatment of superficial transitional cell carcinoma of the bladder in immunosuppressed kidney transplant recipients because of the risk of systemic infection and the likelihood of diminished therapeutic response. [p 372]

37. **a. Prednisone, cyclosporine, sirolimus.** Prednisone, cyclosporine, and sirolimus increase cardiovascular risk because of the hyperlipidemia associated with these drugs. [p 373]

Chapter 11

Physiology and Pharmacology of the Renal Pelvis and Ureter

Robert M. Weiss

Questions

1. During development, the ureteral lumen is obliterated and then recanalizes. Which of the following substances appears to be involved in this recanalization process?

    a. Prostaglandin E_2
    b. Prostaglandin $F_{2\alpha}$
    c. Angiotensin
    d. Calcitonin gene-related peptide (CGRP)
    e. Acetylcholine

2. Caspases are involved in:

    a. smooth muscle relaxation.
    b. smooth muscle contraction.
    c. hysteresis.

d. apoptosis.
   e. calcium sequestration.

3. The resting membrane potential is primarily determined by the distribution of which of the following ions across the cell membrane and the preferential permeability of the cell membrane to that ion?
   a. Potassium
   b. Sodium
   c. Calcium
   d. Chloride
   e. Barium

4. With excitation of the ureteral cell, an action potential is formed. Which of the following pairs of ions is responsible for the upstroke of the action potential?
   a. Potassium and calcium
   b. Sodium and chloride
   c. Calcium and sodium
   d. Potassium and sodium
   e. Calcium and chloride

5. Which of the following must be phosphorylated for smooth muscle contraction to occur?
   a. Actin
   b. Myosin
   c. Calmodulin
   d. Calcium
   e. Troponin

6. The primary site for intracellular storage of calcium is:
   a. mitochondria.
   b. caveolae.
   c. nucleolus.
   d. actin.
   e. endoplasmic reticulum.

7. The second messenger involved in β-adrenergic agonist-induced ureteral relaxation is:
   a. cyclic AMP.
   b. cyclic GMP.
   c. nitric oxide.
   d. inositol 1,4,5-trisphosphate (IP_3).
   e. diacylglycerol (DG).

8. The enzyme that degrades cyclic GMP is:
   a. guanylyl cyclase.
   b. myosin light chain kinase.
   c. phosphodiesterase.
   d. phospholipase C.
   e. nitric oxide synthase (NOS).

9. The enzyme that degrades cyclic AMP is:
   a. adenylyl cyclase.
   b. myosin light chain kinase.
   c. phosphodiesterase.
   d. phospholipase C.
   e. NOS.

10. Nitric oxide causes smooth muscle relaxation. In doing so, it activates which of the following enzymes?
    a. Guanylyl cyclase
    b. Myosin light chain kinase
    c. Phosphodiesterase
    d. Phospholipase C
    e. NOS

11. The substrate for NOS is:
    a. cyclic AMP.
    b. cyclic GMP.
    c. GTP.
    d. L-arginine.
    e. L-citrulline.

12. Inducible NOS (iNOS) is:
    a. nicotinamide adenine dinucleotide phosphate (NADPH) independent and calcium independent.
    b. NADPH independent and calcium dependent.
    c. NADPH dependent and calcium independent.
    d. NADPH dependent and calcium dependent.
    e. nitric oxide dependent and calcium dependent.

13. The enzyme involved in the formation of DG is:
    a. adenylyl cyclase.
    b. guanylyl cyclase.
    c. phosphodiesterase.
    d. protein kinase C (PKC).
    e. phospholipase C.

14. DG increases the activity of which enzyme?
    a. Adenylyl cyclase
    b. Guanylyl cyclase
    c. Phosphodiesterase
    d. PKC
    e. Phospholipase C

15. An agent that prevents re-uptake of norepinephrine in nerve terminals and thus potentiates and prolongs the activity of norepinephrine is:
    a. tyrosine.
    b. monoamine oxidase.
    c. imipramine.
    d. tetramethylammonium.
    e. tetraethylammonium.

16. Norepinephrine is synthesized from:
    a. tyrosine.
    b. arginine.
    c. choline.
    d. cocaine.
    e. imipramine.

17. Which of the following inhibits ureteral and renal pelvic contractile activity?
    a. Substance P
    b. Neurokinin A
    c. Neuropeptide K
    d. Neuropeptide Y
    e. CGRP

18. Which of the following collagen types is associated with ureteral obstruction?
    a. Type I collagen
    b. Type II collagen
    c. Type III collagen
    d. Type IV collagen
    e. Type V collagen

19. The enzyme involved in prostaglandin synthesis is:
    a. phospholipase C.
    b. cyclooxygenase.
    c. protein kinase C.
    d. phosphodiesterase.
    e. ATPase.

20. With ureteral obstruction, prostaglandins are involved in a

process that aids in the preservation of renal function. What is this process?

a. Afferent arteriole vasoconstriction
b. Afferent arteriole vasodilatation
c. Efferent arteriole vasoconstriction
d. Efferent arteriole vasodilatation
e. Glomerular vasoconstriction

21. Which of the following agents could theoretically cause urinary retention?

a. Bethanechol
b. BAY k 8644
c. Prostaglandin $F_{2\alpha}$
d. Verapamil
e. Substance P

22. Which of the following is a β-adrenergic agonist?

a. Cromakalim
b. Physostigmine
c. Propranolol
d. Phenoxybenzamine
e. Isoproterenol

23. Which of the following conditions must be present for urine to pass efficiently from the ureter into the bladder?

a. Intraluminal ureteral contractile pressure must be above 40 cm H_2O.
b. The ureterovesical junction must relax.
c. Intraluminal ureteral contractile pressures must be greater than intravesical baseline pressures.
d. Intravesical contractile pressures must be less than 40 cm H_2O.
e. The bladder must relax just before contraction of the ureter.

24. What is normal baseline or resting ureteral pressure?

a. 0 to 5 cm H_2O
b. 5 to 10 cm H_2O
c. 10 to 15 cm H_2O
d. 15 to 20 cm H_2O
e. 20 to 25 cm H_2O

25. The Laplace equation expresses the relationship between the variables that affect intraluminal pressure. Which of the following conforms with the Laplace relationship?

a. Tension = (radius × wall thickness)/pressure
b. Tension = (radius × pressure)/wall thickness
c. Tension = (wall thickness × pressure)/radius
d. Pressure = (radius × wall thickness)/tension
e. Pressure = (radius × tension)/wall thickness

26. Factors that facilitate ureteral stone passage include:

a. increased hydrostatic pressures proximal to the calculus and relaxation of the ureter in the region of the stone.
b. increased hydrostatic pressures proximal to the calculus and contraction of the ureter in the region of the stone.
c. decreased hydrostatic pressures proximal to the calculus and relaxation of the ureter in the region of the stone.
d. decreased hydrostatic pressures proximal to the calculus and contraction of the ureter in the region of the stone.
e. decreased contractile pressures proximal to the calculus and contraction of the ureter in the region of the stone.

27. Which of the following hormones inhibits ureteral contractility?

a. Bombesin
b. Thyroxine
c. Estrogen
d. Aldosterone
e. Progesterone

28. A drug that has efficacy in managing ureteral colic is:

a. bethanechol.
b. prostaglandin $F_{2\alpha}$.
c. physostigmine.
d. indomethacin.
e. ephedrine.

29. Which of the following is a calcium-binding protein that plays a role in smooth muscle contraction?

a. Connexin43
b. Calmodulin
c. Cromakalim
d. Survivin
e. Myosin

30. The resting or the contractile force developed at any given length, in the ureter, depends on the direction in which the change in length is occurring. This is referred to as:

a. viscoelasticity.
b. creep.
c. hysteresis.
d. stress relaxation.
e. compensatory relaxation.

Answers

1. **c. Angiotensin.** At a point during development, the ureteral lumen is obliterated and then recanalizes. It appears that angiotensin acting through the AT2 receptor is involved in the recanalization process. Knockout mice for the *ATR2* gene have congenital anomalies of the kidney and urinary tract, which include multicystic dysplastic kidneys, megaureters, and ureteropelvic junction obstructions. [p 378]

2. **d. apoptosis.** Programmed cell death, or apoptosis, is involved in branching of the ureteric bud and subsequent nephrogenesis, and inhibitors of caspases, which are factors in the signaling pathway of apoptosis, inhibit ureteral bud branching. [p 378]

3. **a. Potassium.** When a ureteral muscle cell is in a nonexcited or resting state, the electrical potential difference across the cell membrane, the transmembrane potential, is referred to as the resting membrane potential (RMP). The RMP is determined primarily by the distribution of potassium ions (K^+) across the cell membrane and by the permeability of the membrane to potassium ions. [p 378]

4. **c. Calcium and sodium.** When the ureteral cell is excited, its membrane loses its preferential permeability to K^+ and becomes more permeable to calcium ions (Ca^{2+}) that move inward across the cell membrane, primarily through L-type Ca^{2+} channels, and give rise to the upstroke of the action potential. [p 379]

5. **b. Myosin.** The most widely accepted theory suggests that phosphorylation of myosin is involved in the contractile process. [p 382]

6. **e. endoplasmic reticulum.** Calcium release from tightly bound storage sites (i.e., the endoplasmic or sarcoplasmic reticulum) increases the Ca^{2+} concentration in the sarcoplasm. [p 383]

7. **a. cyclic AMP.** Cyclic AMP is believed to mediate the relaxing effects of β-adrenergic agonists in a variety of smooth muscles. [p 384]

8. **c. phosphodiesterase.** Another cyclic nucleotide, cyclic GMP, also can cause smooth muscle relaxation. Cyclic GMP is synthesized from GTP via the enzyme guanylyl cyclase and is degraded to 5'-GMP by a phosphodiesterase. [p 384]

9. **c. phosphodiesterase.** Phosphodiesterase activity that can degrade both cyclic AMP and cyclic GMP has been demonstrated in the canine ureter, and various inhibitors can preferentially inhibit the breakdown of one or the other cyclic nucleotide. [p 384]

10. **a. Guanylyl cyclase.** Nitric oxide released from the nerve activates the enzyme guanylyl cyclase in the smooth muscle cell, with the resultant conversion of guanosine triphosphate to cyclic GMP with resultant smooth muscle relaxation (see Fig. 11–10). [p 385]

11. **d. L-arginine.** NOS converts L-arginine to nitric oxide and L-citrulline in a reaction that requires nicotinamide adenine dinucleotide phosphate (NADPH). [p 385]

12. **c. NADPH dependent and calcium independent.** An inducible NOS isoform, iNOS, is NADPH dependent but Ca^{2+} independent and has been identified in ureteral smooth muscle. [p 385]

13. **e. phospholipase C.** Some actions of α_1-adrenergic and muscarinic cholinergic agonists and a number of other hormones, neurotransmitters, and biologic substances are associated with an increase in intracellular Ca^{2+} and are related to changes in inositol lipid metabolism. These agonists combine with a receptor on the cell membrane, and the agonist-receptor complex, in turn, activates an enzyme, phospholipase C, that leads to the hydrolysis of polyphosphatidylinositol 4,5-bisphosphate, with the formation of two second messengers, IP_3 and DG (see Fig. 11–11). [p 385]

14. **d. PKC.** DG binds to an enzyme, PKC, causes its translocation to the cell membrane, and by reducing the concentration of Ca^{2+} required for PKC activation results in an increase in this enzyme's activity. [p 385]

15. **c. imipramine.** The greatest percentage of the norepinephrine is actively taken up (re-uptake or neuronal uptake) into the neuron. Neuronal re-uptake regulates the duration that norepinephrine is in contact with the innervated tissue and thus regulates the magnitude and duration of the catecholamine-induced response. Agents such as cocaine and imipramine (Tofranil), which inhibit neuronal uptake, potentiate the physiologic response to norepinephrine. [p 389]

16. **a. tyrosine.** Norepinephrine, the chemical mediator responsible for adrenergic transmission, is synthesized in the neuron from tyrosine. [p 389]

17. **e. CGRP.** Tachykinins and CGRP are neurotransmitters released from peripheral endings of sensory nerves. Tachykinins stimulate contractile activity and CGRP inhibits contractile activity. [p 390]

18. **c. Type III collagen.** Increased amounts of collagen type III are seen in a variety of obstructed ureteral states. [p 399]

19. **b. cyclooxygenase.** The "primary" prostaglandins, PGE_1, PGE_2, and $PGF_{2\alpha}$, are synthesized from the fatty acid arachidonic acid by enzymatic reactions involving two cyclooxygenase (COX) isoforms, COX-1 and COX-2. [p 402]

20. **b. Afferent arteriole vasodilatation.** Indomethacin has been employed in the management of ureteral colic. The beneficial effects are probably due to indomethacin's inhibition of the prostaglandin-mediated vasodilatation that occurs subsequent to obstruction. The vasodilatation theoretically would result in an increase in glomerular capillary pressure and subsequent increase in pelviureteral pressure. [p 402]

21. **d. Verapamil.** The calcium channel blockers verapamil, D-600 (a methoxy derivative of verapamil), diltiazem, and nifedipine have been shown to inhibit ureteral activity. These inhibitory effects are accompanied by decreases in action potential duration, number of oscillations on the plateau of the guinea pig action potential, excitability, and rate of rise and amplitude of the action potential. High concentrations of verapamil and D-600 cause a complete cessation of electrical and mechanical activity. Similar inhibition of bladder activity can occur. [p 403]

22. **e. Isoproterenol.** Isoproterenol, a β-adrenergic agonist, depresses contractility. [p 389]

23. **c. Intraluminal ureteral contractile pressures must be greater than intravesical baseline pressures.** The theoretical aspects of the mechanics of urine transport within the ureter were described in detail by Griffiths and Notschaele in 1983; these are depicted in Figure 11–17. At normal flow rates, as the renal pelvis fills, a rise in renal pelvic pressure occurs, and urine is extruded into the upper ureter, which is initially in a collapsed state. The contraction wave originates in the most proximal portion of the ureter and moves the urine in front of it in a distal direction. The urine that had previously entered the ureter is formed into a bolus. To propel the bolus of urine efficiently, the contraction wave must completely coapt the ureteral walls, and the pressure generated by this contraction wave provides the primary component of what is recorded by intraluminal pressure measurements. The bolus that is pushed in front of the contraction wave lies almost entirely in a passive, noncontracting part of the ureter. [pp 391–392]

24. **a. 0 to 5 cm H_2O.** Baseline or resting ureteral pressure is approximately 0 to 5 cm H_2O. [p 392]

25. **b. Tension = (radius $\times$ pressure)/wall thickness.** The Laplace equation expresses the relationship between the variables that affect intraluminal pressure: Pressure = (tension $\times$ wall thickness)/radius. [p 392]

26. **a. increased hydrostatic pressures proximal to the calculus and relaxation of the ureter in the region of the stone.** Two factors that appear to be most useful in facilitating stone passage are an increase in hydrostatic pressure proximal to a calculus and relaxation of the ureter in the region of the stone. [p 399]

27. **e. Progesterone.** Several studies have shown an inhibitory effect of progesterone on ureteral function. Progesterone has been noted to increase the degree of ureteral dilatation during pregnancy and to retard the rate of disappearance of hydrourer in postpartum women. [p 401]

28. **d. indomethacin.** Indomethacin, by reducing pelviureteral pressure and thus pelviureteral wall tension, might eliminate some of the pain of renal colic that is dependent on distention of the upper urinary tract. [p 402]

29. **b. Calmodulin.** With excitation, there is a transient increase in the sarcoplasmic Ca^{2+} concentration from its steady-state concentration of 10^{-8} to 10^{-7} M to a concentration of 10^{-6} M or higher. At this higher concentration, Ca^{2+} forms an active complex with the calcium-binding protein calmodulin. Calmodulin without Ca^{2+} is inactive (see Fig. 11–6). The

calcium-calmodulin complex activates a calmodulin-dependent enzyme, myosin light-chain kinase (see Fig. 11–6). The activated myosin light-chain kinase, in turn, catalyzes the phosphorylation of the 20,000-dalton light chain of myosin (see Fig. 11–7). Phosphorylation of the myosin light chain allows activation by actin of myosin Mg^{2+}-ATPase activity, leading to hydrolysis of ATP and the development of smooth muscle tension or shortening (see Fig. 11–8). [pp 382–383]

30. **c. hysteresis.** Because the ureter is a viscoelastic structure, the resting or contractile force developed at any given length depends on the direction in which change in length is occurring and on the rate of length change. This is referred to as hysteresis; for the ureter, at any given length, the resting force is less and contractile force is greater when the ureter is allowed to shorten than when the ureter is being stretched (see Fig. 11–12). [pp 386–387]

Chapter 12

Pathophysiology of Urinary Tract Obstruction

Fredrick A. Gulmi • Diane Felsen • E. Darracott Vaughan, Jr.

Questions

1. What does the term *obstructive uropathy* refer to, versus the term *hydronephrosis*?

   a. Dilatation of the urinary tract
   b. Damage to the renal parenchyma from obstruction
   c. Obstruction of the urinary tract alone
   d. Dilatation of the renal pelvis only
   e. Obstruction of the ureters only

2. Chronic urinary tract obstruction will result in the which of the following urinary indices?

   a. Increased urinary sodium concentration
   b. Decreased urine osmolality
   c. Decreased urine-to-plasma creatinine ratio
   d. All of the above
   e. None of the above

3. A 36-year-old man with a history of uric acid stones comes into the emergency department with a complaint of flank pain for the last 2 days. He has no associated fever but does have intermittent nausea and vomiting. The patient has a history of asthma and shellfish allergy. He thinks he may have had a reaction to contrast material in the past but is unsure. The emergency department physician ordered a renal sonogram that demonstrated hydronephrosis. What is the next best test?

   a. Intravenous urography
   b. CT with contrast enhancement
   c. Diuretic renography with technetium Tc 99m mercaptoacetyltriglycine (MAG3)
   d. Diuretic renography with diethylenetriamine pentaacetic acid (DTPA)
   e. MRI.

4. A 56-year-old women comes into the emergency department with a complaint of left-sided flank pain for the last 20 hours. She has associated nausea, vomiting, and chills with no fever. Her laboratory data reveal microscopic hematuria, with markedly elevated blood urea nitrogen and creatinine levels. Her kidney, ureter, bladder (KUB) radiograph was negative for any stones. What would the next best test be?

   a. Intravenous urography
   b. Diuretic renography
   c. Conventional CT of the abdomen and pelvis without contrast enhancement
   d. Helical CT of the abdomen and pelvis without contrast enhancement
   e. Duplex Doppler ultrasonography of the kidneys

5. To classify a disease as idiopathic retroperitoneal fibrosis, the physician must have which of the following?

   a. An intravenous urogram
   b. A CT scan of the abdomen and pelvis
   c. Results of biopsy of the retroperitoneum
   d. Ultrasonogram of the abdomen
   e. Bilateral retrograde ureteropyelogram

6. Which of the following is NOT a treatment option in a patient with left ureteral obstruction from biopsy-confirmed idiopathic retroperitoneal fibrosis?

   a. Unilateral left ureterolysis and intraperitonealization of the ureter
   b. Bilateral ureterolysis and intraperitonealization of the ureters
   c. Laparoscopic ureterolysis and intraperitonealization of the ureters
   d. Bilateral ureterolysis and omental wrap of the ureters
   e. Left ureteral stent placement and prednisone therapy

7. The best radiographic test for the diagnosis of pelvic lipomatosis is:

   a. bilateral retrograde ureteropyelography.
   b. intravenous urography.
   c. MRI.
   d. pelvic ultrasonography.
   e. CT of the abdomen and pelvis.

8. The best initial management of the nulliparous patient in the 20th week of gestation with right flank pain associated with nausea, vomiting, and no fever would include:

   a. a right ureteral stent.
   b. intravenous hydration, antimicrobials, and analgesics.

c. an intravenous urogram.
d. right ureteroscopy.
e. a right percutaneous nephrostomy.

9. Which of the following is NOT true of patients with tubo-ovarian abscess?

   a. The ureteral dilatation is usually unilateral.
   b. The ureteral dilatation is usually bilateral.
   c. The ureters are usually deviated laterally.
   d. The most common causative organisms are usually *Neisseria gonorrhoeae* and *Chlamydia trachomatis*.
   e. Patients may be asymptomatic.

10. In the female patient with uterine prolapse, which of the following statements is NOT true?

    a. The majority of patients have hydroureteronephrosis.
    b. Imaging of the upper urinary tracts will usually reveal bilateral hydroureteronephrosis.
    c. Hydroureteronephrosis cannot be caused by compression of the ureters by the levator ani muscles.
    d. Hydroureteronephrosis can be caused by compression of the ureters by the uterine artery and vein.
    e. Surgical correction of the uterine prolapse will usually correct the hydroureteronephrosis.

11. A 55-year-old woman has undergone a total abdominal hysterectomy and bilateral salpingo-oophorectomy for uterine fibroids. On the second postoperative day, she develops fever, left flank pain, nausea, and vomiting. An intravenous urogram demonstrates left hydroureteronephrosis with dilatation into the pelvis and a markedly delayed nephrogram. What would the best management be?

    a. A left percutaneous nephrostomy
    b. A left retrograde ureteropyelogram
    c. Placement of a left ureteral stent
    d. Exploration of the ureter and further management pending intraoperative findings
    e. Observation

12. What is the incidence of ureteral involvement causing ureterohydronephrosis in patients with abdominal aortic aneurysm and periureteral fibrosis?

    a. 2% to 5%
    b. 5% to 10%
    c. 10% to 15%
    d. 15% to 30%
    e. 50% to 70%

13. Treatment options in a patient with an abdominal aortic aneurysm, periureteral fibrosis, and bilateral ureterohydronephrosis may include all of the following except:

    a. aneurysmectomy and bilateral ureterolysis.
    b. initial stent placement to improve renal function and subsequent aneurysmectomy and ureterolysis.
    c. aneurysmectomy alone.
    d. endovascular repair with delayed ureterolysis.
    e. bilateral ureteral stent placement and subsequent endovascular repair.

14. In patients with bilateral aortobifemoral bypass graft placement, which of the following statements is true?

    a. The ureters should be positioned anterior to the graft.
    b. The ureters should be positioned posterior to the graft.
    c. Fibrosis is the primary cause of obstruction.
    d. Compression of the ureters is not a factor in the development of ureteral obstruction.
    e. Devascularization of the ureter is not a factor in the development of ureteral obstruction.

15. Circumcaval ureter is associated with all the following except:

    a. bilaterality.
    b. greater in males than females.
    c. persistence of the subcardinal vein.
    d. persistence of the supracardinal vein.
    e. presentation in the third or fourth decade of life.

16. The usual cutoff point for salvage of a renal unit is what percentage or less of total renal function supplied by that kidney?

    a. 5%
    b. 10%
    c. 15%
    d. 20%
    e. 50%

17. Nonsteroidal anti-inflammatory drugs (NSAIDs) can alleviate renal colic by all of the following mechanisms except:

    a. decreases in pain pathways.
    b. decreases in ureteric contractility.
    c. decreases in renal blood flow.
    d. inhibition of transforming growth factor-β (TGF-β) synthesis.
    e. decreases in diuresis.

18. The persistent decrease in concentrating ability of the kidney in unilateral ureteral occlusion (UUO) is primarily due to:

    a. increased tubular response to cyclic AMP.
    b. inability of proximal tubules to respond to antidiuretic hormone (ADH).
    c. inability of distal tubules to respond to ADH.
    d. increased responsiveness of tubules to ADH.
    e. decreased medullary plasma flow.

19. In classic studies of UUO, renal blood flow was shown to:

    a. increase, then steadily decrease.
    b. remain unchanged.
    c. decrease continually.
    d. increase.
    e. decrease, then steadily increase.

20. Ureteral pressure changes in experimental UUO are characterized by:

    a. an increase followed by a decrease.
    b. a sustained increase.
    c. a decrease, followed by an increase.
    d. no change.
    e. a sustained decrease.

21. The vasoconstrictive phase of UUO is characterized by:

    a. both pre- and postglomerular vasoconstriction.
    b. preglomerular vasoconstriction.
    c. postglomerular vasoconstriction.
    d. afferent arteriolar vasodilatation.
    e. none of the above.

22. Which of the following has(have) been implicated in the initial rise of renal blood flow in UUO?

    a. Eicosanoids and nitric oxide
    b. Thromboxane
    c. Angiotensin II
    d. Endothelin and nitric oxide
    e. Thromboxane and angiotensin II

23. Some investigators have implicated which of the following vasoconstrictor eicosanoids in the decrease in renal blood flow in the third phase of UUO?

a. Thromboxane
b. Prostacyclin
c. Endothelin
d. Platelet-activating factor
e. Angiotensin II

24. Interstitial fibrosis refers to the accumulation of which of the following in the kidney in UUO?

    a. Collagen
    b. Fibroblasts
    c. Insulin-like growth factor
    d. Elastic fibers
    e. Macrophages

25. In obstruction, microscopic changes in the appearance of glomeruli are:

    a. relatively minor.
    b. an immediate occurrence.
    c. significant but delayed.
    d. significant and occur over time.
    e. immediate but resolve with time.

26. Interstitial fibrosis in obstruction may result from:

    a. increased deposition of collagen.
    b. decreased collagen degradation.
    c. increased tissue inhibitor of metalloproteinase (TIMP) activity.
    d. increased TGF-β expression.
    e. all of the above.

27. Which of the following is an approach for decreasing the fibrotic process in UUO?

    a. Use of an angiotensin-converting enzyme inhibitor
    b. Use of an AT2 receptor antagonist
    c. Use of a TGF-β agonist
    d. Use of a nitric oxide synthase inhibitor
    e. Increase in intercellular adhesion molecule 1 expression

28. Nitric oxide has documented effects on all the following in UUO except:

    a. renal tubular apoptosis.
    b. renal blood flow.
    c. tubular proliferation.
    d. tubular phosphate reabsorption.
    e. macrophage infiltration.

29. Chronic bilateral ureteral obstruction (BUO) differs from chronic unilateral UUO in that:

    a. in BUO, renal blood flow goes up, whereas in UUO it goes down.
    b. in BUO, afferent arteriolar constriction does not occur, whereas it does in UUO.
    c. in BUO, ureteral pressure declines, whereas in UUO it remains elevated.
    d. in BUO, atrial natriuretic peptide is not as important as in UUO.
    e. in BUO, postobstructive diuresis is not as important as in UUO.

30. The natriuretic and diuretic actions of atrial natriuretic peptide are caused in part by:

    a. an increase in glomerular filtration rate (GFR).
    b. a decrease in GFR.
    c. a decrease in glomerular capillary ultrafiltration coefficient.
    d. stimulation of glomerular tubular feedback mechanisms.
    e. increased angiotensin II expression.

31. Postobstructive diuresis refers to the marked polyuria occurring after:

    a. BUO.
    b. complete UUO.
    c. partial UUO.
    d. acute UUO.
    e. partial obstruction of a solitary kidney.

32. Pathologic postobstructive diuresis refers to postobstructive diuresis resulting from:

    a. impaired concentrating ability.
    b. changes in aquaporin expression.
    c. increased urea.
    d. decreased prostaglandin excretion.
    e. decreased angiotensin II secretion.

33. The least common but most dangerous form of postobstructive diuresis is termed:

    a. sodium-wasting nephropathy.
    b. potassium-wasting nephropathy.
    c. pathologic sodium reabsorption.
    d. sodium-sparing nephropathy.
    e. postobstructive polyuria.

34. In a patient with normal fluid intake, the accepted definition of polyuria is urine output greater than:

    a. 3 L/day.
    b. 5 L/day.
    c. 10 L/day.
    d. 1 L/day.
    e. 8 L/day.

Answers

1. **a. Dilatation of the urinary tract.** The term *obstructive nephropathy* should be reserved for the damage to the renal parenchyma that results from an obstruction to the flow of urine anywhere along the urinary tract. The term *hydronephrosis* is derived from *hydro* (from the Greek, *hydor*, water), *nephros* (kidney), and *osis* (condition) and is therefore defined as dilatation of the renal pelvis and calyces resulting from obstruction to the flow of urine. Because dilatation of the renal pelvis and calyces can occur without obstruction, this definition is not completely accurate. Hydronephrosis should be used as a descriptive term referring simply to the presence of dilatation of the pelvis and calyces and not to the cause of that dilatation. The terms *obstructive uropathy* and *hydronephrosis* should not be used interchangeably. [p 412]

2. **d. All of the above.** When chronic obstruction is the predominant clinical picture, the urinary diagnostic indices are most often similar to those seen with acute tubular necrosis: an elevated urinary sodium concentration, a decreased urine osmolality, and a decreased urine-to-plasma creatinine ratio. If the obstruction is more acute and not accompanied by renal failure, the urinary indices can resemble those of prerenal azotemia: a low urinary sodium concentration and an increased urine osmolality. [p 413]

3. **c. Diuretic renography with technetium Tc 99m mercaptoacetyltriglycine (MAG3).** The diuretic renogram is becoming more widely utilized than excretory urography for evaluation of the dilated collecting system. It provides a noninvasive measure of the relative renal function and has the ability to wash out the radiopharmaceutical agent from the dilated collecting system. There is a marked reduction in radiation dose in comparison with excretory urography, and there is no potential for contrast material-induced nephrotoxicity. The most widely used radiopharmaceutical agents are (1) tubular tracers ortho-iodohippurate iodine 131 (OIH) and MAG3 and (2) glomerular tracers, namely DTPA. For evaluating obstruction, the radiopharmaceutical agent of choice today is MAG3, because it is more efficiently extracted by the kidney than is DTPA, it delivers a lower dose of radiation to the obstructed kidney than does OIH, and it is excreted by the same portion of the tubule that responds to furosemide. MAG3 has been shown to provide better counting statistics and visualization of the anatomy of obstruction than do OIH and other radiopharmaceutical agents. [p 414]

4. **d. Helical CT of the abdomen and pelvis without contrast enhancement.** Today, unenhanced helical CT is gaining widespread acceptance in many institutions over conventional CT. The images are obtained faster than are those in conventional CT, often in one breath hold. The axial images obtained can be used to create sagittal and/or coronal reformations, adding to the anatomic detail of the urinary tract, and the potential for stone passage. The secondary signs of obstruction on helical CT include (1) hydroureter, (2) perinephric stranding, (3) hydronephrosis, (4) periureteral edema, and (5) renal swelling. Unenhanced helical CT and conventional CT may not differentiate a uric acid stone from a calcium stone, necessitating a KUB to differentiate the stone type. [p 417]

5. **c. Results of biopsy of the retroperitoneum.** Table 12–2 is a list of the possible causes of retroperitoneal fibrosis. These diseases must be ruled out before the process can be labeled as "idiopathic" retroperitoneal fibrosis. Often, biopsy of the retroperitoneal tissue is the only way to confirm the presence or absence of these disease processes before the diagnosis of idiopathic retroperitoneal fibrosis. [p 418]

6. **a. Unilateral left ureterolysis and intraperitonealization of the ureter.** Once malignancy is excluded, ureterolysis can be performed by localizing the ureter in an uninvolved area and tracing it into the fibrotic mass. Extreme care should be taken to prevent a ureterotomy and devascularization of the ureter, as later stricture formation can be troublesome to manage. Once mobilized out of the fibrosis, the ureter can be transposed laterally in a sleeve of peritoneum, wrapped in omentum, or intraperitonealized. If unilateral ureteral involvement is demonstrated upon preoperative exploration, bilateral ureteral transposition or intraperitonealization should be performed, as the contralateral ureter will almost always become involved. Wrapping the ureter with polytetrafluoroethylene vascular graft has been reported, as has successful laparoscopic ureterolysis in six patients with retroperitoneal fibrosis. In patients who are not candidates for surgical intervention, more conservative treatment may be attempted. Once the presence of malignancy is excluded, steroid therapy can be initiated. This is done in combination with the cessation of any medication that may be causative of retroperitoneal fibrosis (methysergide or methyldopa, for example). [p 419]

7. **e. CT of the abdomen and pelvis.** The radiographic appearance of pelvic lipomatosis on an intravenous urogram can range from normal upper tracts to marked bilateral hydroureteronephrosis. Typically, the distal ureter is deviated medially, as opposed to the midureters, with a tapered appearance to the distal intramural ureter. The bladder has a pear-shaped, teardrop-shaped, or gourd-shaped appearance with an elevation of the bladder base. CT can readily diagnose pelvic lipomatosis because of its ability to identify fat, owing to the low attenuation values of fat. CT is also ideally suited for the diagnosis of pelvic lipomatosis, as it can also distinguish the other causes of the pear-shaped bladder listed in Table 12–4. CT can also eliminate the need for a barium enema. MRI can offer more details of anatomic changes resulting from the infiltration of fat into the pelvis (i.e., fat plane dissecting along Denonvilliers' fascia separating the prostate gland and rectum). However, there is little advantage in the typical clinical setting for MRI over CT. [pp 420–421]

8. **b. intravenous hydration, antimicrobials, and analgesics.** Pregnant women can experience nausea, vomiting, back pain, urinary frequency, and dysuria. Such symptoms may also result from ureteral obstruction. The ability to differentiate these symptoms in association with the hydronephrosis of pregnancy is a significant challenge to every clinical urologist. Examination of the patient's urine (preferably a catheterized specimen) with a urine culture may help differentiate obstructive renal colic from pyelonephritis. Initial treatment should consist of intravenous hydration and appropriate antimicrobial therapy, as 50% to 67% of stones will be passed spontaneously. If symptoms worsen despite conservative measures, more invasive treatment may be required, such as ureteral stent placement, percutaneous nephrostomy, or ureteroscopy, with or without lithotripsy. The diagnosis of ureteral obstruction may be aided with a one-shot intravenous pyelogram (see Fig. 12–8). However, because 1 rad of x-ray exposure increases the risk of developing childhood malignancies by 2.4-fold, it would seem prudent to avoid radiating the fetus. Other potential options for the diagnosis of obstruction may be the renal resistive index from Doppler ultrasonography, endoluminal ultrasonography, and MRI. [p 423]

9. **a. The ureteral dilatation is usually unilateral.** A review of findings on excretory urography in 44 cases of tubo-ovarian abscess found 39% associated with ureteral dilatation. The point of obstruction occurred at or just below the pelvic brim in all cases, with 53% bilateral, 35% right-sided, and 12% left-sided. Lateral deviation of the ureter occurred in 23% of the cases, whereas in 14% of the cases the ureter was deviated medially. In the majority of cases (86%), the only finding on excretory urography was a pelvic mass. The finding of medial deviation of the ureter is more characteristic of tubo-ovarian abscess than any other type of pelvic mass. For example, ovarian tumors tend to cause lateral deviation of the ureter. The most likely explanation for this finding is that the inflammation and fibrosis adjacent to the pelvic ureter encase and draw the ureter medially. Pelvic inflammatory disease is usually associated with abdominal pain, fever, and possibly nausea and vomiting. Other symptoms may include vaginal discharge, dyspareunia, and dysuria. On physical examination, there is lower abdominal tenderness, adnexal tenderness, and cervical motion tenderness. The two most common pathogens are *Neisseria gonorrhoeae* and *Chlamydia trachomatis*. Patients with *N. gonorrhoeae* infection tend to have more severe symptoms secondary to the endotoxin produced by the bacteria. Patients with tubo-ovarian abscess may not have any abdominal symptoms upon presentation. Also described were 13 of 44 patients admitted to the hospital with tubo-ovarian abscess who presented for work-up of a pelvic mass with no other signs and symptoms of acute pelvic inflammatory disease. [pp 423–424]

10. **c. Hydroureteronephrosis cannot be caused by compression of the ureters by the levator ani muscles.** One report described 8 of 10 cases of uterine prolapse with hydroureteronephrosis. In this series, 50% of the cases were unilateral and 50% were bilateral ureteral dilatation. Because the association of hydroureteronephrosis with uterine prolapse seems relatively common, imaging of the urinary tract with ultrasonography and/or intravenous urography in these patients is reasonable. This is especially true in patients with higher degrees of prolapse. There are several proposed mechanisms for the development of hydroureteronephrosis in patients with uterine prolapse. These mechanisms include (1) kinking of the urethra and urine stasis in the cystocele (hourglass formation of the bladder); (2) intramural stretching of the bladder wall with compression of the intramural ureter; (3) constriction of the ureter by the uterine artery and vein as the ureter is stretched over these vessels as a result of the descent of the uterus during prolapse; and (4) mechanical compression of the ureters against the soft tissue of the pelvis and the levator ani musculature as the bladder herniates through this muscular support. (5) An additional mechanism is constriction of the ureters by the ligaments of Mackenrodt (cardinal ligaments). The ureters course through these ligaments and with uterine descent they may pull on and constrict the ureters. The surgical correction of the uterine prolapse will improve the hydroureteronephrosis in most cases. [p 426]

11. **d. Exploration of the ureter and further management pending intraoperative findings.** If the injury is recognized intraoperatively or within 3 to 5 days of the surgical procedure, immediate repair can be performed. This may include deligation alone, deligation and ureteroureterostomy, or ureteroneocystostomy if the ligated segment appears ischemic. If the injury is discovered beyond 5 to 7 days postoperatively, placement of a ureteral stent, if possible, may be all that is needed. If unsuccessful, then placement of a percutaneous nephrostomy tube will decompress the obstructed kidney and allow future treatment to be planned. In time, the sutures may dissolve and the periureteral edema may resolve, relieving the obstruction and eliminating the need for further treatment. If these methods are unsuccessful, additional procedures such as ureteroneocystostomy, with or without a psoas hitch, or ureteroureterostomy may be performed. [p 427]

12. **d. 15% to 30%.** The incidence of ureteral involvement in patients with abdominal aortic aneurysm and perianeurysmal fibrosis is 15% to 30%. [p 428]

13. **c. aneurysmectomy alone.** The treatment options in these cases vary from observation alone to aneurysmectomy and ureterolysis. In the past, patients have been treated with observation and steroid administration to reduce the perianeurysmal fibrosis. One study postulated that the periaortic fibrosis would prevent rupture of the aneurysm. Ureterolysis was performed without resection of the aneurysm, allowing for normalization of renal function. Subsequent repair of the aneurysm can be performed at a later time, if the aneurysm increases in size. Some urologists believe that placement of ureteral stents preaneurysmectomy can be performed to improve renal function and overall patient health. Aneurysmectomy can then be performed with concomitant ureterolysis. Another group performed endovascular repair of the aneurysm with regression of fibrosis in 29%, partial regression in 57%, and no regression in 14% of the patients. Initially, they performed ureterolysis in all patients with ureteral obstruction. Subsequently, they have stented the ureters, performed an endovascular repair of the aortic aneurysm, and then removed the stents over time. Only 1 of 11 patients had recurrent ureteral obstruction, perhaps making this treatment modality more favorable in the future. The authors thought that the endovascular stent inhibits the leakage of an insoluble lipid through a thinned arterial wall secondary to atherosclerosis, which promotes perianeurysmal fibrosis. [pp 428–429]

14. **c. Fibrosis is the primary cause of obstruction.** The incidence of hydronephrosis after aortofemoral bypass surgery has been reported to be from 10% to 12%. The most common cause of obstruction is believed to be periureteral fibrosis. However, one study found the most common cause of ureteral obstruction to be compression of the ureter (73% of patients), when the ureter is positioned posterior to the graft limb. However, it was stated that although compression may be the primary cause for obstruction, fibrosis may contribute to the obstruction. Other causes of obstruction include devascularization secondary to extensive dissection and pseudoaneurysms of the vascular anastomosis. [pp 429–430]

15. **d. Persistence of the supracardinal vein.** Normally, the inferior vena cava is formed infrarenally from the supracardinal vein and suprarenally from the subcardinal vein (see Fig. 12–16). If the infrarenal vena cava is formed from the subcardinal vein, which lies ventral to the ureter, then the ureter will develop in a "retrocaval" position. The incidence of circumcaval ureter is 1 in 1000 live births. It is predominantly on the right side. When reported on the left side, it is associated with either partial or complete situs inversus or duplication of the inferior vena cava. Only two cases of a left-sided circumcaval ureter secondary to a persistent left subcardinal vein without situs inversus or caval duplication have been reported. Bilateral circumcaval ureters have also been reported. Patients will usually present in the third to fourth decade of life. The ratio is 3:1 to 4:1 male to female in cadavers, whereas circumcaval ureter occurs 2.8 times more commonly in males than females clinically. [p 431]

16. **b. 10%.** The usual cutoff point for salvage of a renal unit is 10% or less of total renal function being supplied by that kidney. [p 432]

17. **d. inhibition of transforming growth factor-β (TGF-β) synthesis.** NSAIDs have been shown to be as effective as narcotic analgesics in the treatment of colic. NSAID inhibition of eicosanoid synthesis results in decreased eicosanoid-mediated pain pathways, as well as decreases in ureteric contractility, renal pelvic and glomerular capillary pressure, and renal blood flow. [p 433]

18. **c. an inability of distal tubules to respond to ADH.** One study concluded that volume expansion was enhancing an already present defect in water reabsorption either in distal and/or deep nephrons or in collecting ducts of the obstructed kidney. Another study also described an inability of the kidney to concentrate urine after obstruction. This inability to concentrate the urine was associated with an inability of the cortical collecting tubule to respond to either ADH (vasopressin) or cyclic AMP stimulation; there was a 76% reduction in the response of the collecting tubule to either stimulus. [p 434]

19. **a. increase, then steadily decrease.** Hemodynamically, phase 1 is characterized by an initial afferent arteriole vasodilatation followed by an efferent arteriole vasoconstriction in phase 2 and afferent arteriole vasoconstriction in phase 3. The third phase of UUO, the vasoconstrictive phase, is characterized by both pre- and postglomerular vasoconstriction that reduces both renal blood flow and ureteral pressure. [p 436]

20. **a. an increase followed by a decrease.** The first phase is characterized by a rise in both ureteral pressure and renal

blood flow lasting approximately 1 to 1.5 hours. This is followed in phase 2 by a decline in renal blood flow and a continued increase in ureteral pressure lasting until the fifth hour of occlusion. The final phase ensues with a further decline in renal blood flow accompanied by a progressive decrease in ureteral pressure (see Fig. 12–19). [p 436]

21. **a. both pre- and postglomerular vasoconstriction.** The third phase of UUO, the vasoconstrictive phase, is characterized by both pre- and postglomerular vasoconstriction that reduces both renal blood flow and ureteral pressure. [p 436]

22. **a. Eicosanoids and nitric oxide.** The first studies to establish a role for eicosanoids in phase I of UUO were carried out by Allen and coworkers in 1978. They administered a bolus of indomethacin, followed by a continuous infusion for 50 minutes before and during acute UUO in conscious dogs. The intravenous administration of indomethacin caused an immediate decline in both ipsilateral and contralateral renal blood flow before obstruction. After ligation of the ipsilateral ureter, there was a further decline in renal blood flow, without the initial vasodilatation seen in the control group after acute ureteral occlusion. The contralateral renal blood flow after obstruction changed minimally from the initial decrease after the infusion of indomethacin. This decrease in renal blood flow was accompanied by a decrease in ureteral pressure. The data suggested that unopposed renovascular constriction follows from the inhibition of prostaglandin synthesis in the acute UUO model. A number of studies have examined the role of nitric oxide in the hemodynamic response to UUO. In rats, infusion of L-NAME, a nitric oxide synthase inhibitor, after 24 hours of UUO results in a decrease in renal blood flow and an increase in the ratio of renal vascular resistance to total vascular resistance. Administration of L-NMMA before UUO attenuated the initial rise in renal blood flow (see Fig. 12–21A). When the L-NMMA infusion was discontinued, the rise in renal blood flow was restored within 10 minutes. These findings provide evidence for a role of nitric oxide in reducing preglomerular vascular resistance after ureteral occlusion. [pp 437–438]

23. **a. Thromboxane.** Certain workers have implicated thromboxane A2 (TxA2) in the decreased renal blood flow associated with UUO. A decrease in the vasoconstriction post-UUO was demonstrated with administration of imidazole. DP-1904, another TxA2 synthesis inhibitor, decreased renal TxB2 production and increased the ratio of prostacyclin to TxA2 metabolites. Urine volume, glomerular filtration rate, and renal plasma flow were all improved when DP-1904 was given at 4 days after UUO. Using a TxA2 receptor blocker, GR32191, 24 hours after UUO in rats also improved renal function. [p 437]

24. **a. Collagen.** UUO is accompanied by changes in the architecture of the kidney. The most prominent interstitial change is fibrosis, the accumulation of collagens and other extracellular matrix components. [p 439]

25. **a. relatively minor.** Most of the initial microscopic changes are confined to the tubules with little effect on the glomeruli. The glomeruli seem relatively resistant to change except for a slight increase in size and a thickening of Bowman's capsule. The development of hyalinization and connective tissue proliferation are not seen until 231 days of ureteral ligation, and only in relatively few glomeruli. [p 440]

26. **e. all of the above.** In rats studied from 1 to 28 days after UUO, increases in cortical and medullary interstitial space were found; these changes were significant by 7 days after UUO. Collagen III was increased by 3 days in both cortex and medulla, and medullary collagen was further increased by 7 days after UUO. Prominent changes in collagen I were detected at 14 days after UUO. Collagen IV, laminin, and fibronectin also showed prominent changes by 3 days; these components continued to increase through 14 days. Glomerular fibrosis was not prominent, with only small changes in collagen I being found after 14 to 21 days of UUO. Collagen synthesis rates have not been measured in rats in UUO. However, collagen degradation has been examined. In rats with 15 days of UUO, collagenolytic activity of renal tissue from obstructed animals was deceased by a factor of 10 compared with normal and contralateral kidneys. The matrix metalloproteinases (MMPs) are a group of enzymes involved in the degradation of both collagen and other extracellular matrix components. The activity of the MMPs is controlled in part by inhibitors called TIMPs. Beginning at 12 hours after UUO, there was a marked increase in the expression of mRNA for TIMP-1, which continues through 4 days. TIMP-2 was unaffected and TIMP-3 gene expression was actually decreased. Thus, an increase in TIMP-1, which should inhibit the MMPs and therefore collagen degradation, could contribute to the fibrotic response. The expression of TGF-β, a profibrotic cytokine, has been extensively studied in UUO. Increased mRNA expression of TGF-β was found as early as 10 hours after obstruction and was increased through 96 hours. [pp 440–441]

27. **a. Use of an angiotensin-converting enzyme inhibitor.** Various strategies have been used to assess the role of angiotensin II in fibrosis and attempt to ameliorate it. These include angiotensin-converting enzyme inhibitors and angiotensin receptor antagonists, active at either the AT1 or AT2 subtype of angiotensin II receptors. Other constructs have been knockout mice (AT2 receptor) or transgenic mice expressing various copy numbers of the angiotensinogen gene. Decreasing the availability of angiotensin II at the AT1 receptor can be accomplished by either inhibition of angiotensin II synthesis or blockade of the AT1 receptor with specific antagonists. When activation of the AT1 receptor is decreased, fibrosis, smooth muscle A-actin, and TGF-β expression are all decreased. [p 443]

28. **d. tubular phosphate reabsorption.** The administration of arginine and angiotensin-converting enzyme inhibitors has been found to blunt the fibrotic response to UUO. Arginine is a direct precursor to nitric oxide, whereas angiotensin-converting enzyme inhibitors are thought to augment nitric oxide production indirectly by stimulating bradykinin production. Comparable evidence also exists in that the pharmacologic inhibition of nitric oxide synthase during UUO exacerbates the resulting interstitial fibrosis. In iNOS knockout mice, one study demonstrated expanded interstitial volume and increased hydroxyproline and TGF-β, as well as increased macrophage infiltration in the obstructed kidney. Another study demonstrated increased tubular apoptosis and proliferation in iNOS knockout mice. [p 444]

29. **b. in BUO, afferent arteriolar constriction does not occur, whereas it does in UUO.** The triphasic pattern of renal blood flow and ureteral pressure changes that characterizes UUO is not seen after BUO or unilateral obstruction of a solitary kidney. Renal blood flow increases after the first 90 minutes of BUO, as it does with UUO. However, between 90 minutes and 7 hours of BUO, the renal blood flow is significantly lower than the renal blood flow during the same time interval of UUO (see Fig. 12–24A). The decrease is accompanied by an increase in renal vascular resistance during BUO to a greater degree than with UUO (see Fig. 12–24B). However, by 24 hours of BUO, the renal blood flow is as low, and renal vascular resistance as high as with 24 hours of UUO (see Fig. 12–24A, B). However, ureteral

pressure is higher than in UUO. BUO passes through a phase of preglomerular vasodilatation and then a postglomerular vasoconstriction and remains in this state. This explains the progressive and persistent rise in ureteral pressure despite a decrease in renal blood flow and an increase in renal vascular resistance. [pp 445–446]

30. **a. an increase in glomerular filtration rate (GFR).** The natriuretic and diuretic actions of atrial natriuretic peptide have been shown to be caused by (1) an increase in GFR through afferent arteriole vasodilatation and efferent arteriole vasoconstriction, (2) an increase in glomerular capillary ultrafiltration coefficient, and (3) inhibition of the glomerular tubular feedback mechanism. These glomerular hemodynamic effects point to atrial natriuretic peptide as the circulating diuretic and natriuretic substance postulated by previous investigators to explain the observed changes in renal blood flow, ureteral pressure, and glomerular filtration during BUO. [p 448]

31. **a. BUO.** Postobstructive diuresis refers to the marked polyuria that occurs after relief of BUO or obstruction of a solitary kidney. [p 453]

32. **a. impaired concentrating ability.** The diuresis may be classified as physiologic, caused by retained urea, sodium, and water, or pathologic, caused by impairment of concentrating ability or sodium reabsorption. [p 453]

33. **a. sodium-wasting nephropathy.** The least common but most dangerous form of postobstructive diuresis is pathologic sodium loss, which has been termed sodium-wasting nephropathy. Dramatic fractional sodium loss has been reported; it necessitates copious sodium replacement matching output until the patient stabilizes to avoid marked volume depletion and hypotension. [p 454]

34. **a. 3 L/day.** An acceptable definition of polyuria is a urine output greater than 3 L/day in an individual not drinking large amounts of fluid. This amount should be determined through a 24-hour urine collection. [p 456]

Chapter 13

Management of Upper Urinary Tract Obstruction

Stevan B. Streem • Jenny J. Franke • Joseph A. Smith, Jr.

Questions

1. Ureteropelvic junction (UPJ) obstruction in the neonate is most frequently found as a result of:
    a. maternal-fetal ultrasonography.
    b. intravenous urography.
    c. retrograde pyelography.
    d. diuretic renography.
    e. voiding cystourethrography.

2. Which of the following studies can be diagnostic for functional obstruction at the UPJ?
    a. Retrograde pyelography
    b. Diuretic urography
    c. Diuretic renography
    d. Ultrasonography
    e. Three-dimensional helical CT

3. A 62-year-old man presents with left flank pain. Intravenous pyelography reveals delayed excretion and hydronephrosis to the level of a 2.5 cm calculus at the UPJ. Percutaneous stone extraction is accomplished without difficulty, but a postextraction nephrostogram reveals hydronephrosis to the level of the UPJ without residual stone. A follow-up nephrostogram 1 week later is unchanged. What is the next step?
    a. Removal of the nephrostomy tube
    b. Replacement of the nephrostomy tube with an internal stent
    c. Diuretic intravenous pyelography with the nephrostomy tube clamped
    d. Diuretic renography with the nephrostomy tube open
    e. The Whitaker pressure-perfusion test

4. Which of the following clinical situations is most predictive of failure after percutaneous endopyelotomy?
    a. Renal ptosis
    b. History of ipsilateral pyelonephritis
    c. Previous failed open pyeloplasty
    d. Associated renal calculi
    e. Moderate to severe hydronephrosis and crossing vessels

5. Which of the following open or laparoscopic approaches to pyeloplasty is indicated in the case of an associated aberrant crossing vessel?
    a. Foley Y-V plasty
    b. Fenger plasty
    c. Dismembered pyeloplasty
    d. Ureterocalicostomy
    e. Ligation and transection of the crossing vessel

6. A 42-year-old woman underwent left laparoscopic dismembered pyeloplasty over an internal stent. A drain was left in the retroperitoneum. On the first postoperative day, the flank is dry and the Foley catheter is removed. She is discharged home after breakfast. That evening she calls to report that "fluid is coming out of her side" at the site of the drain. What is the next step?
    a. Care by a visiting nurse for frequent dressing changes
    b. Removal of the drain
    c. Insertion of a percutaneous nephrostomy tube
    d. Removal of the internal stent
    e. Replacement of the Foley catheter

7. Of all currently available options for intervention for UPJ

obstruction, which of the following has the highest documented success rate?

   a. Cautery-wire balloon incision
   b. Ureteroscopic laser endopyelotomy
   c. Percutaneous endopyelotomy
   d. Open pyeloplasty
   e. Laparoscopic pyeloplasty

8. A 24-year-old man is referred with persistent right flank pain. His urologic history is significant in that he had undergone an open pyeloplasty 4 years earlier, with recurrence of symptoms shortly thereafter. Follow-up studies at that time showed persistent right UPJ obstruction subsequently managed with an attempt at cautery-wire balloon incision, and then percutaneous antegrade endopyelotomy, both of which failed. At this time, the left kidney is normal. A CT scan shows moderate cortical loss on the affected (right) side. A renogram is performed and reveals 31% differential function on the affected side, and a diuretic study confirms functional obstruction ($T_{1/2} > 22$ min). What is the next step?

   a. Use of a "permanent" internal stent changed every 3 to 4 months
   b. Retrograde balloon dilatation
   c. Another pyeloplasty
   d. Laparoscopic pyeloplasty
   e. Ureterocalicostomy

9. Appropriate indications for the use of a transureteroureterostomy include all of the following except:

   a. invasive adenocarcinoma of the sigmoid colon with involvement of the left distal ureter.
   b. complex urinary tract reconstruction in a 6-year-old boy with posterior urethral valves who is undergoing augmentation ureterocystoplasty.
   c. distal ureteral stricture in a 55-year-old woman status post-definitive radiotherapy for invasive squamous cell carcinoma of the cervix.
   d. gunshot wound to the right lower quadrant with extensive injury to the right distal ureter, cecum, and right lateral bladder wall.
   e. 5 cm distal ureteral stricture in a 72-year-old man with benign prostatic hyperplasia and a small-capacity, trabeculated bladder.

10. When a ureteral substitution is being performed in a patient with a small intrarenal pelvis, the surgeon should be prepared to:

    a. abort the procedure and perform a nephrectomy.
    b. place a permanent nephrostomy tube.
    c. evaluate the patient postoperatively for vitamin B_{12} deficiency.
    d. excise the lower pole parenchyma and perform an ileocalicostomy.
    e. leave a double-J stent in place for 4 months.

11. A 67-year-old man who had had a cystectomy and neobladder 18 months previously for invasive transitional cell carcinoma of the bladder presents with right flank pain, temperature of 102°F, vomiting, and tachycardia. A renal ultrasonographic study reveals moderate to severe right hydronephrosis. What is the next best step?

    a. Perform a right distal ureterectomy and reimplantation
    b. Place a percutaneous nephrostomy tube
    c. Use urine cytology to evaluate the presence of recurrent carcinoma
    d. Schedule in situ extracorporeal shock wave lithotripsy, because the patient's obstruction is likely related to a stone
    e. Convert to a nonrefluxing colon conduit, because there is a clear advantage with respect to preserving renal function

12. The most common cause of retroperitoneal fibrosis is:

    a. idiopathic.
    b. methysergide.
    c. abdominal aortic aneurysm.
    d. multifocal fibrosis.
    e. lymphoma.

13. When a psoas hitch is used, a structure particularly susceptible to injury is the:

    a. obturator nerve.
    b. superior vesicle artery.
    c. psoas minor.
    d. common iliac vein.
    e. genitofemoral nerve.

14. When a distal ureteral stricture is treated, normal bladder capacity and function are critical to the success of all the following except:

    a. ileal ureteral substitution.
    b. psoas hitch.
    c. ureteroneocystostomy.
    d. cold knife incision of the transmural ureter.
    e. extended Boari flap.

15. A 52-year-old man taking atenolol for hypertension presents with a 6-week history of vague back pain and malaise. Abdominal CT demonstrates an aortic diameter of 2.5 cm, a retroperitoneal mass surrounding the great vessels, and bilateral hydronephrosis. The patient's urine is uninfected and his renal function is normal. What is the next step?

    a. Obtain an emergency vascular surgery consultation, as he likely has a leaking abdominal aortic aneurysm
    b. Stop the atenolol, treat the hypertension with another agent, and perform a laparoscopic biopsy of the mass and ureterolysis
    c. Begin anticoagulation to prevent acute thrombosis of the inferior vena cava
    d. Perform a purified protein derivative assay and send urine culture for acid-fast bacteria analysis
    e. Perform a biopsy of a cervical lymph node to rule out lymphoma

Answers

1. **a. maternal-fetal ultrasonography.** The current widespread use of maternal ultrasonography has led to a dramatic increase in the number of asymptomatic newborns' being diagnosed with hydronephrosis, many of whom are subsequently found to have ureteropelvic junction obstruction. [p 464]

2. **c. Diuretic renography.** Provocative testing with a diuretic urogram may allow accurate diagnosis. [p 465]

3. **e. the Whitaker pressure-perfusion test.** When there remains some doubt as to the clinical significance of a dilated collecting system, placement of percutaneous nephrostomy

allows access for pressure perfusion studies. In the pressure perfusion test, as first described by Whitaker in 1973 and then modified in 1978, the renal pelvis is perfused with normal saline or dilute radiographic contrast solution, and the pressure gradient across the presumed area of obstruction is determined. Renal pelvic pressures in excess of 15 to 22 cm are highly suggestive of a functional obstruction. [p 468]

4. **e. Moderate to severe hydronephrosis and crossing vessels.** Consideration of any of the less invasive alternatives to open operative intervention must take into account individual anatomy, including, but not limited to, the degree of hydronephrosis, overall and ipsilateral renal function, and, in some cases, the presence of crossing vessels or concomitant calculi. Although the impact of crossing vessels is controversial, in our opinion, the presence of such vessels is not of and by itself a contraindication to an endopyelotomy. However, significant entanglement of the ureteropelvic junction by crossing vessels can occasionally be identified and, when present, will generally render any endourologic approach unsuccessful. [p 469]

5. **c. Dismembered pyeloplasty.** When aberrant or accessory lower pole vessels are found in association with the UPJ obstruction, a dismembered pyeloplasty allows transposition of the UPJ in relation to these vessels. [p 481]

6. **e. Replacement of the Foley catheter.** If the drain output increases after the Foley catheter has been removed, the Foley catheter should be replaced for 5 to 7 days to eliminate reflux up the stent in the treated ureter and decrease extravasation. [p 488]

7. **d. Open pyeloplasty.** Success rates with most of the alternative less invasive endourologic and laparoscopic approaches have not proved comparable to the rate achieved with standard open pyeloplasty. Open operative intervention for UPJ obstruction provides a widely patent, dependently positioned, well-funneled UPJ. The procedure has stood the test of time and offers a success rate exceeding 95%. [p 469]

8. **e. Ureterocalicostomy.** Anastomosis of the proximal ureter directly to the lower calyceal system has become a well-accepted salvage technique for the failed pyeloplasty. [p 484]

9. **c. distal ureteral stricture in a 55-year-old woman status post-definitive radiotherapy for invasive squamous cell carcinoma of the cervix.** Although the only absolute contraindications are a donor ureter that is too short to reach the contralateral ureter without kinking or tension or a diseased recipient ureter, the relative contraindications include any disease process that may affect both ureters. [p 499]

10. **d. excise the lower pole parenchyma and perform an ileocalicostomy.** In the presence of a scarred or intrarenal pelvis, ileocalicostomy may be preferable. [p 501]

11. **b. Place a percutaneous nephrostomy tube.** Percutaneous nephrostomy drainage is established, and in cases associated with infection or compromised renal function, percutaneous drainage alone is instituted to allow resolution of infection and return to baseline renal function. [p 491]

12. **a. idiopathic.** In the majority of cases, the disease is idiopathic. [p 505]

13. **e. genitofemoral nerve.** Care should be taken to avoid injury to the genitofemoral nerve when placing these sutures. [p 497]

14. **d. cold knife incision of the transmural ureter.** As indicated in the individual sections on these procedures, normal bladder function is essential to the success of ileal ureteral substitution, psoas hitch, Boari flap, and ureteroneocystostomy. [pp 496–499, 500]

15. **b. Stop the atenolol, treat the hypertension with another agent, and perform a laparoscopic biopsy of the mass and ureterolysis.** All patients taking methysergide or any other potentially inciting drug should discontinue it. On occasion, a patient with drug-induced retroperitoneal fibrosis and mild hydronephrosis will improve with discontinuation alone. Clearly, the most definitive means of ruling out malignancy and providing long-term relief of obstruction is biopsy of the mass and ureterolysis. [p 506]

SECTION IV

INFECTIONS AND INFLAMMATIONS OF THE GENITOURINARY TRACT

Chapter 14

Infections of the Urinary Tract

Anthony J. Schaeffer

Questions

1. Acute pyelonephritis is best diagnosed by:
   a. chills, fever, and flank pain.
   b. bacteriuria and pyuria.
   c. focal scar in renal cortex.
   d. delayed renal function.
   e. vesicoureteral reflux.

2. Which one of the following statements is true of nosocomial health care–associated urinary tract infections?
   a. They occur in patients who are hospitalized or institutionalized.
   b. They are caused by common fecal bacteria that are susceptible to most antimicrobials.
   c. They can be suppressed by low-dose antimicrobial therapy.
   d. They are due to reinfection.
   e. They are due to bacterial persistence.

3. The most common cause of unresolved bacteriuria during antimicrobial therapy is:
   a. development of bacterial resistance.
   b. rapid reinfections.
   c. azotemia.
   d. giant staghorn calculi.
   e. initial bacterial resistance.

4. Most recurrent infections in female patients are:
   a. complicated.
   b. reinfections.
   c. due to bacterial persistence.
   d. hereditary.
   e. surgically correctable.

5. Rates of reinfection (i.e., time to recurrence) are influenced by:
   a. bladder dysfunction.
   b. renal scarring.
   c. vesicoureteral reflux.
   d. antimicrobial treatment.
   e. age.

6. Approximately 10% of symptomatic lower urinary tract infections in young, sexually active female patients are caused by:
   a. *Escherichia coli*.
   b. *Staphylococcus saprophyticus*.
   c. *Pseudomonas*.
   d. *Proteus mirabilis*.
   e. *Staphylococcus epidermidis*.

7. The most important bacterial virulence factor is:
   a. hemolysin.
   b. K antigen.
   c. pili.
   d. colicin production.
   e. O serogroup.

8. Phase variation of bacterial pili:
   a. occurs only in vitro.
   b. affects bacterial virulence.
   c. is characteristic of pyelonephritic *E. coli*.
   d. is irreversible.
   e. refers to change in pili length.

9. The first demonstrable biologic difference that has been shown in women susceptible to urinary tract infections is:
   a. increased adherence of bacteria to vaginal cells.
   b. decreased estrogen concentration in vaginal cells.
   c. elevated vaginal pH.
   d. nonsecretor status.
   e. postmenopausal status.

10. The primary bladder defense is:
    a. low urine pH.
    b. low urine osmolarity.
    c. voiding.
    d. Tamm-Horsfall protein (uromucoid).
    e. vaginal mucus.

11. The most reliable urine specimen is obtained by:
    a. urethral catheterization.
    b. catheter aspiration.
    c. midstream voiding.
    d. suprapubic aspiration.
    e. antiseptic periurethral preparation.

12. The validity of a midstream urine specimen should be questioned if microscopy reveals:
    a. squamous epithelial cells.
    b. red blood cells.
    c. bacteria.

59

d. white blood cells.
e. casts.

13. Rapid screening methods for detecting urinary tract infections should be used primarily for:
    a. low-risk asymptomatic patients.
    b. pregnant women.
    c. children.
    d. catheterized patients.
    e. elderly patients.

14. The most accurate test for evaluation of infection in the kidney is:
    a. the Fairley bladder washout test.
    b. ureteral catheterization.
    c. gallium scanning.
    d. CT.
    e. the antibody-coated bacteria test.

15. Urinary tract imaging is NOT usually indicated for recurrent urinary tract infections in:
    a. women.
    b. girls.
    c. men.
    d. boys.
    e. spinal cord injury patients.

16. The most sensitive imaging modality for diagnosing renal abscess is:
    a. ultrasonography.
    b. indium scanning.
    c. gallium scanning.
    d. excretory urography.
    e. CT.

17. Cure of urinary tract infections depends most on antimicrobial:
    a. serum half-life.
    b. serum level.
    c. urine level.
    d. duration of therapy.
    e. frequency of therapy.

18. During the past 5 years, the least development of antimicrobial resistance has been observed for:
    a. ampicillin.
    b. cephalosporins.
    c. nitrofurantoin.
    d. fluoroquinolones.
    e. trimethoprim-sulfamethoxazole (TMP-SMX).

19. The ideal class of drugs for empirical treatment of uncomplicated urinary tract infections is:
    a. aminopenicillins.
    b. aminoglycosides.
    c. fluoroquinolones.
    d. cephalosporins.
    e. nitrofurantoins.

20. The optimal duration of antimicrobial therapy for symptomatic acute uncomplicated cystitis in women is:
    a. 1 day.
    b. 3 days.
    c. 7 days.
    d. 14 days.
    e. 21 days.

21. The optimal antimicrobial for treatment of acute uncomplicated pyelonephritis in women is:
    a. TMP-SMX.
    b. cephalosporin.
    c. aminoglycoside.
    d. fluoroquinolone.
    e. nitrofurantoin.

22. Antimicrobial prophylaxis for transurethral procedures is not indicated for patients with:
    a. valvular heart disease.
    b. prosthetic valves.
    c. unknown urine culture.
    d. sterile urine.
    e. indwelling catheter.

23. Treatment of asymptomatic bacteriuria is indicated for patients who are:
    a. elderly.
    b. catheterized.
    c. pregnant.
    d. confused.
    e. incontinent.

24. The most common predisposing factor for hospital-acquired urinary tract infections is:
    a. surgery.
    b. antimicrobial use.
    c. age.
    d. catheterization.
    e. diabetes mellitus.

25. The most effective measure for reducing catheter-associated urinary tract infection is:
    a. closed drainage.
    b. antimicrobial prophylaxis.
    c. catheter irrigation.
    d. intermittent catheterization.
    e. daily meatal care.

26. The most significant sequela of renal papillary necrosis is renal:
    a. failure.
    b. abscess.
    c. obstruction.
    d. stone.
    e. cancer.

27. The most common cause of acute pyelonephritis in young women is:
    a. vesicoureteral reflux.
    b. P-piliated bacteria.
    c. type 1 piliated bacteria.
    d. recurrent urinary tract infections.
    e. bacterial endotoxin.

28. A patient with acute pyelonephritis, persistent fever, and flank pain for 24 hours warrants:
    a. observation.
    b. CT.
    c. change in antimicrobial therapy.
    d. ultrasonography.
    e. blood cultures.

29. Most patients with chronic pyelonephritis present with:
    a. hypertension.
    b. renal failure.
    c. chronic infection.
    d. flank pain.
    e. no symptoms.

30. The overall mortality rate in emphysematous pyelonephritis is approximately:

    a. 5%.
    b. 10%.
    c. 20%.
    d. 40%.
    e. 60%.

31. In chronic renal abscess, the predominant urographic abnormality is:

    a. calyceal distortion.
    b. renal mass.
    c. calculi.
    d. hydronephrosis.
    e. calyceal amputation.

32. The high mortality rate associated with perinephric abscess is primarily attributed to:

    a. bacterial hemolysis.
    b. diabetes mellitus.
    c. delay in diagnosis.
    d. inappropriate antimicrobial therapy.
    e. inadequate drainage.

33. The primary treatment for a small perirenal abscess in a functioning kidney is:

    a. nephrectomy.
    b. partial nephrectomy.
    c. open surgical drainage.
    d. percutaneous drainage.
    e. retrograde ureteral drainage.

34. The most common bacterial cause of xanthogranulomatous pyelonephritis is:

    a. *E. coli.*
    b. *Pseudomonas.*
    c. *Klebsiella.*
    d. *P. mirabilis.*
    e. *Staphylococcus.*

35. It is hypothesized that the nidus for the Michaelis-Gutmann body is:

    a. renal papillae.
    b. bacterial fragments.
    c. calcium crystals.
    d. macrophages.
    e. uric acid stones.

36. Echinococcosis is rare in/among:

    a. the former Soviet Union.
    b. Eskimos.
    c. Native Americans.
    d. the United States.
    e. Eastern Europe.

37. The prime initiator of bacterial septic shock is:

    a. pili.
    b. lipid A.
    c. exotoxin.
    d. O-side chains.
    e. core oligosaccharides.

38. The most reliable early clinical indicator of septicemia is:

    a. chills.
    b. fever.
    c. hyperventilation.
    d. lethargy.
    e. change in mental status.

39. Urine culture is not routinely recommended for the clinical diagnosis of acute cystitis in:

    a. young women.
    b. elderly women.
    c. children.
    d. men.
    e. patients with hematuria.

40. The drug of choice for uncomplicated cystitis in most young women is:

    a. TMP-SMX.
    b. fluoroquinolone.
    c. penicillin.
    d. cephalosporin.
    e. nitrofurantoin.

41. Nitrofurantoin prophylaxis is effective because of the concentration of the drug in the:

    a. urine.
    b. vaginal mucus.
    c. bowel.
    d. serum.
    e. bladder.

42. The ideal antimicrobial for self-start therapy for a urinary tract infection is:

    a. fluoroquinolone.
    b. cephalosporin.
    c. nitrofurantoin.
    d. TMP-SMX.
    e. tetracycline.

43. Screening for bacteriuria is beneficial in:

    a. pregnant women.
    b. elderly patients.
    c. men.
    d. children.
    e. spinal cord injury patients.

44. Compared with nonpregnant women, pregnant women have a higher prevalence and increased risk from:

    a. asymptomatic bacteriuria.
    b. acute cystitis.
    c. acute pyelonephritis.
    d. recurrent cystitis.
    e. bacterial persistence.

45. Clinical pyelonephritis during pregnancy is most commonly linked to:

    a. maternal sepsis.
    b. maternal anemia.
    c. maternal hypertension.
    d. eclampsia.
    e. congenital malformations.

46. The drug thought to be safe in any phase of pregnancy is:

    a. fluoroquinolone.
    b. nitrofurantoin.
    c. sulfonamide.
    d. penicillin.
    e. tetracycline.

47. The majority of elderly patients with bacteriuria are:

    a. asymptomatic.
    b. febrile.
    c. incontinent.
    d. confused.
    e. dysuric.

62   INFECTIONS AND INFLAMMATIONS OF THE GENITOURINARY TRACT

48. In the absence of obstruction, treatment of asymptomatic bacteriuria in the elderly:

    a. is cost-effective.
    b. prevents renal failure.
    c. reduces mortality.
    d. reduces morbidity.
    e. is unnecessary.

49. In spinal cord injury patients, the bladder drainage technique with the lowest complication rate is:

    a. clean intermittent catheterization.
    b. suprapubic drainage.
    c. indwelling catheter.
    d. condom catheter.
    e. suprapubic pressure.

50. Fournier's gangrene is not associated with scrotal:

    a. pain.
    b. discharge.
    c. crepitation.
    d. erythema.
    e. swelling.

Answers

1. **a. chills, fever, and flank pain.** Acute pyelonephritis is a clinical syndrome of chills, fever, and flank pain that is accompanied by bacteriuria and pyuria, a combination that is reasonably specific for an acute bacterial infection of the kidney. [p 516]

2. **a. They occur in patients who are hospitalized or institutionalized.** Nosocomial or health care–associated urinary tract infections occur in patients who are hospitalized or institutionalized and are caused by *Pseudomonas* and other more antimicrobial-resistant strains. [p 517]

3. **e. initial bacterial resistance.** The most common cause is that the infecting organisms are resistant to the antimicrobial agent selected to treat the infection. [p 518]

4. **b. reinfections.** More than 95% of all recurrent infections in females are reinfections of the urinary tract. [p 519]

5. **d. antimicrobial treatment.** Whether a patient receives no treatment at all, or short-term, long-term, or prophylactic antimicrobial treatment, the risk of recurrent bacteriuria remains the same; antimicrobial treatment appears to alter only the time until recurrence. [p 521]

6. **b. *Staphylococcus saprophyticus*.** *S. saprophyticus* is now recognized as causing approximately 10% of symptomatic lower urinary tract infections in young, sexually active female patients, whereas it rarely causes infection in males and elderly individuals. [p 523]

7. **c. pili.** The bacterial cell structures that seem to be most important for binding of bacteria to epithelial cells are long, filamentous protein appendages called pili or fimbriae. [p 524]

8. **b. affects bacterial virulence.** This process is called phase variation and has obvious biologic and clinical implications. For example, the presence of type 1 pili may be advantageous to the bacteria for adhering to and colonizing the bladder mucosa, but disadvantageous because the pili enhance phagocytosis and killing by neutrophils. [p 525]

9. **a. increased adherence of bacteria to vaginal cells.** These studies established increased adherence of pathogenic bacteria to vaginal epithelial cells as the first demonstrable biologic difference that could be shown in women susceptible to urinary tract infections. [p 526]

10. **c. voiding.** Flow of urine through the urinary tract and voiding are the primary bladder defenses against infection. [p 529]

11. **d. suprapubic aspiration.** A single aspirated specimen reveals the bacteriologic status of the bladder urine without introducing urethral bacteria, which can start a new infection. [p 529]

12. **a. squamous epithelial cells.** The validation of the midstream urine specimen can be questioned if numerous squamous epithelial cells (indicative of preputial, vaginal, or urethral contaminants) are present. [p 531]

13. **a. low-risk asymptomatic patients.** Indirect tests are most useful for screening the urine of asymptomatic patients. [p 531]

14. **b. ureteral catheterization.** Ureteral catheterization allows not only separation of bacterial persistence into upper and lower urinary tracts but also separation of the infection between one kidney and the other. [p 532]

15. **a. women.** Several reports of women patients with recurrent urinary tract infections show, however, that excretory urograms are unnecessary for routine evaluation if women who have special risk factors are excluded. [p 536]

16. **e. CT.** CT and MRI are more sensitive than excretory urography or ultrasonography in the diagnosis of acute focal bacterial nephritis and renal and perirenal abscesses. [p 536]

17. **c. urine level.** The cure of urinary tract infection depends on the antimicrobial levels achieved in the urine, not in the serum. [p 537]

18. **c. nitrofurantoin.** During a 5-year period, the prevalence of resistance to TMP-SMX, ampicillin, and cephalothin increased significantly, whereas resistance to nitrofurantoin and ciprofloxacin remained low. [p 538]

19. **c. fluoroquinolones.** The fluoroquinolones have a broad spectrum of activity that makes them ideal for the empirical treatment of urinary tract infection. [p 541]

20. **b. 3 days.** Compared with 7 or 10 days of therapy, 3-day therapy appears to be optimal because there is no difference in cure rates, side effects are reduced, and the cost is decreased. [p 542]

21. **d. fluoroquinolone.** For patients with outpatient-acquired infections who are sufficiently ill to require hospitalization, a parenteral fluoroquinolone, an aminoglycoside, or an extended-spectrum cephalosporin is recommended. [pp 543–544]

22. **d. sterile urine.** Patients who are known preoperatively to have urinary tract infections should have the infections eradicated before the procedure is started; hence, in these patients, preoperative antimicrobials are therapeutic and not prophylactic. [p 544]

23. **c. pregnant.** Patients at risk for increased morbidity from bacteriuria, such as patients with severe diabetes, pregnant women, and others, should be treated. [p 546]

24. **d. catheterization.** The most common site of hospital-ac-

quired infections is the urinary tract, where approximately 40% of all hospital-acquired infections occur. The most common predisposing factor for these infections is urethral instrumentation, including catheterization. In fact, between 10% and 15% of all hospitalized patients have indwelling catheters. [pp 548–549]

25. **a. closed drainage.** With the advent of closed drainage systems, the average daily rate of acquired bacteriuria has decreased to 4% in males and 10.4% in females (about half the patients received antibiotics with the insertion of the catheter). [p 549]

26. **c. obstruction.** A patient who suffers from an acute ureteral obstruction caused by a sloughed papilla and who has a concomitant urinary tract infection represents a urologic emergency. [p 550]

27. **b. P-piliated bacteria.** If vesicoureteral reflux is absent, a patient bearing the P blood group phenotype may have special susceptibility to recurrent pyelonephritis caused by *E. coli* that have P pili and bind to the P blood group antigen receptors. [p 552]

28. **a. observation.** Most patients have persistent fever and flank pain for several days after initiation of successful antimicrobial therapy. They should be observed; if symptoms persist beyond 72 hours, however, the possibility of perinephric or intrarenal abscesses, urinary tract abnormalities, or obstruction should be considered and radiologic investigation with ultrasonography or CT should be performed. [p 553]

29. **e. no symptoms.** Even when a patient has a radiographically scarred, shrunken kidney with microscopic evidence of inflammation, there is often no recent or remote history of urinary tract infection and no sign of viable bacteria. [p 554]

30. **d. 40%.** Emphysematous pyelonephritis should be considered a complication of severe pyelonephritis rather than a distinct entity. The overall mortality rate is 43%. [p 556]

31. **b. renal mass.** In a more chronic abscess, the predominant urographic abnormalities are those of a renal mass lesion. [p 558]

32. **c. delay in diagnosis.** The mortality rate from perinephric abscesses, as high as 56%, is caused in part by the long delay in making the diagnosis. [pp 560–561]

33. **d. percutaneous drainage.** Although surgical drainage, or nephrectomy if the kidney is nonfunctioning or severely infected, is the classic treatment for perinephric abscesses, renal sonography and CT make percutaneous aspiration and drainage of small perirenal collections possible. [p 562]

34. **d. *P. mirabilis*.** Although review of the literature shows *Proteus* to be the most common organism involved with xanthogranulomatous pyelonephritis, *E. coli* is also common. [p 564]

35. **b. bacterial fragments.** It is hypothesized that bacteria or bacterial fragments form the nidus for the calcium phosphate crystals that laminate the Michaelis-Gutmann bodies. [p 565]

36. **d. the United States.** In the United States the disease is rare, but it is found in immigrants from Eastern Europe or other endemic areas abroad or as an indigenous infection among Native Americans in the Southwest United States and in Eskimos. [p 566]

37. **b. lipid A.** Lipid A, which is bound to the core oligosaccharide, has a highly conserved structure and is responsible for most of the toxicity of endotoxin. [pp 568–569]

38. **c. hyperventilation.** Even before temperature elevation and the onset of chills, bacteremic patients often begin to hyperventilate. Thus, the earliest metabolic change in septicemia is a resultant respiratory alkalosis. [p 570]

39. **a. young women.** In women with symptoms and signs suggesting acute cystitis, and in whom no complicating factors are judged to be present, a urinalysis that is positive for pyuria, hematuria, or bacteriuria or a combination should provide sufficient documentation of urinary tract infections, and a urine culture may be omitted. [pp 573–574]

40. **a. TMP-SMX.** TMP-SMX and TMP are now recommended in areas where the prevalence of resistance to these drugs among *E. coli* strains causing cystitis is less than 20%. [p 574]

41. **a. urine.** Nitrofurantoin, which does not alter the gut flora, is present for brief periods at high concentrations in the urine and leads to repeated elimination of bacteria from the urine, presumably by interfering with bacterial initiation of infection. [p 576]

42. **a. fluoroquinolone.** Fluoroquinolones are ideal for self-start therapy because they have a spectrum of activity broader than that of any of the other oral agents and are superior to many parenteral antimicrobials, including aminoglycosides. [p 578]

43. **a. pregnant women.** Screening for bacteriuria in the first trimester of pregnancy probably represents the only time that screening for bacteriuria in adult women is worthwhile. [p 580]

44. **c. acute pyelonephritis.** The incidence of acute clinical pyelonephritis in pregnant women with bacteriuria is significantly increased compared with that in nonpregnant women. [p 582]

45. **a. maternal sepsis.** Whether clinical pyelonephritis during pregnancy causes an increased risk of prematurity is still unclear, but bacteriuria in the symptomatic or asymptomatic pregnant woman should be treated to avoid pyelonephritis and its possible sequelae, such as sepsis, in the mother. [p 583]

46. **d. penicillin.** Only the penicillins (penicillin, ampicillin, and synthetic penicillins) and cephalosporins, given orally or parenterally, are thought to be safe and effective during any phase of pregnancy. [p 585]

47. **a. asymptomatic.** The majority of elderly subjects with bacteriuria have no urinary tract symptoms. However, other symptoms such as lethargy, confusion, anorexia, and incontinence may be caused by bacteriuria and lead to missed or delayed diagnosis and increased morbidity and mortality. [pp 586–587]

48. **e. is unnecessary.** Until it is determined that elimination of asymptomatic bacteriuria is cost-effective and risk-beneficial and decreases morbidity or lengthens survival, treatment of asymptomatic bacteriuria in the absence of obstruction does not appear to be warranted. [p 588]

49. **a. clean intermittent catheterization.** Although never rigorously compared with indwelling urethral catheterization, clean intermittent catheterization has been shown to decrease lower urinary tract complications by maintaining low intravesical pressure and reducing the incidence of stones. [p 589]

50. **b. discharge.** Early in the course of the illness, the involved area is swollen, erythematous, and tender as the infection begins to involve the deep fascia. Pain is prominent, and fever and systemic toxicity are marked. The swelling and crepitus of the scrotum quickly increase, and dark purple areas develop and progress to extensive gangrene. [pp 590–591]

Chapter 15

Prostatitis and Related Conditions

J. Curtis Nickel

Questions

1. The incidence of chronic prostatitis (diagnoses/symptoms) in population-based studies is approximately:

   a. 1%.
   b. 10%.
   c. 20%.
   d. 30%.
   e. 40%.

2. Which of the following etiologic agents or mechanisms has been definitely confirmed to be associated with prostatic inflammation?

   a. Intraprostatic ductal reflux
   b. Bladder outlet obstruction
   c. Uric acid/urate
   d. Autoimmunity
   e. Enterobacteriaceae spp.

3. The most likely candidate for cryptic infection in category III prostatitis is:

   a. *Chlamydia*.
   b. *Mycoplasma*.
   c. *Corynebacterium*.
   d. coagulase-negative staphylococci.
   e. unknown.

4. The presence of white blood cells (WBCs) in the expressed prostatic secretion (EPS) of patients with category III chronic pelvic pain syndrome (CPPS):

   a. confirms significant prostatic inflammation.
   b. is important only at 10 WBC/hpf.
   c. differentiates category IIIA from category IIIB CPPS.
   d. predicts treatment outcomes.
   e. differentiates CPPS patients from control patients.

5. What is the National Institutes of Health Chronic Prostatitis Symptom Index?

   a. A research tool that is useful only in clinical trials
   b. A tool that is useful for following patients in clinical practice
   c. A tool that can differentiate the various categories of prostatitis
   d. A tool that is useful for the diagnosis of chronic prostatitis
   e. Another invalidated and unreliable clinical symptom index

6. An obese 26-year-old man has an 8-hour history of severe dysuria, stranguria, and suprapubic and perineal pain with fever. On examination, he has suprapubic tenderness, and his prostate is enlarged, boggy, and exquisitely tender. Urinalysis shows pyuria. He continues to complain of symptoms despite insertion of a Foley catheter and has persistent fever following 30 hours of intravenous gentamicin and ampicillin. Culture grew *Escherichia coli*. What is the best next step?

   a. Change antibiotic to a third-generation cephalosporin
   b. Change antibiotic to intravenous ciprofloxacin
   c. Insert a suprapubic tube
   d. Perform an abdominal ultrasonographic examination
   e. Perform a transrectal ultrasonographic examination

7. A 36-year-old man has a 4-month history of dull perineal and suprapubic discomfort, postejaculatory pain, and moderate obstructive voiding symptoms. A preprostatic massage urine sample was sterile, and microscopic evaluation of the sediment showed 2 WBC/hpf. No EPS was obtained during an uncomfortable digital rectal examination. A postprostatic massage urine sample grew 10^2 *Staphylococcus epidermidis* organisms per milliliter, and microscopy of the sediment showed 10 to 12 WBC/hpf. What is the NIH chronic prostatitis (CP)/CPPS classification?

   a. Category I
   b. Category II
   c. Category IIIA
   d. Category IIIB
   e. Category IV

8. A 24-year-old man has an 8-month history of obstructive voiding symptoms and perineal and ejaculatory discomfort. A preprostatic massage urine sample was sterile, and microscopic evaluation of sediment showed 1 WBC/hpf. Microscopy of a minute amount of EPS showed 3 WBC/hpf. A postprostatic massage urine sample was sterile, and microscopy of the sediment showed 2 WBC/hpf. What is the CP/CPPS classification?

   a. Category I
   b. Category II
   c. Category IIIA
   d. Category IIIB
   e. Category IV

9. A 42-year-old man was treated for cystitis but continued to have dysuria, ejaculatory pain, and perineal/testicular discomfort after 7 days of antibiotics. The prostate examination was unremarkable. A midstream urine sample was sterile, but culture of a drop of EPS produced moderate growth of *Enterococcus faecalis*. A postprostatic massage urine sample grew 10^2 *E. faecalis* organisms, and microscopic examination of the sediment showed 12 WBC/hpf. What is the CP/CPPS classification?

   a. Category I
   b. Category II
   c. Category IIIA
   d. Category IIIB
   e. Category IV

10. A 32-year-old man had been successfully treated for an *E. coli* cystitis with trimethoprim-sulfamethoxazole (7-day course) 4 months previously. A recurrence of similar symptoms was again successfully treated with ciprofloxacin (3 days), but no culture was done at this time. The patient presents 3 days after antibiotics were discontinued with continued perineal discomfort, ejaculatory pain, and mild dys-

uria. Pre- and postprostatic massage urine and EPS samples were sterile. Evaluation of the EPS showed 20 WBC/hpf. The prostate felt normal. What is the next best step?

a. Treat with anti-inflammatory agents
b. Wait 4 weeks and repeat the lower urinary tract evaluation
c. Treat with 3 days of nitrofurantoin and then repeat the lower urinary tract evaluation
d. Restart ciprofloxacin and continue therapy for 4 weeks
e. Do a standard Meares/Stamey 4-glass test

11. A 47-year-old man has a 5-year history of perineal and suprapubic pain/discomfort and obstructive voiding symptoms that has not responded to multiple courses of antibiotics, α blockers, anti-inflammatory agents, repetitive prostatic massage, or phytotherapy. The prostate is tender, and the postprostatic massage urine sample was sterile and showed 20 WBC/hpf. The prostate-specific antigen (PSA) value was 1.2 mg/ml. What is the next best step?

a. Incision of bladder neck
b. Transurethral microwave thermal therapy
c. Transrectal ultrasonography
d. Prostate biopsy for culture and histology
e. Video-urodynamics

12. A 28-year-old man has been successfully treated for three episodes of cystitis (cultures not performed). He now presents with a 3-day history of frequency, urgency, dysuria, and suprapubic discomfort. The prostate feels normal and is nontender. An abdominal and pelvic ultrasonographic study had normal results. A midstream culture done 24 hours earlier by his family physician grew 10^5 *E. coli* organisms per milliliter. What is the next best step?

a. A lower urinary tract localization test (2- or 4-glass test)
b. Several days of nitrofurantoin therapy followed by a lower urinary tract localization test (2- or 4-glass test)
c. Fluoroquinolone therapy for 7 days
d. Fluoroquinolone therapy for 4 weeks
e. Transrectal ultrasonography

13. A 37-year-old man has a 3-month history of urinary frequency and urgency and discomfort localized to the perineum, suprapubic area, testicles, and penis. A sterile postprostatic massage urine sample showed 15 WBC/hpf on microscopy. A year earlier, the patient had been successfully treated for moderately severe symptoms with an unspecified antibiotic. He is allergic to many medications, including ciprofloxacin. The symptoms are now a significant bother and affecting his quality of life. The best initial treatment is a trial of:

a. anti-inflammatory agents.
b. nitrofurantoin.
c. trimethoprim-sulfamethoxazole.
d. trimethoprim.
e. tetracycline.

14. A 58-year-old man with a 2-year history of symptomatic recurrent urinary tract infections with *Pseudomonas* (6 to 8 per year) is asymptomatic between treated episodes. *Pseudomonas aeruginosa* is localized to the EPS and postprostatic massage (voided bladder 3, VB3) samples (but not the midstream urine sample, or VB2) during a period when he was asymptomatic. The EPS shows severe pyuria with WBC plugs or aggregates on microscopy. Transrectal ultrasonography shows extensive prostatic calcifications. Cystoscopy results are normal, residual urine is negligible, and the PSA value is 1.0 mg/ml. What is the best treatment?

a. Low-dose prophylactic antibiotics
b. Radical transurethral resection of the prostate (TURP)
c. Radical prostatectomy
d. Repetitive prostatic massage and antibiotics
e. Intraprostatic antibiotic injection

15. A 24-year-old man with a 6-year history of severe perineal pain with irritative and obstructive voiding symptoms has no significant benefits with trimethoprim-sulfamethoxazole, anti-inflammatory agents, α blockers, or phytotherapy. Prostate-specific specimens were sterile and no WBCs were noted on microscopy. The physical examination had normal findings except for anal sphincter spasm and a tender but normal-feeling prostate gland. Video-urodynamics showed a bladder neck/proximal urethra region that opened minimally with detrusor contraction. What is the next best step?

a. 4 weeks of fluoroquinolone therapy
b. Narcotic analgesia
c. Pentosan polysulfate
d. Biofeedback
e. Bladder neck incision

16. A 52-year-old man continues to have high, spiking fever despite suprapubic catheterization and 36 hours of treatment with wide-spectrum intravenous antibiotics. Transrectal ultrasonography confirms a large prostatic abscess. What is the next best step?

a. Transperineal drainage
b. Transrectal drainage
c. Transurethral drainage
d. Percutaneous needle aspiration
e. Transrectal aspiration

17. Clinical improvement has been demonstrated with α blocker therapy in which of the following NIH categories of CP/CPPS?

a. Category II
b. Category IIIA
c. Category IIIB
d. Categories II and III
e. Categories II and IIIA

18. Which of the following is the only therapy that has NOT been evaluated against placebo in a randomized control trial for chronic prostatitis?

a. Finasteride
b. α Blockers
c. Antibiotics
d. Pentosanpolysulfate
e. Allopurinol

19. An asymptomatic 65-year-old man undergoes a prostate biopsy because of an indistinct prostate nodule. The PSA value is 2.2 ng/ml. Pathology reveals extensive glandular and periglandular infiltration with acute and chronic inflammatory cells. What is the next best step?

a. Observation
b. Repeat biopsy with culture
c. Lower urinary tract localization studies
d. Four weeks of antibiotic therapy
e. Cystoscopy

20. Which of the following invasive procedures has been shown to have efficacy compared with placebo-sham therapy in CP/CPPS?

a. Radical TURP
b. Radical prostatectomy
c. Microwave heat therapy
d. Transurethral laser therapy
e. Transurethral balloon dilatation of prostate/bladder neck

Answers

1. **b. 10%.** In a study of an Olmsted County community-based cohort (2113 men from July 1992 through February 1996, a median of 50 months of follow-up) in Minnesota, the overall prevalence of a physician's diagnosis of prostatitis was 11%. Also, in a Lennox and Addington County study in Canada, 9.7% of male respondents, aged 20 to 74 years, reported pain/discomfort in the perineum and/or with ejaculation, plus a total pain score (possible 0 to 21) of greater than or equal to 4. This location and level of pain would be sufficient to lead most physicians to make a diagnosis of chronic prostatitis. [p 604]

2. **e. Enterobacteriaceae spp.** The most common cause of bacterial prostatitis is the Enterobacteriaceae family of gram-negative bacteria. [p 605]

3. **e. unknown.** A careful review of the evidence for and against the role of microorganisms—culturable, fastidious, or nonculturable—leaves the reviewer undecided, and etiologic mechanisms other than microorganisms must be considered. [p 607]

4. **c. differentiates category IIIA from category IIIB CPPS.** The differentiation of the two subtypes of category III CPPS is dependent on cytologic examination of the urine and/or EPS. [p 615]

5. **b. A tool that is useful for following patients in clinical practice.** The National Institutes of Health Chronic Prostatitis Collaborative Research Network developed a reproducible and valid instrument to measure the symptoms and quality of life/impact of chronic prostatitis for use in research protocols as well as in clinical practice. The symptom index has also proved its usefulness in the evaluation and follow-up of patients in general clinical urologic practice. [p 612]

6. **e. Perform a transrectal ultrasonographic examination.** Development of a prostate abscess is best detected with transrectal ultrasonography. Patients with acute bacterial prostatitis are easily diagnosed and successfully treated with appropriate antibiotic therapy, as long as the clinician keeps a high index of suspicion for prostate abscess in patients who fail to respond quickly to the antibiotics. [p 623]

7. **c. Category IIIA.** Diagnosis of category IIIA CP/CPPS, or inflammatory CPPS, is based on the presence of excessive leukocytes in EPS, a postprostatic massage urine sample, or semen. [p 610]

8. **d. Category IIIB.** Diagnosis of category IIIB CP/CPPS, or noninflammatory CPPS, rests on no significant leukocytes being found in similar specimens. [p 610]

9. **b. Category II.** Category I is identical to the acute bacterial prostatitis category of the traditional classification system. Category II is identical to the traditional chronic bacterial prostatitis classification. [p 610]

10. **d. Restart ciprofloxacin and continue therapy for 4 weeks.** The most important clue in the diagnosis of category II, chronic bacterial prostatitis, is a history of documented recurrent urinary tract infections. [p 611]

11. **e. Video-urodynamics.** A wide constellation of irritative and obstructive voiding symptoms is associated with CP/CPPS. Proposed etiologies to account for the persistent irritative and obstructive voiding symptoms include detrusor vesical neck or external sphincter dyssynergia, proximal or distal urethral obstruction, and fibrosis or hypertrophy of the vesical neck. These abnormalities can be clarified and diagnosed by urodynamics, particularly video-urodynamics. [p 616]

12. **b. Several days of nitrofurantoin therapy followed by a lower urinary tract localization test (2- or 4-glass test).** In a patient who has acute cystitis, the localization of bacteria in the EPS or VB3 specimen (postprostatic massage sample) is impossible, and, in this case, the patient can be treated with a short course (1–3 days) of antibiotics such as nitrofurantoin, which penetrates the prostate poorly but eradicates the bladder bacteriuria. Subsequent localization of bacteria in the postprostatic massage urine sample or EPS sample is then diagnostic of category II prostatitis. [p 614]

13. **d. trimethoprim.** Studies of animals with and without infection showed that trimethoprim concentrated in prostatic secretion and prostatic interstitial fluid (exceeding plasma levels), whereas sulfamethoxazole and ampicillin did not. [p 618]

14. **a. Low-dose prophylactic antibiotics.** Prolonged therapy with low-dose prophylactic or suppressive antimicrobials can be considered for recurrent or refractory prostatitis, respectively. [pp 623 and 624]

15. **d. Biofeedback.** On the basis of the possibility that the voiding and pain symptoms associated with CPPS may be secondary to some form of pseudodyssynergia during voiding or repetitive perineal muscle spasm, biofeedback has the potential to improve this process. [p 622]

16. **c. Transurethral drainage.** In patients who fail to respond quickly to antibiotics, a prostatic abscess is optimally drained by the transurethral incision route. [p 623]

17. **d. Categories II and III.** After 1 month of therapy, 40% of category II patients, 47% of category IIIA patients, and 58% of category IIIB patients had resolution of their symptoms. [p 620]

18. **c. Antibiotics.** Studies have generally indicated that approximately 40% of patients with chronic prostatitis have some symptomatic improvement with antimicrobial therapy, but no study in the literature has compared antimicrobial therapy with placebo in nonbacterial prostatitis or prostatodynia patients (CPPS). [pp 619–620]

19. **a. Observation.** Asymptomatic inflammatory prostatitis (category IV) by definition does not require symptomatic therapy. [p 625]

20. **c. Microwave heat therapy.** Although many uncontrolled trials employing heat therapy have shown benefit, three published studies have used sham controls. [p 623]

Chapter 16

Interstitial Cystitis and Related Disorders

Philip Hanno

Questions

1. What condition in men seems to be related to interstitial cystitis (IC)?

   a. Bacterial prostatitis
   b. Hemospermia
   c. Orchitis
   d. Chronic pelvic pain syndrome
   e. Hematuria

2. The definition of interstitial cystitis proposed by the National Institute of Arthritis, Diabetes, Digestive and Kidney Diseases (NIDDK) is best considered:

   a. a de facto definition of the disease.
   b. a diagnostic pathway.
   c. a definition applicable mainly to clinical research studies.
   d. a purely symptom-based description of IC.
   e. a historic document of no current value.

3. Bladder ulceration:

   a. is required to make a diagnosis of IC.
   b. was not considered part of the syndrome when it was initially described by Hunner.
   c. is pathognomonic of IC even in the absence of symptoms.
   d. is synonymous with glomerulation.
   e. is generally found in less than 10% of IC patients.

4. Exclusive use of the NIDDK criteria to diagnose IC would result in:

   a. an accurate depiction of the true prevalence of the condition.
   b. increased diagnostic sensitivity.
   c. increased diagnostic specificity.
   d. a minimum of diagnostic testing and thus medical expenses.
   e. an improved treatment algorithm.

5. IC symptom and problem indices have been validated to:

   a. monitor disease progression or regression with or without treatment.
   b. determine on whom to perform diagnostic testing.
   c. accurately diagnose IC.
   d. determine appropriate candidates for clinical research.
   e. correctly choose who should undergo cystectomy and diversion.

6. Which of the following statements best categorizes the natural history of IC?

   a. The onset is generally insidious, occurring gradually over many years.
   b. The onset is commonly subacute with full development of the symptom complex over a relatively short period of time.
   c. Symptoms occur only after a culture-documented urinary tract infection.
   d. In most patients the symptoms resolve, regardless of treatment, after 1 to 2 years.
   e. Major deterioration in symptom severity is the rule.

7. What percentage of IC patients are men?

   a. 80%
   b. 60%
   c. 40%
   d. 20%
   e. 10%

8. Men with irritative voiding symptoms and pelvic pain should be evaluated for which of the following?

   a. Chronic pelvic pain syndrome
   b. Bacterial prostatitis
   c. Interstitial cystitis
   d. Bladder carcinoma in situ
   e. All of the above

9. Which statement best describes the relationship of IC to bladder cancer?

   a. IC is a premalignant lesion.
   b. IC is often associated with bladder cancer.
   c. A positive urine cytologic result can safely be overlooked in a patient with symptoms of IC.
   d. No reports have documented a relationship of IC to bladder cancer.
   e. Patients with IC should be followed by using urine cytology.

10. The disorder most commonly associated with IC is:

    a. irritable bowel syndrome.
    b. allergy.
    c. lupus.
    d. fibromyalgia.
    e. incontinence.

11. The only animal with a known syndrome that appears to mimic IC is the:

    a. cat.
    b. dog.
    c. giraffe.
    d. rat.
    e. rabbit.

12. The antibiotic of choice in IC is:

    a. doxycycline.
    b. amoxicillin.
    c. gentamicin.
    d. ciprofloxacin.
    e. none.

13. The cell most likely to play a central role in the pathogenesis of IC is the:

    a. granulocyte.
    b. lymphocyte.
    c. mast cell.
    d. eosinophil.
    e. platelet.

14. The clinical test that is said to demonstrate increased bladder epithelial permeability in IC is the:

    a. charcoal test.
    b. myoglobinuria determination.
    c. bladder biopsy.
    d. intravesical potassium chloride (KCl).
    e. 24-hour urine creatinine.

15. The best circumstantial evidence for a urine abnormality in IC comes from what finding?

    a. The absence of pain when a Foley catheter is left indwelling
    b. Relief of symptoms as a result of using narcotic analgesics
    c. Failure of conduit diversion to relieve symptoms
    d. Success with urinary alkalinization
    e. Late occurrence of pain and bowel segment contraction after substitution cystoplasty and continent diversion.

16. The role of histopathology in IC is to:

    a. determine whether the patient has ulcerative or nonulcerative IC.
    b. rule out other diseases that might be the cause of the symptoms.
    c. confirm the diagnosis with pathologic criteria.
    d. help determine the most efficacious treatment modality.
    e. predict prognosis.

17. Which of the following conditions has the least in common with IC?

    a. Vulvodynia
    b. Bacterial prostatitis
    c. Orchialgia
    d. Penile pain
    e. Perineal and rectal pain

18. Urodynamic findings typical of IC include:

    a. uninhibited detrusor contractions.
    b. decreased bladder capacity and hypersensitivity.
    c. increased volume at first urge to void.
    d. abnormal bladder compliance.
    e. obstructed flow patterns.

19. The finding of glomerulations:

    a. is significant only when cystoscopy is performed with the patient under anesthesia.
    b. is sufficient to make a diagnosis of IC.
    c. is present only in patients with IC.
    d. is of no consequence in an asymptomatic patient.
    e. indicates a likelihood of response to laser fulguration of the bladder.

20. A marker for IC is *least* likely to be useful in:

    a. diagnosing the disease in the asymptomatic patient.
    b. stratifying patients in terms of potential response to different treatments.
    c. diagnosing IC when other causes of urinary frequency and pain are found.
    d. helping to establish a prognosis.
    e. confirming the diagnosis in a symptomatic patient.

21. The incidence of short-term spontaneous remission in IC approaches:

    a. 10%.
    b. 30%.
    c. 50%.
    d. 75%.
    e. 100%.

22. Which of the following is potentially both diagnostic and therapeutic?

    a. KCl test
    b. Intravesical heparin
    c. Bladder hydrodistention
    d. Bladder biopsy
    e. Urodynamics

23. Which of the following treatments has been demonstrated in placebo-controlled, blinded trials to increase bladder capacity and decrease urinary frequency?

    a. Amitriptyline
    b. Hydroxyzine
    c. Sodium pentosanpolysulfate
    d. L-Arginine
    e. None of the above

24. Which of the following treatments is targeted to the glycosaminoglycan (GAG) layer of the bladder?

    a. Amitriptyline
    b. Hydroxyzine
    c. Sodium pentosanpolysulfate
    d. Intravesical dimethyl sulfoxide
    e. Hydrodistention

25. Which of the following statements is true of narcotic analgesics?

    a. They have no place in the treatment of a chronic condition such as IC.
    b. They have a therapeutic ceiling limiting their maximum analgesic effect.
    c. They tend to cause diarrhea and sleeplessness.
    d. They generally result in drug addiction when used for chronic pain.
    e. They make patients physically dependent on them.

26. Which of the following is a reasonable surgical procedure to relieve the pain of IC?

    a. Transurethral fulguration of Hunner's ulcer.
    b. Sympathectomy and intraspinal alcohol injections.
    c. Transvesical infiltration of the pelvic plexuses with phenol.
    d. Cystolysis.
    e. Reduction cystoplasty.

27. The most important early step in the management of IC is:

    a. beginning intravesical treatment.
    b. starting therapy with pentosanpolysulfate.
    c. a strict IC diet.
    d. patient education.
    e. physical therapy.

28. The chronic urethral syndrome and IC can be differentiated by:

    a. symptom complex.
    b. response to treatment.
    c. history of urinary tract infection.
    d. response to urethral dilatation.
    e. name only.

Answers

1. **d. Chronic pelvic pain syndrome.** The chronic pelvic pain syndrome in men encompasses what used to be referred to as chronic nonbacterial prostatitis and prostatodynia. There are striking similarities between this poorly defined pain syndrome and IC, including the presence of glomerulations after bladder distention, the chronicity and variability of symptoms, and the lack of pathognomonic findings on diagnostic evaluation. [p 631]

2. **c. a definition applicable mainly to clinical research studies.** The definition of IC proposed by the NIDDK is best considered a definition applicable for use in research studies. It was never meant to define the disease but rather was developed to ensure that patients included in basic and clinical research studies were homogeneous enough that experts could agree on the diagnosis. [p 632]

3. **e. is generally found in less than 10% of IC patients.** Bladder ulceration (so-called Hunner's ulcer) is more appropriately referred to as Hunner's patch and is found in only a small proportion of patients with symptoms of IC, certainly less than 10%. A circumscribed red patch that cracks and bleeds with distention is best appreciated with the patient under anesthesia. [p 633]

4. **c. increased diagnostic specificity.** Exclusive use of the NIDDK criteria to diagnose IC would result in increased specificity and decreased sensitivity. Ninety percent of expert clinicians in the NIDDK database study agreed that patients diagnosed with IC by those criteria had IC. However, 60% of patients diagnosed by these clinicians as having IC did not fulfill the NIDDK criteria. Using the criteria as a basis for diagnosis would probably exclude the majority of patients with this symptom complex from the correct diagnosis. [p 633]

5. **a. monitor disease progression or regression with or without treatment.** IC symptom and problem indices like the one developed by O'Leary and Sant are not intended to diagnose IC. Like the American Urologic Association Symptom Score for benign prostatic hypertrophy, these indices are designed to evaluate the severity of symptoms and to monitor disease progression or regression and response to treatment. [p 633]

6. **b. The onset is commonly subacute with full development of the symptom complex over a relatively short period of time.** Several epidemiologic studies have concluded that the onset of IC is commonly subacute rather than insidious. It presents more like one would expect an infectious disorder to present, rather than like a chronic disease process. Full development of the classic symptom complex takes place over a relatively short period of time. In the majority of cases, it does not progress continuously but reaches its final stage rapidly and then continues without significant change in overall symptoms. [p 634]

7. **e. 10%.** Ten percent of IC patients are men. Whether the chronic pelvic pain syndrome in men and IC are variants of the same disease process is unknown at this time. The female preponderance in occurrence of IC has led investigators to suspect a hormonal component in the etiology, but this has not been worked out. The physiologic changes induced by pregnancy can mitigate the symptoms, but hormone-based therapies have not been shown to be effective. [p 635]

8. **e. All of the above.** IC should be considered in the differential diagnosis of voiding disorders in men accompanied by irritative symptoms and pelvic pain. The standard IC evaluation can be useful in differentiating IC from bladder carcinoma in situ, functional or anatomic bladder outlet obstruction, and bacterial prostatitis. Many men with IC have undergone what has proved to be unnecessary and ill-founded bladder neck surgery. [p 635]

9. **d. No reports have documented a relationship of IC to bladder cancer.** No relationship has ever been shown between IC and the subsequent development of bladder carcinoma. In the 1970s, the Mayo Clinic documented bladder cancer in 12 of 53 men who had been treated for IC, but the association was the result of incorrect diagnosis rather than progression. Urine cytology and cystoscopy have become integral parts of the IC evaluation. [p 635]

10. **b. allergy.** Forty-one percent of IC patients have been diagnosed with allergies, and 45% suffer from allergic symptoms. Fibromyalgia and irritable bowel syndrome are also over-represented in the IC population. Vulvodynia, migraine headaches, endometriosis, chronic fatigue syndrome, incontinence, and asthma have a prevalence similar to that in the general population. Systemic lupus erythematosus can cause bladder symptoms that are difficult to distinguish from IC. [p 635]

11. **a. cat.** The feline urologic syndrome may represent the animal equivalent of IC. Approximately two-thirds of cats with lower urinary tract disease have sterile urine and no evidence of other urinary tract disorders. A portion of these cats experience frequency and urgency of urination, pain, and bladder inflammation. Glomerulations have been found in some of these cat bladders. Other findings similar to IC include bladder mastocytosis, increased histamine excretion, and increased bladder permeability. [p 637]

12. **e. none.** Antibiotics are not indicated for the treatment of IC, nor have they been implicated as a causative factor. Numerous studies have concluded that it is unlikely that active infection is involved in the ongoing pathologic process or that antibiotics have a role to play in treatment. [p 639]

13. **c. mast cell.** Mast cells are strategically localized in the urinary bladder close to blood vessels, lymphatics, nerves, and detrusor smooth muscle. IC appears to be a syndrome with neural, immune, and endocrine components in which activated mast cells play a central, although not primary, role in many patients. [p 640]

14. **d. intravesical potassium chloride (KCl).** The intravesical administration of KCl has been proposed as a diagnostic test for IC. The test compares the sensory nerve provocative ability of sodium versus potassium using a 0.4 M KCl solution. The occurrence of pain and provocation of symptoms constitutes a positive test. Although the test may help determine the contribution of mucosal permeability in the pathogenesis of symptoms of the individual patient, it has not been found to have the sensitivity or specificity necessary for a reliable diagnostic test. [p 642]

15. **e. Late occurrence of pain and bowel segment contraction after substitution cystoplasty and continent diversion.** Substitution cystoplasty and continent diversion both fail in some IC patients because of the development of pain in the bowel segment used or contraction of the bowel segment. Some studies have shown histologic changes in bowel segments used in IC patients similar to those that occur in the IC bladder. Both of these findings provide circumstantial evidence that the urine of IC patients may have toxicity as-

sociated with the symptomatic expression of the disorder. [p 644]

16. **b. rule out other diseases that might be the cause of the symptoms.** The primary value of histopathology in IC is to rule out other diseases that may account for the symptoms. The differentiation between ulcerative and nonulcerative IC is based on endoscopic features. There is no pathognomonic histologic finding for the disorder, nor can histology predict prognosis. Even a severely abnormal microscopic picture does not necessarily indicate a poor prognosis. At this time, no data suggest that the treatment algorithm can be rationally predicated on the basis of the histologic findings. [p 646]

17. **b. Bacterial prostatitis.** IC can be considered one of the pain syndromes of the urogenital and rectal area, all of which are well described but poorly understood. These include vulvodynia, orchialgia, perineal pain, penile pain, and rectal pain. Bacterial prostatitis is a well-understood entity with a known etiology and generally responds to treatment directed at the offending organism. It has no relationship to IC. [p 647]

18. **b. decreased bladder capacity and hypersensitivity.** Cystometry in conscious IC patients generally demonstrates normal function, the exception being decreased bladder capacity and hypersensitivity, perhaps exaggerated by the use of carbon dioxide as a medium. Pain on bladder filling, which reproduces the patient's symptoms, is very suggestive of IC. Bladder compliance in patients with IC is normal, as hypersensitivity would prevent the bladder from filling to the point of noncompliance. [p 648]

19. **d. is of no consequence in an asymptomatic patient.** Glomerulations are not specific for IC, and only when seen in conjunction with the clinical criteria of pain and frequency can the presence of glomerulations be viewed as significant. Glomerulations can be seen after radiation therapy, in patients with bladder carcinoma, after exposure to toxic chemicals or chemotherapeutic agents, and in patients undergoing dialysis or after urinary diversion when the bladder has not filled for extended periods. They have also been reported in the majority of men with prostate pain syndromes. [p 648]

20. **a. diagnosing the disease in the asymptomatic patient.** The search for a marker for IC has expanded in recent years. A blood test, pathologic finding, or clinical test that has appropriate specificity and sensitivity could have some obvious benefits. It might confirm the diagnosis in a patient with other possible reasons to have urinary urgency, frequency, and pain. It might help establish the prognosis for an individual patient or suggest the best treatment algorithm. However, in a disorder defined by its symptoms, one would be ill-advised to make a diagnosis in the asymptomatic patient based on a "marker." [p 649]

21. **c. 50%.** There is a 50% incidence of temporary remission unrelated to therapy, with a mean duration of 8 months. The clinical course of IC is extremely variable, and it can be difficult to differentiate the effects of treatment from the natural history of the disease. [p 650]

22. **c. Bladder hydrodistention.** Bladder hydrodistention with the patient under anesthesia is often the first therapeutic modality employed for IC, frequently as part of the diagnostic evaluation. Between 30% and 50% of patients experience some short-term relief in symptoms after the procedure. About 30% will note a brief exacerbation in their symptoms. A bladder capacity under anesthesia of less than 200 ml is a sign of poor prognosis. [pp 650–651]

23. **e. None of the above.** Few IC medications have been rigorously tested in placebo-controlled trials. No medication has been shown to decrease frequency and increase bladder capacity under those conditions. Sodium pentosanpolysulfate has been put through the most rigorous trials and demonstrated statistically significant improvement in global well-being and pain compared with placebo. [pp 652–654]

24. **c. Sodium pentosanpolysulfate.** The target of sodium pentosanpolysulfate therapy is the GAG layer of the urothelium. This agent is an oral analogue of heparin that is partially excreted in the urine. The proposed mechanism of action is the correction of a GAG dysfunction, thus reversing the abnormal epithelial permeability in some patients. [p 654]

25. **e. They make patients physically dependent on them.** Narcotic analgesics can be very useful in a subset of IC patients with severe disease. Unlike other classes of analgesics, they have no therapeutic ceiling, dosing being limited by tolerance of side effects. They tend to cause constipation and can cause some sedation. Physical dependence is unavoidable, but physical addiction, a chronic disorder characterized by the compulsive use of a substance resulting in physical, psychological, or social harm to the user and the continued use despite that harm, is rare. [p 654]

26. **a. Transurethral fulguration of Hunner's ulcer.** Transurethral fulguration or laser irradiation of Hunner's ulcer can provide symptomatic relief. None of the other procedures listed have any place in the treatment of IC. [p 657]

27. **d. patient education.** Patient education is the most important step in the initial treatment of IC. This condition is incurable, the symptoms wax and wane, and remissions are not uncommon. It lends itself to practitioner abuse, and the uninformed, desperate patient is easy prey. Treatment is symptom-driven, and an informed patient makes the best decisions. [p 659]

28. **e. name only.** The symptomatic manifestations of IC and those of chronic urethral syndrome are indistinguishable. Chronic urethral syndrome is a historical term no longer used in the medical literature. [p 661]

Chapter 17

Sexually Transmitted Diseases

Richard E. Berger • Jay Lee

Questions

1. Which type of epithelium is most often infected by *Neisseria gonorrhoeae* and *Chlamydia trachomatis*?

    a. Columnar epithelium
    b. Transitional cell epithelium
    c. Squamous cell epithelium
    d. None of the above

2. Should sexual partners of patients with urethritis be treated on the basis of culture results or contact, and why or why not?

    a. Yes, to reduce the possibility of reinfection.
    b. Yes, to reduce the possibility of transmission.
    c. Yes, to reduce the possibility of reinfection and transmission.
    d. No, only if culture results are positive, to prevent resistance.

3. What is the percentage of partners of patients with *N. gonorrhoeae* infection who will be symptomatic?

    a. 10% to 20%
    b. 25% to 35%
    c. 40% to 60%
    d. 65% to 75%

4. If you suspect urethritis but cannot detect inflammation, which of the following diagnostic tests should be performed?

    a. Assay of the second void morning sample
    b. Assay of the catheterized sample
    c. Prostate massage
    d. Assay of the early morning void sample

5. Postgonococcal urethritis is most often caused by which of the following organisms?

    a. *C. trachomatis*
    b. *Ureaplasma urealyticum*
    c. *Mycoplasma hominis*
    d. Herpes simplex virus

6. After two episodes of pelvic inflammatory disease (PID), what percentage of women are infertile?

    a. 5%
    b. 15%
    c. 25%
    d. 35%

7. In men younger than 35 years, what is the leading cause of epididymitis?

    a. *N. gonorrhoeae*
    b. *C. trachomatis*
    c. *Escherichia coli*
    d. *Staphylococcus saprophyticus*

8. What percentage of genital ulcers are misdiagnosed on initial examination by an experienced examiner?

    a. 20%
    b. 40%
    c. 60%
    d. 80%

9. Genital vesicles in a non-neural distribution are pathognomonic for which of the following genital ulcer diseases?

    a. Herpes simplex
    b. Chancroid
    c. Syphilis
    d. Lymphogranuloma venereum

10. The diagnosis of chancroid is made by:

    a. polymerase chain reaction (PCR) assay.
    b. tissue culture.
    c. Western blot assay.
    d. Gram stain of the base of the lesion.

11. What is appropriate treatment for an asymptomatic male partner of a woman with cervical warts?

    a. Treatment with acetic acid
    b. Prophylaxis with acyclovir
    c. Treatment of only visible warts
    d. Cystoscopy

Answers

1. **a. Columnar epithelium.** Biologic factors play a part in sexually transmitted diseases (STDs). In early puberty, the columnar epithelium in the uterus extends from the endocervical canal into the vagina and is not protected by cervical mucus. The columnar epithelium is the primary site of invasion for both *C. trachomatis* and *N. gonorrhoeae* organisms. [p 672]

2. **c. Yes, to reduce the possibility of reinfection and transmission.** Because most microbiologic tests have less than 100% sensitivity, and regular partners run a high risk of being infected, they should always be treated regardless of culture result. This practice is especially important for infection with *C. trachomatis,* which has a high infectious, asymptomatic carrier rate. Sexual partners (especially those infected with *Treponema pallidum* [syphilis], *N. gonorrhoeae,* or *C. trachomatis* organisms) should be treated on the basis of contact. If partners are treated only if they become symptomatic, as many as 50% of patients would remain untreated. Furthermore, if cultures of partners are obtained and if the

partner is treated only if the culture is positive, patients will be lost to follow-up, may reinfect their partners, and may have an increased risk of possible serious consequences of their infections. [p 673]

3. **c. 40% to 60%.** Classically, gonococcal urethritis produces urethral discharge and burning on urination. The discharge is usually profuse and purulent, but it may be scant or even absent. Gonococcal urethritis may be asymptomatic in 40% to 60% of the contacts of partners with known gonorrhea. Without treatment, even symptomatic gonorrhea will improve. However, the host may remain a carrier and may be potentially infective. [p 674]

4. **d. Assay of the early morning void sample.** Ideally, a man suspected of having urethritis should be examined after 4 hours of urinary continence so that discharge may be reliably demonstrated. On a Gram stain of a urethral swab, more than four polymorphonuclear leukocytes per field in five 1000× oil immersion fields correlate with urethritis. Alternatively, the presence of 15 or more polymorphonuclear leukocytes in five random 400× fields of the spun sediment of the first-void urine sample correlates with urethritis. The leukocyte esterase urine dipstick test may be useful for screening purposes. A positive test, in the absence of bladder infections, should suggest urethritis, and more specific tests for *N. gonorrhoeae* and *C. trachomatis* should be obtained. When urethritis is suspected but urethral inflammation cannot be detected, the patient should be examined in the early morning before voiding. In one study of 200 men with genitourinary symptoms without urethritis at initial examination, 108 had urethritis diagnosed when examined in the early morning. [pp 675–676]

5. **a. *C. trachomatis*.** Postgonococcal urethritis develops in men who contract gonococcal and chlamydial infection simultaneously and who are treated with penicillin, to which *Chlamydia* is not sensitive. *C. trachomatis* organisms can be recovered from the urethra in 25% to 60% of heterosexual men with nongonococcal urethritis, in 4% to 40% of men with gonorrhea, and in 0% to 7% of men seen in STD clinics without symptoms of urethritis. [p 675]

6. **d. 35%.** PID can lead to serious and permanent consequences, including infertility: after a single episode of PID, 12% of patients will be sterile; after two episodes, 35% will be sterile; and after three attacks, 75% will be sterile. Of women who have had one episode of salpingitis, 25% will incur another. The damage caused by the first occurrence may make the patient more susceptible to further problems. In virtually all cases, PID-caused infertility is due to tubal occlusion. Infertility increases in direct proportion to the severity of the pelvic infection. Infertility is more likely to occur in patients with nongonococcal rather than gonococcal PID. Westrom estimated that of every 29 females born in 1950, one was sterile because of tubal occlusion by the age of 30 years. [p 677]

7. **b. *C. trachomatis*.** Epididymitis caused by sexually transmitted organisms occurs mainly in sexually active males younger than 35 years of age. Conversely, the majority of cases of epididymitis in children and older men are due to the common urinary pathogens. Epididymitis is usually caused by spread of infection from the urethra or bladder (see Table 17–2). The most common cause of epididymitis in each group appears to be the most common cause of genitourinary infection in that group. Although epididymitis is uncommon in children, the most common cause of epididymitis is the coliform organisms that cause bacteriuria. In heterosexual men younger than 35 years, bacteriuria is uncommon, whereas urethritis from *N. gonorrhoeae* and *C. trachomatis* is common. The most common cause of epididymitis in young men, therefore, is the organisms that cause urethritis. [p 678]

8. **b. 40%.** The diagnosis of acute genital ulcers presents a perplexing problem. The initial clinical impressions of even the most experienced specialist in STDs may be incorrect 40% of the time. In only three instances is the presentation of the ulcer pathognomonic: (1) A fixed drug eruption is always triggered by the ingestion of one particular medication. (2) A group of vesicles on an erythematous base that does not follow a neural distribution is pathognomonic for herpes simplex infection. (3) A genital ulcer that develops acutely during sexual activity is diagnostic of trauma. [p 680]

9. **a. Herpes simplex.** Vesicles grouped on an erythematous base that do not follow a neural distribution are pathognomonic for genital herpes. Confirmation of the diagnosis is based on laboratory methods. Papanicolaou (Pap) smears of lesions will demonstrate intranuclear inclusions in 50% to 60% of culture-positive cases. Immunofluorescent techniques reveal 70% of culture-positive cases. Virus isolation by culture is the most sensitive technique for diagnosing herpesvirus infections. Results can be available in 5 days. Serum antibody to herpes simplex virus infections can be measured by a number of methods and is reliable in differentiating type I from type II infection but may be unreliable when both types of infection are present. Polymerase chain reaction for the virus is an excellent noninvasive method. It is far more sensitive than viral cultures or viral antibody determination but requires a high degree of laboratory technical expertise. [p 682]

10. **d. Gram stain of the base of the lesion.** Definitive diagnosis can be made from a Gram stain smear of the base of the lesion. The Gram stain may show gram-negative coccobacilli in chains of clusters with a "school of fish" appearance. Diagnosis can also be made by using selective cultures for *Haemophilus ducreyi*. The optimal culture for *H. ducreyi* may require both supplemented gonococcal base and Mueller-Hinton agar. A PCR method to detect *H. ducreyi* by using primers from a 16S ribosomal RNA gene has been developed but is not in widespread use. [p 684]

11. **c. Treatment of only visible warts.** The goal of treatment is removal of exophytic warts and the amelioration of signs and symptoms, not the eradication of the human papillomavirus (HPV). No therapy has been shown to eradicate HPV. HPV has been found in tissues after laser treatment as well as other treatments. Aceto-whitened areas from the application of 5% acetic acid have been shown to be falsely interpreted as virally infected, and normal areas, not aceto-whitened, have been shown to have virus. Therefore, the benefit of treating patients with subclinical HPV infection has not been demonstrated, and recurrence is usual. The goal with treatment in HPV infection, especially in men, is only to remove exophytic warts and to reduce any signs or symptoms that the patient may have from the wart infection. Because local cure is probably not possible, expensive therapies or toxic therapies that may result in considerable scarring should be avoided when possible. Patients should be made aware that they may infect uninfected partners, and the use of condoms must be recommended. Numerous treatments have been used for warts, and the current Centers for Disease Control and Prevention recommendations are given in Table 17–6. [pp 685 and 686]

Chapter 18

AIDS and Related Conditions

John N. Krieger • John M. Corman

Questions

1. Transmission of HIV infection occurs by all of the following routes except:

    a. blood transfusion.
    b. sexual contact with infected cervical secretions.
    c. perinatal transmission between mother and fetus.
    d. sloughed skin from HIV-positive patients.
    e. sexual contact with infected semen.

2. The flow of genetic information in retroviruses is:

    a. RNA→DNA→RNA→protein.
    b. protein→RNA→DNA→protein.
    c. DNA→RNA→protein.
    d. RNA→protein→DNA.
    e. RNA→DNA→protein.

3. Progression from asymptomatic HIV infection to symptomatic disease occurs at what rate?

    a. 4% to 10% of seropositive persons per year
    b. 10% to 15% of seropositive persons per year
    c. 15% to 20% of seropositive persons per year
    d. 20% to 25% of seropositive persons per year
    e. 25% to 30% of seropositive persons per year

4. Occasional cases of AIDS occurred in the United States and Europe as early as what year?

    a. 1940
    b. 1952
    c. 1964
    d. 1977
    e. 1980

5. What is the probability of infection after receipt of a single-donor blood product documented to be HIV-1-positive?

    a. 20%
    b. 40%
    c. 60%
    d. 80%
    e. 100%

6. What is the risk of acquiring HIV-1 by receiving a single unit of screened donor blood?

    a. 1/100
    b. 1/1000
    c. 1/10,000
    d. 1/100,000
    e. 1/1,000,000

7. What is the risk of HIV infection for an infant of an HIV-seropositive mother?

    a. 1:1
    b. 1:4
    c. 1:5
    d. 1:7
    e. 1:10

8. What is the risk of seroconversion after a needle-stick injury to a health care worker?

    a. 0.1%
    b. 0.3%
    c. 1%
    d. 5%
    e. 10%

9. A 30-year-old healthy, HIV-positive homosexual man has a solid testicular mass. How should evaluation and treatment be modified?

    a. The patient should not receive nephrotoxic preoperative antibiotics.
    b. The patient should undergo a scrotal rather than an inguinal orchiectomy.
    c. The patient should not receive chemotherapy because it is immunosuppressive.
    d. The patient should receive radiation therapy.
    e. No alteration in treatment regimens should occur.

10. What is NOT a generally accepted indication for HIV testing?

    a. Blood donation
    b. Person with history of hepatitis B virus infection
    c. Patient with tuberculosis
    d. Routine preoperative evaluation
    e. Children born to HIV-infected mothers

Answers

1. **d. sloughed skin from HIV-positive patients.** Three modes of transmission have been described for HIV-1: direct sexual contact, exposure to contaminated blood and blood products, and perinatal transmission. Direct contact with semen and cervical secretions is important for sexual transmission of HIV. [pp 703 and 709]

2. **a. RNA→DNA→RNA→protein.** Retroviruses contain their genetic information in RNA. During replication, a copy of the viral RNA is transcribed by the viral DNA polymerase. This process of reverse transcription is the distinctive characteristic of the retroviruses. The viral RNA is transcribed by the reverse transcriptase enzyme into a linear, double-

stranded viral DNA in the host cell cytoplasm. The viral DNA is transported to the nucleus, where it is integrated into the host cell genome to establish infection. The integrated viral DNA (provirus) is transcribed into messenger RNA (mRNA) by the host cell's RNA polymerase. mRNA is translated into structural polypeptide precursors. [pp 694 and 696]

3. **a. 4% to 10% of seropositive persons per year.** The rate at which symptomatic disease develops in seropositive men appears to be approximately 4% to 10% per year of infection. [p 702]

4. **e. 1980.** The AIDS epidemic is usually dated from the 1981 description of *Pneumocystis carinii* pneumonia and Kaposi's sarcoma in previously healthy homosexual men. [p 703]

5. **e. 100%.** The probability of infection after receipt of a single-donor blood product that has been documented to be HIV-1-positive approaches 100%. [p 705]

6. **d. 1/100,000.** The worst-case scenario is that the risk of acquiring HIV-1 by receiving a single unit of blood is less than 1/100,000. [p 705]

7. **b. 1:4.** Pooled data from a variety of large studies suggest that infants born to infected mothers have an approximately 25% risk for acquiring HIV. [p 705]

8. **b. 0.3%.** The risk of seroconversion after a needle-stick injury appears to be approximately 0.3%. [p 710]

9. **e. No alteration in treatment regimens should occur.** The therapeutic dilemma in patients with testicular tumors and HIV-1 infection is that all accepted treatments for testicular neoplasms, except surveillance, may result in additional immune suppression. Furthermore, patients with AIDS often tolerate radiation and chemotherapy poorly. This may require major modifications of standard treatment protocols, resulting in decreased effectiveness. Despite these limitations, most experts recommend that AIDS and HIV-positive patients with testicular neoplasms should receive standard treatment as indicated by the tumor histology and stage. [p 708]

10. **d. Routine preoperative evaluation.** Generally accepted indications for antibody testing include evaluation of blood and organs for tissue donation. In addition, most experts agree that persons at risk for HIV infection should be tested routinely. Such persons include those with a sexually transmitted disease, including hepatitis B; those with a history of intravenous drug use; others who consider themselves at risk for HIV infection; and those with a history of a disease that might be associated with HIV infection. Testing is also recommended for persons who received unscreened blood transfusions after 1977; for all persons with active tuberculosis; for selected women of reproductive age, particularly those living in communities with a high prevalence of HIV infection; and for children born to HIV-infected mothers. [p 711]

Chapter 19

Cutaneous Diseases of the Male External Genitalia

David J. Margolis

Questions

1. What is the most likely diagnosis for an individual with red scaling patches on the elbows and red lesions on the penis?

    a. Psoriasis
    b. Eczema
    c. Bowen's disease
    d. Herpes simplex
    e. Lichen planus

2. Lichen planus may be associated with:

    a. molluscum contagiosum.
    b. a family history of psoriasis.
    c. hepatitis C virus infection.
    d. vigorous sexual activity.
    e. acetaminophen use.

3. Lichen sclerosis is:

    a. a very common skin ailment.
    b. often successfully treated by circumcision.
    c. associated with psoriasis.
    d. associated with scleroderma.
    e. associated with hepatitis C virus infection.

4. Contact dermatitis is best treated by:

    a. a mixture of zinc paste and hydrocortisone.
    b. a high-potency topical steroid.
    c. removing the offending agent.
    d. antihistamines.
    e. vigorous cleansing.

5. A gluten-sensitive enteropathy is associated with:

    a. Hailey-Hailey disease.
    b. erythema multiforme.
    c. psoriasis.
    d. Zoon's balanitis.
    e. dermatitis herpetiformis.

6. Patients with Behçet's disease frequently have all but which one of the following symptoms or signs?

    a. Oral ulcers
    b. Genital ulcers
    c. Uveitis
    d. Arthritis
    e. Asthma

7. Bowenoid papulosis is associated with all but which one of the following?

   a. Sexual activity
   b. Human papillomavirus 16 (HPV-16)
   c. Cervical neoplasia
   d. Invasive carcinoma
   e. Plaques with a verrucous surface

8. The cause of balanoposthitis has been associated with all but which of the following?

   a. Intertrigo
   b. Irritant dermatitis
   c. Bacterial infection
   d. Candidal infection
   e. Circumcision

9. Hidradenitis suppurativa is primarily:

   a. not an infectious disease.
   b. associated with gram-positive organisms.
   c. associated with gram-negative organisms.
   d. associated with lubricant use.
   e. found in patients who are not prone to acne or cysts.

10. Pearly penile papules are:

    a. uncommon.
    b. angiofibroma.
    c. histiocytosis X.
    d. caused by HPV-16.
    e. well treated by oral antibiotics effective against gram-positive organisms.

11. Zoon's balanitis may clinically resemble:

    a. squamous cell carcinoma.
    b. penile melanosis.
    c. wart.
    d. hidradenitis suppurativa.
    e. bug bite.

12. Acanthosis nigricans is associated with:

    a. poor hygiene.
    b. endocrinopathies.
    c. musk dermatitis.
    d. alopecia areata.
    e. psoriasis.

13. Vitiligo can best be described as:

    a. papular.
    b. verrucous.
    c. a hypopigmented patch.
    d. a hyperpigmented patch.
    e. an early cutaneous marker of a visceral carcinoma.

14. The differential diagnosis of psoriasis includes all which of the following?

    a. Lichen planus
    b. Seborrheic dermatitis
    c. Reiter's syndrome
    d. Bowen's disease
    e. Pemphigus vulgaris

15. The differential diagnosis of an aphthous ulcer includes all but which one of the following?

    a. Factitial dermatitis
    b. Syphilis
    c. Herpes simplex
    d. Leukocytoclastic vasculitis
    e. Penile melanosis

Answers

1. **a. Psoriasis.** Lesions appear as red to pink plaques or patches covered with white to gray scale. However, scale may not be present in skin folds and on moist and mucosal surfaces. The diagnosis of genital psoriasis is greatly aided by the discovery of typical red scaling plaques elsewhere on the body. Lesions are most commonly noted on the elbows, knees, scalp, umbilicus, nails, and buttocks. [p 716]

2. **c. hepatitis C virus infection.** This disease may be associated with hepatitis C virus infection. [p 717]

3. **b. often successfully treated by circumcision.** Most males are successfully treated by circumcision. [p 718]

4. **c. removing the offending agent.** Removal of the offending agent is critical. However, identifying the offending agent can be difficult. Some clues may be present on other parts of the body (e.g., nickel dermatitis from a belt buckle, waistband snap, or watch band). Patch testing uninvolved skin to common antigens is often helpful. [p 720]

5. **e. dermatitis herpetiformis.** Dermatitis herpetiformis is an immune-mediated blistering eruption due to immunoglobulin A autoantibodies against the basement membrane. The lesion is an intensely painful burning pruritic papule or vesicle. Lesions are found most frequently on elbows, knees, buttocks, shoulders, and sacrum. A majority of patients suffer from an associated gluten-sensitive enteropathy. [p 721]

6. **e. Asthma.** Behçet's disease is a syndrome characterized by oral and genital ulcers, uveitis, and non-mucous membrane skin lesions of unknown etiology. Individuals may suffer from aneurysms; arthritis; thrombophlebitis; and gastrointestinal, neurologic, and psychiatric problems. [pp 721–722]

7. **d. Invasive carcinoma.** Bowenoid papulosis of the genitalia occurs in sexually active men and women in the third and fourth decades of life. Typically, lesions are multiple, erythematous papules less than 1 cm in diameter. Papules may coalesce to form plaques and may have a verrucous surface. There is a strong causal association between this disorder and HPV-16 infection. Bowenoid papulosis is histologically similar to carcinoma in situ. However, in this disease the atypical keratinocytes do not replace the entire epidermis but are found randomly throughout the epidermis. There is an increased risk of cervical neoplasia in female partners of men with bowenoid papulosis. In men, the disease may regress without treatment, and it has never been reported to progress to invasive squamous cell carcinoma. [p 722]

8. **e. Circumcision.** The cause of balanoposthitis is often never ascertained; when the cause is discovered, it is somewhat dependent on the age of the afflicted individual. The cause in men may be intertrigo, irritant dermatitis, maceration injury, or candidal or bacterial infection. [p 724]

9. **a. not an infectious disease.** Hidradenitis suppurativa is not primarily an infectious disease. [p 724]

10. **b. angiofibroma.** The lesions are histologically angiofibromas. [p 726]

11. **a. squamous cell carcinoma.** Zoon's balanitis must be differentiated from squamous cell carcinoma in situ and other forms of balanitis. [p 727]

12. **b. endocrinopathies.** Patients are frequently bothered only by the "dirty appearance" of this skin lesion. At least five distinct clinical variants exist and have been associated with multiple factors. These factors include heredity; endocrinopathies such as states of insulin resistance; obesity; medications such as niacin; and malignancy of the gastrointestinal tract, prostate, ovaries, and lungs. [p 728]

13. **c. a hypopigmented patch.** Vitiligo is a depigmentation of the skin in which sharply bordered patches of the skin become white. Patches can vary tremendously in size and shape. [p 728]

14. **e. Pemphigus vulgaris.** The differential diagnosis of psoriasis includes seborrheic dermatitis, dermatophyte infection, erythrasma, secondary syphilis, pityriasis rosea, discoid lupus, mycosis fungoides, lichen planus, fixed drug reaction, Reiter's syndrome, pityriasis versicolor, Bowen's disease, and extramammary Paget's disease. [p 716]

15. **e. Penile melanosis.** The differential diagnosis of aphthous ulcer includes syphilis, chancroid, herpes simplex, Crohn's disease, Behçet's disease, granuloma inguinale, lymphogranuloma venereum, factitial dermatitis, Wegener's granulomatosis, and leukocytoclastic vasculitis, and pyoderma gangrenosum. [p 721]

Chapter 21

Tuberculosis and Parasitic Diseases of the Genitourinary System

Warren D. Johnson, Jr. • Christopher W. Johnson • Franklin C. Lowe

Questions

1. Which of the following statements about the epidemiology of tuberculosis is true?
   a. Tuberculosis incidence has increased in the United States during the 1990s.
   b. The incidence of tuberculosis among Asian immigrants is comparable to that for persons born in the United States.
   c. Tuberculosis occurrence is decreasing worldwide.
   d. Tuberculosis occurs predominantly in patients with acquired immunodeficiency syndrome (AIDS) late in the course of their disease (CD4$^+$ T-cell count of <200 cells/mm^3).
   e. Globally, tuberculosis is the most common opportunistic infection in AIDS patients.

2. The spread of *Mycobacterium tuberculosis* is least dependent on which of the following?
   a. Size of the bacillary inoculum inhaled
   b. Infectivity of the mycobacterial strain
   c. Duration of exposure to the source case
   d. Immune status of the source case
   e. Immune status of the exposed individual

3. Which of the following statements regarding tuberculosis is correct?
   a. Humans are not the only reservoir for the organism.
   b. Renal tuberculosis is usually caused by the activation of a prior blood-borne metastatic renal infection.
   c. Epididymitis is a rare presenting symptom of genitourinary tuberculosis.
   d. Transmission of genital tuberculosis from male to female is common.
   e. Renal tuberculosis is most common in children younger than 5 years of age.

4. Which one of the following conditions is least likely to reactivate a dormant *M. tuberculosis* infection?
   a. Human immunodeficiency virus (HIV) infection
   b. Collagen-vascular disease
   c. Immunosuppressive therapy
   d. Allergic asthma
   e. Diabetes

5. The Centers for Disease Control and Prevention (CDC) has recommended defining a positive tuberculin reaction of 5 mm or greater induration for all the following except:
   a. HIV-infected patients.
   b. recent close contacts of a person who has active tuberculosis.
   c. a person with a chest film showing granulomas from prior tuberculosis.
   d. a person receiving chemotherapy for psoriasis.
   e. an intravenous drug abuser.

6. The radiologic test that is most useful for evaluating the anatomic manifestations of genitourinary tuberculosis is:
   a. ultrasonography.
   b. intravenous pyelography.
   c. computed tomography (CT).
   d. magnetic resonance imaging (MRI).
   e. retrograde pyelography.

7. All of the following features of genitourinary tuberculosis can be seen on an intravenous urogram except:

a. infundibular stenosis.
   b. renal calcifications.
   c. ureteral stricture.
   d. "thimble" bladder.
   e. vesicoureteral reflux.

8. Which is the following antituberculous drugs is bacteriostatic?

   a. Isoniazid (INH)
   b. Rifampicin
   c. Pyrazinamide
   d. Streptomycin
   e. Ethambutol

9. Six-month regimens of antibiotic therapy are effective for most forms of tuberculosis except which of the following?

   a. Pulmonary
   b. Genitourinary
   c. Osteomyelitis (Pott)
   d. Nodal (tuberculous lymphadenitis [scrofula])
   e. Concomitant pulmonary and genitourinary

10. Hepatic toxicity from INH is:

    a. preventable with vitamin B_6.
    b. irreversible.
    c. evident almost immediately after initiation of therapy.
    d. manifested by hyperbilirubinemia.
    e. possibly normalized after 3 to 4 months of therapy.

11. Which of the following statements regarding surgery for genitourinary tuberculosis is correct?

    a. Patients should have at least 4 to 6 weeks of extensive chemotherapy before surgery.
    b. Lack of renal calcification is not a contraindication to partial nephrectomy.
    c. Open surgical drainage of an abscess is useful.
    d. There is no indication for an epididymectomy in the modern era of effective chemotherapy.
    e. Strictures at the ureteropelvic junction are common and frequently require endopyelotomy.

12. Which of the following statements about *Schistosoma haematobium* and its life cycle is false?

    a. Worm pairs are principally located in the perivesical venous plexus in humans.
    b. It is a digenetic blood fluke.
    c. Human infection is acquired by exposure to salt water that harbors infected snails.
    d. Worm pairs have life spans estimated between 3 and 6 years and can spawn as many as 600,000 eggs.
    e. The sexual reproductive phase occurs in vesical and pelvic venules (adult worms) and the asexual reproductive phase occurs (sporocyst) in host snails.

13. When one evaluates a patient for *S. haematobium* infection, which one of the following statements is correct?

    a. An active infection can be diagnosed by the presence of laterally spined eggs in the urine, feces, or tissues.
    b. An active infection has the full complement of egg stages present.
    c. a history of living or traveling in the Middle East, South America, or Africa means that the patient has been to endemic areas.
    d. The intensity of infection is inversely related to the egg burden found in tissues or body fluids.
    e. Calculating the number of eggs per 10 ml of urine is the most sensitive and specific way to determine the intensity of the infection.

14. The human host response to *S. haematobium* is characterized by which one of the following?

    a. T-cell—dependent host responses modulate granuloma formation.
    b. The granulomatous host response to the schistosome eggs does not cause the pathologic response.
    c. Eosinophil-mediated killing is effective against adult worms.
    d. It is postulated that HIV-positive patients with lower $CD4^+$ T-cell counts have higher egg burdens than patients with normal $CD4^+$ T-cell counts.
    e. A "sandy patch" is a granulomatous ulcer.

15. Which one of the following is the most common presentation of acute *S. haematobium* disease?

    a. Katayama fever.
    b. Swimmers' itch.
    c. A calcified bladder.
    d. Hematuria and terminal dysuria.
    e. Obstructive uropathy.

16. Bilharzial bladder cancer is a known sequela of *S. haematobium* infection. Which of the following statements is not correct?

    a. The bladder cancer is often manifested at ~ 40 to 50 years of age.
    b. Squamous cell carcinoma accounts for 60% to 90% of the cancers.
    c. Nitrates, nitrite, N-nitroso compounds, and tryptophan metabolites have been identified in elevated amounts in the urine of patients with bilharzial bladder cancer.
    d. More than 95% of the squamous cell carcinomas are poorly differentiated and have a poor prognosis.
    e. Patients are frequently treated with an anterior pelvic exenteration and a urinary diversion.

17. A 43-year-old woman from Madagascar has schistosomal obstructive uropathy (SOU). What might you expect to find at her work-up?

    a. SOU usually obstructs the ureters symmetrically.
    b. The egg burden would be highest at the distal end of the ureter.
    c. The obstruction would likely be at the ureteropelvic junction.
    d. If untreated, hydronephrosis could progress to hydroureter.
    e. There is no change in ureteral function until radiologically demonstrable disease is noted.

18. A 24-year-old man who had recently come from Syria had been previously diagnosed with urinary schistosomiasis. He had not received any treatment. His medical records from Syria noted that he had *S. haematobium* infection and an intravenous pyelogram had demonstrated severe hydroureter on the left with a segmental distal ureteral lesion and delayed excretion. He has a normal creatinine level. He should be initially managed with:

    a. cystoscopy with ureteral stent placement.
    b. cystoscopy with ureteral stent placement and intravesical medical therapy.
    c. percutaneous nephrostomy tube placement followed by medical therapy.
    d. partial ureterectomy with primary ureteroureterostomy.
    e. medical management with oral praziquantel.

19. Filarial disease can be characterized by all of the following except:

a. Elephantiasis of the limbs, chyluria, fever, localized lymphangitis, and hydrocele formation are seen.
b. *Wuchereria bancrofti* accounts for fewer than half of human lymphatic filariasis cases.
c. Obstructive lymphatic disease occurs in patients who are repeatedly infected.
d. The female mosquito (*Culex pipiens*) is the vector.
e. After inoculation, larvae travel through the lungs via blood before settling in their ultimate destination, large lymphatic vessels.

20. A 34-year-old shepherd from Spain has dull bilateral flank pain and intermittent microscopic hematuria. You suspect that a parasite may be responsible for the patient's complaints. If you are correct, which of the following statements would be valid?

a. Hanging groin, or scrotal elephantiasis, may ultimately develop.
b. Metronidazole is a first-line treatment option.
c. Ivermectin is a first-line treatment option.
d. Thick-walled fluid-filled cysts with calcified walls are diagnostic.
e. Needle aspiration of any lesion is indicated before initiating therapy.

Answers

1. **e. Globally, tuberculosis is the most common opportunistic infection in AIDS patients.** Studies in New York showed that among patients with both tuberculosis and AIDS, almost two thirds had developed tuberculosis within 6 months of their diagnosis of AIDS. Human immunodeficiency virus (HIV) infection is a cofactor with one of the highest risk ratios for the development of tuberculosis in people already infected with *Mycobacterium tuberculosis*. [p 745]

2. **d. Immune status of the source case.** The probability that a person will become infected depends on the duration of exposure to source case, the size of the bacillary inoculum inhaled, and infectivity of the mycobacterial strain. The probability of a competent host developing active tuberculosis after *M. tuberculosis* infection is 5% to 10% over the person's lifetime. Virtually all AIDS patients with a positive purified protein derivative (PPD) test result will develop active tuberculosis during their lifetime unless antituberculous prophylaxis is offered or another fatal opportunistic infection develops. [p 746]

3. **b. Renal tuberculosis is usually caused by the activation of a prior blood-borne metastatic renal infection.** Genitourinary tuberculosis is usually caused by metastatic spread of organisms through the blood stream during the initial infection. Later, active disease results from the reactivation of that initial infection, probably because of failure of the local immune response. [p 746]

4. **d. Allergic asthma.** Most persons will control an initial infection and develop no clinical illness. They will have dormant bacilli, which may begin to multiply and produce disease years later. This may occur after debilitating disease, trauma, collagen-vascular disease, immunosuppressive therapy, diabetes, and AIDS. [p 746]

5. **e. an intravenous drug abuser.** For persons who are at highest risk for developing active TB if they are infected with *M. tuberculosis* (e.g., persons with HIV infection, who are receiving immunosuppressive therapy, who have had recent close contact with persons with infectious TB, or who have abnormal chest radiographs consistent with prior TB), 5 mm or greater of induration is considered positive. For other persons with an increased probability of recent infection or with other clinical conditions that increase the risk for progression to active TB, 10 mm or greater of induration is considered positive. These include recent immigrants (within the last 5 years) from high-prevalence countries; injection drug users; residents and employees of high-risk congregate settings (including health care workers with exposure to TB); mycobacteriology laboratory personnel; persons with clinical conditions such as silicosis, diabetes mellitus, chronic renal failure, leukemias and lymphomas, carcinoma of the head or neck and lung, weight loss of ≥10% ideal body weight, gastrectomy, and jejunoileal bypass; and children younger than 4 years of age or infants, children, and adolescents exposed to adults in high-risk categories. [pp 751–752]

6. **b. intravenous pyelography.** The introduction of the high-dose intravenous urogram has been a major advance in the investigation of renal tract pathology, and its use is now standard practice. [pp 752–753]

7. **e. vesicoureteral reflux.** The renal lesion may appear as a distortion of a calyx (Fig. 21–6), as a calyx that is fibrosed and completely occluded (lost calyx from infundibular stenosis), as multiple small calyceal deformities, or as severe calyceal and parenchymal destruction. Calcification may be present. Tuberculous ureteritis is manifested by dilatation above a ureterovesical stricture or, if the disease is more advanced, by a rigid fibrotic ureter with multiple strictures. The intravenous urogram can give valuable information about the condition of the bladder, which may be small and contracted (thimble bladder). [pp 753–754]

8. **e. Ethambutol.** The first-line antituberculous drugs are INH, rifampicin, pyrazinamide, streptomycin, and ethambutol. The first four drugs are bactericidal. [p 755]

9. **c. Osteomyelitis (Pott).** There is now abundant evidence that 6-month regimens are effective for most forms of tuberculosis, with the exception of disseminated tuberculosis, tuberculous osteomyelitis, and tuberculous meningitis. [p 757]

10. **e. possibly normalized after 3 to 4 months of therapy.** INH is associated with hepatic toxicity in 10% to 20% of patients, usually in the form of asymptomatic elevations in transaminase levels. This occurs after 6 to 8 weeks of therapy and may normalize with continued INH treatment. Patients are advised to discontinue INH if they develop symptoms suggestive of hepatitis (fatigue, nausea, anorexia) because severe hepatic necrosis has been reported. Peripheral neuropathy in patients taking higher than standard INH doses is due to enhanced pyridoxine excretion and is prevented by daily supplemental oral pyridoxine (vitamin B_6). [p 755]

11. **a. Patients should have at least 4 to 6 weeks of extensive chemotherapy before surgery.** If surgery is required, it is scheduled as an elective procedure, and the patient is admitted 4 to 6 weeks after the start of the intensive course of chemotherapy. The aims are (1) to treat the active disease, (2) to make the patient noninfectious as soon as possible,

and (3) to preserve the maximal amount of renal tissue. [p 758]

12. **c. Human infection is acquired by exposure to salt water that harbors infected snails.** Human infection is acquired by exposure to fresh (not salt) water that harbors the infected snails. [p 764]

13. **c. a history of living or traveling in the Middle East, South America, or Africa means that the patient has been to endemic areas.** Transmission of *S. haematobium* occurs throughout the African continent, including the islands of Madagascar and Mauritius. It is also found in southern Yemen, Yemen, Saudi Arabia, Lebanon, Syria, Turkey, Iraq, and Iran. [pp 765–766]

14. **a. T-cell–dependent host responses modulate granuloma formation.** The perioval granulomas of all schistosomes are T-cell–dependent host responses and are modulated by that system. [p 767]

15. **d. Hematuria and terminal dysuria.** The classic clinical presentation of "active" bilharziasis is hematuria and terminal dysuria. [p 769]

16. **d. More than 95% of the squamous cell carcinomas are poorly differentiated and have a poor prognosis.** More than 40% of squamous cell carcinomas associated with urinary schistosomiasis are well differentiated (grade 1) or perhaps verrucous carcinomas that are exophytic and carry a good prognosis. [p 777]

17. **b. The egg burden would be highest at the distal end of the ureter.** Ureteral egg burdens correlate with egg burdens of the entire urinary tract and are highest at the distal end, adjacent to the bladder, progressively diminishing proximally, except for uncommon focal involvement of the upper ureter in the "second or third lumbar" and "fifth lumbar" segmental lesions. [p 778]

18. **e. medical management with oral praziquantel.** In general, surgery is reserved for complications that have not responded to adequate medical treatment within a reasonable follow-up time (e.g., SOU) or for those mandating immediate intervention such as intractable bladder hemorrhage. [p 772]

19. **b. *Wuchereria bancrofti* accounts for fewer than half of human lymphatic filariasis cases.** *W. bancrofti* accounts for 90% of cases of human lymphatic filariasis and is widespread throughout the tropics. [p 780]

20. **d. Thick-walled fluid-filled cysts with calcified walls are diagnostic.** Diagnosis can be made by radiography or CT that shows a thick-walled, fluid-filled spherical cyst, often with a calcific cyst wall. [p 787]

Chapter 22

Fungal and Actinomycotic Infections of the Genitourinary System

Gilbert J. Wise

Questions

1. During the decade of 1980 through 1990, 344,610 cases of different infection were reported to the National Nosocomial Infections Surveillance System. What percentage of infections were caused by fungi?
    a. 1% to 2%
    b. 3% to 4%
    c. 6% to 8%
    d. 10% to 12%
    e. 14% to 16%

2. What is the most prevalent underlying disease associated with a single episode of candiduria?
    a. Malignancy
    b. Malnutrition
    c. Urinary tract disease
    d. Diabetes mellitus
    e. Collagen disease

3. An effective treatment for vulvovaginal candidiasis is:
    a. vinegar douches.
    b. amphotericin B vaginal inserts.
    c. itraconazole.
    d. oral fluconazole (150 mg).
    e. saline vaginal irrigations.

4. All of the following are major predisposing factors for renal candidal infection in pediatric patients except:
    a. indwelling intravascular catheters.
    b. broad-spectrum antibiotics.
    c. prematurity.
    d. low birth weight.
    e. maternal diabetes mellitus.

5. The appropriate imaging study for a pediatric patient with oliguria and fungal elements in the urine is:
    a. nuclide renal scan.
    b. voiding cystourethrogram.
    c. intravenous pyelogram.
    d. renal sonogram.
    e. spiral CT scan.

6. Treatment for bladder-confined ("local") candidal infection may utilize all of the following except:

a. oral flucytosine.
b. oral fluconazole.
c. bladder irrigations of amphotericin B.
d. intravenous amphotericin B.
e. ketoconazole.

7. Aspergillosis has the greatest predilection for which genitourinary structure?

    a. Adrenal gland
    b. Bladder
    c. Testes
    d. Kidney
    e. Prostate gland

8. In AIDS patients, which genitourinary organ becomes the "reservoir" for *Cryptococcus* after treatment of cryptococcal meningitis?

    a. Kidney
    b. Adrenal gland
    c. Epididymis
    d. Testes
    e. Prostate gland

9. Which genitourinary organ or structure is vulnerable to disseminated mucormycosis?

    a. Testes
    b. Epididymis
    c. Kidney
    d. Prostate gland
    e. Bladder

10. A predisposing condition for systemic blastomycosis is:

    a. prostate carcinoma.
    b. bladder carcinoma.
    c. hematologic malignancy.
    d. colon carcinoma.
    e. metastatic testicular carcinoma.

11. What is the primary site of infection by *Coccidioides immitis*?

    a. Skin
    b. Pulmonary system
    c. Gastrointestinal tract
    d. Genitourinary system
    e. Nasopharyngeal system

12. Generalized histoplasmosis has the greatest predilection for which of the following genitourinary structures?

    a. Prostate gland
    b. Kidney
    c. Bladder
    d. Testes
    e. Adrenal gland

13. Paracoccidioidomycosis is prevalent in:

    a. the western Unites States.
    b. South America.
    c. the Great Lakes region.
    d. Central America.
    e. Africa.

14. The drug of choice for the treatment of actinomycosis is:

    a. penicillin.
    b. amphotericin B.
    c. fluconazole.
    d. itraconazole.
    e. flucytosine.

15. Amphotericin B may cause an adverse reaction in the:

    a. oropharynx.
    b. gastrointestinal tract.
    c. peripheral nervous system.
    d. retina.
    e. kidney.

16. Ketoconazole has a limited role in the treatment of urinary fungal infections because of:

    a. renal toxicity.
    b. poor excretion by the kidney.
    c. liver toxicity.
    d. poor in vivo antifungal activity.
    e. a high degree of fungal drug resistance.

17. Itraconazole is NOT effective in the treatment of infection with which organism?

    a. *Aspergillus*
    b. *Blastomyces*
    c. *Coccidioides*
    d. *Candida*
    e. *Histoplasma*

18. Fluconazole may cause an adverse reaction in the:

    a. kidney.
    b. testes.
    c. adrenal gland.
    d. liver.
    e. myocardium.

Answers

1. **c. 6% to 8%.** Fungi caused 27,200 infections (7.9%), of which *Candida* accounted for 22,000 (6.2%). [p 797]

2. **d. Diabetes mellitus.** In a multicenter study of 861 patients with a *documented single episode* of candiduria, the major associated illnesses included diabetes mellitus in 336 patients (39%), urinary tract disease in 325 patients (37.7%), malignancy in 191 patients (22.2%), and malnutrition in 146 patients (17%). [p 798]

3. **d. oral fluconazole (150 mg).** Oral fluconazole (as a single 150 mg dose) is as effective as intravaginal clotrimazole in the treatment of vulvovaginal candidiasis. [p 799]

4. **e. maternal diabetes mellitus.** Indwelling intravascular catheters, broad-spectrum antibiotics, prematurity, and low birth weight have been associated with the development of renal candidal infection in infants. [p 801]

5. **d. renal sonogram.** Renal sonography is crucial for diagnosis in such a case; it often demonstrates hydronephrosis with fungal accretions in the collecting system. [p 801]

6. **e. ketoconazole.** The imidazoles miconazole and ketoconazole are poorly excreted by the kidney and have low urinary concentrations. The success rate in the treatment of urinary candidal infection ranges from 40% to 50%. [pp 803–804]

7. **d. Kidney.** Postmortem studies of 98 patients with aspergillosis showed that aspergilli infected the pulmonary tract in 92 patients (94%), the gastrointestinal tract in 21 (23%), the brain in 19 (21%), the liver in 12 (13%), and the kidney in

12 (13%). The testes and adrenal gland were involved in one patient each. The infected kidneys demonstrated multiple small focal abscesses, vascular occlusion by fungi, and multiple renal infarcts. [p 806]

8. **e. Prostate gland.** In AIDS patients, the prostate gland has become a "reservoir" for *Cryptococcus* following treatment for cryptococcal meningitis. [p 809]

9. **c. Kidney.** Renal involvement with and without associated disseminated disease has been reported. Renal zygomycosis (mucormycosis) may cause acute illness with signs of sepsis (i.e., fever, chills, tachycardia, and decreased urinary output), often associated with fungus-induced obstructive uropathy and renal infection. [pp 809–810]

10. **c. hematologic malignancy.** Blastomycosis has become more prevalent in immunocompromised patients. Predisposing conditions or factors have included chronic corticosteroid use, hematologic malignancy, solid tumor requiring cytotoxic or radiation therapy, having received a solid organ or bone marrow transplant, HIV-positive status, end-stage renal or hepatic disease, and pregnancy. [p 811]

11. **b. Pulmonary system.** After inhalation of the arthroconidia, the patient may develop an asymptomatic and transient pulmonary infection. A more virulent infection occurs in some cases, with radiographic changes indicative of pulmonary infiltration or cavitation. [p 812]

12. **e. Adrenal gland.** The liver, spleen, and lymph nodes are major sites of extrapulmonary histoplasmosis. However, the genitourinary tract is often involved in disseminated infection. In a postmortem study of 17 patients with generalized histoplasmosis, the adrenal gland was infected in 14 patients (82%), the kidney in 3 (18%), and the prostate gland in 1 (6%). [p 814]

13. **b. South America.** *Paracoccidioides brasiliensis* causes a chronic granulomatous disease known as South American blastomycosis (paracoccidioidomycosis) that can mimic tuberculosis or histoplasmosis. Indigenous to South America, it is rare in the Northern Hemisphere. [p 816]

14. **a. penicillin.** In renal actinomycotic infections, nephrectomy has been the treatment of choice; however, long-term antibiotic treatment (6 weeks of parenteral penicillin at 12 million U/day and 1 year of oral penicillin at 1.2 g/day) has resolved a renal infection without the need for surgery. [p 817]

15. **e. kidney.** Amphotericin B nephrotoxicity is characterized by hematuria, pyuria, cylindruria, proteinuria, and electrolyte imbalance. Amphotericin B may exacerbate the nephrotoxic effects of other agents, such as cisplatin. [p 818]

16. **b. poor excretion by the kidney.** Because of poor renal excretion, ketoconazole has low urinary levels that may be insufficient to inhibit many fungal species; thus, it has a limited role in the treatment of fungi that may infect the urinary collecting system and bladder. [p 819]

17. **d. *Candida*.** Itraconazole is effective in the treatment of infections caused by *Aspergillus, Blastomyces, Coccidioides, Histoplasma,* and *Sporothrix*. [p 820]

18. **d. liver.** Fluconazole may affect the liver or steroidogenesis but to a lesser degree than the imidazoles do. [p 821]

SECTION V

VOIDING FUNCTION AND DYSFUNCTION

Chapter 23

Physiology and Pharmacology of the Bladder and Urethra

Michael B. Chancellor • Naoki Yoshimura

Questions

1. Sacral-evoked response testing measures nerve conduction time via which of the following pathways?

    a. Somatic afferent, sympathetic efferent
    b. Somatic afferent, somatic efferent
    c. Sympathetic afferent, somatic efferent
    d. Sympathetic afferent, parasympathetic efferent
    e. Parasympathetic afferent, sympathetic efferent

2. During the resting state, bladder smooth muscle electrical activity is characterized by:

    a. a concentration of K^+ ions higher on the outside of the cell membrane.
    b. a concentration of Na^+ ions higher on the inside of the cell membrane.
    c. the cell membrane preferentially permeable to K^+.
    d. the cell membrane preferentially permeable to Na^+.
    e. the inside of the cell membrane positive with respect to the outside.

3. Two weeks after complete C6 spinal cord injury (SCI), a 31-year-old woman has a urodynamic study that demonstrates detrusor areflexia. What is the most likely urodynamic finding 2 years later?

    a. Detrusor hyperreflexia
    b. Detrusor areflexia
    c. Detrusor hyperreflexia with detrusor-sphincter dyssynergia
    d. Detrusor areflexia with decreased bladder compliance
    e. Detrusor areflexia with detrusor-sphincter dyssynergia

4. Urinary tract smooth muscle contractility is inhibited by:

    a. propranolol.
    b. nifedipine.
    c. phenylephrine.
    d. acetylcholine.
    e. substance P.

5. Phosphodiesterase inhibitors cause smooth muscle relaxation by inhibiting:

    a. calmodulin binding.
    b. production of cyclic GMP.
    c. production of cyclic AMP.
    d. degradation of phospholipase C.
    e. degradation of cyclic GMP.

6. The most common urodynamic finding in sacral level spinal cord injury is:

    a. detrusor hyperreflexia.
    b. detrusor hyperreflexia with detrusor–external sphincter dyssynergia.
    c. detrusor areflexia.
    d. poor detrusor compliance.
    e. normal urodynamics.

7. During physiologic filling, bladder compliance is most affected by:

    a. perivesical ganglia activity.
    b. peripheral nerve activity.
    c. sacral spinal cord activity.
    d. suprasacral spinal cord activity.
    e. bladder wall viscoelasticity.

8. When the hypogastric nerve is stimulated, the primary neurotransmitter released at the ganglionic level is:

    a. acetylcholine.
    b. ATP.
    c. dopamine.
    d. norepinephrine.
    e. prostaglandin $F_{2\alpha}$.

9. Pudendal nerve block may be useful in the treatment of neuropathic bladder dysfunction in patients with:

    a. lower motor lesions with spastic bladder.
    b. lower motor lesions with spastic sphincter.
    c. upper motor lesions with atonic bladder.
    d. upper motor lesions with spastic sphincter.
    e. upper motor lesions with vesicoureteral reflux.

10. Postganglionic sympathetic nerve fibers to the bladder release:

    a. acetylcholine.
    b. epinephrine.
    c. nitric oxide.

d. norepinephrine.
e. vasoactive intestinal polypeptide (VIP).

11. The bladder contraction and simultaneous urethral relaxation during voiding are coordinated by a reflex center located in the:

    a. hypothalamus.
    b. basal ganglia.
    c. medulla.
    d. pons.
    e. thoracic cord.

12. The sudden rise in detrusor pressure seen at the onset of carbon dioxide cystometry is due do:

    a. tonic contraction of the bladder.
    b. phasic contraction of the bladder.
    c. viscoelastic properties of the bladder.
    d. sacral reflex arc.
    e. bladder-urethral reflex arc.

13. The first event to occur with normal micturition is:

    a. relaxation of the bladder neck.
    b. relaxation of the prostate and prostatic capsule.
    c. relaxation of the external striated sphincter.
    d. contraction of the bladder body.
    e. contraction of the bladder trigone.

14. In patients with hypersensitive bladder dysfunction, intravesical capsaicin instillation may potentially benefit the patient by blockade of:

    a. the glycosaminoglycan receptor.
    b. serotonin reuptake.
    c. A-delta fiber afferents.
    d. C-fiber afferents.
    e. the tachykinin receptor.

15. Bladder painful sensations are conveyed by which nerve(s)?

    a. Hypogastric
    b. Pelvic
    c. Pudendal
    d. Pelvic and hypogastric
    e. Pelvic and pudendal

16. Smooth muscle contraction results from phosphorylation of which of the following proteins?

    a. Actin
    b. Caldesmon
    c. Desmin
    d. G protein
    e. Myosin

17. Neurally mediated relaxation of the urethra during voiding occurs by release of:

    a. nitric oxide from sympathetics.
    b. nitric oxide from parasympathetics.
    c. VIP from sympathetics.
    d. VIP from parasympathetics.
    e. neuropeptide Y from sympathetics.

18. Influx of which ion or chemical is responsible for generation of action potential by bladder smooth muscle cells?

    a. Calcium
    b. Potassium
    c. Sodium
    d. Chloride
    e. Nitric oxide

19. Efflux of which ion or chemical results in relaxation of the bladder smooth muscle cells?

    a. Calcium
    b. Potassium
    c. Sodium
    d. Chloride
    e. Nitric oxide

20. The decrease in bladder compliance is due to what change in connective tissue component?

    a. Decrease in elastin
    b. Decreased in type I collagen
    c. Decrease in type II collagen
    d. Increase in type III collagen
    e. Increase in type V collagen

21. Acetylcholine binds predominately to which of the five muscarinic receptor(s) to induce bladder contraction?

    a. M_1
    b. M_2
    c. M_1 and M_2
    d. M_2 and M_3
    e. M_2 and M_4

22. Substance P is located in which type(s) of nerves?

    a. Afferent
    b. Efferent
    c. Afferent and efferent
    d. A-delta fibers
    e. Spinal cord interneurons

23. Which hormone increases α-adrenergic receptors density in the urethra?

    a. Luteinizing hormone–releasing hormone
    b. Dihydrotestosterone
    c. Testosterone
    d. Estrogen
    e. Testosterone and estrogen

24. The most important excitatory neurotransmitter in the central nervous system to facilitate micturition is:

    a. acetylcholine.
    b. γ-aminobutyric acid.
    c. norepinephrine.
    d. glutamate.
    e. serotonin.

25. The central nervous system neurotransmitter that inhibits micturition is:

    a. acetylcholine.
    b. substance P.
    c. norepinephrine.
    d. glutamate.
    e. serotonin.

26. What is the function of delta and mu opioid receptors in the spinal cord?

    a. They do not participate in the micturition reflex.
    b. They enhance bladder sensation.
    c. They inhibit descending pontinespinal signaling.
    d. They stimulate bladder contraction.
    e. They inhibit bladder contraction.

27. The nerves that trigger normal micturition are:

    a. sympathetic nerves.
    b. myelinated A-delta afferent nerves.
    c. unmyelinated C afferent nerves.
    d. both A-delta and C-fiber afferent nerves.
    e. none of the above.

84 VOIDING FUNCTION AND DYSFUNCTION

28. The receptor that intravesical capsaicin acts on is:
    a. muscarinic.
    b. glutamatergic.
    c. nitrogenergic.
    d. purinergic.
    e. vanilloid.

29. The nerve that triggers uninhibited bladder contractions induced by a spinal micturition reflex in the cat model of chronic spinal cord transection is:
    a. sympathetic.
    b. A-delta.
    c. C fiber.
    d. both A-delta and C fibers.
    e. none of the above.

Answers

1. **b. Somatic afferent, somatic efferent.** Sacral-evoked response testing or measurement of sacral latency is accomplished by electrical stimulation of the skin of the penis while recording activity of the bulbocavernosus muscle. Both the afferent and efferent limbs of this reflex arc are somatic nerves. At present, no clinically useful neurophysiologic study exists that directly measures nerve conduction over autonomic nerves, which supply the lower urinary tract or penis. [pp 846–848]

2. **c. the cell membrane preferentially permeable to K$^+$.** During the resting state, the cell membrane is preferentially permeable to K$^+$. The tendency of K$^+$ is to move from the inside of the cell, where it is more concentrated, to the outside of the cell membrane. This outward migration of K$^+$ creates an electrical gradient across the cell membrane, with the inside of the cell membrane being negative with respect to the outside. [pp 837–838]

3. **c. Detrusor hyperreflexia with detrusor-sphincter dyssynergia.** After SCI, patients generally develop a spinal shock phase that lasts approximately 4 weeks. During spinal shock, the detrusor is areflexic. In patients with complete high SCI, the long-term urodynamic manifestation is most commonly detrusor hyperreflexia with detrusor-sphincter dyssynergia. Incomplete SCI generally demonstrates detrusor hyperreflexia with or without detrusor sphincter-dyssynergia. In up to 15% of cervical SCI cases, detrusor areflexia may be a permanent finding. The variability of urodynamic findings in SCI emphasizes the need for careful urodynamic evaluation and follow-up in all SCI patients. [p 870]

4. **b. nifedipine.** Phenylephrine is an α-adrenergic agonist, acetylcholine is a muscarinic cholinergic agonist, and substance P is a tachykinin. All three agents stimulate smooth muscle contractility. Propranolol is a β-adrenergic antagonist and blocks the inhibitory effects of β-adrenergic agonists such as isoproterenol. Nifedipine is a calcium channel blocker and inhibits the inward movement of calcium across the cell membrane that is needed for the upstroke of the smooth muscle action potential and for supplying the calcium that is required for contractility. [pp 837–839]

5. **e. degradation of cyclic GMP.** Cyclic GMP is a second messenger for nitric oxide that activates protein kinases, promoting smooth muscle relaxation. Cyclic GMP is degraded to GMP by phosphodiesterase. A phosphodiesterase inhibitor potentiates the effect of cyclic GMP. Ca^{2+} binding to calmodulin is the first step in the initiation of smooth muscle contraction that activates myosin light chain kinase. [pp 860–861]

6. **c. detrusor areflexia.** Sacral level spinal injury most commonly results in cauda equina injury. This lower motor neuron injury presents as paralysis of bladder. Only a small number of patients with detrusor areflexia have poor detrusor compliance. [pp 870–871]

7. **e. bladder wall viscoelasticity.** The elastic and viscoelastic properties of the bladder are the main determinants of compliance during filling. Although neurogenic influences may be operative in late stages of filling, it is clearly these passive properties that are the main determinants of the pressure-volume curve. When these properties are destroyed, as in fibrosis of the bladder wall, markedly decreased compliance results. [p 834]

8. **a. acetylcholine.** All preganglionic efferent autonomic fibers release acetylcholine, whether they are anatomically parasympathetic or sympathetic. The term *cholinergic* refers to all those receptor sites where acetylcholine is a primary neurotransmitter, including the autonomic ganglion cells, the neuromuscular junctions of somatic nerve fibers, and the junction of all postganglionic parasympathetic fibers. Cholinergic receptor sites are divided into two major classes: muscarinic and nicotinic. Muscarinic sites include all autonomic effector cells. *Nicotinic* is applied to the receptor sites on autonomic ganglia, such as those referred to in this question, and the motor end plates of skeletal muscle. [p 846]

9. **d. upper motor lesions with spastic sphincter.** The pudendal nerve innervates the striated muscle sphincter. Temporary (lidocaine) or permanent (alcohol) block of the pudendal nerve may inhibit detrusor-sphincter dyssynergia. This form of treatment has not been popular, however, because complete bilateral blockade of the pudendal nerves is not easy and has the side effect of impotence. [pp 870–871]

10. **d. norepinephrine.** Postganglionic sympathetic nerves are traditionally noradrenergic and release norepinephrine. Other substances released include neuropeptide Y and ATP. Vasoactive intestinal polypeptide (VIP) often coexists with acetylcholine in parasympathetic postganglionics. However, "sympathetic" does not *always* mean "noradrenergic," because in some tissues (e.g., sweat glands) sympathetics release acetylcholine. [pp 846–848]

11. **d. pons.** The center for integration and coordination of bladder and urethral activity during voiding is located in the pons (the pontine micturition center), as determined on the basis of animal electrophysiologic studies and lesioning or positron emission tomography in humans. The basal ganglia and medulla seem to be involved in modulation of detrusor activity and perhaps in facilitation of detrusor contractility but not in integration of bladder and urethral response. [p 854]

12. **c. viscoelastic properties of the bladder.** Sudden stretch of detrusor muscle strips in vivo preparations or in human bladder during cystometry causes a sudden rise in pressure that is due entirely to passive viscoelastic properties of the bladder. Clinically, this rise in pressure may stimulate a detrusor contraction. Because the phenomenon is a passive one, it does not require intact innervation. [p 834]

13. **c. relaxation of the external striated sphincter.** Synchronous pressure-flow electromyographic studies have demonstrated that the initiation of micturition reflex is character-

ized by a sudden and complete relaxation of the striated external sphincter followed by detrusor contraction, opening of the bladder neck, and uroflow. [p 851]

14. **d. C-fiber afferents.** Capsaicin inhibits C-fiber afferent activity because vanilloid receptors, which bind to capsaicin, are predominantly located in C fibers. Although there are solid animal studies of capsaicin blockade of bladder inflammation, clinical data are scant. Only uncontrolled trials suggest that bladder hypersensitivity and pain are mediated by C-fiber afferents and that the symptoms are improved with intravesical capsaicin therapy. [p 864]

15. **d. Pelvic and hypogastric.** Bladder pain caused by overdistention is mediated by the hypogastric nerve. Bladder pain from inflammatory stimuli is mediated by pelvic nerves. [pp 847–848]

16. **e. Myosin.** Phosphorylation of myosin by myosin light chain kinase results in smooth muscle contraction. This process is crucial for contraction of the ureter, vas deferens, bladder, and corporeal smooth muscle. [p 836]

17. **b. nitric oxide from parasympathetics.** During voiding, active contraction of the bladder occurs through parasympathetically mediated cholinergic contraction. In addition, parasympathetically mediated urethral smooth and striated muscle relaxation occurs. An abundance of experimental data indicate that nitric oxide is responsible for this relaxation. [p 860]

18. **a. Calcium.** Influx of calcium results in action potential generation in smooth muscle cells. [pp 837–838]

19. **b. Potassium.** Efflux of potassium causes hyperpolarization and results in smooth muscle relaxation. [pp 837–838]

20. **d. Increase in type III collagen.** An increase in type III collagen results in decreased bladder compliance. [p 840]

21. **d. M_2 and M_3.** Binding of acetylcholine to predominantly M_2 and M_3 muscarinic receptors results in bladder contraction. [p 857]

22. **a. Afferent.** Substance P is located exclusively in afferent nerves. [pp 861–862]

23. **d. Estrogen.** Only estrogen has been shown to increase the number of α-adrenergic receptors. [p 863]

24. **d. glutamate.** Glutamate plays an essential role as an excitatory neurotransmitter in the central nervous system to facilitate voiding. Glutamate is facilitatory at the levels of bladder afferents and spinal neurons, descending projection from the pons, within the pons, and in the brain. [pp 866–867]

25. **e. serotonin.** Serotonin acts as a neurotransmitter in the spinal cord to inhibit micturition. [p 864]

26. **e. They inhibit bladder contraction.** Delta and mu opioid receptors in the spinal cord and the brain regulate the micturition threshold volume and inhibit bladder contraction. [pp 868–869]

27. **b. myelinated A-delta afferent nerves.** A-delta myelinated pelvic nerve afferents are responsible for triggering normal micturition. C fibers are unmyelinated afferent nerves. [pp 851–852]

28. **e. vanilloid.** Capsaicin acts on the vanilloid receptors. A high dose of capsaicin causes depletion of substance P and other tachykinins from capsaicin-sensitive unmyelinated C fibers and re-reduces sensory nerve function in the bladder wall. [pp 864–865]

29. **c. C fiber.** After spinal cord transection, unmyelinated C-fiber afferents in the pelvic nerve trigger a spinal micturition reflex in the cat. In the rat, C-fiber afferents are responsible for nonvoiding uninhibited bladder contractions, although voiding bladder contractions are still dependent on A-delta fiber afferent nerves. [p 864]

Chapter 24

Pathophysiology and Categorization of Voiding Dysfunction

Alan J. Wein

Questions

1. Which of the following best describes normal bladder behavior during the filling-storage phase of the micturition cycle?

    a. Low compliance due to elastic properties
    b. High compliance due to elastic properties
    c. Low compliance due to elastic and viscoelastic properties
    d. High compliance due to elastic and viscoelastic properties
    e. High compliance due to a low relaxation coefficient of the lamina propria

2. A patient who has significantly and urodynamically dangerous decreased compliance because of a replacement by collagen of other components of the stroma is generally best managed by:

    a. pharmacologic manipulation.
    b. hydraulic distention.
    c. nerve section.
    d. augmentation cystoplasty.
    e. neuromodulation.

3. The primary effect of the spinal sympathetic reflexes that are evoked in animals during bladder filling and that facilitate bladder filling-storage is:

    a. neurally mediated stimulation of the α-adrenergic receptors in the area of the smooth sphincter.
    b. neurally mediated stimulation of the β-adrenergic receptors in the bladder body smooth musculature.

c. direct inhibition of detrusor motor neurons in the sacral spinal cord.
d. neurally mediated inhibition of cholinergic receptors in the area of the bladder body.
e. neurally mediated sympathetic modulation of cholinergic ganglionic transmission.

4. The organizational center for the micturition reflex in an intact neural axis is:
   a. the pontine mesencephalic formation in the brain stem.
   b. the frontal area of the cerebral cortex.
   c. the parietal area of the cerebral cortex.
   d. the cerebellum.
   e. the sacral spinal cord.

5. Involuntary bladder contractions are most commonly seen in association with:
   a. sacral spinal cord neurologic disease or injury.
   b. infrasacral neurologic disease or injury.
   c. suprasacral neurologic disease or injury.
   d. peripheral nerve neurologic disease or injury.
   e. interstitial cystitis.

6. In the Bors-Comarr system of classification, the term *unbalanced*, when applied to a patient with an upper motor neuron (UMN) lesion, implies:
   a. a cerebellar lesion.
   b. involuntary bladder contractions during filling.
   c. an areflexic bladder.
   d. decreased bladder compliance during filling.
   e. sphincter dyssynergia.

7. In the Bors-Comarr system, a patient with post-cerebrovascular accident voiding dysfunction characterized by urgency, frequency, and urge incontinence would most commonly be characterized as having a(an):
   a. UMN lesion, complete, balanced.
   b. UMN lesion, complete, imbalanced.
   c. lower motor neuron (LMN) lesion, complete, imbalanced.
   d. LMN lesion, incomplete, balanced.
   e. UMN lesion/LMN lesion, complete, balanced.

8. In the Bradley classification system, a patient with post-cerebrovascular accident voiding dysfunction characterized by urgency, frequency, and urge incontinence would most commonly be characterized as having a:
   a. loop 1 lesion.
   b. loop 2 lesion.
   c. loop 3 lesion.
   d. loop 4A lesion.
   e. loop 4B lesion.

9. In the Lapides classification system, a patient with post-cerebrovascular accident voiding dysfunction characterized by urgency, frequency, and urge incontinence would most commonly be characterized as having a:
   a. sensory neurogenic bladder.
   b. motor paralytic bladder.
   c. uninhibited neurogenic bladder.
   d. reflex neurogenic bladder.
   e. autonomous neurogenic bladder.

10. A reflex neurogenic bladder, as described in the Lapides system classification, is characteristically seen in which of the following situations?
    a. Following traumatic spinal cord injury between the sacral spinal cord and the brain stem.
    b. Following traumatic spinal cord injury between the sacral spinal cord and conus medullaris.
    c. Following a cerebrovascular accident in a patient with insulin-dependent diabetes mellitus.
    d. In a patient with non–insulin-dependent diabetes mellitus.
    e. In a patient with multiple sclerosis.

11. In the urodynamic classification system, a patient with post–cerebrovascular accident voiding dysfunction characterized by urgency, frequency, and urge incontinence would most commonly be characterized as having:
    a. detrusor areflexia, striated sphincter dyssynergia, smooth sphincter dyssynergia.
    b. detrusor hyperreflexia, striated sphincter synergia, smooth sphincter synergia.
    c. detrusor hyperreflexia, striated sphincter dyssynergia, smooth sphincter synergia.
    d. detrusor areflexia, striated sphincter synergia, smooth sphincter dyssynergia.
    e. detrusor hyperreflexia, striated sphincter synergia, smooth sphincter dyssynergia.

12. In the International Continence Society classification of voiding dysfunction, what does the term *unstable detrusor* indicate?
    a. The presence of involuntary detrusor contractions during the filling phase of micturition that are spontaneous
    b. The presence of involuntary detrusor contractions during the filling phase of micturition that are provoked
    c. The presence of involuntary detrusor contractions during the filling phase of micturition that are due to neurologic disease
    d. The presence of involuntary detrusor contractions during the filling phase of micturition that are not due to neurologic disease
    e. No significant rises in detrusor pressure during the filling phase of micturition in a psychotic patient

Answers

1. **d. High compliance due to elastic and viscoelastic properties.** The normal adult bladder response to filling at a physiologic rate is an almost imperceptible change in intravesical pressure. During at least the initial stages of bladder filling, after unfolding of the bladder wall from its collapsed state, this very high compliance (Δ volume/Δ pressure) of the bladder is due primarily to its elastic and viscoelastic properties. Elasticity allows the constituents of the bladder wall to stretch to a certain degree without any increase in tension. Viscoelasticity allows stretch to induce a rise in tension followed by a decay (stress relaxation) when the filling (stretch stimulus) slows or stops. [p 889]

2. **d. augmentation cystoplasty.** The viscoelastic properties of the stroma (bladder wall less smooth muscle and epithelium) and the urodynamically relaxed detrusor muscle account for the passive mechanical properties and normal bladder compliance seen during filling. The main components of stroma are collagen and elastin. When the collagen component increases, compliance decreases. This can occur with various

types of injury, chronic inflammation, bladder outlet obstruction, and neurologic decentralization. Once decreased compliance occurs because of a replacement by collagen of other components of the stroma, it is generally unresponsive to pharmacologic manipulation, hydraulic distention, or nerve section. Most often, under those circumstances, augmentation cystoplasty is required to achieve satisfactory reservoir function. [pp 889–890]

3. **e. neurally mediated sympathetic modulation of cholinergic ganglionic transmission.** Does the nervous system affect the normal bladder response to filling? At a certain level of bladder filling, spinal sympathetic reflexes facilitatory to bladder filling-storage are clearly evoked in animals, a concept developed over the years by deGroat and associates, who have also cited indirect evidence to support such a role in humans. This inhibitory effect is thought to be mediated primarily by sympathetic modulation of cholinergic ganglionic transmission. Through this reflex mechanism, two other possibilities exist for promoting filling-storage. One is neurally mediated stimulation of the predominantly α-adrenergic receptors in the area of the smooth sphincter, the net result of which would be to cause an increase in resistance in that area. The second is neurally mediated stimulation of the predominantly β-adrenergic receptors (inhibitory) in the bladder body smooth musculature, which would cause a decrease in bladder wall tension. McGuire has also cited evidence for direct inhibition of detrusor motor neurons in the sacral spinal cord during bladder filling that is due to increased afferent pudendal nerve activity generated by receptors in the striated sphincter. Good evidence also seems to exist to support a tonic inhibitory effect of other neurotransmitters on the micturition reflex at various levels of the neural axis. Bladder filling and consequent wall distention may also release autocrine-like factors that themselves influence contractility (nitric oxide, prostaglandins, and peptides, for example). [p 890]

4. **a. the pontine mesencephalic formation in the brain stem.** Although the origin of the parasympathetic neural outflow to the bladder, the pelvic nerve, is in the sacral spinal cord, the actual organizational center for the micturition reflex in an intact neural axis is in the brain stem, and the complete neural circuit for normal micturition includes the ascending and descending spinal cord pathways to and from this area and the facilitatory and inhibitory influences from other parts of the brain. [p 890]

5. **c. suprasacral neurologic disease or injury.** Involuntary contractions (IVCs) are most commonly seen associated with suprasacral neurologic disease or following suprasacral neurologic injury; however, they may also be associated with aging, inflammation or irritation of the bladder wall, bladder outlet obstruction, or stress urinary incontinence, or they may be idiopathic. [p 891]

6. **e. sphincter dyssynergia.** This system applies only to patients with neurologic dysfunction and considers three factors: (1) the anatomic localization of the lesion; (2) the neurologic completeness or incompleteness of the lesion; and (3) a designation as to whether lower urinary tract function is balanced or unbalanced. The latter terms are based solely on the percentage of residual urine relative to bladder capacity. *Unbalanced* signifies the presence of greater than 20% residual urine in a patient with a UMN lesion or 10% in a patient with an LMN lesion. This relative residual urine volume was ideally meant to imply coordination (synergy) or dyssynergia between the smooth and striated sphincters of the outlet and the bladder, during bladder contraction or during attempted micturition by abdominal straining or the Credé method. [p 893]

7. **a. UMN lesion, complete, balanced.** In this system, *UMN bladder* refers to the pattern of micturition that results from an injury to the suprasacral spinal cord after the period of spinal shock has passed, assuming that the sacral spinal cord and the sacral nerve roots are intact and that the pelvic and pudendal nerve reflexes are intact. *LMN bladder* refers to the pattern resulting if the sacral spinal cord or sacral roots are damaged and the reflex pattern through the autonomic and somatic nerves that emanate from these segments is absent. This system implies that if skeletal muscle spasticity exists below the level of the lesion, the lesion is above the sacral spinal cord and is by definition a UMN lesion. This type of lesion is characterized by IVCs during filling. If flaccidity of the skeletal musculature below the level of a lesion exists, an LMN lesion is assumed to exist, implying detrusor areflexia. Exceptions occur and are classified in a mixed lesion group characterized either by IVCs with a flaccid paralysis below the level of the lesion or by detrusor areflexia with spasticity or normal skeletal muscle tone neurologically below the lesion level. *UMN lesion, complete, imbalanced* implies a neurologically complete lesion above the level of the sacral spinal cord that results in skeletal muscle spasticity below the level of the injury. IVC occurs during filling, but a residual urine volume of greater than 20% of the bladder capacity is left after bladder contraction, implying obstruction in the area of the bladder outlet during the involuntary detrusor contraction. This obstruction is generally due to striated sphincter dyssynergia, typically occurring in patients who are paraplegic and quadriplegic with lesions between the cervical and the sacral spinal cord. Smooth sphincter dyssynergia may be seen as well in patients with lesions above the level of T6, usually in association with autonomic hyperreflexia (see Chapter 26). *LMN lesion, complete, imbalanced* implies a neurologically complete lesion at the level of the sacral spinal cord or of the sacral roots, resulting in skeletal muscle flaccidity below that level. Detrusor areflexia results, and whatever measures the patient may use to increase intravesical pressure during attempted voiding are not sufficient to decrease residual urine to less than 10% of bladder capacity. [p 893]

8. **a. loop 1 lesion.** Bradley's "loop system" of classification is a primarily neurologic system based on his conceptualization of central nervous system control of the lower urinary tract that identifies four neurologic "loops." Dysfunctions are classified according to the loop affected, as follows:

   Loop 1 consists of neuronal connections between the cerebral cortex and the pontine-mesencephalic micturition center; this coordinates voluntary control of the detrusor reflex. Loop 1 lesions are seen in conditions such as brain tumor, cerebrovascular accident or disease, and cerebral atrophy with dementia. The final result is characteristically IVC.

   Loop 2 includes the intraspinal pathway of detrusor muscle afferents to the brain stem micturition center and the motor impulses from this center to the sacral spinal cord. Loop 2 is thought to coordinate and provide for a detrusor reflex of adequate temporal duration to allow complete voiding. Partial interruption by spinal cord injury results in a detrusor reflex of low threshold and in poor emptying with residual urine. Spinal cord transection of loop 2 acutely produces detrusor areflexia and urinary retention—spinal shock. After this has passed, IVC results.

   Loop 3 consists of the peripheral detrusor afferent axons and their pathways in the spinal cord; these terminate by synapsing on pudendal motor neurons that ultimately innervate periurethral striated muscle. Loop 3 was thought to provide a neurologic substrate for coordinated reciprocal action of the bladder and striated sphincter. Loop 3 dys-

function could be responsible for detrusor-striated dyssynergia or involuntary sphincter relaxation.
Loop 4 consists of two components. Loop 4A is the suprasacral afferent and efferent innervation of the pudendal motor neurons to the periurethral striated musculature. Loop 4B consists of afferent fibers from the periurethral striated musculature that synapse on pudendal motor neurons in Onuf's nucleus, the segmental innervation of the periurethral striated muscle. Loop 4 provides for volitional control of the striated sphincter. [p 894]

9. **c. uninhibited neurogenic bladder.** Lapides contributed significantly to the classification and care of the patient with neuropathic voiding dysfunction by slightly modifying and popularizing a system originally proposed by McLellan in 1939. Lapides' classification differs from that of McLellan in only one respect, and that is the division of the group "atonic neurogenic bladder" into sensory neurogenic bladder and motor neurogenic bladder. This remains one of the most familiar systems to urologists and nonurologists because it describes in recognizable shorthand the clinical and cystometric conditions of many types of neurogenic voiding dysfunction. An uninhibited neurogenic bladder was described originally as resulting from injury or disease to the "corticoregulatory tract." The sacral spinal cord was presumed to be the micturition reflex center, and this corticoregulatory tract was believed to normally exert an inhibitory influence on the sacral micturition reflex center. A destructive lesion in this tract would then result in overfacilitation of the micturition reflex. Cerebrovascular accident, brain or spinal cord tumor, Parkinson's disease, and demyelinating disease were listed as the most common causes in this category. The voiding dysfunction is most often characterized symptomatically by frequency, urgency, and urge incontinence, and urodynamically by normal sensation with IVC at low filling volumes. Residual urine is characteristically low unless anatomic outlet obstruction or true smooth or striated sphincter dyssynergia occurs. The patient can generally initiate a bladder contraction voluntarily but is often unable to do so during cystometry because sufficient urine storage cannot occur before IVC is stimulated. [pp 894–895]

10. **a. Following traumatic spinal cord injury between the sacral spinal cord and the brain stem.** Reflex neurogenic bladder describes the post–spinal shock condition that exists after complete interruption of the sensory and motor pathways between the sacral spinal cord and the brain stem. Most commonly, this occurs in traumatic spinal cord injury and transverse myelitis, but it may occur with extensive demyelinating disease or any process that produces significant spinal cord destruction as well. Typically, there is no bladder sensation and there is inability to initiate voluntary micturition. Incontinence without sensation generally results because of low-volume IVC. Striated sphincter dyssynergia is the rule. This type of lesion is essentially equivalent to a complete UMN lesion in the Bors-Comarr system. [p 895]

11. **b. detrusor hyperreflexia, striated sphincter synergia, smooth sphincter synergia.** When exact urodynamic classification is possible, this system provides a truly precise description of the voiding dysfunction that occurs. If a normal or hyperreflexic detrusor exists with coordinated smooth and striated sphincter function and without anatomic obstruction, normal bladder emptying should occur.

    Detrusor hyperreflexia is most commonly associated with neurologic lesions above the sacral spinal cord. Striated sphincter dyssynergia is most commonly seen after complete suprasacral spinal cord injury, following the period of spinal shock. Smooth sphincter dyssynergia is seen most classically in autonomic hyperreflexia (see Chapter 26), when it is characteristically associated with detrusor hyperreflexia and striated sphincter dyssynergia.
    Detrusor areflexia may be secondary to bladder muscle decompensation or to various other conditions that produce inhibition at the level of the brain stem micturition center, sacral spinal cord, bladder ganglia, or bladder smooth muscle. Patients with a voiding dysfunction secondary to detrusor areflexia generally attempt bladder emptying by abdominal straining, and their continence status and the efficiency of their emptying efforts are determined by the status of their smooth and striated sphincter mechanisms. [p 896]

12. **d. The presence of involuntary detrusor contractions during the filling phase of micturition that are not due to neurologic disease.** Normal bladder function during filling-storage implies no significant rises in detrusor pressure (stability). Overactive detrusor function indicates the presence of "involuntary detrusor contractions during the filling phase, which may be spontaneous or provoked and which the patient cannot completely suppress," that is, the patient is trying to inhibit micturition if sensation is present. If contractions are due to neurologic disease, the term *detrusor hyperreflexia* is used; if not, the term *unstable detrusor* is applied. Bladder sensation can be categorized only in qualitative terms as indicated. Bladder capacity and compliance (Δ volume/ Δ pressure) are cystometric measurements. [p 896]

Chapter 25

The Neurourologic Evaluation

George D. Webster • Michael L. Guralnick

Questions

1. A patient complains of urinary frequency, urgency, and nocturia. He is best described as having:

    a. obstructive symptoms.
    b. irritative symptoms.
    c. prostatism.
    d. storage symptoms.
    e. voiding symptoms.

2. Urinary continence in a neurologically intact male with an involuntary bladder contraction is maintained by:

a. volitional contraction of the distal sphincter mechanism.
b. reflex contraction of the distal sphincter mechanism.
c. volitional contraction of the proximal sphincter mechanism.
d. reflex contraction of the proximal sphincter mechanism.
e. none of the above.

3. A woman who complains of unconscious leakage may have all of the following except:

   a. bladder instability.
   b. intrinsic sphincter deficiency.
   c. vesicovaginal fistula.
   d. urge incontinence.
   e. overflow incontinence.

4. All of the following statements about symptom scores such as the International Prostate Symptom Score (IPSS) and International Continence Society (ICS) male questionnaire are true except for which one?

   a. They have been validated psychometrically.
   b. They help assess the severity and degree of bother of lower urinary tract symptoms.
   c. They do not correlate well with urodynamic indices.
   d. They help differentiate between patients who have obstruction and those who do not.
   e. They are not sex specific.

5. Which of the following statements is false? Bladder diaries are useful because they:

   a. allow for quantitation of urinary output.
   b. help determine whether excessive frequency is due to low capacity or to polyuria.
   c. often correlate well with the patient's subjective estimate of urinary frequency.
   d. assist in the planning of behavioral therapy.
   e. help document triggers for urinary incontinence.

6. Which of the following statements about the bulbocavernosus reflex (BCR) is true?

   a. It tests the integrity of L5-S1 cord segments.
   b. Its absence confirms the presence of a neurologic lesion.
   c. It is the contraction of the gluteus muscles in response to the squeezing of the glans.
   d. It may be maintained in patients with incomplete sacral lesions.
   e. None of the above.

7. All of the following are indicated in the routine work-up of a patient with a neurogenic bladder except:

   a. an upper urinary tract study such as an ultrasonogram or renal scan.
   b. assessment of reflexes.
   c. cystoscopy.
   d. urinalysis.
   e. serum creatinine assay.

8. Which of the following statements is true about urodynamics?

   a. If the study does not demonstrate unstable contractions, the patient does not have detrusor instability.
   b. A study showing detrusor instability proves that it is the cause of the patient's symptoms.
   c. If a study does not reproduce the patient's symptoms, it is not diagnostic.
   d. It is best to initially use the most sophisticated urodynamics test to make a diagnosis.
   e. None of the above.

9. Clear indications for urodynamic study include all of the following except:

   a. persistent LUTS despite presumably adequate therapy.
   b. patients in whom therapy may be hazardous.
   c. women with mixed incontinence after prior anti-incontinence procedures.
   d. a patient with a spinal cord injury.
   e. children with isolated nocturnal enuresis.

10. All of the following statements about patient preparation and precautions are true except which one?

    a. Urodynamics should be deferred in patients with a urinary tract infection.
    b. Ideally, patients should not have an indwelling Foley catheter before the study.
    c. Ideally, drugs that affect bladder function should be stopped before the study.
    d. Routine antibiotic prophylaxis is needed for all patients.
    e. Patient cooperation is crucial for a successful test.

11. Which of the following statements about autonomic dysreflexia is false?

    a. It is an exaggerated sympathetic response to visceral stimulation.
    b. If a patient experiences it during a urodynamic study, the bladder should be emptied immediately.
    c. It occurs in patients with spinal cord lesions above T6.
    d. Pretreatment with an α-blocker or calcium channel blocker may be helpful.
    e. It manifests with sweating, headache, hypertension, and flushing below the level of the lesion.

12. Which of the following statements is true regarding cystometrography (CMG)?

    a. The reference point for external transducers is the umbilicus.
    b. Pressures should be zeroed to atmospheric pressure.
    c. It is the measurement of intravesical pressure during voiding.
    d. Air bubbles in the pressure lines cause increases in pressure measurement.
    e. None of the above.

13. Which of the following statements about fluid factors that affect CMG is false?

    a. Rapid fill rates can produce instability.
    b. Alkaline fluids may result in increased bladder capacity.
    c. Acidic fluids may inhibit unstable contractions.
    d. Rapid fill rates are those that are faster than 100 ml/min.
    e. Fluid temperature should be as close to body temperature as possible.

14. Which of the following statements about detrusor pressure (P_{det}) is true?

    a. It is determined with single-channel urodynamics.
    b. It is the component of bladder pressure created by extravesical forces.
    c. It is calculated by adding intravesical pressure (P_{ves}) and abdominal pressure (P_{abd}).
    d. True changes in P_{det} are independent of changes in P_{ves}.
    e. None of the above.

15. The following variables are routinely measured by CMG except:

    a. capacity.
    b. compliance.
    c. sensation.

d. instability.
e. obstruction.

16. Which of the following statements is true of compliance?
    a. It is the change in volume for given change in pressure.
    b. It is a measure of outlet resistance.
    c. Measured compliance is affected by fill rate.
    d. The normal pressure rise during the course of a CMG test is 50 cm H_2O.
    e. None of the above.

17. An unstable bladder contraction:
    a. is defined as an involuntary pressure rise of greater than 20 cm H_2O.
    b. is always demonstrated in patients with urge incontinence.
    c. is called *detrusor hyperreflexia* in neurologically intact patients.
    d. may be inhibited by a patient with sensory urgency.
    e. is always symptomatic.

18. Which of the following statements about provocative testing and pitfalls in CMG is false?
    a. Bethanechol testing is unreliable in diagnosing neurogenic bladder.
    b. The ice water test is used to differentiate upper motor neuron lesions from lower motor neuron lesions.
    c. Vesicoureteral reflux may decrease measured bladder compliance.
    d. If the bladder outlet is incompetent, it may be necessary to occlude it with a Foley catheter for accurate measurement.
    e. None of the above.

19. Which of the following statements about detrusor leak point pressure (DLPP) is true?
    a. DLPP is the lowest pressure causing urine leakage with abdominal straining.
    b. DLPP is a reflection of resistance of the urethra to the bladder.
    c. DLPP less than 20 is associated with a high risk of upper tract damage.
    d. DLPP is not affected by catheter size.
    e. detrusor pressure determines bladder outlet resistance.

20. Which of the following statements about Valsalva leak point pressure (VLPP) is true?
    a. A normally positioned and functioning urethra can be caused to leak by straining.
    b. A low VLPP means that stress incontinence is the sole cause of incontinence.
    c. There is good correlation between VLPP and maximum urethral closing pressure (MUCP).
    d. VLPP is the highest abdominal pressure that causes incontinence.
    e. None of the above.

21. All of the following cause a high VLPP except:
    a. prolapse.
    b. patient anxiety.
    c. poor bladder compliance.
    d. large catheter size.
    e. all of the above cause high VLPP.

22. Which of the following statements about uroflow is true?
    a. The uroflow pattern of a plateau with a prolonged flow time is diagnostic of bladder outlet obstruction.
    b. Q_{max} is affected by age in patients of both sexes.
    c. A difference in Q_{max} on repeated testing may be spurious.
    d. All voids of less than 150 ml should be discarded.
    e. A flow rate of greater than 15 ml/s rules out bladder outlet obstruction.

23. Which of the following statements about pressure-flow studies is true?
    a. Catheter size does not seem to be important.
    b. If a patient is unable to void, he has bladder areflexia.
    c. After-contractions are more common in patients with instability than in patients without instability.
    d. Normal postvoid residual rules out bladder outlet obstruction.
    e. Bladder outlet obstruction can be diagnosed only if P_{det} is greater than 100 cm H_2O.

24. Which of the following is true of the Abrams-Griffith nomogram?
    a. It is based on preoperative and postoperative urodynamic data.
    b. It clearly divides patients into obstructed versus unobstructed groups.
    c. It can help grade the degree of obstruction by calculating the Abrams-Griffith (AG) number.
    d. It has been validated for use in both men and women with obstruction.
    e. It is based on the detrusor contractility being the only important variable in diagnosing bladder outlet obstruction.

25. Which of the following is true of Schafer's method?
    a. It is based on a model of the urethra as a rigid tube.
    b. It essentially describes the relationship between pressure and flow during the period of maximal urethra resistance.
    c. It is based on empirical and theoretical data.
    d. It involves calculation of linear passive urethral resistance relation (PURR), which allows for grading obstruction into eight grades.
    e. It involves the use of two outlet parameters, urethral collapsibility and cross-sectional area.

26. Which of the following is true of the ICS nomogram?
    a. It is based on the fact that the various models of urethral resistance are different.
    b. It allows for continuous grading of obstruction by calculating the bladder outlet obstruction index (BOOI).
    c. It is essentially identical to the Schafer nomogram in appearance.
    d. It is intended for use in females with possible bladder outlet obstruction.
    e. It relies solely on flow rate, obviating the need for invasive testing.

27. Ambulatory urodynamics is thought to be advantageous over conventional urodynamics because:
    a. it predominantly uses natural filling and allows the subject to reproduce normal activities.
    b. it does not require much patient compliance.
    c. it is less likely to document insignificant detrusor instability.
    d. it can better classify patients as obstructed versus unobstructed.
    e. it tends to exaggerate the magnitude of low bladder compliance.

28. Advantages of video-urodynamics include:
    a. the ability to determine the presence and location of obstruction.
    b. the ability to determine the significance of an open bladder neck.

c. the ability to diagnose detrusor sphincter dyssynergy.
d. the ability to determine the significance of vesicoureteral reflux.
e. all of the above.

29. Which statement about kinesiologic sphincter electromyography (EMG) is true?

    a. It determines whether the bladder and external sphincter are coordinated.
    b. It diagnoses neuropathy.
    c. It measures latency responses.
    d. It tests the integrity of peripheral nervous pathways.
    e. It requires the use of an oscilloscope.

30. Detrusor sphincter dyssynergy (DSD):

    a. is the technical term for dysfunctional voiding in neurologically impaired patients.
    b. is the term for delayed sphincter relaxation in patients with Parkinson's disease.
    c. typically occurs in patients with suprasacral cord injuries.
    d. is the relaxation of the bladder neck that occurs during a detrusor contraction.
    e. is the normal response of the external sphincter during unstable bladder contraction.

31. On neurophysiologic testing, neuropathy is implied by:

    a. polyphasic potentials that constitute greater than 15% of all activity.
    b. high amplitude potentials.
    c. negative sharp waves.
    d. monophasic potentials.
    e. all of the above.

Answers

1. **d. storage symptoms.** *Voiding symptoms* is the term used to replace *obstructive symptoms* and includes the symptoms of hesitancy, slow stream, intermittency, straining to void, terminal dribbling, and a feeling of incomplete emptying. *Storage symptoms* replaces the term *irritative symptoms* for the symptoms of frequency, nocturia, urgency, and urge incontinence. [p 901]

2. **a. volitional contraction of the distal sphincter mechanism.** With an involuntary bladder contraction, the bladder neck automatically opens and continence must be maintained by the volitional contraction of the distal sphincter mechanism. [p 901]

3. **d. urge incontinence.** In some patients, incontinence occurs in the absence of any obvious increase in intra-abdominal pressure, without an urge to void or any conscious recognition that leakage is occurring. This is called unconscious incontinence and may be secondary to unstable bladder contractions, intrinsic sphincter deficiency, overflow incontinence, or extraurethral incontinence, such as that caused by a fistula. [pp 901–902]

4. **d. They help differentiate between patients who have obstruction and those who do not.** Although the IPSS has been formally validated with both clinimetric and psychometric principles, the symptoms it grades are not specific to benign prostatic hyperplasia and are also common in women. Furthermore, although the system tests the degree to which symptoms are present and bothersome, they do not correlate with urodynamic indices such as the presence of detrusor instability or bladder outlet obstruction. In fact, symptomatic patients with bladder outlet obstruction do not have significantly different scores from those who are not obstructed (who have detrusor dysfunction). [p 902]

5. **c. often correlate well with the patient's subjective estimate of urinary frequency.** A 3- to 5-day voiding diary is one of the most helpful tools in the assessment of voiding dysfunction. From this record, the total 24-hour urinary output, number of voids, voiding interval, diurnal distribution, timing and triggers for incontinence, and functional bladder capacity may be determined. In fact, it may be more reliable than the patient's own history, as there is often no correlation between the number of voids per patient history compared with the number documented on a voiding diary. [p 902]

6. **d. It may be maintained in patients with incomplete sacral lesions.** The normal BCR is the contraction of the anal sphincter and bulbocavernosus muscles in response to such maneuvers as placing an examining finger in the patient's rectum and then either squeezing the glans penis or clitoris or pulling on an indwelling Foley catheter. This is primarily a test of the integrity of spinal cord segments S2-S4. Thirty percent of neurologically intact females have an absent BCR, and patients with incomplete sacral lesions may maintain the reflex and thus the presence or absence of the reflex does not establish the diagnosis of a neurologic lesion. [pp 903–904]

7. **c. cystoscopy.** In the routine evaluation of a patient with a neurogenic bladder, an assessment of reflexes, a urinalysis, a serum creatinine assay, and a baseline upper tract imaging study (intravenous pyelogram, ultrasonogram, or renal scan) are indicated. Endoscopic evaluation of the lower urinary tract is not indicated in the routine screening of patients with neurogenic bladder. [pp 904–905]

8. **c. If a study does not reproduce the patient's symptoms, it is not diagnostic.** The goal in performing a urodynamic study is to answer specific questions related to the patient's storage and voiding functions. Nitti noted three important principles: (1) a study that does not duplicate the patient's symptoms is not diagnostic; (2) failure to record an abnormality does not rule out its existence; and (3) not all abnormalities detected are clinically significant. [p 905]

9. **e. children with isolated nocturnal enuresis.** Clear indications for some type of urodynamic investigation, however, include patients with persistent LUTS despite presumed appropriate therapy and patients in whom potential therapy may be hazardous (one would want to be sure of the correct diagnosis prior to instituting such therapy). Other indications for some type of urodynamic investigation include women with recurrent incontinence in whom surgery is planned, those with a confusing mix of stress and urge symptoms, and those with associated voiding problems. All neurologically impaired patients who have neurogenic bladder dysfunction should undergo urodynamic study to characterize the nature of the detrusor and sphincter problem and to determine prognosis and management. Children with isolated nocturnal enuresis rarely have abnormalities that are identified by routine laboratory-based urodynamic investigations. [pp 905–906]

10. **d. Routine antibiotic prophylaxis is needed for all patients.** Urodynamic studies are invasive and have been associated with morbidity, including urinary retention, hematuria, urinary tract infection, and pain. Although these effects are not common, patients need to be counseled about them and may be asked to sign a consent form. Studies should be deferred in the presence of urinary tract infection and ideally should not be performed after recent instrumentation (e.g., cystoscopy). Urinary tract infection and indwelling catheters may result in altered bladder dynamics (e.g., loss of compliance, reduced capacity) that may not otherwise exist. Patients who are catheter dependent ideally should have the catheter removed and have clean intermittent catheterization for a period of time before the urodynamic study is undertaken. Many pharmacologic agents can significantly affect detrusor or sphincteric function, and either patients should stop these medications or their impact on the urodynamic study should be taken into account. Parenteral antibiotic prophylaxis is necessary in patients at risk, such as those with rheumatic heart disease, mitral valve prolapse, prosthetic heart valves and joints, and so on. Routine oral prophylactic antibacterial drugs are not necessary. However, those patients requiring multiple instrumentation or those at high risk for urinary tract infection are usually treated for 24 to 48 hours after the completion of the study. Patient cooperation is crucial, and it is important that the patient be as relaxed as possible to avoid the artifactual effects of anxiety. [p 906]

11. **e. It manifests with sweating, headache, hypertension, and flushing below the level of the lesion.** Autonomic dysreflexia is an exaggerated sympathetic nervous system response to afferent visceral stimulation that occurs in patients with high neurologic lesions above the sympathetic outflow tract (at or above T6). It manifests with symptoms such as sweating, headache, flushing above the level of the lesion, severe (possibly life-threatening) hypertension, and reflex bradycardia. If the patient begins to experience these symptoms during a urodynamic study, the bladder should be emptied immediately and the patient given an antihypertensive, such as sublingual nifedipine (10 mg) or intravenous hydralazine if the condition does not resolve rapidly. In patients with a known diagnosis of autonomic dysreflexia, blood pressure should be monitored throughout the test and pretreatment with sublingual nifedipine or an α-blocking agent may be used. [p 906]

12. **b. Pressures should be zeroed to atmospheric pressure.** Cystometry is the measurement of intravesical pressure during the course of bladder filling. When external transducers are used, the reference point is the superior edge of the pubic symphysis. All systems should be zeroed to atmospheric pressure, and it is crucial that there are no air bubbles in any of the transducers or tubing that could otherwise cause pressure dampening or dissipation. [pp 906–907]

13. **c. Acidic fluids may inhibit unstable contractions.** An alkaline pH (>8.5) has been noted to increase bladder capacity in patients with instability, whereas an acidic solution (pH < 3.5) can provoke instability in otherwise stable bladders. [p 907]

14. **e. None of the above.** A shortcoming of single-channel cystometry is that the measured P_{ves} represents a summation of the pressure caused by bladder wall events (e.g., detrusor contraction, P_{det}), and the pressure caused by extravesical sources (e.g., abdominal straining, P_{abd}). Thus, when there is a rise in bladder pressure recorded using single-channel cystometry (P_{ves}), one cannot be sure whether this is due to a bladder contraction or to increases in intra-abdominal pressures that are transmitted to the bladder, or both. The use of multichannel cystometry, whereby a catheter that records abdominal pressure is used in addition to an intravesical catheter, allows for the determination of the contributions of the individual components of P_{ves}, P_{det}, and P_{abd}. Because P_{det} is the component of P_{ves} that is created by the contractile forces within the bladder wall, it is the critical pressure to measure. However, it cannot be measured directly; it is rather obtained by subtracting the abdominal pressure from the total vesical pressure ($P_{det} = P_{ves} - P_{abd}$), which is done electronically. P_{abd} is generally recorded by a catheter placed in the rectum. The rectum is close to the bladder and thus theoretically the intra-abdominal pressure experienced by both should be similar. A change in either P_{abd} or P_{det} should be accompanied by a change in P_{ves}. If P_{abd} changes independently of P_{ves}, then the subtracted P_{det} will also change, but this will be an artifact (poor pressure transmission, rectal contraction); true detrusor pressure cannot change in the absence of a change in P_{ves}. [pp 907–908]

15. **e. obstruction.** During the course of cystometry, information is sought regarding four bladder characteristics: (1) capacity, (2) sensation, (3) compliance, and (4) the occurrence of involuntary contractions. [pp 908–909]

16. **c. Measured compliance is affected by fill rate.** Bladder compliance is defined as the change in bladder pressure for a given change in volume. It is a measure of bladder elasticity and reflects the sum of two forces: a mechanical force proportional to the amount of collagen present in the bladder wall and a neuromuscular force called tonus. The measured compliance is also variably dependent on the fill rate. Customarily, the pressure rise during the course of CMG in the normal bladder will be only 6 to 10 cm H_2O (see Fig. 25–3). [p 909]

17. **d. may be inhibited by a patient with sensory urgency.** The unstable bladder is one that can be demonstrated to contract either spontaneously or with provocative maneuvers during filling cystometry while the patient is trying to inhibit micturition. When it occurs in a patient with neurologic disease (e.g., spinal cord injury, cerebrovascular accident, demyelinating disease), it is called detrusor hyperreflexia; in the absence of neurologic disease, it is called detrusor instability (DI). Patients with urgency and urge incontinence in whom unstable bladder contractions can be demonstrated cystometrically are said to have motor urge incontinence. If the same symptoms are present with a stable bladder cystometrically, it is called sensory urgency. It is probable that sensory and motor urgency are conditions in the same spectrum and that patients with sensory urgency are better able to inhibit the unstable contractions during a urodynamic study. The absence of documented instability on CMG does not rule out its existence. As many as 40% of people with motor urge incontinence will not demonstrate DI on CMG. [p 909]

18. **c. Vesicoureteral reflux may decrease measured bladder compliance.** The bethanechol supersensitivity test was originally described by Lapides and colleagues to try to distinguish between a neurogenic and a myogenic cause in a patient with an acontractile bladder. It is based on the observation that after an organ is deprived of its nerve supply, it develops hypersensitivity to the normal excitatory neurotransmitters for that organ. The test has been shown to be unreliable, however. A positive test by itself does not indicate a neurogenic bladder and a negative test does not rule it out. The ice water test was first described by Bors and Blinn in 1957 as a way to differentiate upper from lower motor neuron lesions. It is based on the principle that mucosal temperature receptors can elicit a spinal reflex contraction of the detrusor, a reflex that is normally inhibited by

supraspinal centers. On cystometry, if the bladder outlet is incompetent, urine may leak around the filling catheter, and a low bladder compliance may be not be diagnosed because the bladder is never adequately filled (e.g., spinal dysraphism, severe intrinsic sphincter deficiency in an older woman). In this scenario, the CMG test should be repeated using a Foley catheter for bladder filling, with the distended catheter balloon pulled down to occlude the bladder neck. In patients with massive reflux, large volumes of the filling solution reflux into the dilated upper tracts and a low capacity–low compliance detrusor may be missed because of this "pop-off" mechanism. [pp 910–911]

19. **b. DLPP is a reflection of resistance of the urethra to the bladder.** DLPP is defined as the lowest bladder pressure (in the absence of a detrusor contraction) at which leakage occurs across the urethra. As such, it is a reflection of the resistance of the urethra to the bladder and a measure of the storage pressures in the bladder (i.e., compliance). An important concept in urodynamics is the fact that bladder outlet resistance is the main determinant of detrusor pressure. If the outlet resistance is high, a higher bladder pressure will be needed to overcome this resistance and cause leakage. McGuire's group found that in myelodysplastic patients (who have elevated outlet resistance due to fixed external sphincters), those with DLPP values greater than 40 cm H_2O were at significantly higher risk for upper tract deterioration (hydronephrosis, reflux) than those with DLPP values less than 40 cm H_2O. Catheter size has not been standardized for the test, but it appears that catheter size can affect the results. [p 911]

20. **e. None of the above.** VLPP or abdominal leak point pressure is the lowest abdominal pressure that causes leakage of urine across the urethra in the absence of a bladder contraction. Whereas the detrusor pressure tends to force the urethral sphincter open, the abdominal pressure will not open a urethral sphincter if the urethra is normally positioned and closed. If leakage is caused by an increase in abdominal pressure, then the urethra must be abnormal. If there is no leakage at high pressures (>150 cm H_2O), then the urethra is unlikely to be the cause of the patient's incontinence and rather the bladder is the more likely culprit. However, the converse is not true (i.e., a low VLPP does not rule out a significant detrusor-related component to the incontinence). A poor correlation between VLPP and MUCP has been noted by several authors, which is not surprising because the MUCP is a reflection of the urethral resistance to detrusor pressure and as such is more related to the DLPP than to the VLPP. [pp 911–912]

21. **c. poor bladder compliance.** There is evidence that VLPP is affected by catheter size, and anterior vaginal wall prolapse (i.e., cystocele) may artificially elevate the VLPP. Other potential artifacts are related to patient anxiety and cooperation. [pp 912–913]

22. **c. A difference in Q_{max} on repeated testing may be spurious.** The flow pattern, that is, the shape of the flow tracing, can sometimes be used to make a presumptive diagnosis, although it cannot be used to make a definitive diagnosis. The typical obstructed flow pattern has a plateau-shaped curve with a prolonged flow time, sustained low flow rate, and increased time to Q_{max}. This is not diagnostic of outlet obstruction because detrusor hypocontractility can give a similar tracing. Furthermore, a high flow rate (>15 ml/s) does not rule out bladder outlet obstruction. In men, Q_{max} decreases with age, whereas in women it is not influenced by age. It has been documented that 40% of men have a difference in Q_{max} of at least 2 ml/s between voids, and 20% of men may have a difference of at least 4 ml/s. Thus, it has been recommended by some that multiple flow rates be recorded to increase the likelihood that a representative flow is achieved. The volume voided probably has the greatest effect on peak flow rate, and it is generally accepted that voided volumes of less than 150 ml generate inaccurate flow patterns and parameters. However, voids of less than 150 ml can provide useful information (particularly in truly obstructed patients) and thus should not be discarded. [pp 913–917]

23. **c. After-contractions are more common in patients with instability than in patients without instability.** Catheter size may influence the results of pressure-flow studies, and the larger the catheter, the greater the chance that the catheter will cause some degree of outlet obstruction. Failure to void during a pressure-flow study does not in and of itself indicate a functional abnormality, as many patients find it difficult to void in the setting of the urodynamic laboratory. Postvoid residual urine is the volume of urine remaining in the bladder immediately after voiding. Although the testing situation often leads to inefficient voiding and a falsely elevated residual urine volume, the absence of residual urine does not exclude infravesical obstruction or bladder dysfunction. Postmicturition contraction (after-contraction) is a reiteration of the detrusor contraction after flow has ceased, and its magnitude is typically greater than that of the micturition pressure at maximum flow. After-contractions are not well understood, but they seem to be more common in patients with unstable or hypersensitive bladders. There is no consensus regarding a critical value for pressure and flow that is diagnostic for obstruction. Outlet obstruction is suggested by a pressure-flow study in which low flow occurs despite a detrusor contraction of adequate force, duration, and speed, regardless of the actual numerical values. [pp 917–919]

24. **c. It can help grade the degree of obstruction by calculating the Abrams-Griffiths (AG) number.** The degree of obstruction can be graded by using the AG number, which is derived from the equation for the slope of the line that divides the obstructed group from the equivocal group on the AG nomogram and is calculated by the formula AG number = $P_{det}Q_{max} - 2Q_{max}$. [p 920]

25. **e. It involves the use of two outlet parameters, urethral collapsibility and cross-sectional area.** On the basis of the position and slope of the PURR, two outlet parameters were characterized: P_{muo} (where the curve intersects the pressure axis), which reflects the collapsibility of the urethra or the degree of compressive obstruction, and the cross-sectional area of the flow controlling zone (represented by the slope of the PURR), which reflects the extensibility of the urethra or the degree of constrictive obstruction. [p 920]

26. **b. It allows for continuous grading of obstruction by calculating the bladder outlet obstruction index (BOOI).** A continuous grading of obstruction is possible by calculating the BOOI, which is essentially the AG number, given by the formula: BOOI = $P_{det}Q_{max} - 2Q_{max}$. [pp 921–922]

27. **a. it predominantly uses natural filling and allows the subject to reproduce normal activities.** Ambulatory urodynamic monitoring (AUM) is defined as any functional test of the lower urinary tract predominantly utilizing natural filling of the urinary tract and reproducing the subject's normal activity. As such, the unphysiologic nature of conventional urodynamics (filling by rapid infusion through a catheter, monitoring in a laboratory setting) is avoided, and the patient may move about and continue with the activities of daily living that may trigger the presenting symptoms (e.g., urgency, incontinence). However, the patient must play an active role in the performance of AUM because the test is not confined to a laboratory with staff monitoring. This reli-

ance on patient compliance may a source of significant error. Studies have shown that AUM is more sensitive than conventional CMG in the detection of unstable detrusor contractions, in both symptomatic and asymptomatic subjects, and furthermore that AUM can detect DI in patients in whom CMG is nondiagnostic. However, the significance of this increased detection of DI is unclear given the high incidence found in asymptomatic patients. Studies have shown that in neurogenic patients, filling pressures with AUM tend to be significantly lower than those with conventional CMG, and patients with hydronephrosis and high end filling pressures (and low compliance) on CMG were found to have normal filling pressures on AUM. Instead, these patients were found to have increased phasic detrusor activity on AUM that correlated with the presence of upper tract changes. It has therefore been hypothesized that the high end filling pressure (and thus low compliance) seen on conventional CMG may in fact be an artifact related to the high phasic activity on AUM being converted to low compliance by the more rapid (and unphysiologic) filling of conventional CMG. AUM has not been clearly demonstrated to better classify patients as having obstructed versus unobstructed conditions. [pp 922–923]

28. **e. all of the above.** Simultaneous fluoroscopic screening of the bladder outlet during voiding and while pressure-flow data are being recorded helps to identify the site of the obstruction as being at the bladder neck, prostatic urethra, or distal sphincter mechanism (see Fig. 25–22). It is particularly useful in the identification of bladder neck dysfunction and in the identification of dyssynergia of the proximal and distal sphincter mechanisms in neurogenic patients; in determining whether an open bladder neck in the absence of a detrusor contraction in a woman with stress incontinence may be a sign of intrinsic sphincter deficiency; and in identifying and characterizing pathology that can be associated with complex voiding dysfunction including reflux, diverticula, fistulas, and stones. [pp 923–925]

29. **a. It determines whether the bladder and external sphincter are coordinated.** Clinically, the most important information obtained from sphincter EMG is whether there is coordination or discoordination between the external sphincter and the bladder. [pp 925–926]

30. **c. typically occurs in patients with suprasacral cord injuries.** DSD typically occurs in patients with suprasacral spinal cord injury in which there is an interruption of the spino-bulbar-spinal pathways that normally coordinate the detrusor and sphincter muscles. [p 926]

31. **a. polyphasic potentials that constitute greater than 15% of all activity.** Normal muscle may have up to 15% of its activity in the form of such polyphasic potentials; however, when the amount of polyphasic activity is significantly greater than this, neuropathy is implied. [p 927]

Chapter 26

Neuromuscular Dysfunction of the Lower Urinary Tract and Its Treatment

Alan J. Wein

Questions

1. What is the general pattern of voiding dysfunction secondary to neurologic lesions above the level of the brain stem?
   a. Involuntary bladder contractions, smooth sphincter dyssynergia, striated sphincter synergy.
   b. Involuntary bladder contractions, smooth sphincter synergy, striated sphincter synergy.
   c. Involuntary bladder contractions, smooth sphincter synergy, striated sphincter dyssynergia.
   d. Detrusor hypocontractility, smooth sphincter synergy, striated sphincter synergy.
   e. Detrusor areflexia, smooth sphincter synergy, striated sphincter synergy.

2. What is the general pattern of voiding dysfunction that results from complete lesions of the spinal cord above the level of S2 after recovery from spinal shock?
   a. Involuntary bladder contractions, smooth sphincter dyssynergia, striated sphincter synergy.
   b. Involuntary bladder contractions, smooth sphincter synergy, striated sphincter synergy.
   c. Involuntary bladder contractions, smooth sphincter synergy, striated sphincter dyssynergia.
   d. Detrusor hypocontractility, smooth sphincter synergy, striated sphincter synergy.
   e. Detrusor areflexia, smooth sphincter synergy, striated sphincter synergy.

3. Which of the following is the most common long-term expression of lower urinary tract dysfunction after a cerebrovascular accident (CVA)?
   a. Detrusor areflexia
   b. Lack of sensation of filling
   c. Impaired bladder contractility
   d. Striated sphincter dyssynergia
   e. Detrusor hyperreflexia

4. Urinary incontinence is most likely to occur in a patient following a CVA if which of the following areas is affected?
   a. Internal capsule
   b. Basal ganglia

c. Thalamus
d. Cerebellum
e. Hypothalamus

5. In a post-CVA patient who exhibits urgency and frequency but no incontinence, the state of striated sphincter activity can most commonly be best described as:

   a. uninhibited relaxation.
   b. dyssynergia.
   c. fixed voluntary tone.
   d. pseudodyssynergia.
   e. myotonus.

6. You are asked to evaluate and treat a 65-year-old man who has sustained a stroke but who is otherwise in good health. He has symptoms of hesitancy, straining to void, urgency, and frequency. The optimal next step in management is:

   a. anticholinergic therapy.
   b. transurethral resection of the prostate.
   c. transurethral incision of the bladder neck and prostate.
   d. clean intermittent catheterization.
   e. full urodynamic evaluation.

7. When considering the subject of voiding dysfunction associated with brain tumors, which of the following areas is more likely to be associated with urinary retention than with urinary incontinence?

   a. Pituitary gland
   b. Cerebellum
   c. Posterior fossa
   d. Hypothalamus
   e. Frontal cortex

8. The most common pattern of micturition in children and adults who have only cerebral palsy (CP) (no other complicating neurologic conditions) is:

   a. abnormal filling/storage because of detrusor hyperreflexia; normal emptying.
   b. normal filling/storage; normal emptying.
   c. normal filling/storage; abnormal emptying because of striated sphincter dyssynergia.
   d. normal filling/storage; abnormal emptying because of smooth sphincter dyssynergia.
   e. abnormal filling/storage because of detrusor hyperreflexia; abnormal emptying because of striated sphincter dyssynergia.

9. Deficiency of which of the following compounds in the nigrostriatal pathway accounts for most of the classic clinical motor features of Parkinson's disease (PD)?

   a. Dopamine
   b. Norepinephrine
   c. Acetylcholine
   d. Serotonin
   e. L-Dopa

10. The most common urodynamic abnormality found in patients with voiding dysfunction secondary to PD is:

    a. impaired sensation during filling.
    b. striated sphincter dyssynergia.
    c. striated sphincter bradykinesia.
    d. detrusor hyperreflexia.
    e. impaired detrusor contractility.

11. Shy-Drager syndrome is commonly characterized clinically by all of the following except:

    a. hypertension.
    b. anhydrosis.
    c. cerebellar dysfunction.
    d. voiding dysfunction.
    e. erectile dysfunction.

12. Which of the following is more common in patients with PD than in patients with multiple system atrophy (MSA)/Shy-Drager syndrome?

    a. Intrinsic sphincter deficiency
    b. Evidence of striated sphincter denervation on an electromyogram
    c. Decreased compliance
    d. Incontinence after transurethral resection of the prostate
    e. Disease diagnosis preceding voiding and erectile symptoms

13. The lesions seen in multiple sclerosis most commonly affect which of the following locations in the nervous system?

    a. Thoracic spinal cord
    b. Sacral spinal cord
    c. Cervical spinal cord
    d. Lumbar spinal cord
    e. Midbrain

14. Which of the following urodynamic findings is least common in patients with multiple sclerosis and voiding dysfunction?

    a. Detrusor hyperreflexia
    b. Detrusor areflexia
    c. Impaired detrusor contractility
    d. Striated sphincter dyssynergia
    e. Smooth sphincter dyssynergia

15. Which of the following most accurately reflects the number of patients with HIV/AIDS, overall, with moderate or severe voiding problems?

    a. 15% or less
    b. 15% to 25%
    c. 25% to 40%
    d. 40% to 60%
    e. 60% to 80%

16. The sacral spinal cord terminates in the cauda equina at approximately the spinal column level of:

    a. T10.
    b. L1.
    c. L2.
    d. L3.
    e. S1.

17. In spinal shock, findings generally include all of the following except:

    a. acontractile bladder.
    b. areflexic bladder.
    c. open bladder neck.
    d. absent guarding reflex.
    e. maximal urethral closure pressure above normal.

18. All of the following are risk factors for upper urinary tract deterioration in a patient with a suprasacral spinal cord injury except:

    a. high-pressure storage.
    b. high detrusor leak point pressure.
    c. chronic bladder overdistention.
    d. high abdominal leak point pressure.
    e. vesicourethral reflux with infection.

19. The presence of true detrusor striated sphincter dyssynergia implies:

    a. a neurologic lesion between the pons and the sacral spinal cord.

b. a neurologic lesion between the cerebral cortex and the pons.
c. a neurologic lesion between the cervical and the sacral spinal cord.
d. a neurologic lesion between the sacral spinal cord and the striated sphincter.
e. normal sensation in the presence of involuntary bladder contractions.

20. Which of the following is least characteristic as a finding in autonomic hyperreflexia?
    a. Headache before bladder contraction
    b. Hypertension
    c. Flushing above the level of the lesion
    d. Tachycardia
    e. Sweating above the level of the lesion

21. Which of the following drugs or types of agents is not among those used for the treatment of, or prophylaxis for, autonomic hyperreflexia?
    a. Phentolamine
    b. Propranolol
    c. Ganglionic blockade
    d. Nifedipine
    e. Terazosin

22. In a male patient with detrusor striated sphincter dyssynergia, a high detrusor leak point pressure, high-pressure vesicoureteral reflux, and beginning upper urinary tract deterioration, which of the following is least likely, as an isolated procedure, to halt or reverse the upper tract changes?
    a. Ureteral reimplantation
    b. Augmentation cystoplasty
    c. Dorsal root ganglionectomy
    d. Anticholinergic therapy and intermittent catheterization
    e. Sphincterotomy

23. In a patient with voiding dysfunction secondary to myelomeningocele who has slightly decreased compliance, detrusor areflexia, and low-pressure moderate to severe vesicoureteral reflux, which of the following urodynamic changes would be most likely after ureteral reimplantation alone?
    a. Compliance further decreased
    b. Voiding pressure decreased
    c. Valsalva leak point pressure decreased
    d. Maximum urethral closure pressure decreased
    e. Maximum bladder capacity increased

24. The symptoms of voiding dysfunction in a child with tethered cord syndrome present most commonly after which of the following precipitating factors?
    a. Urinary tract infection
    b. Meningitis
    c. Puberty
    d. Cystoscopy
    e. Growth spurt

25. A classic "sensory neurogenic bladder" (Lapides classification system) is most commonly produced by:
    a. herpes zoster.
    b. herpes simplex.
    c. transverse myelitis.
    d. pernicious anemia.
    e. sacral spinal cord injury.

26. Patients who have voiding dysfunction secondary to lumbar disc disease most commonly present with which of the following symptoms and urodynamic findings?
    a. Retention; involuntary bladder contractions
    b. Incontinence; involuntary bladder contractions
    c. Retention; decreased bladder compliance
    d. Difficulty voiding; normal bladder compliance
    e. Incontinence; normal bladder compliance

27. The combination that best describes the type of permanent voiding dysfunction that can occur after radical pelvic surgery is:
    a. exertional (or stress) incontinence; detrusor areflexia.
    b. urge incontinence; detrusor areflexia.
    c. reflex incontinence; detrusor areflexia.
    d. urge incontinence; detrusor hyperreflexia.
    e. exertional (or stress) incontinence; hyperreflexia.

28. What is optimal management for a 65-year-old man who has had a first occurrence of urinary retention after radical pelvic surgery?
    a. Anticholinergic therapy
    b. Clean intermittent catheterization
    c. Transurethral resection of the prostate
    d. External sphincterotomy
    e. Bethanechol chloride

29. The urodynamic parameter most likely to differentiate urinary retention due to prostatic obstruction from urinary retention due to the neurologic changes caused by diabetes is:
    a. uroflow.
    b. residual urine volume.
    c. bladder compliance.
    d. vesical pressure.
    e. detrusor pressure.

30. Detrusor striated sphincter dyssynergia would be least expected to occur with which of the following conditions?
    a. Multiple sclerosis
    b. Spinal cord injury
    c. Stroke
    d. Autonomic hyperreflexia
    e. Transverse myelitis

31. Differentiation of bladder neck obstruction from dysfunctional voiding is most easily and accurately made by:
    a. filling cystometry.
    b. voiding cystometry.
    c. cystourethroscopy.
    d. flowmetry and residual urine determination.
    e. video-urodynamic study.

32. Which of the following is the most specific study to make the diagnosis of the Fowler syndrome?
    a. Striated sphincter needle EMG recording
    b. Striated sphincter patch EMG recording
    c. Neurologic examination
    d. Spinal MRI examination
    e. Detrusor pressure/urinary flow recording

33. Which of the following has proved to be successful in treating the urologic manifestations of the Fowler syndrome?
    a. Estrogen therapy
    b. Progesterone therapy
    c. Baclofen therapy
    d. Botulinum toxin injection therapy
    e. Neuromodulation

34. There is an increased incidence of urinary incontinence after prostatectomy in men with:

a. hyperthyroidism.
b. myasthenia gravis.
c. schizophrenia.
d. gastroparesis.
e. Isaacs' syndrome.

35. Endometriosis affects the bladder in what percentage of all cases?

    a. 60% to 65%
    b. 40% to 45%
    c. 20% to 25%
    d. 10% to 15%
    e. 1% to 2%

36. The effects of administration of anticholinergic agent to an individual with an overactive bladder include all except:

    a. increased total bladder capacity.
    b. depressed amplitude of involuntary bladder contractions.
    c. increased warning time.
    d. increased volume to the first involuntary bladder contraction.
    e. increased mean volume voided.

37. Which of the following muscarinic receptor subtypes is most common in human detrusor smooth muscle?

    a. M_1
    b. M_2
    c. M_3
    d. M_4
    e. M_5

38. Which of the following muscarinic receptor subtypes is predominantly responsible for the mediation of bladder contraction in human detrusor smooth muscle?

    a. M_1
    b. M_2
    c. M_3
    d. M_4
    e. M_5

39. The use of anticholinergic agents to treat overactive bladder is limited by their lack of uroselectivity. Which of the following is not a recognized side effect of anticholinergic agents?

    a. Dry mouth
    b. Constipation
    c. Cognitive dysfunction
    d. Bradycardia
    e. Blurred vision

40. As a therapeutic anticholinergic agent, propantheline bromide is:

    a. receptor specific.
    b. tissue specific.
    c. poorly absorbed from the gastrointestinal tract.
    d. a tertiary ammonium compound.
    e. more effective than oxybutynin.

41. Oxybutynin exerts its clinical effects on the urinary bladder primarily by:

    a. calcium channel blockade.
    b. local anesthetic activity.
    c. inhibition of norepinephrine uptake.
    d. M_3 receptor blockade.
    e. M_1 receptor blockade.

42. The Committee on Pharmacologic Treatment of the 1st International Consultation on Incontinence assessed which of the following agents as lacking pharmacologic and/or physiologic evidence of efficacy and as lacking evidence of clinical efficacy as judged by good-quality randomized trials?

    a. Dicyclomine
    b. Flavoxate
    c. Trospium
    d. Tolterodine
    e. Oxybutynin

43. Terodiline is an agent that seemed quite effective for the treatment of overactive bladder but has been withdrawn from use because of reports of what?

    a. Dry mouth
    b. Cognitive dysfunction
    c. Cardiac toxicity
    d. Constipation
    e. Asthma

44. Potassium channel openers would be expected to be particularly effective in treating overactive bladder due to which of the following specific causes?

    a. Lack of suprapontine inhibition
    b. Descending spinal cord column injury
    c. Ascending spinal cord column injury
    d. Denervation supersensitivity (myogenic)
    e. Increased afferent input from the periphery

45. Which of the following pharmacologic actions of imipramine is least prominent?

    a. Sedative, on a central basis
    b. Block reuptake of norepinephrine in presynaptic nerve endings
    c. Block reuptake of serotonin in presynaptic nerve endings
    d. Antihistaminic, by blocking H1 receptors
    e. Direct anticholinergic, on bladder smooth muscle

46. Which of the following combinations of pharmacologic agents for the treatment of overactive bladder is theoretically most attractive?

    a. Oxybutynin and propantheline
    b. Oxybutynin and trospium
    c. Imipramine and doxepin
    d. Dicyclomine and flavoxate
    e. Tolterodine and imipramine

47. Which of the following is not listed as a common side effect of imipramine?

    a. Peripheral anticholinergic effects
    b. Weakness, fatigue
    c. Priapism
    d. Cardiac arrhythmia
    e. Hepatic dysfunction

48. Resiniferatoxin, as compared with capsaicin, exhibits which of the following properties?

    a. Greater desensitization at lower concentrations
    b. More early noxious side effects when administered intravesically
    c. More late side effects when administered intravesically
    d. Blockade of only A fiber–mediated contraction
    e. Nonvanilloid compound (capsaicin is a vanilloid)

49. The quoted rate of bladder rupture secondary to therapeutic overdistention of the bladder is:

    a. 20% to 25%.
    b. 10% to 20%.
    c. 5% to 10%.
    d. 1% to 4%.
    e. <1%.

50. The conclusions drawn from experiments in the cat to study the effects of peripheral electrical stimulation as a therapeutic modality to inhibit bladder contractility have proposed all the following except one as potential mechanisms involved in this effect. Which mechanism is least likely to be involved?

    a. Inhibitory pudendal to pelvic nerve reflex
    b. Sympathetic inhibition of parasympathetic ganglion cell activity
    c. Sympathetic induced β-adrenergic relaxation of the bladder body
    d. Pudendal to hypogastric nerve reflex
    e. Antimuscarinic effect on bladder smooth muscle

51. Sacral root neural stimulation (neuromodulation) has been reported as capable of treating all of the following entities except:

    a. pelvic pain.
    b. idiopathic urinary retention.
    c. detrusor hyperreflexia.
    d. detrusor instability.
    e. smooth sphincter dyssynergia.

52. Pick the combination of stimulation frequencies, as used in electrical stimulation of peripheral nerves, for inhibiting bladder contractility on the one hand and increasing outlet resistance on the other.

    a. 20 to 50 Hz; 5 to 10 Hz
    b. 10 to 30 Hz; 60 to 80 Hz
    c. 60 to 80 Hz; 10 to 30 Hz
    d. 5 to 10 Hz; 20 to 50 Hz
    e. 100 to 200 Hz; 200 to 500 Hz

53. Which of the following conditions or diagnoses is least likely to be benefited by neuromodulation via sacral root stimulation?

    a. Urge incontinence
    b. Detrusor hyperreflexia
    c. Detrusor instability
    d. Detrusor hypocontractility
    e. Pelvic pain

54. Subarachnoid block generally accomplishes all but which of the following?

    a. Conversion of somatic spasticity to flaccidity
    b. Conversion of bladder hyperreflexia to areflexia
    c. Abolishing of autonomic hyperreflexia
    d. Completion of peripheral sensory loss where incomplete
    e. Improvement of reflexogenic erections

55. Which of the following represents the most devastating complication of subtrigonal infiltration of the pelvic plexus with phenol to treat urgency incontinence?

    a. Rectal fistula
    b. Urinary retention
    c. Vaginal fistula
    d. Decreased bladder compliance
    e. Stress incontinence

56. Which of the following most closely approximates the percentage of improvement (incontinence episodes or amount of urine lost) to be expected with behavioral therapy for "genuine" stress urinary incontinence?

    a. 85%
    b. 70%
    c. 55%
    d. 40%
    e. 25%

57. α-Adrenergic agonists, in general, produce all but which of the following?

    a. An increase in maximum urethral pressure
    b. An increase in maximum urethral closure pressure
    c. A contraction of urethral smooth muscle
    d. A decrease in maximal bladder capacity
    e. An increase in bladder outlet resistance

58. The side effects of the α-adrenergic agonists include all of the following except:

    a. tremor.
    b. palpitations.
    c. hypertension.
    d. somnolence.
    e. respiratory difficulties.

59. Which of the following agents has been reported to increase stroke risk in young women within 3 days of taking their first dose?

    a. Phenylpropanolamine
    b. Ephedrine
    c. Pseudoephedrine
    d. Midodrine
    e. Norephedrine

60. In theory, which of the following agents, from the standpoint of potential efficacy and safety, would be preferred for the treatment of stress incontinence in a hypertensive individual?

    a. Ephedrine
    b. Propranolol
    c. Phenylpropanolamine
    d. Pseudoephedrine
    e. Norephedrine

61. In a 70-year-old woman with urinary incontinence, which of the following is the most favorable characteristic for the use of an external urethral occlusion device?

    a. Moderate sphincteric incontinence
    b. Overactive bladder
    c. Cognitive impairment
    d. Moderate mixed incontinence
    e. Massive obesity

62. The problems described as being associated with unstimulated graciloplasty include all but the which of the following?

    a. Unsatisfactory sustained muscle contraction
    b. Passive obstruction
    c. Fibrosis of the muscle
    d. Active obstruction by tetanic muscle contraction
    e. Necessity for prolonged leg adduction

63. Which of the following statements is false with respect to DDAVP?

    a. It is classically used to test nocturnal enuresis.
    b. It is classically used to treat diabetes insipidus.
    c. It can be given orally or intranasally at the same doses.
    d. It suppresses urine production for 7 to 12 hours.
    e. It can be used in both children and adults.

64. Relative contraindications to the use of DDAVP include all but which of the following?

    a. Hypertension
    b. Liver disease
    c. Crohn's disease

d. Heart disease
e. Obstructive uropathy

65. Of the following, which is the main advantage of continuous suprapubic drainage over urethral drainage?

    a. It is more comfortable.
    b. There is less risk of carcinoma.
    c. It is easier to replace.
    d. There is less bacteriuria.
    e. It obviates detrusor-related leakage.

66. In a patient for whom it has been decided that a urinary diversion is indicated, which of the following constitutes a clear indication for an ileal conduit over an ileovesicostomy?

    a. Progressive hydronephrosis
    b. Recurrent urosepsis
    c. Ureterovesical obstruction
    d. Incontinence
    e. Retention

67. The most significant complication that has been associated with the use of an external collecting device in the paraplegic male is:

    a. urine leakage.
    b. penile pressure necrosis.
    c. upper tract decompensation.
    d. visibility.
    e. urinary infection.

68. All of the following accurately describe the factors associated with the Credé maneuver except which statement?

    a. Funneling of the bladder outlet generally occurs.
    b. Increases in outlet resistance may occur.
    c. Vesicoureteral reflux is a relative contraindication.
    d. It is easier in a thin than in an obese individual.
    e. It is most effective when outlet resistance is decreased.

69. In a young female paraplegic, the most effective way of initiating a bladder reflex contraction by "trigger voiding" is:

    a. squeezing the clitoris.
    b. digital rectal stimulation.
    c. pulling the skin of the pubis.
    d. pinching the skin of the thigh.
    e. rhythmic suprapubic manual pressure.

70. With regard to bethanechol chloride, the least objective evidence exists to support which of the following statements?

    a. It has relatively selective in vitro action on urinary bladder and bowel.
    b. It has little or no nicotinic action.
    c. It is cholinesterase resistant.
    d. It causes in vitro contraction of bladder smooth muscle.
    e. It facilitates bladder emptying.

71. What oral dose of bethanechol chloride is required to produce the same urodynamic effects, at least in a denervated bladder, at the subcutaneous dose of 5 mg?

    a. 200 mg
    b. 100 mg
    c. 50 mg
    d. 25 mg
    e. 10 mg

72. Direct electrical stimulation of the bladder often results in all of the following except:

    a. pelvic musculature contraction.
    b. erection.
    c. defecation.
    d. bladder neck opening.
    e. ejaculation.

73. All of the following statements regarding the use of the Brindley device are true except which one?

    a. It requires intact neural pathways between the sacral cord and the bladder.
    b. Sacral posterior rhizotomy is generally performed.
    c. Myogenic decompensation is a contraindication.
    d. Electrodes are applied extradurally to sacral roots S2 to S4.
    e. It utilizes the principle of post-stimulation voiding.

74. With respect to α-adrenergic receptors versus β-adrenergic receptors in the lower urinary tract, all but which of the following statements are true?

    a. The α receptors are more prominent in the bladder base than are β receptors.
    b. The α_1 receptors are more common than α_2 receptors.
    c. The α receptors are less prominent in the bladder body than are β receptors.
    d. Bladder smooth muscle contraction is mediated predominantly by α_1 receptors.
    e. Urethral smooth muscle contraction is mediated predominantly by α_1 receptors.

75. Which of the following α-adrenergic blocking agents has significant antagonistic properties at both α_1- and α_2-receptor sites?

    a. Prazosin
    b. Terazosin
    c. Phenoxybenzamine
    d. Doxazosin
    e. Tamsulosin

76. Which of the following side effects is more common with tamsulosin than with either terazosin or doxazosin?

    a. Dizziness
    b. Asthenia
    c. Postural hypotension
    d. Palpitations
    e. Retrograde ejaculation

77. Which of the following agents or classes of agents, when administered systemically, will selectively relax the striated musculature of the pelvic floor?

    a. The benzodiazepines
    b. Dantrolene
    c. Baclofen
    d. Botulinum toxin
    e. None of the above

78. Which of the following is the most widely distributed inhibitory neurotransmitter in the mammalian central nervous system?

    a. γ-Aminobutyric acid (GABA)
    b. Glycine
    c. Glutamate
    d. Dopamine
    e. Norepinephrine

79. Baclofen (Lioresal) acts to decrease striated sphincter activity by which of the following mechanisms?

    a. Facilitating neuronal hyperpolarization through the GABA$_A$ receptor.
    b. Activating the GABA$_B$ receptor and depressing monosynaptic and polysynaptic excitation of motor neurons and interneurons in the spinal cord.
    c. Inhibiting excitation-contraction coupling in skeletal mus-

cle by decreasing calcium release from the sarcoplasmic reticulum.
d. Inhibiting excitation-contraction coupling by preventing calcium entry into the cell.
e. Inhibiting acetylcholine release at the neuromuscular junction.

80. The preferred site(s) of surgical sphincterotomy, when carried out transurethrally, is(are) which of the following?

   a. 11 and 1 o'clock
   b. 3 and 9 o'clock
   c. 12 o'clock
   d. 5 and 7 o'clock
   e. 6 o'clock.

81. Which of the following is the most reliable urodynamic parameter to predict the risk of upper tract complications after sphincterotomy?

   a. Residual urine volume
   b. Maximum urethral pressure
   c. Valsalva leak point pressure
   d. Detrusor leak point pressure
   e. Maximum urethral closure pressure

Answers

1. **b. Involuntary bladder contractions, smooth sphincter synergy, striated sphincter synergy.** Neurologic lesions above the level of the brain stem that affect micturition generally result in involuntary bladder contractions with smooth and striated sphincter synergy. Sensation and voluntary striated sphincter function are generally preserved. Areflexia may occur, however, either initially or as a permanent dysfunction. [p 935]

2. **c. Involuntary bladder contractions, smooth sphincter synergy, striated sphincter dyssynergia.** Patients with complete lesions of the spinal cord between spinal cord level T6 and S2, after they recover from spinal shock, generally exhibit involuntary bladder contractions without sensation, smooth sphincter synergy, but striated sphincter dyssynergia. Those with lesions above T6 may experience, in addition, smooth sphincter dyssynergia and autonomic hyperreflexia. [p 935]

3. **e. Detrusor hyperreflexia.** The most common long-term expression of lower urinary tract dysfunction after a CVA is detrusor hyperreflexia. Sensation is variable but is classically described as generally intact, and thus the patient has urgency and frequency with hyperreflexia. [p 937]

4. **a. Internal capsule.** Previous descriptions of the voiding dysfunction after a CVA have all cited the preponderance of detrusor hyperreflexia with coordinated sphincter activity. It is difficult to reconcile this with the relatively high incontinence rate that occurs, even considering the probability that a percentage of these patients had an incontinence problem before the CVA. Tsuchida and co-workers in 1983 and Khan and associates in 1990 made early significant contributions in this area by correlating the urodynamic and CT pictures after CVA. They reported that patients with lesions in only the basal ganglia or thalamus have normal sphincter function. This means that when an impending involuntary contraction or its onset was sensed, these patients could voluntarily contract the striated sphincter and abort or considerably lessen the effect of an abnormal micturition reflex. The majority of patients with involvement of the cerebral cortex and/or internal capsule were unable to forcefully contract the striated sphincter under these circumstances. [p 937]

5. **d. pseudodyssynergia.** Some authors have described striated sphincter dyssynergia in 5% to 21% of patients with brain disease and voiding dysfunction. This is incompatible with accepted neural circuitry. I agree with those who believe that true detrusor-striated sphincter dyssynergia does not occur in this situation. Pseudodyssynergia may indeed occur during urodynamic testing of these patients. This refers to an electromyographic (EMG) sphincter "flare" during filling cystometry, which is secondary to attempted inhibition of an involuntary bladder contraction by voluntary contraction of the striated sphincter. [p 937]

6. **e. full urodynamic evaluation.** Poor flow rates and high residual urine volumes in a male with pre-CVA symptoms of prostatism generally indicate prostatic obstruction, but a full urodynamic evaluation is advisable before committing a patient to mechanical outlet reduction primarily to exclude detrusor hyperactivity with impaired contractility as a cause of symptoms. [pp 937–938]

7. **c. Posterior fossa.** The areas that are most frequently involved with associated micturition dysfunction are the superior aspects of the frontal lobe. When voiding dysfunction occurs, it generally consists of detrusor hyperreflexia and urinary incontinence. These individuals may have a markedly diminished awareness of all lower urinary tract events and, if so, are totally unable to even attempt suppression of the micturition reflex. Smooth and striated sphincter activity is generally synergic. Pseudodyssynergia may occur during urodynamic testing. Fowler in 1999 reviewed the literature on frontal lobe lesions and bladder control. She cited instances of resection of a tumor relieving the micturition symptoms for a period of time, raising the question of whether the phenomenon of tumor-associated bladder hyperreflexia was a positive one (activating some system) rather than a negative one (releasing a system from control). Urinary retention has also been described in patients with space-occupying lesions of the frontal cortex, in the absence of other associated remarkable neurologic deficits. Posterior fossa tumors may be associated with voiding dysfunction (32% to 70%, based on references cited by Fowler). Retention or difficulty voiding is the rule, with incontinence being rarely reported. [pp 938–939]

8. **b. normal filling/storage; normal emptying.** Most children and adults with only CP have urinary control and what seems to be normal filling/storage and normal emptying. The actual incidence of voiding dysfunction is somewhat vague, because the few available series report findings predominantly in those who present with voiding symptoms. One study estimated that a third or more of children with CP are so affected. When an adult with CP presents with an acute or subacute change in voiding status, however, it is most likely unrelated to CP. [p 939]

9. **a. Dopamine.** PD is a neurodegenerative disorder of unknown cause that affects primarily the dopaminergic neurons of the substantia nigra but also heterogeneous populations of neurons elsewhere. The most important site of pathology is the substantia nigra pars compacta, the origin of the dopa-

minergic nigrostriatal tract to the caudate nucleus and putamen. Dopamine deficiency in the nigrostriatal pathway accounts for most of the classic clinical motor features of PD. [p 939]

10. **d. detrusor hyperreflexia.** The most common urodynamic finding is detrusor hyperreflexia. The pathophysiology of detrusor hyperreflexia most widely proposed is that the basal ganglia normally have an inhibitory effect on the micturition reflex, which is abolished by the cell loss in the substantia nigra. [p 940]

11. **a. hypertension.** Some practitioners consider Shy-Drager syndrome as late-stage MSA. Shy-Drager syndrome is characterized clinically by orthostatic hypotension, anhydrosis, and varying degrees of cerebellar and parkinsonian dysfunction. [p 941]

12. **e. Disease diagnosis preceding voiding and erectile symptoms.** One study compared the clinical features of 52 patients with probable MSA and 41 patients with PD. Of patients with MSA, 60% had their urinary symptoms precede or present with their symptoms of parkinsonism. Of patients with PD, 94% had been diagnosed for several years before the onset of urinary symptoms. In patients with MSA, urinary incontinence was a significant complaint in 73%, whereas 19% had only frequency and urgency without incontinence. Sixty-six percent of the patients with MSA had a significant postvoid residual volume (100 to 450 ml). In patients with PD, frequency and urgency were the predominant symptoms in 85%, and incontinence was the primary complaint in 15%. In only 5 of 32 patients with PD in whom residual urine volume was measured was it significant. Ninety-three percent of the men with MSA questioned about erectile function reported erectile failure, and in 13 of 27 of these the erectile dysfunction preceded the diagnosis of MSA. Seven of the 21 men with PD had erectile failure, but in all these men the diagnosis of erectile dysfunction followed the diagnosis of PD by 1 to 4 years. The initial urinary symptoms of MSA are urgency, frequency, and urge incontinence, occurring up to 4 years before the diagnosis is made, as does erectile failure. Cystourethrography or videourodynamic studies generally reveal an open bladder neck (intrinsic sphincter deficiency), and many patients exhibit evidence of striated sphincter denervation on motor unit electromyography. The smooth and striated sphincter abnormalities predispose women to sphincteric incontinence and make prostatectomy hazardous in men. [p 941]

13. **c. Cervical spinal cord.** The demyelinating process most commonly involves the lateral corticospinal (pyramidal) and reticulospinal columns of the cervical spinal cord. [p 941]

14. **e. Smooth sphincter dyssynergia.** Detrusor hyperreflexia is the most common urodynamic abnormality detected, occurring in 34% to 99% of cases in reported series. Of the patients with hyperreflexia, 30% to 65% have coexistent striated sphincter dyssynergia. Up to 60% of those with hyperreflexia may have impaired detrusor contractility, a phenomenon that can considerably complicate treatment efforts. Bladder areflexia may also occur; reports of its frequency vary but generally average from 5% to 20%. Generally, the smooth sphincter is synergic. [p 942]

15. **a. 15% or less.** How common are voiding problems overall in patients with HIV infection and AIDS? One study prospectively investigated voiding function in 77 men and 4 women with HIV infection or AIDS consecutively attending an outpatient clinic. Eight of these (10%) had moderate subjective voiding problems, whereas two (2%) had severe problems. The authors thought that in only 4% of patients did the nature of the disturbance warrant urodynamic examination and concluded that urinary voiding symptoms are only a modest problem; overall in an HIV/AIDS population, neuropathic bladder dysfunction is rare and mostly occurs in the late stages of the disease. [p 943]

16. **c. L2.** Spinal column (bone) segments are numbered by the vertebral level, and these have a different relationship to the spinal cord segmental level at different locations. The sacral spinal cord begins at about spinal column level T12-L1. The spinal cord terminates in the cauda equina at approximately the spinal column level of L2. [p 944]

17. **c. open bladder neck.** Spinal shock includes a suppression of autonomic activity as well as somatic activity, and the bladder is acontractile and areflexic. Radiologically, the bladder has a smooth contour with no evidence of trabeculation. The bladder neck is generally closed and competent unless there has been prior surgery or in some cases or thoracolumbar and presumably sympathetic injury. The smooth sphincter mechanism seems to be functional. Some EMG activity may be recorded from the striated sphincter, and the maximum urethral closure pressure is lower than normal but still maintained at the level of the external sphincter zone; however, the normal guarding reflex is absent and there is no voluntary control. [p 945]

18. **d. high abdominal leak point pressure.** As with all patients with neurologic impairment, a careful initial evaluation and periodic follow-up evaluation must be performed to identify and correct the following risk factors and potential complications: bladder overdistention, high pressure storage, high detrusor leak point pressure, vesicoureteral reflux, stone formation (lower and upper tracts), and complicating infection, especially in association with reflux. [p 948]

19. **a. a neurologic lesion between the pons and sacral spinal cord.** A diagnosis of striated sphincter dyssynergia implies a neurologic lesion that interrupts the neural axis between the pontine-mesencephalic reticular formation and the sacral spinal cord. [p 948]

20. **d. Tachycardia.** Symptomatically, autonomic hyperreflexia is a syndrome of exaggerated sympathetic activity in response to stimuli below the level of the lesion. The symptoms are pounding headache, hypertension, and flushing of the face and body above the level of the lesion with sweating. Bradycardia is a usual accompaniment, and tachycardia or arrhythmia may be present. [p 950]

21. **b. Propranolol.** Acutely, the hemodynamic effects of this syndrome may be managed with parenteral ganglionic or α-adrenergic blockade or with parenteral chlorpromazine. Sublingual nifedipine has been reported to be capable of alleviating this syndrome when given during cystoscopy (10 to 20 mg) and of preventing it when given orally 30 minutes before cystoscopy (10 mg). This presumably prevents smooth muscle contraction through its calcium antagonist properties and thereby prevents the increase in peripheral vascular resistance normally seen with sympathetic stimulation. The use of sublingual nifedipine has been prohibited in our particular medical center, and doubtless in some others as well. It should be noted in this regard that it has been reported that the sublingual absorption of nifedipine is negligible, and that the favorable therapeutic results obtained from such administration are probably due to swallowing the drug. van Harten and colleagues believed that if a fast onset of action of nifedipine is desired, the patient should be instructed to bite the capsule and swallow the contents with water, thereby rapidly achieving therapeutic plasma levels of the drug. Steinberger and colleagues recommended oral prophylaxis with 20 mg of nifedipine before electroejaculation and found that this markedly lowered pressure rises during treatment. [p 951]

22. **a. Ureteral reimplantation.** The best initial treatment for reflux in a patient with voiding dysfunction secondary to neurologic disease or injury is to normalize lower urinary tract urodynamics as much as possible. Depending on the clinical circumstances, this may be by pharmacotherapy, urethral dilatation (in the myelomeningocele patient), neuromodulation, deafferentation, augmentation cystoplasty, or sphincterotomy. If this fails, the question of whether to operate on such patients for correction of the reflux or to correct the reflux while performing another procedure (e.g., augmentation cystoplasty) is not an easy one, because correction of reflux in an often very thickened bladder may not be an easy task. [p 951]

23. **a. Compliance further decreased.** One must also remember the potential artefact that significant reflux can introduce into urodynamic studies. Measured bladder capacity may be less and measured pressures at given inflow volumes may be less than those after reflux correction. The apparent significance of detrusor hyperactivity may thus be underestimated. [p 951]

24. **e. Growth spurt.** One study pointed out that, whereas children often develop symptoms of tethered cord after growth spurts, in adults the presenting symptoms often follow activities that stretch the spine, such as sports or motor vehicle accidents. [p 953]

25. **d. pernicious anemia.** Although syphilitic myelopathy is disappearing as a major neurologic problem, involvement of the spinal cord dorsal columns and posterior sacral roots can result in a loss of bladder sensation and large residual urine volumes and therefore can be a cause of sensory neurogenic bladder. Another spinal cord cause of the classic sensory bladder is the now uncommon pernicious anemia. [p 953]

26. **d. Difficulty voiding; normal bladder compliance.** A study reported on findings in 114 patients with lumbar disc protrusion who were prospectively studied. The authors found detrusor areflexia in 31 (27.2%) and normal detrusor activity in the remaining 83. All 31 patients with detrusor areflexia reported difficulty voiding with straining. Patients with voiding dysfunction generally present with these symptoms or in urinary retention. The most consistent urodynamic finding is that of a normally compliant areflexic bladder associated with normal innervation or findings of incomplete denervation of the perineal floor musculature. [p 954]

27. **a. exertional (or stress) incontinence; detrusor areflexia.** When permanent voiding dysfunction occurs after radical pelvic surgery, the pattern is generally one of a failure of voluntary bladder contraction, or impaired bladder contractility, with obstruction by what seems urodynamically to be residual fixed striated sphincter tone, which is not subject to voluntarily induced relaxation. Often, the smooth sphincter area is open and nonfunctional. Decreased compliance is common in these patients, and this, with the "obstruction" caused by fixed residual striated sphincter tone, results in both storage and emptying failure. These patients often experience leaking across the distal sphincter area and, in addition, are unable to empty the bladder, because although intravesical pressure may be increased, there is nothing that approximates a true bladder contraction. The patient often presents with urinary incontinence that is characteristically most manifest with increases in intra-abdominal pressure. This is usually most obvious in females, as the prostatic bulk in males often masks an equivalent deficit in urethral closure function. Alternatively, patients may present with variable degrees of urinary retention. [p 955]

28. **b. Clean intermittent catheterization.** The temptation to perform a prostatectomy should be avoided unless a clear demonstration of outlet obstruction at this level is possible. Otherwise, prostatectomy simply decreases urethral sphincter function and thereby may result in the occurrence or worsening of sphincteric urinary incontinence. Most of these dysfunctions will be transient, and the temptation to "do something" other than perform clean intermittent catheterization initially after surgery in these patients, especially in those with little or no pre-existing history of voiding dysfunction, cannot be too strongly discouraged. [p 955]

29. **e. detrusor pressure.** Detrusor contractility is classically described as being decreased in the end-stage diabetic bladder. Current evidence points to both sensory and motor neuropathy as being involved in the pathogenesis, the motor aspect per se contributing to the impaired detrusor contractility. The typically described classic urodynamic findings include impaired bladder sensation, increased cystometric capacity, decreased bladder contractility, impaired uroflow, and, later, increased residual urine volume. The main differential diagnosis, at least in men, is generally bladder outlet obstruction, because both conditions commonly produce a low flow rate. Pressure/flow urodynamic studies easily differentiate the two. [p 956]

30. **c. Stroke.** True detrusor sphincter dyssynergia should exist only in patients who have an abnormality in pathways between the sacral spinal cord and the brain stem pontine micturition center, generally due to neurologic injury or disease. [pp 957–958]

31. **e. video-urodynamic study.** Objective evidence of outlet obstruction in these patients is easily obtainable by urodynamic study. Once obstruction is diagnosed, it can be localized at the level of the bladder neck by video-urodynamic study, cystourethrography during a bladder contraction, or micturitional urethral profilometry. [p 959]

32. **a. Striated sphincter needle EMG recording.** The Fowler syndrome refers particularly to a syndrome of urinary retention in young women in the absence of overt neurologic disease. The typical history is that of a young woman between the ages of 20 and 30 years who has found herself unable to void over the preceding 12 hours. MRI studies of the brain and the entire spinal cord are normal. On concentric needle electrode examination of the striated muscle of the urethral sphincter, however, Fowler and associates described a unique EMG abnormality. This abnormal activity, localized to the urethral sphincter, consists of a type of activity that would be expected to cause inappropriate contraction of the muscle. Sphincter activity consists of two components: complex repetitive discharges and decelerating bursts. This abnormal activity impairs sphincter relaxation. [p 960]

33. **e. Neuromodulation.** Fowler reported that efforts to treat this condition by hormonal manipulation, pharmacologic therapy, or injections of botulinum toxin have been unsuccessful. She indicated, however, that preliminary results suggest that this condition is highly responsive to neuromodulation, even in women who have had retention for many months or years. [p 960]

34. **b. myasthenia gravis.** Any neuromuscular disease that affects the tone of the smooth or striated muscle of the distal sphincter mechanism can predispose an individual patient to a greater chance of urinary incontinence after even a well-performed transurethral or open prostatectomy. Myasthenia gravis is an autoimmune disease caused by autoantibodies to acetylcholine nicotinic receptors. This leads to neuromuscular blockade and hence weakness in a variety of striated muscle groups. The incidence of incontinence after prostatectomy is indeed greatly increased in patients with this disease. [p 962]

35. **e. 1% to 2%.** Endometriosis involving the urinary tract occurs in approximately 1% to 2% of all cases; the percentage of these cases affecting the bladder ranges from 84% to 90%. [p 964]

36. **c. increased warning time.** Atropine and atropine-like agents will depress normal bladder contractions and involuntary bladder contractions of any cause. In such patients, the volume to the first involuntary bladder contraction will generally be increased, the amplitude of the involuntary bladder contraction decreased, and the total bladder capacity increased. However, although the volume and pressure thresholds at which an involuntary bladder contraction is elicited may increase, the warning time (the time between the perception of an involuntary bladder contraction about to occur and its occurrence) and the ability to suppress are not increased. [p 967]

37. **b. M_2.** On the basis of existing knowledge, it is now recommended that the designations M_{1-5} be used to describe both the pharmacologic subtypes and the molecular subtypes of muscarinic acetylcholine receptors. The human urinary bladder smooth muscle contains a mixed population of M_2 and M_3 subtypes, with M_2 receptors being predominant (80% of the total muscarinic receptor population). [p 967]

38. **c. M_3.** The minor population of M_3 receptors is generally accepted at this time as being primarily responsible for the mediation of bladder contraction. [p 967]

39. **d. Bradycardia.** In general, drug therapy for lower urinary tract dysfunction is hindered by a concept that can be expressed in one word: uroselectivity. The clinical utility of available antimuscarinic agents is limited by their lack of selectivity, responsible for the classic peripheral anticholinergic side effects of dry mouth, constipation, blurred vision, tachycardia, and effects on cognitive function. [p 968]

40. **c. poorly absorbed from the gastrointestinal tract.** Propantheline bromide (Pro-Banthīne, others) was the classically described oral agent for producing an antimuscarinic effect in the lower urinary tract. It is a nonselective muscarinic antagonist. Propantheline is a quaternary ammonium compound, all of which are poorly absorbed after oral administration. There seems to be little difference between the antimuscarinic effects of propantheline on bladder smooth muscle and the effects of other classic antimuscarinic agents. [p 968]

41. **d. M_3 receptor blockade.** Although the agents with mixed actions do relax smooth muscle in vitro by musculotropic activity and do have some local anesthetic properties, it is generally accepted that the clinical effects, at least of oxybutynin, occur solely through muscarinic blockade, as the other effects occur at much higher concentrations than its antimuscarinic actions. Oxybutynin chloride (Ditropan) is a potent muscarinic receptor antagonist with some degree of selectivity for M_3 and M_1 receptors. [p 970]

42. **b. Flavoxate.** Flavoxate hydrochloride (Urispas) is a compound that was thought originally to be a weak anticholinergic agent but to have a direct inhibitory action in addition. One study cited references showing no anticholinergic effect of the compound, but moderate calcium antagonist activity, local anesthetic properties, and the ability to inhibit phosphodiesterase. The drug failed to achieve a "recommended" assessment by Andersson and colleagues, who thought that cogent evidence of pharmacologic and/or physiologic efficacy was lacking for this agent, as was evidence for its efficacy in good-quality randomized controlled trials. [p 973]

43. **c. Cardiac toxicity.** Questions were raised about the occurrence of a rare arrhythmia (torsades de pointes) in patients taking terodiline simultaneously with antidepressants or antiarrhythmic drugs. One study reported a prolongation of AT and QTc intervals and a reduction of heart rate in elderly patients taking 12.5 mg twice daily of terodiline. These effects were apparent after 1 week but not 1 day of therapy. They also reported four cases of polymorphic ventricular tachycardia in four patients (three older than 80 years of age) receiving the drug. They advised avoiding use of the drug in patients with cardiac disease requiring cardioactive drugs, in patients with hypokalemia, or in combination with other drugs that can prolong the QT interval such as tricyclic antidepressants or antipsychotics. After further reports of apparent cardiac toxicity, the drug was voluntarily withdrawn by the manufacturer. [p 974]

44. **d. Denervation supersensitivity (myogenic).** Potassium channel openers efficiently relax various types of smooth muscle, including detrusor smooth muscle, by increasing potassium efflux, resulting in membrane hyperpolarization. This hyperpolarization reduces the opening probability of ion channels (primarily calcium) involved in membrane depolarization, with subsequent relaxation or inhibition of contraction. What makes potassium channel openers so attractive is that theoretically these drugs may be active during the filling/storage phase of micturition, abolishing bladder hyperactivity, yet with no effect on normal bladder contraction. If, as has been suggested, certain types of bladder overactivity may be secondary to the effects of denervation supersensitivity on the smooth muscle, potassium channel openers might be a particularly attractive alternative for the treatment of involuntary bladder contractions in such circumstances. [p 974]

45. **e. Direct anticholinergic, on bladder smooth muscle.** All of these agents possess various degrees of at least three major pharmacologic actions: (1) they have central and peripheral anticholinergic effects at some, but not all, sites; (2) they block the active transport system in the presynaptic nerve ending, which is responsible for the reuptake of the released amine neurotransmitters norepinephrine and serotonin; and (3) they are sedatives, an action that occurs presumably on a central basis but is perhaps related to antihistaminic properties. Imipramine has prominent systemic anticholinergic effects but has only a weak antimuscarinic effect on bladder smooth muscle. A strong direct inhibitory effect on bladder smooth muscle does exist, however, which is neither anticholinergic nor adrenergic. [p 976]

46. **e. Tolterodine and imipramine.** In my experience, the effects of imipramine on the lower urinary tract are often additive to those of the atropine-like agents, and consequently a combination of imipramine and an antimuscarinic or an antispasmodic is sometimes especially useful for decreasing bladder contractility. If imipramine is used in conjunction with an atropine-like agent, it should be noted that the anticholinergic side effects of the drugs may also be additive. [p 977]

47. **c. Priapism.** The most frequent side effects of the tricyclic antidepressants are those attributable to their systemic anticholinergic activity. Allergic phenomena (including rash), hepatic dysfunction, obstructive jaundice, and agranulocytosis may also occur, but rarely. Central nervous system side effects may include weakness, fatigue, parkinsonian effect, fine tremor noted most in the upper extremities, manic or schizophrenic picture, and sedation, probably from an antihistaminic effect. Postural hypotension may also be seen, presumably on the basis of selective blockade (a paradoxical effect) of α_1-adrenergic receptors in some vascular smooth muscle. Tricyclic antidepressants can also cause excess sweating of obscure cause and a delay of orgasm or orgas-

mic impotence, whose cause is likewise unclear. They can also produce arrhythmias and interact in deleterious ways with other drugs, and so caution must be observed in their use in patients with cardiac disease. [p 977]

48. **a. Greater desensitization at lower concentrations.** Resiniferatoxin is a vanilloid and is in fact an ultrapotent analogue of capsaicin, 1000 times more potent but with minimal initial excitatory effect. It may induce desensitization in concentrations that are so low that no noxious effects are elicited. [p 979]

49. **c. 5% to 10%.** Therapeutic overdistention involves prolonged stretching of the bladder wall using a hydrostatic pressure equal to systolic blood pressure. Improvement, when it occurs, is generally attributable to ischemic changes in the nerve endings or terminals in the bladder wall. Potential complications include bladder rupture (5% to 10%), hematuria, and retention. [pp 980–981]

50. **e. Antimuscarinic effect on bladder smooth muscle.** Peripheral (anal, perineal, vaginal) electrical stimulation for this purpose, when effective, seems to be mediated primarily by an inhibitory pudendal to pelvic nerve reflex. In addition to the inhibitory pudendal to pelvic nerve reflex, in cats the depression of bladder contractility involves a pudendal to hypogastric nerve reflex, with further inhibition mediated through sympathetic inhibition of parasympathetic ganglionic cell transmission and perhaps through a β-adrenergic effect on the bladder smooth muscle itself. There may also be cortical inhibition, the mechanism of which is uncertain. Such stimulation will also, at least in cats, increase outlet resistance through an α-adrenergic effect on the smooth musculature of the bladder neck and proximal urethra. [p 982]

51. **e. smooth sphincter dyssynergia.** Tanagho and Schmidt, who deserve enormous credit for their persistent progressive work in this field, shifted emphasis to the sacral roots as the site of electrostimulation and were among the first to suggest that their technique could be used not only for inhibiting detrusor contractility but also to facilitate detrusor contractility in cases of idiopathic urinary retention, to treat pelvic pain syndromes, and to augment striated sphincter activity for the treatment of sphincteric incontinence. The mechanisms of action of sacral root stimulation (neuromodulation) for the treatment of various types of voiding dysfunction are not exactly known, and any theory must be able to explain why, under certain circumstances, this single therapy is capable of treating bladder overactivity, idiopathic urinary retention, and pelvic pain. [p 982]

52. **d. 5 to 10 Hz; 20 to 50 Hz.** For the inhibition of bladder contractility by peripheral electrical stimulation, stimulation frequencies in the range of 5 to 10 Hz (low) have been used, whereas frequencies in the range of 20 to 50 Hz (high) have been used to increase outlet resistance. [pp 982–983]

53. **e. Pelvic pain.** It has been pointed out that when evaluating reported results, it is crucial to look at the response rate for subchronic sacral modulation, and then the results in those in whom implantation has been carried out, recognizing that the latter represent an already selected series. Also, patients most likely to benefit are those with detrusor hyperactivity or detrusor hypocontractility, whereas those with pain syndromes are less likely to benefit. [p 983]

54. **e. Improvement of reflexogenic erections.** Historically, very central (subarachnoid block) type of interruption was not used solely for urologic indications but, rather, to convert a state of severe somatic spasticity to flaccidity and to abolish autonomic hyperreflexia. As a by-product, bladder hyperreflexia was converted acutely to areflexia. The flaccid bladder that resulted generally required additional therapy to empty, or required clean intermittent catheterization. The obvious disadvantage of this type of procedure is a lack of selectivity, with unintended motor or sensory loss other than related to the bladder. Impotence was very common in males, and in those patients with some residual motor or sensory function, these functions were often significantly altered or lost. [p 985]

55. **c. Vaginal fistula.** Transvesical infiltration of the pelvic plexus with phenol aims to produce a chemical neurolysis whose results parallel the surgical approaches outlined in the text. The potential risks of this procedure include urinary retention and vaginal fistula. [p 987]

56. **c. 55%.** Although behavioral therapy has not received the favorable attention that it deserves in the urologic literature as a successful modality of treatment in "anatomic" or "genuine" stress urinary incontinence, it has been increasingly obvious that the recent literature is remarkably consistent in describing at least a significant improvement rate in 50% to 65% of the patients so treated. [p 987]

57. **d. A decrease in maximal bladder capacity.** The bladder neck and proximal urethra contain a preponderance of α_1-receptor sites, which, when stimulated, produce smooth muscle contraction. The static infusion urethral pressure profile is altered by such stimulation, which produces an increase in maximum urethral pressure and maximum urethral closure pressure. Various orally administered pharmacologic agents are available that produce α-adrenergic stimulation. Generally, outlet resistance is increased to a variable degree by such an action. [p 988]

58. **d. somnolence.** Potential side effects of all of these agents include blood pressure elevation, anxiety, and insomnia due to stimulation of the central nervous system; headache; tremor; weakness; palpations; cardiac arrhythmias; and respiratory difficulties. They should be used with caution in patients with hypertension, cardiovascular disease, or hyperthyroidism. [p 988]

59. **a. Phenylpropanolamine.** Most recently, the Food and Drug Administration has asked manufacturers to voluntarily stop selling phenylpropanolamine-containing drugs and replace the ingredient with a safer alternative. This request, which, it was hinted, may be replaced by a ban, was based on a study reported by Kernan and colleagues in 2000 in the *New England Journal of Medicine*. In commenting on this article, the *Medical Letter* (Abramowicz and Zuccotti, 2000) noted that no case-control studies were available on the safety of phenylephrine, ephedrine, or pseudoephedrine but did note that case reports have associated ephedra alkaloids with hypertension, stroke, seizures, and death. The *Medical Letter* concluded: "Phenylpropanolamine may not be the only alpha-adrenergic agonist that can cause serious adverse effects when taken systemically in over-the-counter products marketed for nasal congestion or weight loss." [pp 989–990]

60. **b. Propranolol.** Theoretically, β-adrenergic blocking agents might be expected to "unmask" or potentiate an α-adrenergic effect, thereby increasing urethral resistance. Such treatment has been suggested as an alternative treatment to α-agonists in patients with sphincteric incontinence and hypertension. [p 990]

61. **a. Moderate sphincteric incontinence.** The ideal patient for such a device would be one with pure sphincteric incontinence, mild to moderate, without significant bladder overactivity or decreased compliance, who desires active involve-

ment in her treatment program, who desires immediate results, and who has the body habitus, manual dexterity, and cognitive ability to apply or insert the device and remove it. [p 992]

62. **d. Active obstruction by tetanic muscle contraction.** One 1998 study described unstimulated graciloplasty as an innovative idea, but one that was associated with a number of problems: (1) the need for uncomfortable prolonged adduction of the leg to maintain sphincteric contraction; (2) unsatisfactory sustained muscle contraction due to the high content of fast-twitch, non–fatigue-resistant fibers; (3) loss of resting tension after dissection of the muscle, resulting in reduced contractility; (4) passive obstruction; (5) and the risk of fibrosis because the minor pedicles supplying the caudal segment of the gracilis are severed. [p 993]

63. **c. It can be given orally or intranasally at the same doses.** The synthetic antidiuretic hormone peptide analogue DDAVP (1-deamino-8-D-arginine vasopressin) has been utilized for the symptomatic relief of refractory nocturnal enuresis in both children and adults. The drug can conveniently be administered by intranasal spray at bedtime (dose, 10 to 40 μg) or as an oral preparation (dose, 100 to 400 μg) and effectively suppresses urine production for 7 to 12 hours. [p 994]

64. **e. Obstructive uropathy.** Asplund and colleagues excluded from their 1999 study, dealing with nocturnal polyuria in the elderly, patients with heart disease and/or hypertension, liver disease, Crohn's disease, and primary polydipsia, and these disorders seem reasonable to consider as relative contraindications for other patients as well. [pp 994–995]

65. **a. It is more comfortable.** Occasionally, more often in females than in males, an indwelling catheter is a last resort type of therapy for long-term bladder drainage. Virtually all such patients have bacteriuria after a certain period. A contracted fibrotic bladder may be the ultimate result. Bladder calculi may form on the catheter or on the retention balloon. Urethral complications are relatively uncommon in females when proper care is exercised, but bladder spasm may occur, producing urinary incontinence around the catheter. The temptation to use a larger bore catheter with a larger capacity balloon should be resisted, as the continuous use of such a drainage system combined with some pressure on the catheter may cause erosion of the bladder neck. A suprapubic catheter may be initially more comfortable and obviates urethral complications in the male, the main advantage of this type of continuous drainage over longer periods of time. Use of a suprapubic catheter does not, however, obviate urethral leakage with detrusor contraction, nor does it provide better drainage or less leakage in patients with sphincteric incontinence. When blockage or dislodgment occurs, nursing personnel may be reluctant to change this type of catheter without a physician's assistance. [pp 995–996]

66. **c. Ureterovesical obstruction.** Supravesical diversion is now rarely indicated in any patient with only voiding dysfunction. Indications may include (1) progressive hydronephrosis and intractable upper tract dilatation (which may be due to obstruction at the ureterovesical junction caused by a trabeculated thick bladder or to vesicoureteral reflux that does not respond to conservative measures); (2) recurrent episodes of urosepsis; and (3) intractable filling/storage or emptying failure when clean intermittent catheterization is impossible. In view of the success of cutaneous vesicostomy in children, cutaneous incontinent diversion at the level of the bladder can be accomplished without the need for ureteral reimplantation by an ileovesicostomy or "chimney" procedure. Another advantage to the ileovesicostomy over a bowel conduit is that it is easier to reverse if such a situation arises. [pp 997–998]

67. **b. penile pressure necrosis.** External collecting devices for the male (a condom or Texas catheter) are generally successful, insofar as urine collection is concerned, but are unacceptable to many patients because of the visible equipment required and the leaks of often foul-smelling urine that can result. Because many patients with neurogenic lower urinary tract dysfunction have impairment of sensation, it is easy for these devices to cause severe pressure necrosis of the penis down to and including the urethra. Maintaining an external urinary collecting device is a major problem in some spinal cord injury patients because of the inability to maintain a device during a vigorous voiding contraction, often associated with inadequate penile length, and because of recurrent lacerations of the penile skin dictating temporary use of a Foley catheter. [p 998]

68. **a. Funneling of the bladder outlet generally occurs.** The Credé maneuver (manual compression of the bladder) is most effective in patients with decreased bladder tone who can generate an intravesical pressure greater than 50 cm H_2O with this maneuver and in whom outlet resistance is borderline or decreased. The Credé maneuver obviously requires adequate hand control. Straining at the time the Credé maneuver is applied is generally counterproductive because this increases intra-abdominal pressure and causes bulging of the abdominal wall, which then tends to lift the compressing hands off the fundus of the bladder. If the proper reflex arcs are intact, this also causes striated sphincter contraction. The Credé maneuver is obviously much easier in a patient with a lax, lean abdominal wall than in a person with a taut or obese one, and it is more readily performed in a child than an adult. Such "voiding" is unphysiologic and is resisted by the same forces that normally resist stress incontinence. Adaptive changes (funneling) of the bladder outlet generally do not occur with external compression maneuvers of any kind. As referred to previously, increases in outlet resistance (via a reflex mechanism) may actually occur. If adequate emptying does not occur, other types of therapy to decrease outlet resistance may be considered; however, these may adversely affect urinary continence. Vesicoureteral reflux is a relative contraindication to external compression or the Valsalva maneuver, especially in patients capable of generating a high intravesical pressure by doing so. [pp 998–999]

69. **e. rhythmic suprapubic manual pressure.** In most types of spinal cord injury or disease characterized by detrusor hyperreflexia, manual pressure sometimes provokes a reflex bladder contraction. Such "trigger voiding" is sometimes induced by pulling of the skin or hair of the pubis, scrotum, or thigh; squeezing of the clitoris; or digital rectal stimulation. According to the classic reference, the most effective method of initiating a reflex contraction is rhythmic suprapubic manual pressure (seven or eight pushes every 3 seconds). Such activity is thought to produce a summation effect on the tension receptors in the bladder wall, resulting in an afferent neural discharge that activates the bladder reflex arc. Ideally, the contractions thus produced will be sustained and of adequate magnitude. [p 999]

70. **e. It facilitates bladder emptying.** Many acetylcholine-like drugs exist, but only bethanechol chloride (Urecholine, Duvoid, others) exhibits a relatively selective in vitro action on the urinary bladder and gut with little or no nicotinic action. Bethanechol chloride is cholinesterase resistant and causes an in vitro contraction of smooth muscle from all areas of the bladder. Although it has been reported to increase gas-

trointestinal motility and has been used in the treatment of gastroesophageal reflux, and although anecdotal success in specific patients with voiding dysfunction seems to occur, there is little or no evidence to support its success in facilitating bladder emptying in series of patients when the drug was the only variable. [p 1000]

71. **a. 200 mg.** It is generally agreed that, at least in a "denervated" bladder, an oral dose of 200 mg is required to produce the same urodynamic effects as a subcutaneous dose of 5 mg. [p 1001]

72. **d. bladder neck opening.** The spread of current to other pelvic structures whose stimulus thresholds are lower than that of the bladder has often resulted in (1) abdominal, pelvic, and perineal pain; (2) a desire to defecate or defecation; (3) contraction of the pelvic and leg muscles; and (4) erection and ejaculation in males. It has also been noted that the increase in intravesical pressure was generally not coordinated with bladder neck opening or with pelvic floor relaxation and that other measures to accomplish these ends could be necessary. [p 1003]

73. **d. Electrodes are applied extradurally to sacral roots S2 to S4.** Prerequisites for such usage were described in one study as (1) intact neural pathways between the sacral cord nuclei of the pelvic nerve and the bladder, and (2) a bladder that is capable of contracting. The chief application is in patients with inefficient or no reflex micturition after spinal cord injury. Simultaneous bladder and striated sphincter stimulation is obviated by sacral posterior rhizotomy, usually complete, which also (1) eliminates reflex incontinence and (2) improves low bladder compliance, if present. Electrodes are applied intradurally to sacral roots 2, 3, and 4, but the pairs can be activated independently. The current Brindley stimulator utilizes the principle of poststimulus voiding, a term first introduced by Jonas and Tanagho to obviate this. Relaxation time of the striated sphincter after a stimulus train is shorter than the relaxation time of the detrusor smooth muscle. When interrupted pulse trains are used, voiding is achieved between the pulse trains due to the sustained high intravesical pressure. [p 1004]

74. **b. The α_1 receptors are more common than α_2 receptors.** The smooth muscle of the β bladder base and proximal urethra contains predominantly α-adrenergic receptors, although β receptors are present. The bladder body contains both varieties of adrenergic receptors, with the β variety being more common. The human lower urinary tract contains more α_2- than α_1-adrenergic receptors, but prostatic smooth muscle contraction and human lower urinary tract smooth muscle contraction are mediated largely, if not exclusively, by α_1 receptors. [p 1006]

75. **c. Phenoxybenzamine.** Phenoxybenzamine (Dibenzyline) was the α-adrenolytic agent originally used for the treatment of voiding dysfunction. It and phentolamine have blocking properties at both α_1- and α_2-receptor sites. Prazosin hydrochloride (Minipress) was the first potent selective α_1 antagonist used to lower outlet resistance. Terazosin (Hytrin) and doxazosin (Cardura) are two highly selective postsynaptic α_1 blockers. Most recently, alfuzosin and tamsulosin (Flomax), both highly selective α_1 blockers, have appeared and are marketed solely for the treatment of benign prostatic hyperplasia because of some reports suggesting preferential action on prostatic rather than vascular smooth muscle. [pp 1007–1008]

76. **e. Retrograde ejaculation.** Available data suggest that retrograde ejaculation and rhinitis are more common with tamsulosin, whereas dizziness and asthenia are more common with terazosin and doxazosin. [p 1008]

77. **e. None of the above.** There is no class of pharmacologic agents that will selectively relax the striated musculature of the pelvic floor. [p 1009]

78. **a. γ-Aminobutyric acid (GABA).** GABA and glycine have been identified as major inhibitory transmitters in the central nervous system. GABA is the most widely distributed inhibitory neurotransmitter in the mammalian central nervous system. GABA appears to mediate the inhibitory actions of local interneurons in the brain and presynaptic inhibition within the spinal cord. [p 1009]

79. **b. Activating the $GABA_B$ receptor and depressing monosynaptic and polysynaptic excitation of motor neurons and interneurons in the spinal cord.** Benzodiazepines potentiate the action of GABA by facilitating neuronal hyperpolarization through the $GABA_A$ receptor. Baclofen (Lioresal) depresses monosynaptic and polysynaptic excitation of motor neurons and interneurons in the spinal cord by activating $GABA_B$ receptors. Dantrolene (Dantrium) exerts its effects by a direct peripheral action on skeletal muscle. It is thought to inhibit the excitation-induced release of calcium ions from the sarcoplasmic reticulum of striated muscle fibers, thereby inhibiting excitation-contraction coupling and diminishing the mechanical force of contraction. Botulinum A toxin (Botox) is an inhibitor of acetylcholine release at the neuromuscular junction of somatic nerves on striated muscle. [pp 1009–1010]

80. **c. 12 o'clock.** The 12 o'clock sphincterotomy, originally proposed by Madersbacher and Scott in 1975, remains the procedure of choice for a number of reasons. The anatomy of the striated sphincter is such that its main bulk is anteromedial. The blood supply is primarily lateral, and thus there is little chance of significant hemorrhage with a 12 o'clock incision. There is some disagreement about the rate of postoperative erectile dysfunction in those individuals who preoperatively have erections. Estimates utilizing the 3 o'clock and 9 o'clock technique vary from 5% to 30%, but, whatever the true figure is, it is clear that most would agree that this complication is far less common (approximately 5%) with incision in the anteromedial position. [pp 1011–1012]

81. **d. Detrusor leak point pressure.** One 1995 study reported long-term follow-up (time from last sphincterotomy 2 to 30 years, mean 11) in a group of 63 patients. The authors considered detrusor leak point pressure as the most reliable urodynamic parameter to predict the risk of upper tract complications after sphincterotomy. A later 1998 study likewise concluded that a detrusor leak point pressure of higher than 40 cm H_2O is a valid indicator of failure of sphincterotomy. [p 1012]

Chapter 27

Urinary Incontinence: Pathophysiology, Evaluation, and Management Overview

Jerry G. Blaivas • Asnat Groutz

Questions

1. Bladder accommodation allows:

   a. urethral sphincter contraction during bladder filling.
   b. urethral sphincter relaxation during bladder emptying.
   c. low, constant detrusor pressure during bladder filling.
   d. low, constant detrusor pressure during bladder emptying.
   e. normal sensation during bladder filling.

2. Normal urethral sphincter function is the result of:

   a. urethral position.
   b. periurethral support and compression.
   c. watertight apposition of the urethral lumen.
   d. neural control.
   e. all of the above.

3. Where in the central nervous system is the micturition reflex center located?

   a. Right hemisphere
   b. Left hemisphere
   c. Cerebellum
   d. Corpus callosum
   e. Pons

4. All of the following statements regarding urinary incontinence are correct except which one?

   a. Extraurethral incontinence is the most common cause.
   b. The symptom indicates the patient's statement of involuntary urine loss.
   c. The sign is the objective demonstration of incontinence.
   d. The condition is demonstrated by clinical or urodynamic techniques.
   e. The condition may be presumed or definite.

5. Detrusor instability is defined as:

   a. involuntary detrusor contraction due to a neurologic disorder.
   b. involuntary detrusor contraction not due to a neurologic disorder.
   c. idiopathic involuntary detrusor contractions.
   d. involuntary detrusor contraction due to a psychiatric disorder.
   e. none of the above.

6. All of the following statements regarding female sphincteric incontinence are correct except which one?

   a. In urethral hypermobility, the basic abnormality is a weakness of pelvic floor support.
   b. Intrinsic sphincter deficiency denotes an intrinsic malfunction of the urethral sphincter.
   c. Urethral hypermobility and intrinsic sphincter deficiency may coexist in the same woman.
   d. Most women with urethral hypermobility are incontinent.
   e. The normal urethra is intended to remain closed no matter what the degree of stress or rotational descent.

7. Detrusor external sphincter dyssynergia:

   a. is usually caused by neurologic lesions above the pons.
   b. is seen exclusively in patients with neurologic lesions between the pontine and sacral micturition centers.
   c. is seen exclusively in patients with multiple sclerosis.
   d. is characterized by an acontractile detrusor.
   e. may be diagnosed in neurologically intact patients.

8. Female stress urinary incontinence may be caused by:

   a. stress-induced involuntary detrusor contractions.
   b. unequal movement of the anterior and posterior walls of the proximal urethra.
   c. impaired suburethral-supporting layer.
   d. intrinsic malfunction of the urethral sphincter.
   e. all of the above.

9. Risk factors for intrinsic sphincter deficiency (ISD) include:

   a. neurologic parasympathetic injury.
   b. elective cesarean section.
   c. previous anti-incontinence surgery.
   d. chemotherapy.
   e. all of the above.

10. Vaginal delivery may cause:

    a. stress urinary incontinence.
    b. anal incontinence.
    c. urogenital prolapse.
    d. partial denervation of the pelvic floor.
    e. all of the above.

11. Pretreatment evaluation of urinary incontinence should consist of at least:

    a. cystometry and pressure-flow studies.
    b. video-urodynamics.
    c. perineal electromyography.
    d. cystoscopy.
    e. urethral profilometry.

12. Patient history:

    a. is important in assessing the characteristics and severity of incontinence.
    b. enables a reliable differentiation between sphincteric incontinence and detrusor overactivity.

c. enables the diagnosis of bladder outlet obstruction.
d. enables the diagnosis of low bladder compliance.
e. enables a reliable differentiation between intrinsic sphincter dysfunction and hypermobility-related sphincteric incontinence.

13. All of the following medications may cause or aggravate urinary incontinence except:

    a. parasympathomimetics.
    b. sympathomimetics.
    c. sympatholytic agents.
    d. diuretics.
    e. hormone replacement therapy.

14. The sacral dermatomes are evaluated by assessing all of the following except:

    a. anal sphincter tone.
    b. genital sensation.
    c. the bulbocavernosus reflex.
    d. anal sphincter control.
    e. the ice water test.

15. The bulbocavernosus reflex:

    a. is not detectable in up to 30% of otherwise normal men.
    b. if absent in women almost always indicates association with a neurologic lesion.
    c. is checked by sudden squeezing of the glans penis or clitoris.
    d. is usually absent in patients with sphincteric incontinence.
    e. is detectable in 90% of normal women.

16. Which of the following defines urethral hypermobility by the Q-tip test?

    a. A resting or straining angle of more than 10 degrees from the horizontal
    b. A resting or straining angle of more than 30 degrees from the horizontal
    c. A resting or straining angle of more than 50 degrees from the horizontal
    d. It cannot be determined by the Q-tip test.
    e. Extrusion of the Q-tip with straining

17. Which is the least reliable parameter in the micturition diary?

    a. Total number of micturition episodes
    b. Daytime micturition episodes
    c. Nocturnal micturition episodes
    d. Total number of incontinence episodes
    e. All parameters considered equally reliable

18. Which weight gain is considered to be normal in the 24-hour pad test?

    a. Up to 1 g
    b. Up to 2 g
    c. Up to 4 g
    d. Up to 6 g
    e. Up to 8 g

19. The most precise diagnostic tool for the evaluation of micturition disorders is:

    a. history and physical examination.
    b. multichannel video-urodynamics.
    c. ambulatory urodynamics.
    d. dynamic urethral pressure profile.
    e. urethrocystoscopy.

20. Urogenital prolapse may cause all of the following except:

    a. overt sphincteric incontinence.
    b. masked sphincteric incontinence.
    c. bladder outlet obstruction.
    d. anal incontinence.
    e. voiding difficulties.

21. Continent patients with urogenital prolapse should undergo:

    a. preoperative urodynamic evaluation without prolapse reduction.
    b. preoperative urodynamic evaluation with and without prolapse reduction.
    c. transvaginal repair of the prolapse only.
    d. a routine prophylactic anti-incontinence procedure during prolapse repair.
    e. urethrocystoscopy.

22. Common side effects of anticholinergic agents include:

    a. dry mouth.
    b. diarrhea.
    c. tremor.
    d. supraventricular bradycardia.
    e. postural hypotension.

23. Surgical management of refractory urge incontinence may include all of the following except:

    a. collagen injections.
    b. sacral root neuromodulation.
    c. augmentation enterocystoplasty.
    d. detrusor myectomy.
    e. urinary diversion.

24. The most successful and durable treatment of female stress urinary incontinence is:

    a. pelvic floor exercise.
    b. electrical stimulation.
    c. collagen injection.
    d. colposuspension, or pubovaginal sling surgery.
    e. vaginal wall sling.

25. The most successful and durable treatment of persistent post-prostatectomy incontinence is:

    a. α-adrenergic agonists.
    b. electrical stimulation.
    c. collagen injection.
    d. pubovaginal sling surgery.
    e. a sphincter prosthesis.

Answers

1. **c. low, constant detrusor pressure during bladder filling.** During bladder filling, detrusor pressure remains nearly constant because of a special property of the bladder known as *accommodation*. Accommodation accounts for the nearly flat cystometric curve that is seen during normal bladder filling. [p 1028]

2. **e. all of the above.** The principles underlying the functional components of the sphincter are (1) watertight apposition of the urethral lumen, (2) compression of the wall around the lumen, (3) structural support to keep the proximal urethra from moving during increases in pressure, (4) a means of compensating for abdominal pressure changes (pressure transmission), and (5) neural control. [p 1028]

3. **e. Pons.** The micturition reflex is normally under voluntary

control and is organized in the rostral brain stem (the pontine micturition center). [p 1029]

4. **a. Extraurethral incontinence is the most common cause.** Urinary leakage usually occurs through the urethra. Loss of urine from a source other than the urethra is defined as extraurethral incontinence. It may be due to urinary fistula or ectopic ureter. These topics are discussed in detail elsewhere in the text and will not be recounted here. The International Continence Society further differentiated between incontinence as a symptom, a sign, and a condition. The symptom indicates the patient's (or caregiver's) statement of involuntary urine loss. The sign is the objective demonstration of incontinence, and the condition is the urodynamic demonstration of urine loss. The Urodynamics Society suggested a modified definition for conditions causing urine loss. According to this definition "the condition is the pathophysiology underlying incontinence as demonstrated by clinical or urodynamic techniques . . . . Conditions may be presumed or definite. Definite conditions are documented by urodynamic techniques. Presumed conditions are documented clinically." [p 1029]

5. **b. involuntary detrusor contraction not due to a neurologic disorder.** The term *detrusor instability* should be used to denote involuntary detrusor contractions that are not due to neurologic disorders. [p 1030]

6. **d. Most women with urethral hypermobility are incontinent.** Many women with urethral hypermobility remain continent. [p 1031]

7. **b. is seen exclusively in patients with neurologic lesions between the pontine and sacral micturition centers.** Detrusor external sphincter dyssynergia is seen exclusively in patients with neurologic lesions between the brain stem (pontine micturition center) and the sacral spinal cord (sacral micturition center). [p 1034]

8. **e. all of the above.** Until recently, the commonly held view was that loss of structural urethral support results in varying degrees of descent of the bladder neck and urethra and that the resultant urethral hypermobility is the proximate cause of stress urinary incontinence. More recent investigations have challenged the traditional hypermobility concept. In a series of elegant MRI studies of the pelvic floor, stress incontinence was found to occur when there was unequal movement of the anterior and posterior walls of the bladder neck and proximal urethra during stress; the urethral lumen is literally pulled open as the posterior wall moves away from the anterior wall. [pp 1034–1035]

9. **c. previous anti-incontinence surgery.** Conditions associated with an increased risk of ISD include previous urethral or periurethral surgery (such as anti-incontinence surgery or urethral diverticulectomy), which may result in postoperative ISD as a result of periurethral fibrosis, scarring, or denervation. The prevalence of ISD after two or more failed anti-incontinence operations was found to be as high as 75%. [p 1036]

10. **e. all of the above.** Labor and delivery have long been known as the major risk factors for stress incontinence, urogenital prolapse, and anal incontinence. [p 1036]

11. **a. cystometry and pressure-flow studies.** Any urodynamic evaluation should consist of at least cystometry and detrusor pressure–uroflow studies. [p 1037]

12. **a. is important in assessing the characteristics and severity of incontinence.** The patient's history is important in assessing the characteristics and severity of incontinence as well as its impact on the quality of life. It is also important in identifying risk factors and/or transient causes of incontinence. However, the patient's history alone is not an accurate tool in the diagnosis of sphincteric incontinence or detrusor overactivity and should not be used as the sole determinant of diagnosis or treatment. [p 1037]

13. **e. hormone replacement therapy.** Medications are a rare cause of urinary incontinence. Sympatholytic agents such as clonidine, phenoxybenzamine, terazosin, and doxazosin may cause or worsen stress incontinence. Sympathomimetics and tricyclic antidepressants such as ephedrine, pseudoephedrine, and imipramine may increase bladder outlet obstruction and contribute to urinary retention and overflow incontinence. Diuretics, although they do not cause incontinence, may aggravate incontinence symptoms. Women should be asked about menopausal status and the use of estrogen replacement therapy. [p 1038]

14. **e. the ice water test.** The sacral dermatomes are evaluated by assessing anal sphincter tone and control, genital sensation, and the bulbocavernosus reflex. [p 1038]

15. **c. is checked by sudden squeezing of the glans penis or clitoris.** The bulbocavernosus reflex is checked by suddenly squeezing the glans penis or clitoris and feeling (or seeing) the anal sphincter and perineal muscles contract. Alternatively, the reflex may be initiated by suddenly pulling the balloon of the Foley catheter against the bladder neck. The absence of this reflex in men is almost always associated with a neurologic lesion, but the reflex is not detectable in up to 30% of otherwise normal women. [p 1038]

16. **b. A resting or straining angle of more than 30 degrees from the horizontal.** Hypermobility is defined as a resting or straining angle of greater than 30 degrees from the horizontal. [p 1038]

17. **c. Nocturnal micturition episodes.** The nocturnal micturition episodes were found to have the lowest correlation value in the test-retest analysis. [p 1039]

18. **e. Up to 8 g.** A weight gain of up to 8 g for a 24-hour pad test is considered normal. [p 1039]

19. **b. multichannel video-urodynamics.** Synchronous measurement and display of urodynamic parameters with radiographic visualization of the lower urinary tract is the most precise diagnostic tool for evaluating disturbances of micturition. [p 1041]

20. **d. anal incontinence.** Urogenital prolapse may (1) cause bladder outlet obstruction, (2) impede micturition assisted by abdominal straining, (3) mask sphincteric incontinence, or (4) cause sphincteric incontinence. [p 1042]

21. **b. preoperative urodynamic evaluation with and without prolapse reduction.** We find preoperative urodynamic evaluation, with and without prolapse reduction, to be essential in making the correct diagnosis of masked stress incontinence in clinically continent women with urogenital prolapse. We believe that the decision to perform a concomitant prophylactic anti-incontinence procedure should be tailored to individual urodynamic findings. [p 1043]

22. **a. dry mouth.** Common side effects include dry mouth, blurred vision, and constipation. Occasionally, supraventricular tachycardia may occur. [p 1044]

23. **a. collagen injections.** If conservative techniques fail, neuromodulation and denervation procedures have been recommended, although there is little documentation of long-term efficacy of the denervation procedures, and many of the techniques are associated with considerable morbidity and, for practical purposes, have been abandoned. Further, despite an initial short-term response, the long-term results are dominated by the development of low bladder compliance or re-

current detrusor overactivity. Sacral root neuromodulation, a relatively new treatment modality for refractory voiding and storage symptoms, has been shown to be effective in patients with refractory urge incontinence, urgency/frequency syndrome, and idiopathic nonobstructive retention. In the great majority of patients with refractory detrusor instability, augmentation enterocystoplasty is effective. There have been several reports of successful short-term outcomes after detrusor myectomy, and in some patients with severe refractory incontinence, a urinary diversion by ileal loop or continent reservoir may be indicated. [pp 1044–1045]

24. **d. colposuspension, or pubovaginal sling surgery.** A wide variety of surgical techniques have been devised for the treatment of stress urinary incontinence, but only the Burch colposuspension and autologous fascial pubovaginal sling have sufficient studies that document long-term efficacy. [p 1046]

25. **e. a sphincter prosthesis.** The most successful surgical treatment is the implantation of a sphincter prosthesis, which has a reported success rate of 80% to 90%. [p 1047]

Chapter 28

Post-prostatectomy Incontinence

Victor W. Nitti

Questions

1. Which of the following is true about post–radical prostatectomy incontinence?
   a. During the past 10 years, its incidence has increased.
   b. During the past 10 years, its incidence has likely decreased but its prevalence has likely increased.
   c. During the past 10 years, both the incidence and the prevalence have decreased.
   d. Reported incidence rates have been consistent in the literature.
   e. Its incidence is similar to that for incontinence after transurethral resection of the prostate (TURP).

2. After prostatectomy, the most important structure or tissue in maintaining urinary continence is the:
   a. smooth muscle of the bladder neck.
   b. rhabdosphincter.
   c. paraurethral skeletal muscle (including the levator ani complex).
   d. fast-twitch (type II) skeletal muscle fibers.
   e. proximal urethral sphincter.

3. The incidence of sphincter dysfunction in post–radical prostatectomy incontinent patients is:
   a. less than 20%.
   b. 20% to 30%.
   c. 40% to 50%.
   d. 0% to 70%.
   e. greater than 80%.

4. Which of the following is(are) a risk factor(s) for developing incontinence after radical prostatectomy?
   a. Prior radiation of the prostate
   b. Prior TURP
   c. Surgical stage
   d. a and b
   e. a, b, and c

5. Which of the following statements is NOT true regarding the evaluation of the post-prostatectomy incontinent patient?
   a. The timing and extent of evaluation are usually determined by the degree of bother to the patient.
   b. Simple treatments, such as pelvic floor exercises, may be instituted with a minimal work-up.
   c. Insertion of an artificial urinary sphincter should be preceded by a complete urodynamic work-up.
   d. History is unreliable in predicting the presence of sphincter insufficiency (as in stress incontinence).
   e. Evaluation should routinely include the determination of postvoid residual urine volume.

6. Which of the following statements is most accurate concerning urodynamics and sphincter dysfunction after radical prostatectomy?
   a. Abdominal leak point pressure provides an accurate quantitative assessment of sphincter function in post-prostatectomy incontinent patients.
   b. Urethral pressure profilometry provides an accurate quantitative assessment of sphincter function in post-prostatectomy incontinent patients.
   c. Abdominal leak point pressure correlates well with treatment outcomes for post-prostatectomy incontinent patients.
   d. Urethral pressure profilometry correlates well with treatment outcomes for post-prostatectomy incontinent patients.
   e. Sphincter dysfunction is defined as the loss of urine with an increase in abdominal pressure and the absence of a detrusor contraction, regardless of any quantitative values.

7. In urodynamic testing of the post-prostatectomy incontinent patient, which of the following is true?
   a. The diagnosis of detrusor instability can be made only if the unstable contraction has a magnitude of 15 cm H_2O.
   b. Impaired compliance and detrusor instability are mutually exclusive.
   c. The presence of detrusor instability is diagnostic for bladder dysfunction as the principal cause of incontinence.
   d. Sphincter dysfunction may be missed with a urethral catheter present.
   e. Video-urodynamics is necessary to accurately diagnose sphincter dysfunction.

8. Which of the following statements is false regarding the treatment of post–radical prostatectomy bladder dysfunction?
   a. Its treatment is similar to that for other causes of bladder dysfunction.
   b. Pharmacologic (anticholinergic) therapy is a first line of treatment.
   c. Pelvic floor exercises have been shown to have a role.
   d. Augmentation cystoplasty is contraindicated.
   e. The role of neuromodulation has not been defined.

9. Which of the following is the least effective treatment for post-prostatectomy sphincter dysfunction?
   a. Pelvic floor exercises
   b. α-Agonist medication
   c. Periurethral bulking agents
   d. Artificial urinary sphincter
   e. Bulbourethral sling

10. Which of the following is true about the artificial urinary sphincter?
    a. It should never be implanted in cases in which there is coexisting bladder dysfunction.
    b. It has been shown to offer the best long-term success rate for the treatment of post-prostatectomy incontinence secondary to sphincter dysfunction.
    c. High rates of reoperation make the artificial urinary sphincter (AUS) impractical for widespread use.
    d. Success rates are comparable to those for collagen injection.
    e. Patient satisfaction rates are approximately 50%.

Answers

1. **b. During the past 10 years, its incidence has likely decreased but its prevalence has likely increased.** The incidence of incontinence after radical prostatectomy has been a source of controversy in recent years, as reported rates have varied greatly. The incidence has likely declined in the past decade, owing to advances in surgical technique and to earlier recognition of lower stage disease in younger patients. Despite this, the prevalence of post-prostatectomy incontinence has likely risen, paralleling the increase in surgical procedures performed annually. [p 1053]

2. **b. rhabdosphincter.** The rhabdosphincter is a concentric muscular structure consisting of longitudinal smooth muscle and slow-twitch (type I) skeletal muscle fibers, which can maintain resting tone and preserve continence. [p 1055]

3. **e. greater than 80%.** Several rather recent studies have concluded that sphincter, not bladder, dysfunction is the main cause of post–radical prostatectomy incontinence. In these studies, the incidence of sphincteric dysfunction ranged from 88% to 98.5%, with associated bladder dysfunction in 26% to 46% of cases. Bladder dysfunction was the sole cause of incontinence in only 1.5% to 4% of cases. [p 1057]

4. **a. Prior radiation of the prostate.** Patients who have undergone prior radiation for prostate cancer are at high risk for developing incontinence after radical prostatectomy. Rates of significant incontinence after salvage prostatectomy range from 57% to 64%. This result has prompted some physicians to recommend urinary diversion at the time of salvage radical prostatectomy. [p 1059]

5. **d. History is unreliable in predicting the presence of sphincter insufficiency (as in stress incontinence).** Many studies have stressed the lack of reliability of symptoms and have emphasized the importance of urodynamic testing to determine the exact cause of incontinence. Although this is true, there is still valuable information to be gained from a careful history. The symptom of stress incontinence is highly predictive of the presence of sphincter dysfunction. One study found that 67 of 71 men with post-prostatectomy incontinence secondary to sphincter dysfunction complained of the symptom of stress incontinence. Similarly, another study found a 95% positive predicative value and a 100% negative predicative value for the symptom of stress incontinence and sphincter dysfunction. [p 1060]

6. **e. Sphincter dysfunction is defined as the loss of urine with an increase in abdominal pressure and the absence of a detrusor contraction, regardless of any quantitative values.** Sphincter dysfunction is defined as the demonstration of loss of urine with a rise in abdominal pressure, in the absence of a rise in detrusor pressure. [p 1061]

7. **d. Sphincter dysfunction may be missed with a urethral catheter present.** In post-prostatectomy incontinent patients with any degree of anastomotic scarring, abdominal (or Valsalva) leak point pressure can be affected, or stress incontinence may not be demonstrated with a urethral catheter in place. [p 1061]

8. **d. Augmentation cystoplasty is contraindicated.** In cases of severe, bothersome bladder dysfunction that has failed to respond to the simpler methods of treatment, augmentation cystoplasty should be considered. [p 1063]

9. **b. α-Agonist medication.** Controlled studies of these agents for post–radical prostatectomy incontinence are lacking. Our own clinical experience would suggest that these agents have minimal, if any, effect on post-prostatectomy sphincter insufficiency and are of limited utility. [p 1065]

10. **b. It has been shown to offer the best long-term success rate for the treatment of post-prostatectomy incontinence secondary to sphincter dysfunction.** The AUS has been shown to be the most effective long-term treatment for post-prostatectomy incontinence secondary to sphincter dysfunction. The prototype artificial sphincter developed by American Medical Systems was introduced in 1972, and refinements led to the development of the AMS 800, which remains the model in use today. Follow-up of greater than 10 years confirms its safety and efficacy. Contemporary series evaluating incontinence management focusing on self-reported patient satisfaction and quality of life data have shown social continence rates of approximately 80% and satisfaction rates of 90% with the AUS. [p 1065]

Chapter 29

Urinary Incontinence: Nonsurgical Management

Christopher K. Payne

Questions

1. Urinary urge incontinence has been associated with an increased risk of:

   a. bladder cancer.
   b. stroke.
   c. renal failure.
   d. Alzheimer's disease.
   e. falls and fractures.

2. Nonsurgical treatments for urinary incontinence are usually the preferred first-line interventions for all of the following reasons except which one?

   a. Pelvic floor rehabilitation is superior to surgery for stress incontinence.
   b. Urinary incontinence is not a uniformly progressive disease.
   c. Nonsurgical treatments are safe and reversible.
   d. Patients often request nonsurgical treatments.
   e. Medical therapies are very effective for patients with overactive bladder (OAB) and urge incontinence.

3. Which of the following is an example of behavioral therapy?

   a. Use of a pessary to correct a cystocele
   b. Use of incontinence pads
   c. Vaginal electromyographic (EMG) biofeedback training
   d. Discussion of normal bladder and sphincter function
   e. Use of oxybutynin on an as-needed basis

4. Which of the following statements is NOT an accurate description of the results of behavioral therapy?

   a. When behavioral therapy is combined with pharmacologic treatment of urge incontinence, approximately 50% of patients will maintain good results after the drug is discontinued.
   b. Fantyl and colleagues demonstrated that behavioral approaches are equally effective for stress and urge incontinence.
   c. Behavioral therapy is equally successful with cystometrogram-negative, cystometrogram-positive, and neurogenic patients with OAB symptoms.
   d. Burgio demonstrated that behavioral therapy is as effective as medication for patients with urge incontinence and mixed incontinence.
   e. Outpatient behavioral therapy is as successful as intensive inpatient regimens.

5. Accurate statements about pelvic floor exercise therapy (Kegel) include which of the following?

   a. Kegel exercises were initially described as using biofeedback training.
   b. Pelvic muscle exercises are rarely effective in postmenopausal women.
   c. Approximately 50% of incontinent women cannot properly contract the pelvic muscles on command.
   d. a and c.
   e. All of the above.

6. Which of the following is not a type of pelvic floor biofeedback training?

   a. Verbal coaching
   b. Vaginal cones
   c. Pressure perineometer
   d. Perineal EMG patches
   e. Stoller afferent nerve stimulator (SANS) therapy

7. Which of the following statements most accurately describes passive pelvic floor therapies (electrical and magnetic stimulation)?

   a. Patient motivation is the key to successful outcome.
   b. Restoration of continence results from conversion of urethral skeletal muscle to predominantly fast-twitch fibers.
   c. Magnetic stimulation is more effective than electrical stimulation.
   d. Patients with mixed incontinence are not candidates for these therapies.
   e. High-frequency stimulation (50 to 100 Hz) is thought to be most effective for stress incontinence.

8. Which of the following is NOT true of vaginal electrical stimulation therapy?

   a. Electrical stimulation is superior to sham therapy.
   b. Electrical stimulation decreased stress incontinent episodes by 42% in a prospective controlled trial.
   c. The optimal regimen for stimulation is twice per day in the induction phase.
   d. Electrical stimulation can theoretically improve both stress and urge incontinence.
   e. Long-term durability of stimulation results are uncertain.

9. What is Neotonus electromagnetic therapy?

   a. A simple, one-time office procedure performed with the patient under local anesthesia and sedation
   b. The most effective nonsurgical treatment for female stress incontinence
   c. A much better tolerated therapy than vaginal electrical stimulation
   d. A reasonable choice for the incontinent patient who is unable to identify the pelvic floor muscles
   e. An ineffective therapy if a patient has detrusor instability

10. The literature analysis conducted by the Berghmans group supports which of the following statements?

    a. Pelvic floor exercises are effective in treating stress incontinence.
    b. Pelvic floor exercises are effective in treating urge incontinence.
    c. Biofeedback training is superior to pelvic floor exercises alone in treatment of stress incontinence.
    d. Vaginal or rectal electrical stimulation is superior to sham stimulation in treatment of urge incontinence.
    e. Drugs are more effective than is bladder (re)training for urge incontinence.

11. A 60-year-old woman requests medical therapy for stress urinary incontinence. She had had an abdominal hysterectomy for fibroids 12 years before. She has no other medical problems, is normotensive, and notes dryness with intercourse. What should the practitioner suggest?

    a. The current first-line medical therapy for female stress urinary incontinence, phenylpropanolamine, 50 mg twice daily.
    b. The α-agonist pseudoephedrine in a long-acting formulation, once each morning
    c. Because the patient is postmenopausal, conjugated estrogens at 0.625 mg/day
    d. Vaginal estrogen cream
    e. b and d.

12. Which of the following statements about tolterodine is NOT true?

    a. Tolterodine is a new compound with antimuscarinic pharmacology.
    b. Tolterodine produces bladder selectivity through specific muscarinic subtype affinity.
    c. Urinary incontinence episodes are reduced by 40% to 60%, the same as with oxybutynin.
    d. The most common side effects are dry mouth and constipation.
    e. In long-term follow-up, more than 50% of patients continued treatment for a full year.

13. Which of the following statements accurately describes the oxybutynin products available for treatment of OAB?

    a. The extended-release formulation had superior efficacy to the immediate release in the Anderson study.
    b. Central nervous system events are the most common limiting side effects in clinical studies.
    c. The extended-release product is created by converting an alcohol side group to an ester.
    d. Once stabilized with an immediate-release preparation, a patient's dosage can be converted to an extended-release formulation at one half the dose daily.
    e. Both formulations should be dose titrated.

14. Which of the following is true in a comparison of tolterodine, oxybutynin immediate release, and oxybutynin extended release?

    a. There is no significant difference in efficacy among the three drugs.
    b. Tolterodine is much more expensive.
    c. The extended-release form of oxybutynin prevents the drug from crossing the blood-brain barrier.
    d. They simply represent different preparations of the same underlying compound.
    e. The combination of tolterodine with one of the oxybutynin preparations increases efficacy while minimizing side effects.

15. When reviewing clinical trials of anticholinergic agents for treatment of OAB, one must consider that:

    a. forced dose titration increases efficacy while minimizing adverse events.
    b. forced dose titration increases both efficacy results and adverse events.
    c. medically "naive" patients (no prior exposure to anticholinergic agents) increase efficacy results.
    d. medically "experienced" patients (screened for tolerating anticholinergic agents) produce better efficacy.
    e. although study design differences preclude efficacy comparisons from different trials, one may compare adverse events across studies because the definitions are very similar.

16. Which of the following statements is true of imipramine?

    a. It improves bladder neck closure and bladder contractility.
    b. It improves continence through α- and β-blocking effects.
    c. It can be combined with standard anticholinergics because it does not cause dry mouth.
    d. It is contraindicated for patients with renal insufficiency.
    e. It may improve bladder capacity and compliance additively with anticholinergics.

17. When devices for stress incontinence are considered, which of the following statements is most correct?

    a. Meatal-based products are the most likely to achieve dryness.
    b. Urethral stents are the easiest to use and the best tolerated.
    c. Urethral stents are contraindicated in the sexually active female.
    d. Bladder neck support devices are ideal for patients with intrinsic sphincter deficiency.
    e. Most devices are advantageous in that they can be used on an as-needed basis.

18. When a patient with mixed incontinence is evaluated for possible surgical therapy, which of the following devices will predict the response of the patient to an operation?

    a. A urethral meatal adhesive device
    b. A urethral stent
    c. A bladder neck support device
    d. None of the above
    e. All of the above

19. The next consideration after a patient fails to respond to conservative treatment of OAB should be:

    a. transvaginal cystolysis.
    b. endoscopic bladder transection.
    c. sacral nerve stimulation.
    d. endoscopic injection of alcohol.
    e. a Foley catheter.

20. With regard to percutaneous nerve evaluation (PNE), which of the following statements is true?

    a. Proper localization is confirmed by the motor response of buttock clenching and ipsilateral foot rotation.
    b. Proper localization is confirmed by a sensory response radiating across the pelvis.
    c. The most common complication is an inconclusive test caused by lead migration.
    d. A positive test will be obtained in 75% to 90% of properly selected patients.

e. a positive test must be reconfirmed with a second PNE before a permanent implant is considered.

21. Appropriate patients for consideration of sacral nerve stimulation include all of the following except:

    a. a 40-year-old woman with 20 years of urge frequency symptoms, but no incontinence, refractory to medical therapy.
    b. a 62-year-old stroke patient with detrusor hyperreflexia still having leakage despite oxybutynin treatment.
    c. a 59-year-old woman with type II diabetes and urge incontinence who failed to respond to medications and biofeedback.
    d. a 70-year-old man with urgency, nocturia, and overflow incontinence after a technically satisfactory transurethral resection of the prostate for chronic retention.
    e. a healthy 75-year-old woman with detrusor hyperreflexia and impaired contractility.

22. The surgical placement of a permanent sacral nerve stimulator:

    a. may be done with the patient under general or regional anesthesia.
    b. may produce better results than the test stimulation, as the lead has four separate electrodes that can be programmed.
    c. is associated with a 10% reoperation rate.
    d. is associated with infection of the device requiring removal, the most common complication.
    e. is nearly universally effective when the PNE (test stimulation) has demonstrated at least 50% improvement.

23. Which of the following statements is true of sacral nerve stimulation?

    a. It cannot be used in patients with neurogenic bladder.
    b. It is most often effective at S3 in OAB patients.
    c. It works through activation of bladder efferents.
    d. It creates a permanent "re-education" of the pelvic floor.
    e. It can be used to chronically rehabilitate an end-stage fibrotic bladder.

24. In comparing the various forms of electrical stimulation for urinary incontinence, which of the following is true?

    a. Only InterStim is indicated for treatment of stress urinary incontinence.
    b. The PerQ SANS device is advantageous for chronic stimulation.
    c. Vaginal electrical stimulation is potentially most useful for mixed incontinence.
    d. All of the above.
    e. None of the above.

25. Treatment planning for the incontinent female requires all of the following except:

    a. knowledge of the patient's goals and preferences.
    b. assessment of urethral support and pelvic anatomy.
    c. assessment of pelvic muscle strength.
    d. voiding diary.
    e. filling cystometry.

26. The maximum voided volume on a bladder diary correlates with which of the following urodynamic parameters?

    a. Compliance
    b. Valsalva leak point pressure
    c. Detrusor leak pressure
    d. Cystometric capacity
    e. Residual urine

27. When pelvic floor function in a stress incontinent female is considered, which of the following statements is true?

    a. Those with absent voluntary contraction have intrinsic sphincter deficiency and should be treated with a pubovaginal sling or periurethral injections.
    b. Those with absent contraction are probably best served by biofeedback training.
    c. Those with a weak contraction cannot benefit from pelvic floor exercises alone.
    d. Those with strong baseline contraction will benefit from passive stimulation.
    e. Those with strong baseline contraction cannot benefit from surgery because the urethral closure is already high.

28. Relative indications for surgical treatment of female stress incontinence include all of the following except:

    a. patient preference.
    b. prolapse beyond the hymenal ring.
    c. good pelvic muscle function.
    d. failure to respond to medical therapy.
    e. more severe leakage, with minimal activity.

29. Which of the following statements is true of pessaries?

    a. They are only for prolapse and are not useful in the treatment of stress incontinence.
    b. They may unmask occult stress incontinence in 50% of cystocele patients.
    c. They are contraindicated when urge incontinence is present.
    d. They must be used continuously and are associated with a high incidence of vaginal erosions.
    e. They are indicated only for those too ill to be considered for surgical correction.

30. An 82-year-old woman with diabetes and coronary artery disease presents for evaluation of incontinence. She says that she "leaks all the time" but sounds as though she has both stress and urge incontinence symptoms. She uses six to eight pads per day. On the first visit, a urinary tract infection is diagnosed and treated. On return, she is slightly improved but still using multiple pads. The physical examination reveals about 30 degrees of bladder neck hypermobility and a stage 1 rectocele without other pelvic organ prolapse. The voluntary pelvic muscle contraction is 0/5. The catheterization postvoid residual is 15 ml, and the urine sample for urinalysis is clear. A voiding diary demonstrates 10 voids in 24 hours, with a maximal void volume of 180 ml and a 24-hour void volume of 1100 ml. She is intolerant of anticholinergic medications, and you therefore request urodynamic testing. The cystometrogram shows compliant filling with no sensation to 125 ml, when there is sudden urgency and leakage with a 5 cm H_2O contraction. The Valsalva leak point pressure is 110 cm H_2O at 100 ml. Voiding is normal. What would be the best course of action at this point?

    a. Fluid restriction and Kegel exercises
    b. Use of a Femsoft urethral stent
    c. Pelvic floor biofeedback combined with vaginal electrical stimulation
    d. Percutaneous nerve evaluation and possible placement of an InterStim device
    e. Pubovaginal sling procedure

Answers

1. **e. falls and fractures.** In multivariate analysis, weekly or more frequent urge incontinence has been shown to be associated with an increased risk of falls (odds ratio 1.26) and fractures (relative hazard 1.34) in a group of elderly community-dwelling women. [p 1069]

2. **a. Pelvic floor rehabilitation is superior to surgery for stress incontinence.** Urinary incontinence is not an inexorably progressive disease. A moderate delay in surgical therapy does not make such treatment more difficult. As is amply documented in the chapter, "conservative" therapies are effective, well tolerated, and safe. They are preferred by many patients. It seems proper to counsel women who might appropriately choose surgery that, although surgery is the single most effective treatment for stress urinary incontinence, there is a 40% to 50% chance that they can avoid an operation and be satisfied with the outcome by going through pelvic floor training. [pp 1070 and 1086]

3. **d. Discussion of normal bladder and sphincter function.** Behavioral therapy begins with instruction about normal lower urinary tract anatomy and function. [p 1070]

4. **c. Behavioral therapy is equally successful with cystometrogram (CMG)-negative, CMG-positive, and neurogenic patients with OAB symptoms.** Long-term cure/improve rates for CMG-negative, reduced compliance, idiopathic instability, and neurogenic groups of patients were 94%, 90%, 90%, and 50%, respectively; the corresponding relapse rates were 6%, 42%, 44%, and 100%. [p 1071]

5. **d. a and c.** Half of patients are unable to perform a proper contraction with simple instructions. Kegel routinely employed a perineometer with his patients in one of the first documented uses of biofeedback in medicine. [p 1072]

6. **e. Stoller afferent nerve stimulator (SANS) therapy.** Biofeedback is any method of training a patient to control a bodily function by providing the patient with information about that function. With incontinence, the patient hopes to gain control of and strengthen the pelvic muscles. The information can be relayed to the patient orally after digital biofeedback from examination, through the sensation of vaginal cones, or with mechanized equipment emitting audio or visual signals that correlate with muscle activity. [pp 1073 and 1083]

7. **e. High-frequency stimulation (50 to 100 Hz) is thought to be most effective for stress incontinence.** High-frequency stimulation (usually 50 to 100 Hz) of the pelvic floor muscles is used to treat stress urinary incontinence by directly stimulating a contraction. [p 1073]

8. **c. The optimal regimen for stimulation is twice per day in the induction phase.** There was no difference in outcome between daily stimulation and every-other-day stimulation. [p 1073]

9. **d. A reasonable choice for the incontinent patient who is unable to identify the pelvic floor muscles.** Until data on the durability of response with advanced techniques exist, biofeedback, electrical stimulation, and electromagnetic therapy are all potential competitive treatment options for rehabilitation of the pelvic floor when Kegel exercises are insufficient. [p 1074]

10. **a. Pelvic floor exercises are effective in treating stress incontinence.** There is strong evidence that pelvic floor muscle exercises are effective in treating stress urinary incontinence, but there is no evidence that pelvic floor muscle exercises with biofeedback are more effective than pelvic floor muscle exercises alone. It was also found that "there is strong evidence to suggest that electrostimulation is superior to sham electrostimulation" but that limited existing data show "no difference between electrostimulation and other physical therapies." A second article from the same Berghman group examined treatments for urge incontinence. Eight of 15 trials were considered to be of adequate quality for analysis. The authors concluded that there is "weak evidence to suggest that bladder (re)training is more effective than no treatment . . . and drug therapy." There was not sufficient evidence to conclude that electrical stimulation was superior to sham stimulation, and the data were insufficient to evaluate pelvic floor exercises with or without biofeedback. [p 1074]

11. **e. b and d.** The interaction between α-agonists and estrogens should be explored, as small controlled studies suggest synergy between the two. [pp 1075–1076]

12. **b. Tolterodine produces bladder selectivity through specific muscarinic subtype affinity.** Tolterodine is a new compound, a competitive muscarinic receptor antagonist. In a cat model, the compound demonstrated selectivity for detrusor contractility over salivary gland secretion that is not related to receptor subtype affinity. [p 1076]

13. **e. Both formulations should be dose titrated.** Both oxybutynin preparations require dose titration. [p 1077]

14. **a. There is no significant difference in efficacy among the three drugs.** The bottom line is that neither drug was able to demonstrate efficacy superiority to conventional, immediate-release oxybutynin. [p 1077]

15. **b. forced dose titration increases both efficacy results and adverse events.** The oxybutynin design employed a forced dosed titration. This might be expected to have enhanced efficacy results but it would similarly increase adverse events. [p 1077]

16. **e. It may improve bladder capacity and compliance additively with anticholinergics.** Imipramine is the drug of choice to add to standard anticholinergics to produce an additive effect on OAB. [p 1077]

17. **e. Most devices are advantageous in that they can be used on an as-needed basis.** Among the advantages of vaginal support devices are that they (1) are potentially applicable to the majority of the incontinent population (those with pure stress or mixed incontinence and urethral hypermobility), (2) do not require specific testing such as urodynamics, (3) can be used as needed for predictable stress incontinence (as can the other devices), and (4) have minimal side effects. [pp 1079–1080 and 1087]

18. **c. A bladder neck support device.** When stress incontinence is suspected to be the primary component, a short-term trial of one of the vaginal support devices may clarify the picture. [p 1089]

19. **c. sacral nerve stimulation.** Whereas very few OAB patients had been considered candidates for surgical reconstruction, the majority of patients who function independently in a community setting could be considered candidates for neuromodulation, greatly expanding the number of patients who can reasonably be offered surgical therapy. [p 1081]

20. **c. The most common complication is an inconclusive test

caused by lead migration. Complications were minimal, with 9.9% of patients experiencing lead migration, which prevented adequate stimulation, 2.6% suffering temporary pain related to stimulation, 0.8% experiencing skin irritation, and 0.6% having an adverse change in bowel or voiding function. [p 1082]

21. **d. a 70-year-old man with urgency, nocturia, and overflow incontinence after a technically satisfactory transurethral resection of the prostate for chronic retention.** Patients with end-stage, small, contracted bladders cannot respond and must have augmentation or diversion. Neurogenic patients were excluded from the clinical trials but can be successfully treated if the bladder has not progressed to "end-stage" fibrosis. Neuromodulation cannot work when the peripheral nerves are destroyed, as may happen with sacral spinal cord injury, radical pelvic surgery, or spinal cord tumor. It is also doomed to failure when the bladder is areflexic because of myogenic damage from chronic overdistention. Nonetheless, the many neurogenic bladder patients, including those with suprasacral spinal cord injuries, stroke, and multiple sclerosis, could be considered for treatment when the primary problem is detrusor hyperreflexia, the bladder capacity is adequate, and the peripheral nerves are intact. [p 1083]

22. **b. may produce better results than the test stimulation, as the lead has four separate electrodes that can be programmed.** A quad lead with four separate electrodes is positioned in the foramen used during the PNE. The four leads can be programmed externally; the quad lead increases the likelihood of proximity to the nerve and good functional results. [p 1082]

23. **b. It is most often effective at S3 in OAB patients.** In the case of an OAB patient, S3 afferent nerve stimulation inhibits detrusor activity at the level of the sacral spinal cord, decreasing detrusor instability and urge incontinence. [p 1081]

24. **c. Vaginal electrical stimulation is potentially most useful for mixed incontinence.** The role of dual stimulation for mixed incontinence has not been adequately evaluated; this treatment would seem to be ideal for such patients using the high frequency for the sphincter and low frequency for the bladder. [pp 1073 and 1089]

25. **e. filling cystometry.** The clinician needs three primary pieces of information to develop a treatment plan for a given patient: the type of incontinence, the baseline voiding diary, and an assessment of anatomy, with particular emphasis on pelvic floor muscle strength and function. [p 1085]

26. **d. Cystometric capacity.** The largest voided volume on a diary has been shown to correlate with the cystometric capacity defined by urodynamic testing. [p 1085]

27. **b. Those with absent contraction are probably best served by biofeedback training.** Patients with inappropriate or absent baseline function need some form of biofeedback just to get started with treatment. [p 1086]

28. **d. failure to respond to medical therapy.** Patients who might logically benefit from immediate surgery would include those who have significant associated prolapse (beyond the hymenal ring) that may be corrected at the same time, those who are highly motivated to be completely dry or who have high levels of physical stress because of lifestyle or occupation, those with relatively severe stress incontinence, and especially those with good pelvic floor function on initial examination. [p 1086]

29. **b. They may unmask occult stress incontinence in 50% of cystocele patients.** Elevation of a cystocele will unmask occult sphincteric incompetence in more than 50% of patients who are continent with the prolapse. [p 1089]

30. **c. Pelvic floor biofeedback combined with vaginal electrical stimulation.** The mixed incontinence patient can usually benefit from each form of conservative treatment: behavioral, pelvic floor, and medical therapies. Pelvic floor rehabilitation is probably the most important treatment in this patient group, and there may be a special role for electrical stimulation because, at least theoretically, stimulation may specifically improve both urethral and bladder function. [p 1089]

Chapter 30

Vaginal Reconstructive Surgery for Sphincteric Incontinence and Prolapse

Sender Herschorn • Lesley K. Carr

Questions

1. Which one of the following factors can most likely explain the higher prevalence of urinary incontinence in the United States compared with Europe?

   a. Different definitions of urinary incontinence
   b. Lack of validation of the results
   c. Older ages surveyed
   d. More detailed questionnaires in Europe
   e. Different availability of therapy

2. Incidence rates of urinary incontinence are more difficult to ascertain than prevalence rates because of which requirement?

   a. Test-retest reliability
   b. Increased awareness of the problem

c. Knowledge of the natural history of incontinence
   d. Repeated surveys of the same population
   e. Different definitions of incontinence

3. In the study from Oregon by Olsen and colleagues in 1997, what was the lifetime risk of a woman undergoing a single operation for prolapse or incontinence by the age of 80?

   a. 2%
   b. 11%
   c. 33%
   d. 56%
   e. 74%

4. Which one of the following factors shows the strongest epidemiologic link to urinary incontinence?

   a. Menopause
   b. Obesity
   c. Episiotomy
   d. Chronic respiratory problems
   e. Pregnancy and childbirth

5. Which of the following muscles is NOT part of the levator ani?

   a. Pubococcygeus
   b. Puboanalis
   c. Puborectalis
   d. Ileococcygeus
   e. Coccygeus

6. The arcus tendineus runs from the:

   a. pubic rami to ischial spine.
   b. ischial spine to anterior coccyx.
   c. ischial tuberosity to lateral coccyx.
   d. surface of superior rami to ilia.
   e. vaginal apex to sacrum.

7. Which of the following supportive structures is formed by fusion of the ileococcygeus and pubococcygeus muscles behind the rectum?

   a. Cardinal ligaments
   b. Arcus tendineus fasciae pelvis
   c. Levator plate
   d. Perineal membrane
   e. Puborectalis fascia

8. Which of the following statements about the urogenital diaphragm (perineal membrane) is NOT true?

   a. It closes the urogenital hiatus below the pelvic diaphragm.
   b. It is contiguous with a parallel perianal diaphragm.
   c. It has a sphincter-like effect at the distal vagina.
   d. It contributes to continence with connections to periurethral striated muscles.
   e. It is the structural support for the distal urethra.

9. Central cystoceles result from:

   a. detachment of the paravaginal support from the arcus tendineus fasciae pelvis.
   b. breakage of the pubourethral ligaments.
   c. separation of the pubocervical fascia from the pubis.
   d. widening of the urogenital hiatus.
   e. weakness of the anterior vaginal wall or fascia.

10. What is the role of the cardinal and uterosacral ligaments?

    a. They support the uterine fundus to the lateral pelvic sidewalls.
    b. They are the major source of support for the proximal ladder base.
    c. They hold the uterus and upper vagina in place on the levator plate.
    d. They provide urethral support and closure.
    e. They support the rectum via attachment to lateral prerectal fascia.

11. Which of the following defects is usually seen with level I defects?

    a. Urethrocele
    b. Cystocele
    c. Rectocele
    d. Vault prolapse
    e. Descending perineal syndrome

12. Which of the following enteroceles is most commonly seen?

    a. Posterior (between vagina and rectum)
    b. Anterior (between bladder and vagina)
    c. Lateral (pudendal)
    d. Congenital
    e. Post–Burch procedure

13. Which of the following symptoms consistently correlates with the severity of pelvic organ prolapse?

    a. Stress incontinence
    b. Anal incontinence
    c. Dyspareunia
    d. Low back pain
    e. None of the above

14. A 65-year-old woman presents with severe anterior compartment prolapse. She mentioned that her complaint of stress incontinence had improved in the previous year. Which of the following statements about her evaluation is true?

    a. It is not necessary to ascertain any further lower urinary tract symptoms.
    b. Occult or potential stress incontinence should be elicited.
    c. Cystoscopy and urodynamic studies must be performed.
    d. MRI studies will provide a definitive diagnosis.
    e. Transvaginal ultrasonography has been shown to help in this situation.

15. What has the voiding diary, or frequency-volume chart, been shown to do?

    a. Predict the outcome of stress incontinence surgery
    b. Confirm the result of the pad test
    c. Reflect symptoms most accurately
    d. Be independent of the patient's willingness to complete the diary
    e. Check the validity of incontinence questionnaires

16. What is the reported prevalence of severe hydronephrosis in patients with pelvic organ prolapse?

    a. <1%
    b. 5% to 10%
    c. 12% to 18%
    d. 20% to 25%
    e. >30%

17. Urethral axis testing is helpful because:

    a. the deflection angle correlates with the severity of incontinence.
    b. it assesses the degree of urethral hypermobility.
    c. it is sensitive to deflection from concomitant uterine prolapse.
    d. it predicts the outcome of treatment.
    e. it confirms radiologic results.

18. On speculum examination of the vaginal vault of a woman after a hysterectomy, dimples seen at the 3 and 9 o'clock positions are the location of:

    a. level 3 supports.
    b. pubocervical fascia.
    c. cardinal uterosacral ligaments.
    d. arcus tendineus fasciae pelvis.
    e. lateral rectal fascia.

19. In the Pelvic Organ Prolapse Quantification (POPQ) system for pelvic organ prolapse, which fixed structure is the reference point for prolapse?
    a. Hymenal ring
    b. Introitus
    c. Perineal body
    d. Ischial spine
    e. Genital hiatus

20. In the POPQ system, the genital hiatus is measured from:
    a. ischial spine to ischial spine.
    b. the anterior hymenal ring to the anterior pouch of Douglas.
    c. the midplane of the vagina to the introitus.
    d. the anterior fornix to the urethral meatus.
    e. the middle of urethral meatus to the posterior hymeneal ring.

21. In the POPQ system for prolapse, stage I is seen when:
    a. there is essentially complete vaginal eversion.
    b. no prolapse is demonstrated.
    c. the most distal portion of the prolapse is 1 cm or less proximal or distal to the hymenal plane.
    d. the most distal portion of the prolapse is more than 1 cm above the level of the hymen.
    e. the most distal portion of the prolapse protrudes more than 1 cm below the hymen but protrudes no further than 2 cm less than the total vaginal length.

22. Which of the following statements about MRI of pelvic organ prolapse is true?
    a. T1-weighted images give clearer soft tissue discrimination.
    b. It is more sensitive than cystocolpoproctography.
    c. Fast spin echo T2-weighted sequences yield the clearest pictures.
    d. It is more operator dependent than is ultrasonographic imaging.
    e. It is the procedure of choice for assessing the degree of pelvic organ prolapse.

23. In the original Raz (1981) modification of the Pereyra needle suspension, all but which one of the following steps were new?
    a. Cystoscopic verification
    b. Entry into the retropubic space
    c. Digital guidance of the ligature carrier
    d. Placement of helical sutures into the periurethral connective tissue
    e. Urethrolysis if required

24. The tension-free vaginal tape (TVT) procedure is thought to work by:
    a. abolishing bladder neck hypermobility.
    b. augmenting midurethral support.
    c. obstructing the urethra.
    d. improving urethral apposition.
    e. causing a periurethral inflammatory reaction.

25. How is bleeding from vaginal veins during the performance of a vaginal suspension for stress incontinence usually treated?
    a. Blood transfusion
    b. Laparotomy
    c. Angiographic embolization
    d. Vaginal sutures and packing
    e. Cystoscopy and suture removal

26. Which of the following procedures has the highest reported incidence of postoperative retention?
    a. Sling procedures
    b. The TVT procedure
    c. Vaginal needle suspension (Raz)
    d. Vaginal suspension with bone anchors
    e. Anterior repair

27. Culdoplasty refers to which of the following?
    a. Obliteration of the vaginal lumen
    b. Resection of the vagina
    c. Suspension of the vaginal wall
    d. Incision into the (posterior) cul-de-sac (pouch of Douglas)
    e. Surgical obliteration of the cul-de-sac (pouch of Douglas)

28. Regarding the natural history of untreated pelvic organ prolapse, which of the following statements is true?
    a. Occult weaknesses always surface eventually.
    b. There is good correlation of symptoms and physical findings.
    c. Epidemiologic data are lacking.
    d. Broad consensus exists on an adequate work-up.
    e. Physical findings rather than symptoms determine the morbidity.

29. Preparation of the vagina with which of the following may be beneficial before pelvic organ prolapse surgery?
    a. Ring pessary
    b. Estrogen cream
    c. Kegel exercises
    d. Antibiotic solution
    e. Topical lidocaine

30. What is involved in the maneuver to support the posterior aspect of a large cystocele during anterior colporrhaphy?
    a. Imbricating the pubocervical fascia
    b. Supporting the repair with mesh
    c. Extending the repair to or through the arcus tendineus fasciae pelvis
    d. Incorporating the precervical or cardinal-uterosacral complex
    e. Repairing the concomitant rectocele

31. The paravaginal repair can be used to repair which of the following anterior wall defects?
    a. Lateral
    b. Central
    c. Combined
    d. Posterior
    e. Distal

32. The addition of which of the following techniques to a four- or six-corner suspension will specifically address a concomitant moderate or large central cystocele?
    a. Paravaginal repair
    b. Bone anchors
    c. Goalpost incision
    d. Cardinal ligament suturing
    e. Anterior colporrhaphy

33. The difficulty in comparing results of reported series of needle suspensions combined with anterior colporrhaphy is most likely from:
    a. incomplete reporting.
    b. variations in surgical technique.

c. lack of follow-up.
d. different methods of assessment.
e. different populations of patients.

34. Which of the following has been proposed as a cause of enterocele formation after a Burch procedure for stress urinary incontinence?

    a. Denervation of the vaginal wall
    b. Pelvic hematoma
    c. Urinary obstruction
    d. Alteration of the vaginal axis
    e. Effacement of the perineum

35. Vault evisceration after vaginal hysterectomy is treated by:

    a. vaginal packing.
    b. endoscopic manipulation.
    c. bed rest and intravenous fluids.
    d. immediate surgery.
    e. sterile pessary.

36. Which structure or structures travel just beneath the sacrospinous ligament and should be avoided during a sacrospinous ligament vault suspension?

    a. Pudendal vessels
    b. Hypogastric vessels
    c. Genitofemoral nerve
    d. Sciatic nerve
    e. Inferior gluteal artery

37. The main vaginal site of recurrent pelvic relaxation after sacrospinous ligament vault suspension has been reported to be in which structure?

    a. The vault
    b. The posterior wall
    c. The perineum
    d. The anterior wall
    e. The enterocele

38. Which of the following vaginal vault suspension procedures has the greatest likelihood of associated ureteral injury?

    a. Sacrospinous ligament suspension
    b. Ileococcygeus suspension
    c. Uterosacral ligament suspension
    d. Abdominal sacral colpopexy
    e. Laparoscopic sacral colpopexy

39. A successful rectocele repair may accomplish all but which of the following?

    a. Narrowing of the posterior aspect of the vaginal canal
    b. Plication of the prerectal and pararectal fascias
    c. Narrowing of the vaginal caliber
    d. Narrowing of the posterior aspect of the levator (urogenital) hiatus with levator plication
    e. Prevention of recurrent incontinence after anterior suspension.

40. Which of the following is thought to cause dyspareunia after traditional rectocele repair?

    a. Persistence of enterocele
    b. Constipation
    c. Levator plication during the procedure
    d. Unrecognized rectal injury
    e. Persistence of the descending perineum syndrome

Answers

1. **b. Lack of validation of the results.** Epidemiologic studies conducted in the United States, the majority of which did not validate the results of interviews or questionnaires, tended to have higher prevalence estimates (37% in 13 studies) than European (26% in 19 studies) and British (28.7% in 8 studies) series. In about one third of the non-U.S. studies, the data were verified with other tests such as clinical examination, pad tests, and urodynamics. [p 1093]

2. **d. Repeated surveys of the same population.** Incidence rates have been more difficult to ascertain because they require repeated surveys of the same population. [p 1093]

3. **b. 11%.** Olsen and co-workers, on the basis of chart reviews from a large managed care population in Oregon, reported that the lifetime risk of undergoing a single operation for prolapse or incontinence by age 80 was 11.1%. [p 1094]

4. **e. Pregnancy and childbirth.** Vaginal delivery is a major factor for the development of pelvic floor dysfunction in the majority of women. Most studies demonstrate a link between urinary incontinence and parity, although the level of risk is variable and may fade with age. [p 1094]

5. **e. Coccygeus.** The levator ani and coccygeus muscles that are attached to the inner surface of the minor pelvis form the muscular floor of the pelvis. With their corresponding muscles from the opposite side, they form the pelvic diaphragm (see Fig. 30–3). The levator ani is composed of two major muscles from medial to lateral: pubococcygeus and ileococcygeus. [p 1096]

6. **a. pubic rami to ischial spine.** The arcus tendineus of the levator ani is a dense connective tissue structure that runs from the pubic ramus to the ischial spine and courses along the surface of the obturator internus muscle. [p 1096]

7. **c. Levator plate.** This median raphe between the anus and the coccyx is called the levator plate, the shelf on which the pelvic organs rest. It is formed by the fusion of the ileococcygeus and the posterior fibers of the pubococcygeus muscles. In the standing position, the levator plate is horizontal and supports the rectum and upper two thirds of vagina above it. [p 1097]

8. **b. It is contiguous with a parallel perianal diaphragm.** The urogenital diaphragm bridges the gap between the inferior pubic rami bilaterally and the perineal body. It closes the urogenital (levator) hiatus, supports and has a sphincter-like effect at the distal vagina, and contributes to continence because it is attached to periurethral striated muscles. It also provides structural support for the distal urethra. The posterior triangle, around the anus, does not have a corresponding diaphragm or membrane. [p 1098]

9. **e. weakness of the anterior vaginal wall or fascia.** Weaknesses in the central part of the anterior vaginal wall or fascia give rise to cystoceles from a central defect. [p 1101]

10. **c. They hold the uterus and upper vagina in place on the levator plate.** The cardinal and uterosacral ligaments hold the uterus and upper vagina in their proper place over the levator plate. [p 1102]

11. **d. Vault prolapse.** Level I, or apical, defects are thought to be caused by loss of normal support of the upper paracol-

pium and parametrium and are associated with uterine prolapse, vaginal vault prolapse, and possibly enterocele. [p 1104]

12. **a. Posterior (between vagina and rectum).** The posterior type is located between the vagina and the rectum and is most common. [p 1105]

13. **e. None of the above.** Symptoms caused by pelvic organ prolapse have not been systematically characterized or absolutely established. [p 1106]

14. **b. Occult or potential stress incontinence should be elicited.** This phenomenon has been termed occult or potential stress incontinence and should be elicited when therapy is being considered. [p 1107]

15. **e. Check the validity of incontinence questionnaires.** They have been shown to exhibit test-retest reliability for incontinent episodes and have been used to check the validity of questionnaires. [p 1108]

16. **a. <1%.** The prevalence of hydronephrosis in patients with pelvic organ prolapse is also low. One study reported mild to moderate hydronephrosis in 6.8% and severe hydronephrosis in 0.9% of 323 patients with pelvic organ prolapse. The severe cases were seen only with uterine procidentia. [p 1109]

17. **b. it assesses the degree of urethral hypermobility.** Urethral axis testing does not diagnose any form of incontinence because continent women may demonstrate rotational descent of the urethra. Although it has been shown to be reproducible, it has not been compared with other radiologic methods. However, it may be helpful in assessing the amount of hypermobility. In women with large defects, the urethra may be compressed by the large bulge when the patient strains, impairing assessment of mobility and stress incontinence. [p 1110]

18. **c. cardinal uterosacral ligaments.** After hysterectomy, the vaginal cuff will have dimples at the 3 and 9 o'clock areas, at the locations of the cardinal uterosacral ligament attachments. [p 1111]

19. **a. Hymenal ring.** The POPQ system assigns negative numbers (in centimeters) to structures that have not prolapsed beyond the hymen and positive numbers to structures that protrude, with the plane of the hymen defined as 0 (see Fig. 30–18). The hymen was selected as the reference point rather than the introitus because it is more precisely identified. [p 1112]

20. **e. the middle of urethral meatus to the posterior hymeneal ring.** The genital hiatus is measured from the middle of the urethral meatus to the posterior hymeneal ring. [p 1112]

21. **d. the most distal portion of the prolapse is more than 1 cm above the level of the hymen.** Stage I is defined as when the most distal portion of the prolapse is more than 1 cm above the level of the hymen. [p 1113]

22. **c. Fast spin echo T2-weighted sequences yield the clearest pictures.** MRI provides multiplanar images, does not use ionizing radiation, usually does not require a contrast medium, and is relatively non–operator dependent. T1-weighted sequences can be obtained in a shorter time, resulting in less motion artefact, and are used as the initial imaging sequence. T2-weighted images have clearer soft tissue contrast discrimination. Two groups of investigators showed that MRI was not as sensitive as contrast radiographic imaging with cystocolpoproctography in detecting cystoceles and enteroceles, whereas rectoceles were imaged equally. MRI may be very helpful in patients with complex organ prolapse to supplement the physical examination. Its clinical utility in comparison with physical examination and in the decision for surgical management has yet to be demonstrated. [p 1114]

23. **a. Cystoscopic verification.** In 1981, Raz described a modification of the Pereyra procedure (see Fig. 30–22). The technique employed an inverted U-shaped vaginal incision to improve access. It also was the first to open the retropubic space sharply by detaching the periurethral connective tissue from the arcus tendineus. Opening the retropubic space facilitates blind passage of the ligature carrier from the abdomen to the vaginal incision by allowing finger guidance, permitting urethrolysis if required, and allowing placement of helical sutures into the abdominal and vaginal sides of the periurethral connective tissue, which results in a more secure purchase of tissue. [p 1116]

24. **b. augmenting midurethral support.** Another technique focusing on the midurethral continence mechanism is the tension-free vaginal tape procedure. The procedure does not seem to abolish urethral hypermobility as assessed by pre- and postoperative cotton-tipped applicator tests. [p 1118]

25. **d. Vaginal sutures and packing.** Bleeding from vaginal veins may be brisk but can generally be controlled with electrocautery or absorbable stitches. Bleeding from the retropubic dissection may be more problematic and is often a result of dissection too far laterally into the obturator fossa. Temporary vaginal packing along with digital compression can slow bleeding. Suture ligatures may be required to stop bleeding. Vaginal closure with packing may tamponade bleeding that is not too brisk or flowing freely into the retropubic space. Rarely, an abdominal approach may be required to control bleeding. Transfusion requirement for suspensions is estimated at 1%. [p 1119]

26. **a. Sling procedures.** Postoperative complications from stress incontinence surgery are not unique to transvaginal suspension techniques. Many result from an increased urethral resistance or relative obstruction and as such are thought to be more common after sling-type procedures. Three-year follow-up with 50 consecutive women showed an 86% cure rate with no mesh rejection or permanent retention. [pp 1118 and 1119]

27. **e. Surgical obliteration of the cul-de-sac (pouch of Douglas).** Colpocleisis is obliteration of the vaginal lumen (LeFort—denudation of anterior and posterior vaginal mucosal strips with approximation of anterior and posterior walls). Colpectomy refers to resection of vagina; colpopexy, suspension of the vaginal wall; culdotomy, incision into the (posterior) cul-de-sac (pouch of Douglas); and culdoplasty, surgical obliteration of the cul-de-sac to treat or prevent enterocele. [p 1120]

28. **c. Epidemiologic data are lacking.** As yet, no consensus or guidelines exist regarding which tests constitute an adequate work-up for patients before surgery, nor are the functional deficits and symptoms caused by pelvic organ prolapse and pelvic floor dysfunction well characterized or absolutely established. It is therefore important for the surgeon to fully evaluate the patient clinically and record all of the symptoms and physical findings in a standardized manner. Because the various forms of organ prolapse are interrelated owing to shared support mechanisms, it is generally recommended that all defects be repaired at the same time, because occult weaknesses in other sites or new support defects may be acquired. Although this approach is definitely supported by clinical experience and the reported occurrence of prolapse after retropubic urethropexy and vaginal vault suspension, there is a lack of epidemiologic data on the natural history of untreated pelvic organ prolapse. [p 1120]

29. **b. Estrogen cream.** In postmenopausal women, estrogen therapy has been widely proposed for the preparation of the vagina before surgery and is known to improve vascularity and total skin collagen content. A practical regimen is a 6-week preoperative course of vaginal estrogen cream. [p 1120]

30. **d. Incorporating the precervical or cardinal-uterosacral complex.** In the posterior aspect, approximating stitches can be placed in the pericervical fascia or cardinal-uterosacral ligament complex for additional support. [p 1121]

31. **a. Lateral.** Lateral defects, causing mild to moderate cystoceles, can be repaired abdominally with a paravaginal repair. [p 1123]

32. **e. Anterior colporrhaphy.** For moderate to large cystoceles, Raz and co-workers combined anterior colporrhaphy with the previously described four-corner suspension. [p 1124]

33. **b. variations in surgical technique.** The difficulty in assessing and comparing results may stem from variations in the surgical procedures. As mentioned earlier, Raz and colleagues, in addition to modifying the incision, substantially modified the suspension by limiting the retropubic dissection to the level of the urethra rather than from the urethra to the ischial spine. They also modified the suture placement and added a piece of absorbable mesh above the colporrhaphy. [p 1124]

34. **d. Alteration of the vaginal axis.** Ventral fixation of the vagina, such as a Burch procedure, may also cause widening of the cul-de-sac, with resultant enterocele formation. [p 1125]

35. **d. immediate surgery.** Vaginal evisceration is a rare but life-threatening surgical emergency that can arise after vaginal or abdominal hysterectomy or enterocele repair. The evisceration repair operation can be done vaginally, abdominally, or by combined approach. [p 1127]

36. **a. Pudendal vessels.** Many important structures are in proximity and must be avoided during the procedure. The hypogastric vessels lie superior and medial. The sciatic nerve and inferior gluteal artery exit the pelvis through the lower part of the greater sciatic foramen. The pudendal vessels and nerve and the nerve to the obturator internus travel around the ischial spine and re-enter the pelvis through the lesser sciatic foramen, below the pelvic diaphragm. The sutures are placed 1.5 to 3 cm medial to the ischial spine, to avoid injury to the pudendal nerves and vessels, and through the substance of the ligament. [pp 1127–1128]

37. **d. The anterior wall.** Recurrent pelvic relaxation developed in 109 (18%) patients, including 81 anterior vaginal wall defects, 32 vaginal vault eversions, 24 posterior vaginal wall prolapses, and 56 defects at unspecified or multiples sites. Reoperations were performed in 7 of 81 patients with anterior defects, 20 of 32 with vault eversion, and 4 of 24 with posterior wall prolapse. The relatively high recurrence or new onset of anterior vaginal prolapse was mentioned earlier and ranges from 22% to 92%. It may be due to exaggerated retroversion of the vagina with exposure of the anterior wall to greater abdominal pressure or possibly a neuropathic lesion caused by the vaginal dissection. [p 1128]

38. **c. Uterosacral ligament suspension.** Intraoperative ureteral injury has been reported as high as 11%, underscoring the importance of performing intraoperative cystoscopy. If ureteral obstruction is suspected, the ipsilateral uterosacral stitches should be replaced or additional maneuvers, such as retrograde and stent, may be required. [p 1129]

39. **e. Prevention of recurrent incontinence after anterior suspension.** The aims of traditional posterior colporrhaphy for the repair of rectocele are to (1) plicate the prerectal and pararectal fascias in the midline, (2) narrow the posterior aspect of the levator hiatus with levator plication, and (3) repair the perineal body (perineorrhaphy). The repair effectively narrows the vaginal caliber. The perineorrhaphy closes the genital hiatus, elongates the vagina, and gives inferior support to the rectocele repair. However, there is no evidence that rectocele repair helps to support the anterior wall or to prevent recurrent incontinence after a suspension. [p 1130]

40. **c. Levator plication during the procedure.** Dyspareunia or apareunia has been reported in 21% to 50% of patients and is thought to be secondary to levator plication or excessive tightness of the introitus or vagina. [p 1131]

Chapter 31

Retropubic Suspension Surgery for Female Incontinence

George D. Webster • Michael L. Guralnick

Questions

1. Genuine stress urinary incontinence refers to:
   a. incontinence that is demonstrated at a clinical examination.
   b. incontinence secondary to a weak urethra.
   c. incontinence secondary to hypermobility of the urethral vesicle junction.
   d. incontinence that is demonstrated urodynamically.
   e. incontinence occurring in the absence of urgency symptoms.

2. All of the following may be indications for retropubic repair of stress incontinence except which scenario?
   a. A patient who needs a concomitant hysterectomy that cannot be performed vaginally
   b. A patient with chronic obstructive pulmonary disease and stress incontinence
   c. A patient with a lateral defect cystocele and genuine stress incontinence

d. A patient with type III stress incontinence
e. A patient with urethral descent with straining and stress incontinence

3. Retropubic suspension procedures act to:
   a. recreate the normal continence mechanism.
   b. restore the bladder neck and proximal urethra to a fixed retropubic position.
   c. provide a slinglike compression of the urethra during straining.
   d. correct a central defect cystocele that is an etiologic factor in incontinence.
   e. strengthen the external sphincter.

4. Which of the following statements is true regarding retropubic procedures for incontinence?
   a. It is important to avoid dissecting the old retropubic adhesions from prior incontinence procedures, as these may contribute to continence.
   b. Nonabsorbable sutures are better than absorbable sutures for retropubic suspension procedures.
   c. It may be necessary to open the bladder to facilitate identification of the bladder margins and bladder neck.
   d. A urethral Foley catheter is preferred for bladder drainage because it is more comfortable and associated with fewer urinary tract infections and earlier resumption of voiding.
   e. The retropubic space must be drained after the procedure to prevent bleeding.

5. Which of the following statements is true regarding the Marshall-Marchetti-Krantz (MMK) procedure?
   a. It is important to elevate the mid-urethra and external sphincter.
   b. One should try to incorporate full-thickness urethral wall with each suture to get secure fixation.
   c. The urethra is elevated to the iliopectineal ligament to maintain it in a fixed retropubic position.
   d. A better than 80% cure rate can be expected in the short term.
   e. Long-term results appear durable.

6. Which of the following is true of the Burch procedure?
   a. It is appropriate only for patients with adequate vaginal mobility and capacity.
   b. It requires extensive dissection of the proximal urethra to ensure adequate mobility.
   c. It is important to make sure that the vaginal wall is closely approximated to Cooper's ligament.
   d. Long-term results are disappointing.
   e. The repair is performed to the arcus tendineus fasciae pelvis bilaterally.

7. Laparoscopic retropubic urethropexy is advantageous because:
   a. it is technically simple to perform.
   b. it is associated with good long-term results.
   c. it is less costly to perform than standard procedures.
   d. it is associated with short hospitalization and recovery times.
   e. it provides access for repair of an associated central defect cystocele.

8. What is the most common complication after an MMK procedure?
   a. Bleeding
   b. Urinary retention
   c. Urinary tract infection
   d. Wound-related complications
   e. Pneumonia

9. All of the following are thought to cause postoperative voiding dysfunction except:
   a. bladder denervation.
   b. pre-existing detrusor dysfunction.
   c. overcorrection of the urethral axis.
   d. urethral fixation by sutures.
   e. detrusor sphincter dyssynergy.

10. Which of the following statements is true regarding urinary obstruction after retropubic suspension procedures?
    a. It does not occur after paravaginal repair.
    b. It is predicted by a preoperatively small, poorly compliant bladder.
    c. Women with postoperative voiding problems are easily identified by urodynamic studies.
    d. A history of voiding symptoms and new-onset irritative symptoms as well as a retropubically angulated urethra usually suggests obstruction.
    e. None of the above.

11. Which of the following statements is true regarding detrusor instability (DI) and anti-incontinence suspension procedures?
    a. Preoperative DI contraindicates a retropubic suspension because it increases the risk of postoperative DI.
    b. The Burch procedure is associated with a higher risk for postoperative DI than is a needle suspension.
    c. The management of postoperative DI consists of behavioral therapy and anticholinergic medication.
    d. Pre-existing DI rarely resolves after surgical correction of stress urinary incontinence in patients with mixed incontinence.
    e. New-onset DI after a suspension procedure performed for stress urinary incontinence invariably resolves within 3 months.

12. Obliteration of the cul-de-sac in retropubic suspension procedures is used to prevent what?
    a. Central defect cystocele
    b. Lateral defect cystocele
    c. Rectocele
    d. Enterocele
    e. Urethrocele

Answers

1. **c. incontinence secondary to hypermobility of the urethral vesicle junction.** Hypermobility of the bladder neck and proximal urethra results from weakening or loss of their supporting elements (ligaments, fasciae, and muscles), which in turn results from aging, hormonal changes, childbirth, and prior surgery. When this is the cause of incontinence, it is called anatomic or genuine stress incontinence. [p 1140]

2. **d. A patient with type III stress incontinence.** Several specific indications are suggested for a retropubic approach for the correction of anatomic stress incontinence, with the most obvious being a patient who requires concomitant abdominal surgery that cannot be performed vaginally. This may include hysterectomy, enterocele repair, or vaginal cuff suspension by sacral colpopexy when these, by their nature,

are deemed inappropriate for vaginal performance. Limited vaginal capacity and mobility, such as that following a prior vaginal incontinence procedure, has also been proposed as an indication for a retropubic approach. In the face of prior failed incontinence procedures, the existence of significant intrinsic sphincter deficiency must be suspected, even if hypermobility exists, and consideration given to performing a pubovaginal sling, although retropubic suspensions may be successful in this scenario as well. Furthermore, when true type III stress urinary incontinence exists (i.e., a fixed, nonfunctional proximal urethra), a retropubic suspension procedure is not indicated because there is no hypermobility to correct and the main problem is that of intrinsic sphincter deficiency, which is better served by a pubovaginal sling, collagen injections, or an artificial sphincter. [p 1141]

3. **b. restore the bladder neck and proximal urethra to a fixed retropubic position.** Retropubic procedures act to restore the bladder neck and proximal urethra to a fixed, retropubic position and are used when hypermobility is thought to be causative in the stress incontinence. [p 1140]

4. **c. It may be necessary to open the bladder to facilitate identification of the bladder margins and bladder neck.** If difficulty is encountered in the identification of the bladder neck, the bladder may be partially filled or even opened to identify its limits, and an assistant's examining finger in the vagina may help identify the vaginal wall. [pp 1141–1142]

5. **d. A better than 80% cure rate can be expected in the short term.** Short-term and medium-term results with the MMK have been good. Jarvis' meta-analysis of studies in the literature noted subjective continence in 88.2% (range 72% to 100%) of 2460 patients with 1 to 72 months of follow-up and objective continence in 89.6% (range 71% to 100%) of 384 patients with 3 to 12 months of follow-up. [p 1142]

6. **a. It is appropriate only for patients with adequate vaginal mobility and capacity.** The Burch retropubic colposuspension, which has undergone few modifications since its original description, is appropriate only if the patient has adequate vaginal mobility and capacity to allow the lateral vaginal fornices to be elevated toward and approximated to Cooper's ligament on either side. [pp 1142–1144]

7. **d. it is associated with short hospitalization and recovery times.** Proposed advantages of the laparoscopic approach include improved intraoperative visualization, less postoperative pain, shorter hospitalization, and quicker recovery times. [p 1146]

8. **d. Wound-related complications.** A review of the MMK literature (2712 patients) noted an overall complication rate of 21%, with wound complications and urinary infections accounting for the majority of complications (5.5% and 3.9%, respectively). Direct surgical injury to the urinary tract occurred in only 1.6% and genitourinary tract fistulas occurred in 0.3% overall. [p 1146]

9. **e. detrusor sphincter dyssynergy.** Postoperative voiding difficulty after any type of cystourethropexy is not uncommon and may arise because of pre-existing detrusor dysfunction, or perhaps because of denervation resulting from extensive perivesical dissection. In most cases, however, it is the result of overcorrection of the urethral axis owing to sutures' being inappropriately placed or excessively tightened. [pp 1146–1147]

10. **d. A history of voiding symptoms and new-onset irritative symptoms as well as a retropubically angulated urethra usually suggests obstruction.** Temporary voiding difficulty has been noted in up to 17% of patients after a paravaginal fascial repair, also termed the vagino-obturator shelf procedure, and chronic (more than 2 years) voiding difficulty has been noted in up to 11% of patients after the paravaginal repair. Women with postcystourethropexy voiding problems who have obstruction often do not exhibit the classic urodynamic features of obstruction. However, the history of postoperative voiding symptoms and associated new-onset bladder irritative symptoms, and a finding of a retropubically angulated and fixed urethra, generally indicate that obstruction does exist. [pp 1146–1147]

11. **c. The management of postoperative DI consists of behavioral therapy and anticholinergic medication.** For those patients in whom postoperative bladder instability symptoms persist, management should include anticholinergic therapy and behavioral modification. In intractable cases, surgical techniques including neuromodulation, augmentation cystoplasty, and detrusor myectomy may be indicated. [p 1147]

12. **d. Enterocele.** The Burch procedure, because of lateral vaginal elevation, may aggravate posterior vaginal wall weakness predisposing to enterocele. The incidence varies between 3% and 17%, and because of this, prophylactic obliteration of the cul-de-sac of Douglas is sometimes considered when retropubic suspensions are performed. [p 1147]

Chapter 32

Pubovaginal Slings

Edward J. McGuire • Quentin J. Clemens

Questions

1. Type III stress urinary incontinence is characterized by all of the following except:

   a. an open bladder neck at rest.
   b. a low abdominal leak point pressure.
   c. maximal urethral closure pressure (MUCP) less than 20 cm H_2O.
   d. severe incontinence.
   e. poor treatment response to bladder neck suspension procedures.

2. Which of the following conditions is not commonly associated with loss of proximal urethral closing function?
   a. Myelodysplasia
   b. Abdominoperineal resection
   c. Cervical spinal cord injury
   d. Radical hysterectomy
   e. Pelvic fracture

3. Which of the following is not an indication for a sling procedure?
   a. Postpartum stress incontinence associated with genital prolapse
   b. Stress incontinence associated with a urethral diverticulum
   c. Stress incontinence associated with poor urethral function on abdominal leak point pressure testing
   d. Recurrent stress incontinence after one or more prior procedures
   e. Type III stress incontinence associated with diminished bladder compliance

4. All of the following statements describe characteristics of diminished bladder compliance except which one?
   a. It may be diagnosed with a careful history and physical examination.
   b. It is associated with chronic bladder catheterization.
   c. It is evaluated by the cystometrogram, a sensitive and accurate test.
   d. It is frequently associated with type III stress incontinence.
   e. It should be treated before treatment of urethral dysfunction.

5. Which of the following does not affect the measurement of abdominal leak point pressure?
   a. Urethral hypermobility
   b. Bladder volume
   c. Diminished compliance
   d. Presence of a large cystocele
   e. Catheter size

6. Which of the following statements is false?
   a. A normal urethra will not leak when a Valsalva maneuver is used.
   b. Urethral pressure measurements correlate closely with abdominal leak point pressure recordings.
   c. Changes in abdominal leak point pressure correlate with symptomatic changes in incontinence severity.
   d. New urge incontinence occurs in 5% to 15% of patients after pubovaginal sling surgery.
   e. Among patients with urge incontinence symptoms preoperatively, urge incontinence persists in approximately 25% of patients after pubovaginal sling surgery.

7. With regard to bladder injury during pubovaginal sling surgery, which of the following statements is true?
   a. If a bladder injury occurs, a urethral catheter should be left in place for 14 to 21 days.
   b. Intravesical clamp passage can be avoided by passing the tip of the clamp in the pubic periosteum.
   c. Aggressive bladder mobilization with a finger may prevent bladder injury by releasing retropubic scar tissue.
   d. Most bladder injuries occur at the trigone.
   e. Large bladder injuries are best treated with catheter drainage because the injury is extraperitoneal.

8. A compressive, as opposed to a previously supportive, sling is most indicated in which of the following situations?
   a. MUCP = 60 cm H_2O, urethral hypermobility
   b. Valsalva leak point pressure (VLPP) > 90 cm H_2O, urethral hypermobility
   c. VLPP = 60 cm H_2O, positive Q-tip test
   d. High-grade vaginal prolapse with occult stress incontinence
   e. VLPP < 60 cm H_2O, minimal urethral mobility

9. Which of the following statements regarding autologous fascia lata for use as sling material is false?
   a. It is obtained from the iliotibial tract.
   b. Its use results in increased procedure duration.
   c. It provides greater tension per surface area.
   d. It requires repositioning of the patient after harvest.
   e. It is generally obtainable as large unscarred pieces of fascia.

10. Synthetic sling material, as opposed to autologous and allograft fascia, is associated with:
    a. a higher incidence of erosion and infection.
    b. a greater chance of disease transmission.
    c. lower cost.
    d. a greater ease of tension adjustment.
    e. superior performance over time.

Answers

1. **c. maximal urethral closure pressure (MUCP) less than 20 cm H_2O.** Type III stress incontinence, an expansion of Green's types I and II, refers to stress incontinence associated with little or no urethral mobility but an open nonfunctional proximal urethra. By video-urodynamic evaluation, type III stress incontinence is defined by an open bladder neck and proximal urethra at rest, or a urethra that leaks at a low abdominal pressure. An MUCP of less than 20 cm is generally accepted as indicative of intrinsic sphincter deficiency (ISD). [p 1152]

2. **c. Cervical spinal cord injury.** In addition to information suggesting that ISD and type III stress incontinence are conditions that may be resistant to standard operative procedures, there are other examples of loss of proximal urethral closing function in which severe, unremitting, abdominal pressure-driven incontinence occurs. By video-urodynamic studies, the appearance and function of the urethra in these conditions are similar, if not identical, to type III stress incontinence. Most myelodysplastic children and adults (85%) have a congenital neural condition associated with total lack of proximal urethral closing function. Occasionally, patients develop loss of proximal urethral function after abdominoperineal resection for rectal carcinoma, after radical hysterectomy for carcinoma of the cervix, after pelvic fracture, and in association with a spinal cord injury at a T12-L1 level. [pp 1152 and 1153]

3. **e. Type III stress incontinence associated with diminished bladder compliance.** Recurrent stress incontinence after one or more prior procedures, especially when the most recent procedure was a retropubic suspension, was the usual indica-

tion for slings before the description of the low-pressure or poorly functional urethra. Stress incontinence associated with a low-pressure urethra defined by urethral pressure profile testing, and poor urethral function defined by measuring the abdominal pressure required to drive urine across the urethra, are the currently accepted indications for a sling. There are additional indications for sling procedures, including stress incontinence in association with a urethral diverticulum or when that condition develops after repair of a urethral diverticulum. Some surgeons use slings for virtually any kind of stress incontinence. [pp 1153 and 1156]

4. **a. It may be diagnosed with a careful history and physical examination.** A low-compliance bladder refers to a bladder that abnormally gains pressure with volume increments. This creates a situation in which at some point vesical pressure and proximal urethral pressure become equal. At that point, type III stress incontinence exists, but the expulsive force is actually detrusor pressure and not abdominal pressure. A treatment that increases urethral resistance will have no effect on the leakage unless the driving force for the leakage, detrusor pressure, is also treated. Low-compliance bladders can develop as a late effect of radiation therapy, occasionally after certain kinds of chemotherapy, after prolonged chronic catheter drainage, and with obstructive uropathy (structural or neurogenic) and bladder decentralization syndromes, as for example those occasionally associated with radical pelvic extirpative surgery. A cystometrogram is a sensitive and accurate method to determine whether a low-compliance bladder is present. If identified, this condition must be treated before treatment of putative urethral dysfunction is undertaken. [pp 1156 and 1157]

5. **a. Urethral hypermobility.** Leak point pressures vary with subject position, catheter size, bladder volume, and subjective effort. Vaginal prolapse, for example, interferes with leak point pressure testing, apparently because the abdominal pressure is dissipated in the prolapse and this makes the urethra appear in better condition than it really is. In the absence of prolapse, leak point pressure testing can be valuable to establish at what pressure this occurs. Selection of patients whose urethral function is so poor as to be reparable only with a compressive operative procedure may not always require urodynamics, especially video-urodynamics, but the tests are quite useful in cases in which urethral failure is not so obvious and in cases in which low bladder compliance could be a problem. [pp 1156 and 1157]

6. **b. Urethral pressure measurements correlate closely with abdominal leak point pressure recordings.** How best to identify the condition of stress incontinence and ISD or the various types of urethral dysfunction within the broader diagnosis of stress incontinence remains controversial. Gynecologists tend to use urethral pressure profilometry, whereas urologists use leak point pressures. The two measurements do not correlate very well. [pp 1156 and 1157]

7. **b. Intravesical clamp passage can be avoided by passing the tip of the clamp in the pubic periosteum.** A Crawford clamp is placed from above through the defect in the transversalis fascia lateral to the rectus muscle. The tip of the clamp should be in contact with the pubis at all times to ensure that inadvertent bladder injury does not occur. If a prior bladder neck suspension has been performed, the bladder may be densely adherent to the lateral pelvic sidewall, and clamp passage must then be subperiosteal. If a bladder injury is suspected, cystoscopy is performed with a 70-degree lens. The clamp should be kept in place so that any injury will be obvious at cystoscopy. Bladder injuries occur near the dome of the bladder, at the 11-o'clock and 1-o'clock positions. In the event of a small bladder injury, the clamp is removed and passed again, extravesical passage is confirmed with cystoscopy, and the procedure is completed. Larger injuries must be formally repaired before the procedure can continue. [pp 1158 and 1159]

8. **e. VLPP < 60 cm H$_2$O, minimal urethral mobility.** The degree of sling tension that is required to achieve continence varies for different types of patients. Patients with urethral hypermobility and a reasonable degree of urethral function (VLPP > 90 cm H$_2$O) require slings that increase urethral support; these slings can be quite loose. Slings for patients with high-grade pelvic prolapse and occult stress incontinence also require no tension. For more severe ISD (VLPP < 90 cm H$_2$O) with periurethral and perivesical scarring, such as often occurs following a prior bladder neck suspension, a degree of tension on the sutures is required to prevent urethral mobility and attain continence. When urethral function is very poor (VLPP < 60 cm H$_2$O) and mobility is minimal, a compressive sling is required. [p 1159]

9. **c. It provides greater tension per surface area.** Fascia lata may be harvested for use as the sling material instead of rectus fascia. Use of this technique allows the surgeon to obtain a large piece of fascia that is not compromised by scarring from previous surgery. Furthermore, a smaller abdominal incision is performed for sling passage than that used for obtaining a rectus fascial strip. Disadvantages of this technique include the wider operative field, the potential morbidity of the lateral thigh incision, and the requirement for patient repositioning after fascial harvest. The graft is obtained from the iliotibial tract. [p 1160]

10. **a. a higher incidence of erosion and infection.** In an effort to decrease surgical morbidity and hospitalization time, various tissues have been used as a substitute for autologous fascia. To date, the most commonly used tissue has been allograft fascia lata. This fascia is procured by licensed tissue banks after donors are screened for sepsis, cancer, drug addiction, hepatitis, collagen vascular disease, rabies, Creutzfeldt-Jakob disease, and syphilis. With regard to surgical technique, the only difference between autograft and allograft sling placement is the use of a smaller midline suprapubic incision for the latter. The use of a smaller incision may also result in shorter operative time and less postoperative discomfort, although these benefits must be weighed against the increased cost of the allograft. Many synthetic material slings have been described in the literature. The surgical technique is essentially the same as that for cadaveric fascia lata slings except that synthetic material rather than donor tissue is used for the sling. These slings carry no risk of disease transmission but are more prone to erosion and infection. [pp 1160 and 1161]

Chapter 33

Injection Therapy for Urinary Incontinence

Rodney A. Appell

Questions

1. What urodynamics parameter is affected in the treatment by injectable materials?
   a. Q_{max}—maximal flow rate
   b. P_{abd}—abdominal leak point pressure
   c. P_{det}—voiding detrusor pressure
   d. P_{ur}—maximal urethral closure pressure
   e. All of the above

2. When are injectables most successful?
   a. When the patient has intrinsic sphincteric deficiency (ISD)
   b. When the patient has detrusor instability
   c. When the patient has hypersensitivity
   d. All of the above
   e. None of the above

3. What factor most influences the positive results of treatment with injectables?
   a. Bladder capacity
   b. Viability of tissue at the injection site
   c. Cause of the incontinence
   d. Volume of injectable agent used
   e. Leak point pressure

4. What is the correct site for injections for incontinence in men?
   a. Bulbous urethra
   b. Site is irrelevant
   c. Anastomotic line in post–radical prostatectomy patients
   d. Verumontanum in postresection patients
   e. Proximal to the external sphincter.

5. How is postoperative urinary retention best handled?
   a. Self-catheterization with a small catheter
   b. A Foley catheter for 24 hours
   c. Trochar cystotomy
   d. Acute urethral dilatation with sounds
   e. α-Blockers

6. What is the primary disadvantage to the use of injectables?
   a. Cost
   b. Allergic responses
   c. Need for reinjections
   d. Need for special equipment for injection
   e. Pain and bleeding immediately after the procedure

7. What is the most common complication from injection therapy?
   a. Transient urinary retention
   b. Irritative voiding symptoms
   c. Urinary tract infection
   d. Extravasation of injectable material
   e. Sepsis

8. What is the purpose of cross linking bovine collagen with glutaraldehyde (GAX)?
   a. To reduce the infection rate
   b. To prevent urethral inflammation
   c. To prevent extravasation of collagen
   d. To reduce the volume needed to gain urethrothelial coaptation
   e. To minimize immunoreactivity and increase resistance to collagenase

9. Suprapubic transvesical injections are routinely used in which of the following circumstances?
   a. In females who cannot tolerate local anesthesia for intraurethral injections
   b. In any male patient
   c. In males or females with bladder neck contracture
   d. In males with unsuccessful transurethral attempts or with scarred urethras
   e. In patients with mixed incontinence problems (ISD and detrusor instability)

10. The optimal bulking agent has to meet all of the following standards except:
    a. simple (easy) administration.
    b. no special equipment.
    c. no migration to other areas.
    d. easy quantification of material per patient per injection session.
    e. no degradation (must be inert).

11. The concept of implantable balloons for incontinence is less appealing than that of an injectable bulking agent for all of the following reasons except which one?
    a. They require more difficult placement.
    b. They do not allow adjustments over time.
    c. Implantation requires special equipment.
    d. Regional or general anesthesia is required for manipulation.
    e. Surgery is required for removal or replacement.

12. Results have been similar thus far for bulking agents with the exception of:
    a. silicone.
    b. polytetrafluoroethylene (PTFE; Teflon).
    c. autologous fat.
    d. GAX-collagen.
    e. zirconium-carbon beads.

13. In reviewing data for male patients who have been treated with injectable materials, a major difficulty in interpreting data has been:

    a. differentiating neurogenic disease patients from post-prostatectomy patients.
    b. determining the number of injections required to reach dryness.
    c. assessing the duration of dryness once it has been attained.
    d. differentiating post–radical prostatectomy patients from benign prostatic hyperplasia patients.
    e. conversion of patients from ISD as the cause of incontinence to overactive bladder problems.

14. One of the causes of failure to attain a good result initially in women is:

    a. instrumentation of the injected portion of the urethra.
    b. overinjection (too much injectable material).
    c. underinjection (too little injectable material).
    d. inexact placement of injectable material.
    e. urinary tract injection.

15. Which of the following materials has now been proved unsafe as an injectable agent?

    a. PTFE (Teflon)
    b. Silicone
    c. Zirconium-carbon beads
    d. All of the above
    e. None of the above

16. The disadvantage of periurethral injection over transurethral injection is:

    a. more bleeding.
    b. infection.
    c. longer learning curve.
    d. more extrusion of bulking material.
    e. sexual dysfunction.

Answers

1. **b. P_{abd}—abdominal leak point pressure.** One does not wish to increase resistance to P_{det} just to obviate stress incontinence produced by increases in P_{abd}. Injectable materials can be used successfully in patients because they dramatically improve the ability of the urethra to resist increases in P_{abd} without changing voiding pressure or the P_{det} at the time of leakage. [p 1172]

2. **a. When the patient has intrinsic sphincteric deficiency (ISD).** The ideal patient for the use of injectables is one with poor urethral function (ISD), normal bladder capacity and compliance, and good anatomic support. Contraindications to injectables include active urinary tract infection, untreated detrusor overactivity, and known hypersensitivity to the proposed injectable agent. [p 1173]

3. **b. Viability of tissue at the injection site.** Bladder neck contracture must be recognized and addressed before injectable therapy, and previous radiation therapy may limit the ability to do bulking without rupture of the urothelium, thus reducing the ability to coapt the walls of the urethra. [p 1173]

4. **e. Proximal to the external sphincter.** The needle must be positioned proximal to the external sphincter, as injection into the sphincter has been associated with sphincter spasm and failure. To be effective, any injectable material must be injected into the urethra superior to the external sphincter. [pp 1175 and 1176]

5. **a. Self-catheterization with a small catheter.** If urinary retention should occur, clean intermittent catheterization should be utilized with a small 10-Fr to 14-Fr catheter. [p 1177]

6. **c. Need for reinjections.** Long-term results (>5 years) for all of these injectable procedures are scarce in the literature, and patients having been so treated have been followed for only short periods. The data available also do not take into consideration the reinjection rates, which run as high as 22% with collagen at 2 years after dryness is attained. This factor ultimately affects the cost of this therapy. [pp 1182–1183]

7. **b. Irritative voiding symptoms.** Irritative voiding symptoms develop in 20% of patients after injection of PTFE. More recent reports describe surprisingly high rates of irritative voiding symptoms. Corcos and Fournier in 1999 demonstrated a 10% rate of de novo urgency and frequency, whereas Steele and colleagues in 2000 stated that 50% of patients developed some degree of de novo detrusor overactivity. [p 1181]

8. **e. To minimize immunoreactivity and increase resistance to collagenase.** Cross linking with GAX results in a fibrillar collagen with resistance to collagenase digestion and significantly enhances persistence with stabilization preventing syneresis. GAX-collagen is a highly purified 35% suspension of bovine collagen in a phosphate buffer containing at least 95% of type I collagen and 1% to 5% of type III collagen prepared by selective hydrolysis of the nonhelicoidal amino-terminal and carboxy-terminal segments (telopeptides) of the collagen molecules, which has the effect of decreasing the antigenicity and increasing the duration of the implant within the human body by increasing its resistance to collagenase. [pp 1173–1174]

9. **d. In males with failed transurethral attempts or with scarred urethras.** A newer method of injecting collagen in men by using a suprapubic antegrade approach is being employed. This approach has been described as using a flexible cystoscope placed through a suprapubic cystotomy. The antegrade approach has the advantage of direct visualization of the bladder neck and the injection of material into more supple, less scarred urethra. [p 1175]

10. **b. no special equipment.** The optimal substance has to be inert and nondegradable. It must encapsulate and remain where injected, and it must neither lose bulk nor gain it (syneresis). It must not be too viscous, so that it can be injected with standard cystoscopic equipment used for other purposes under local anesthesia in an outpatient setting to help keep the procedure safe and cost-effective. In addition, more accurate techniques for determining the quantity of material to inject in an individual must be developed to get the optimal result in a single treatment session. [p 1183]

11. **b. They do not allow adjustments over time.** Early experience with implantable microballoons (called Urovive) placed intraurethrally via a periurethral approach is encouraging; however, continued changes in the delivery device have de-

layed clinical trials in the United States. Another implantable balloon designed to have its volume adjusted once implanted via a completely periurethral approach (called ACT) is presently undergoing trials outside the United States. This balloon is placed completely outside the urethra at the level of the bladder neck and then filled through a port that remains accessible in the patient's labium, much like a pump mechanism from an artificial urinary sphincter. A disadvantage thus far has been the requirement for general or regional anesthesia for implantation. [p 1184]

12. **c. autologous fat.** Reports of studies with autologous fat have had less than impressive results. It appears that autologous fat undergoes a rapid rate of reabsorption because of its high water content. [pp 1179–1180]

13. **d. differentiating post–radical prostatectomy patients from benign prostatic hyperplasia patients.** On the male side, those patients with incontinence after prostatic resection for benign prostatic hyperplasia have often not been distinguished from those who have had a radical prostatectomy. For those with post–radical prostatectomy incontinence, it is often unclear which approach (retropubic or perineal) was employed. There has been very little in the way of objective reporting, with mostly subjective patient statements of cure, improvement, or failure. In addition, mixed techniques of injection and instrumentation are often intertwined. [p 1178]

14. **a. instrumentation of the injected portion of the urethra.** An effort should be made to avoid using instrumentation of the urethra and the risk of compressing the freshly placed implant by the endoscope. [p 1177]

15. **e. None of the above.** After injection of PTFE, the particles are noted to be found within lymphatics and blood vessels. Particles have also been found 1 year after injection in the pelvic lymph nodes, lungs, brain, kidneys, and spleen of animal models. [p 1182]

16. **c. longer learning curve.** There is a trade-off: the periurethral approach decreases bleeding complications, which hamper visualization and extrusion of the injected material, but is associated with a much longer learning curve than the transurethral approach. [p 1175]

Chapter 34

Implantation of the Artificial Genitourinary Sphincter

John J. Smith, III • David M. Barrett

Questions

1. The principle of delayed activation in artificial urinary sphincter implantation refers to:
    a. waiting for the device to cycle.
    b. the time it takes for the device to open.
    c. implantation of separate nonconnected components at one operation.
    d. postponement of the operation of the device for 6 to 8 weeks.
    e. the time it takes the device to close.

2. What is the most common cause of urinary retention in the immediate postoperative period?
    a. Edema
    b. Cuff erosion
    c. Change in bladder function
    d. Early activation
    e. Recurrent stricture

3. Where is the most common site of cuff placement in male patients with incontinence after prostatectomy?
    a. Anterior urethra
    b. Anastomosis
    c. Bulbous urethra
    d. Bladder neck
    e. None of the above

4. Why has the cuff erosion rate decreased since 1987?
    a. Routine deactivation at night
    b. Narrow-backed cuff design
    c. Delayed deactivation
    d. Less pressure in the reservoir
    e. Leaving the bulbocavernosus muscle intact

5. A 12-year-old boy with myelodysplasia underwent implantation of an artificial urinary sphincter 3 years ago. He now has recurrent incontinence. What is the next step in his work-up?
    a. Excretory urography to assess the components of the device and upper tracts
    b. Cystoscopy to rule out erosion
    c. Urodynamic evaluation to measure leak point pressure and assess functional bladder capacity
    d. MRI to rule out tethered cord
    e. Open surgery to replace the cuff

6. A female patient has an artificial urinary sphincter placed via the transvaginal route and after operation has continuous leakage after activation. She should be evaluated for:
    a. cuff erosion.
    b. mechanical failure of the device.
    c. vesicovaginal fistula.
    d. overflow incontinence.
    e. de novo urge incontinence.

7. Which of the following is(are) a definitive contraindication to implantation of an artificial urinary sphincter?
   a. Detrusor sphincter dyssynergia
   b. Low-volume detrusor hyperreflexia
   c. Unstable urethral stricture disease at the cuff site
   d. Future pregnancy
   e. a, b, and c

8. Recurrent incontinence develops 5 years after implantation of an artificial urinary sphincter in an adult male patient. Evaluation of the pump mechanism is normal, and urodynamic studies reveal no detrusor instability. What is the next step in making the diagnosis?
   a. Use of an ohmmeter to measure resistance
   b. Cystoscopy
   c. Exploration of the device, decision on cuff size, increase in balloon pressure, or use of a tandem cuff
   d. Augmentation cystoplasty
   e. Retrograde urethrography

9. Tenderness, swelling, and erythema develop around the pump 2 weeks after implantation of an artificial urinary sphincter. What is the next step?
   a. Cystoscopy
   b. Exploration and explantation
   c. Antibiotics
   d. Sitz bath
   e. Incision, drainage, and observation

10. When a penile prosthesis and an artificial urinary sphincter are placed simultaneously, which device should be placed first?
    a. Artificial urinary sphincter
    b. Penile prosthesis
    c. Foley catheter
    d. Hegar dilators
    e. Suprapubic tube

Answers

1. **d. postponement of the operation of the device for 6 to 8 weeks.** The device is tested and then deactivated for 6 to 8 weeks. This delayed activation ensures no undue tissue trauma during the healing phase. [p 1189]

2. **a. Edema.** An additional early complication is urinary retention. This predicament is nearly always the result of postoperative edema. [p 1192]

3. **c. Bulbous urethra.** In the male patient, the bulbous urethra is the most common site of implantation. Exposure is obtained through a midline perineal incision. [p 1189]

4. **b. Narrow-backed cuff design.** In 1987, American Medical Systems (Pfizer) introduced a narrow-backed cuff to improve the transmission of cuff pressure to the underlying tissue and decrease the possibility of erosion. [p 1188]

5. **c. Urodynamic evaluation to measure leak point pressure and assess functional bladder capacity.** In patients with neurogenic voiding dysfunction, urinary retention or overflow incontinence may represent a change in bladder function, which would necessitate a new urodynamic evaluation. [p 1192]

6. **c. vesicovaginal fistula.** The female patient with persistent incontinence should be evaluated to rule out vesicovaginal fistula. [p 1192]

7. **e. a, b, and c.** An artificial urinary sphincter is contraindicated in patients with poor bladder compliance, low-volume detrusor hyperreflexia, detrusor sphincter dyssynergia, and unstable recurrent urethral stricture or diverticular disease. [p 1188]

8. **c. Exploration of the device, decision on cuff size, increase in balloon pressure, or use of a tandem cuff.** If urodynamic evaluation confirms the lack of urethral resistance, treatment can be approached a number of ways. Balloon reservoir pressure can be increased to the next higher category. A reduction in size of the cuff can be accomplished, or a more proximal location can be used. Brito and associates as well as other investigators have advocated the use of tandem cuffs. [p 1192]

9. **b. Exploration and explantation.** Usually the first sign of infection is pain. Often this is noted by the patient in the region of the scrotal pump. Some surgeons have tried local drainage. In most instances, the periprosthetic infection requires the explant of all components of the sphincter mechanism. [p 1192]

10. **a. Artificial urinary sphincter.** For simultaneous procedures, the sphincter should be placed first. The components can be connected, tested, and deactivated before insertion of the penile prosthesis. [p 1191]

Chapter 35

Surgery for Vesicovaginal Fistula, Urethrovaginal Fistula, and Urethral Diverticulum

Roger Dmochowski

Questions

1. All of the following are important in the diagnostic considerations for vesicovaginal fistulas except:

    a. evaluation of the upper urinary tracts, including either a contrast study or sonography.
    b. biopsy of the fistula site in the patient who has previously been treated for pelvic malignancy.
    c. retrograde pyelography in the presence of a vesicovaginal fistula site close to the ureteral orifice on that side.
    d. diagnostic laparoscopy to evaluate the contiguous pelvic organs.
    e. instillation of intravesical dyes to facilitate identification of the fistula site.

2. Which of the following represents the best management technique for vesicovaginal fistulas?

    a. Prolonged urethral catheter drainage with oral anticholinergic paralysis of the bladder
    b. Cystoscopic electrofulguration of the fistula site followed by 2 weeks of catheter drainage
    c. Tension-free, nonoverlapping closure of vaginal and vesical components with viable interposition tissue
    d. Colpocleisis
    e. A modified Latzko technique with overlapping suture lines

3. Which of the following is true regarding the appropriate timing for fistula repair?

    a. A waiting period of 3 to 6 months is mandatory.
    b. Induration and fibrosis associated with excessive inflammatory response around the fistula site indicate fistula site maturity.
    c. Timing of the procedure should be individualized for each patient.
    d. The best time period for surgical management of fistulas is within the 7- to 14-day time frame.
    e. Fistulas identified in the immediate postoperative period (24 to 48 hours) should be observed for several weeks before surgical correction is attempted.

4. All of the following represent important considerations in the transvaginal surgical management of vesicovaginal fistulas except:

    a. lateral dissection away from the fistula tract to facilitate resection of the fistula site for ease of closure.
    b. advancement of the vaginal wall flap to avoid overlapping closure lines.
    c. circumscription of the fistula tract to facilitate oversewing.
    d. complete excision of the fistula tract, on both the vaginal and the bladder sides.
    e. relaxing incisions posteriorly to facilitate exposure to the fistula site.

5. The best interposition tissue to be used in any fistula closure is:

    a. omentum.
    b. fibrofatty labial fat pad.
    c. gracilis muscle.
    d. rectus abdominis.
    e. the local graft with best viability and mobility to the surgical area.

6. Postoperative management of vesicovaginal fistulas includes all of the following except:

    a. continuous urinary catheter drainage for 10 to 14 days.
    b. ingestion of anticholinergic agents for bladder paralysis until catheter removal.
    c. judicious use of antibiotics, including perioperative coverage.
    d. immediate reoperation if vaginal urinary drainage begins after removal of the drainage catheters.
    e. use of belladonna and opium suppositories in conjunction with oral anticholinergic agents.

7. An often unforeseen complicating factor in urethral and bladder neck reconstruction is:

    a. the indurated inner fibrotic nature of the periurethral tissues.
    b. stress incontinence.
    c. unappreciated bladder compliance and storage abnormalities.
    d. the need for routine use of interpositional tissues.
    e. uninterrupted catheter drainage.

8. The most important factor to consider when contemplating urethral reconstruction in the presence of a damaged urethra is:

    a. the amount of urethral loss and extension into the bladder neck.
    b. the equality of the labial tissues.
    c. the size of the paraurethral reconstruction flaps.
    d. the presence or absence of stress incontinence.
    e. the type of injury that produced the urethral loss.

9. The most important consideration in bladder neck closure is:

    a. the volume of bladder capacity.
    b. access to labial interposition tissue.

c. the size of the bladder neck defect.
d. the significance of incontinence.
e. complete circumferential dissection of the bladder neck to allow tension-free layered closure, best accomplished by disruption of the endopelvic fascia.

10. All of the following are associated with the clinical presentation of a urethral diverticulum except which one?
    a. The triad of dyspareunia, postvoid urinary dribbling, and dysuria
    b. A tender and fluctuant anterior vaginal wall mass located in the midline
    c. Recurrent urinary tract infections
    d. An asymptomatic patient
    e. A lateral anterior vaginal wall mass associated with hydronephrosis on the ipsilateral side seen on an intravenous urogram.

11. All of the following modalities may assist in the diagnosis of urethral diverticulum except which one?
    a. MRI of the periurethral tissues
    b. Transvaginal or endoluminal urethral ultrasonography
    c. Cystoscopy
    d. Voiding cystourethrography with or without the double-balloon technique
    e. Intravenous urography

12. In counseling the patient with a urethral diverticulum regarding the surgical outcomes, all of the following statements are true except which one?
    a. The patient will need uninterrupted urethral and suprapubic catheter drainage for 10 days to 2 weeks.
    b. A recurrent diverticulum may be identified postoperatively.
    c. A urethral stricture may result from overaggressive urethral closure.
    d. Urethral vaginal fistulas occurring postoperatively will always close with observation.
    e. The patient may still experience recurrent urinary tract infections.

13. Closure of a urethral diverticulum includes:
    a. dissection of the periurethral fascia on all cases.
    b. overlapping urethral and vaginal suture lines.
    c. tubular ligation of the diverticulum into the anterior vaginal wall.
    d. meticulous dissection of the periurethral fascia off the underlying diverticular sac followed by resection of the sac and closure of the periurethral fascia.
    e. mobilization of the diverticular cavity and incorporation into urethral closure.

Answers

1. **d. diagnostic laparoscopy to evaluate the contiguous pelvic organs.** Any diagnostic algorithm for lower genitourinary fistulas should include an assessment of ureteral integrity, either with intravenous urography or with retrograde pyelography. In the patient with a prior history of pelvic malignancy (cervical, uterine, vaginal), biopsy of the fistula tract is crucial in determining appropriate therapeutic approaches. [p 1197]

2. **c. Tension-free, nonoverlapping closure of vaginal and vesical components with viable interposition tissue.** All suture lines should be watertight, tension-free, and nonoverlapping and should exist in an uninfected environment. If the repair is tenuous, interpositional graft materials are indicated. [p 1200]

3. **c. Timing of the procedure should be individualized for each patient.** More recently, surgeons have advocated an individualized approach without an observational period. [p 1200]

4. **d. complete excision of the fistula tract, on both the vaginal and the bladder sides.** The flap is usually oriented anteriorly for fistulas located at the cuff; however, posterior flaps may also be used depending on the location of the fistula. The fistula tract is circumscribed but should not be widely excised. [p 1200]

5. **e. the local graft with best viability and mobility to the surgical area.** Reconstructive techniques have been described utilizing a variety of interpositional tissues including fibrofatty labial interposition tissues; anterior or posterior bladder flaps (autografts); myocutaneous flaps including rectus, sartorius, gluteus, and gracilis muscle; and combined myocutaneous flaps as adjuncts to repair of the complex vesicovaginal fistula. [p 1202]

6. **d. immediate reoperation if vaginal urinary drainage begins after removal of the drainage catheters.** Patient management after a vaginal, abdominal, or combined fistula repair approach is similar. Uninterrupted urinary drainage with large urethral and suprapubic catheters is crucial, as is bladder paralysis obtained either with oral or intrarectal anticholinergics, or both. Intravenous or oral antibiotics may be used as long as the urinary catheters are in place, but they must be used for the immediate perioperative period. Catheter drainage should be used for 10 to 14 days postoperatively before a voiding cystourethrogram to confirm fistula tract closure. Anticholinergics should be discontinued for approximately 24 to 48 hours before the voiding cystourethrography is performed. If the closure is confirmed and the patient is able to void once the urethral catheter is removed, then the suprapubic catheter may be subsequently removed. If spontaneous urinary loss persists, catheter drainage may be maintained for as long as 6 weeks as an adjunct to bladder decompression. [p 1203]

7. **c. unappreciated bladder compliance and storage abnormalities.** Evaluation of the bladder is important to exclude involvement of the bladder neck and/or trigone. Even in the presence of a seemingly normal trigone, a renal ultrasonographic study or intravenous pyelogram is a recommended screening examination to exclude occult upper tract abnormality. A voiding cystourethrogram obtained at the time of simultaneous cystometrography (video-urodynamics) in the standing position will identify concomitant vesicovaginal fistula involvement and the possibility of stress incontinence and/or compliance or detrusor instability abnormalities. [p 1204]

8. **a. the amount of urethral loss and extension into the bladder neck.** Complete reconstruction is necessary for large fistulas with extensive loss, including those that involve the bladder neck. The type of incontinence procedure necessitated will be indicated by the preoperative evaluation, although the pubovaginal sling represents potentially the best option, given the fact that this procedure both has beneficial

effects on urethral function (closure) and provides an interpositional tissue. [p 1204]

9. **e. complete circumferential dissection of the bladder neck to allow tension-free layered closure, best accomplished by disruption of the endopelvic fascia.** Bladder neck closure should accomplish a tension-free circumferential closure of the remnant urethra at the bladder neck by compete disruption of the endopelvic fascia at the bladder neck, and layered inverting closure of the urethral stump. [p 1206]

10. **e. a lateral anterior vaginal wall mass associated with hydronephrosis on the ipsilateral side seen on an intravenous urogram.** Careful physical examination will, according to Davis, often reveal the diagnosis in up to 63% of the cases. An anterior vaginal wall mass or fullness is often identified and compression of this may result in discharge of purulence or blood from the urethra. There may also be tenderness only on direct palpation of the urethra. The differential diagnosis of anterior vaginal wall masses includes ureterocele, Gärtner's duct cyst, müllerian remnant cysts, vaginal wall inclusion cysts, and urethral vaginal neoplasm. [pp 1208–1209]

11. **e. Intravenous urography.** Upper urinary tract evaluation should be performed if there is concern regarding the presence of an ectopic ureterocele. Any nonmidline anterior vaginal wall mass should be evaluated as possibly representing an ectopic ureterocele, and this entity should be diligently excluded with contrast delineation of the lower ureter in question. [p 1209]

12. **d. Urethral vaginal fistulas occurring postoperatively will always close with observation.** As with all vaginal surgery, counseling should include the risk of infection, bleeding, recurrent diverticulum, fistula, urinary incontinence, and urethral stenosis from overzealous resection of diverticulum. [p 1212]

13. **d. meticulous dissection of the periurethral fascia off the underlying diverticular sac followed by resection of the sac and closure of the periurethral fascia.** Once excision is complete, vertical urethral mucosal closure is carried out in a running, locking manner with a 4-0 polyglycolic acid suture. Care should be taken to avoid excessive tension on the urethral wall during closure to avoid compromise of the integrity of the urethral lumen with resultant stricture or fistula formation risk. A second-layer closure of the urethral wall is also attempted using similar suture. The periurethral fascia is then closed with a running transverse 3-0 polyglycolic acid suture as a second layer. Any dead space should be obliterated and meticulous hemostasis obtained. [p 1212]

Chapter 36

Geriatric Incontinence and Voiding Dysfunction

Neil M. Resnick • Subbarao V. Yalla

Questions

1. In people older than 65 years of age, what is the prevalence of urinary incontinence?

   a. 1% to 10%
   b. 15% to 30%
   c. 35% to 50%
   d. 55% to 75%
   e. 75% to 100%

2. In demented elderly patients, incontinence:

   a. is inevitable.
   b. is virtually always due to detrusor hyperreflexia.
   c. is unlikely to respond to therapy.
   d. is multifactorial and often reversible.
   e. treatment should focus primarily on preventing skin breakdown.

3. Urinary incontinence in older people is usually:

   a. brought to a physician's attention by the patient.
   b. detected by the patient's primary physician.
   c. obvious to the urologist.
   d. detected by the physician but ignored.
   e. unknown to any physician.

4. In older patients, uninhibited bladder contractions:

   a. are rarely seen in asymptomatic patients.
   b. are primarily due to a central nervous system pathologic lesion.
   c. are almost always the cause of the patient's incontinence.
   d. are inevitable with dementia.
   e. may not be the cause of the incontinence.

5. After the history and physical examination, evaluation of the incontinent older patient should include which of the following?

   a. Cystoscopy
   b. Video-urodynamics
   c. Postvoid residual (PVR) assessment
   d. Urinary cytology
   e. Assessment of prostate size in a male

6. Which of the following occurs as part of normal aging?

   a. Urinary incontinence
   b. A small increase in serum creatinine concentration
   c. Uninhibited detrusor contractions
   d. Increase in bladder capacity
   e. No change in urinary flow rate

7. What is the cornerstone of treatment for persistent urge incontinence?

a. Behavioral therapy
   b. Flavoxate
   c. Oxybutynin
   d. Tolterodine
   e. Imipramine

8. Acute urinary retention in an older man:

   a. indicates the need for surgical decompression.
   b. is treated effectively with α-adrenergic blockers.
   c. can be seen with detrusor hyperactivity with impaired contractility.
   d. is treated effectively with bethanechol.
   e. always requires treatment of the underlying urinary tract abnormality.

9. Incontinence management products (e.g., garments and pads):

   a. are reimbursed by insurance companies.
   b. should include menstrual pads.
   c. generally cost less than $1 per day.
   d. should be chosen according to the type of incontinence rather than its severity.
   e. should be tailored to the individual.

10. The voiding diary completed by an 83-year-old woman bothered by daytime incontinence discloses 800 ml of output between 8 AM and 11 PM, and 1500 ml from 11 PM to 8 AM. What should the next step be?

    a. Have her repeat the diary with a record of fluid intake.
    b. Prescribe furosemide at 7 PM to reduce nocturnal excretion.
    c. Have her use pressure gradient stockings to minimize peripheral edema.
    d. All of the above
    e. None of the above

11. Cystometry in a 78-year-old man reveals detrusor overactivity. If behavioral methods fail, the next step is to prescribe a bladder relaxant (true or false).

12. Anticholinergic agents should always be discontinued or substituted in an older patient with incontinence (true or false).

Answers

1. **b. 15% to 30%.** Although its prevalence increases with age, incontinence is abnormal at any age. Even among residents of nursing homes, where the average age is 85 years and dementia and immobility affect more than half of residents, incontinence prevalence is 40% to 60%. More impressive is the fact that incontinence affects only slightly more than 50% of the most severely demented nursing home residents, provided that they can transfer themselves from a bed to a chair and do not have other contributing factors. Even if they do, many of the factors fall into the category of transient incontinence and are reversible. Thus, incontinence is never the norm, no matter how old or frail the individual. [p 1218]

2. **d. is multifactorial and often reversible.** Incontinence is never normal, even in a patient with dementia. Detrusor overactivity (DO) is the most common type of lower urinary tract dysfunction among demented incontinent nursing home residents, but it is also the most common dysfunction among their continent peers. Moreover, incontinence in 40% of these individuals is not associated with DO but with obstruction (in men), stress incontinence (in women), or a combination of an outlet and a detrusor problem, and the cause does not correlate with either the presence or the severity of dementia. Thus, it is no longer tenable to attribute incontinence a priori to DO. Because incontinence in the elderly is usually multifactorial, involving urinary tract as well as non–urinary tract contributions, it is often treatable. Even among nursing home patients, studies have documented more than a 50% reduction in incontinent episodes overall and full daytime continence in nearly 40% of residents. Particularly among demented individuals, nonurinary factors are prevalent and commonly include medication use, depression, fecal impaction, urinary tract infection, atrophic vaginitis, and disorders of fluid excretion. It is important to prevent skin breakdown, but this should not be the primary approach to the incontinent nursing home resident. [pp 1219, 1222, 1223, and 1228]

3. **e. unknown to any physician.** Despite the fact that incontinence is so common and amenable to therapy, most patients do not mention it to a physician. Reasons include embarrassment, misperception that it is a normal part of aging, belief that it is untreatable, fear of complications associated with its evaluation and treatment, or misconception that only major surgery can cure it. Moreover, when patients do mention it, most physicians either dismiss it as a normal part of aging or merely check a urinalysis. With newer undergarments and pads that better absorb and deodorize, physicians may be unaware of the problem unless they ask about it. [p 1218]

4. **e. may not be the cause of the incontinence.** It is important to realize that involuntary bladder contractions are commonly found in even continent, neurologically intact elderly people; the prevalence ranges in various studies between 5% and 50%. This fact underscores the concept that such contractions are a risk factor for urinary incontinence but not necessarily sufficient to cause it. Moreover, even when such contractions are the major contributor to urinary incontinence, they may be due to a urethral abnormality. More than half of individuals with obstruction and approximately 25% of those with stress incontinence have associated DO that usually remits with correction of the urethral abnormality alone. The proportion of elderly individuals in whom DO remits is likely lower, but clearly it is insufficient merely to identify involuntary contractions on cystometry and attribute the incontinence to them. To be considered the cause of the urinary incontinence, such contractions must reproduce the patient's type of leakage and urethral abnormalities must be excluded. This is particularly important because a bladder relaxant medication prescribed for DO that is actually due to obstruction may precipitate acute retention. [pp 1219–1222]

5. **c. Postvoid residual (PVR) assessment.** Determining the PVR is essential in all incontinent older individuals, not only because retention can mimic other causes of urinary incontinence, but also because knowledge of the PVR will affect therapy. For instance, an older woman with DO and PVR of 200 ml would be treated differently from a woman

with DO and PVR of 5 ml. The rest of the diagnostic evaluation depends on the need for diagnostic certainty. In many older adults, the empirical approach outlined in the chapter will be appropriate. However, if surgical correction is contemplated, or if the risk of empirical therapy exceeds the benefit, further testing is warranted. Cytology is indicated when bladder carcinoma is suspected and would be treated if found (i.e., not in a bedfast, demented patient). Cystoscopy has many indications, but it is not routinely required for evaluation of incontinence, nor is it alone sufficient to detect or exclude prostatic obstruction. Palpated prostate size correlates poorly with the presence of obstruction. [pp 1225–1226]

6. **c. Uninhibited detrusor contractions.** Incontinence is never part of normal aging; even at 90 years of age, at least half of people are continent. Although renal function declines in most older adults, there is no change in serum creatinine value, owing to a balanced and concomitant decrease in muscle mass. Involuntary detrusor contractions are quite common in continent and even asymptomatic elderly people but are rarely seen during routine cystometry in younger people. Bladder capacity may decrease in the elderly, but there is no evidence for an increase. Flow rate declines, not only because obstruction becomes more likely in aging men but also because contractility appears to decrease in both sexes. [pp 1218–1219]

7. **a. Behavioral therapy.** Behavioral therapy is the cornerstone of treatment for DO, although the type of therapy must be tailored to the individual. Bladder retraining attempts to restore a normal voiding pattern by progressively lengthening the voiding interval. Scheduled toileting aims to reduce incontinence by frequent voiding, which reduces total bladder volume and the chance of triggering involuntary bladder contractions. Prompted voiding works by regularly and frequently reminding cognitively impaired residents of the need to void. The role of medications is to supplement behavioral therapy, but only if needed. By reducing bladder irritability, such agents allow the bladder to hold more urine before spasming. Even when continence is restored by these drugs, however, DO is still generally demonstrable. Furthermore, if the drug increases residual urine more than total bladder capacity, it may paradoxically decrease functional capacity, allowing the persistent involuntary contraction to occur at more frequent intervals. Thus, before it is decided that drug therapy has failed, PVR should be remeasured. Except for flavoxate, each of the agents listed has been proved effective in randomized controlled trials that included substantially or even solely elderly people. [p 1228]

8. **c. can be seen with detrusor hyperactivity with impaired contractility.** The differential diagnosis for urinary retention goes beyond urethral obstruction, particularly in the elderly. Patients with underactive detrusor or detrusor hyperactivity with impaired contractility may also develop urinary retention. In addition, fecal impaction, pain (e.g., after hip replacement), and medications with urinary tract side effects (e.g., anticholinergics, sedating antihistamines, decongestants, opiates) may induce acute urinary retention, particularly in patients with underlying bladder weakness or obstruction. Thus, the bladder should be decompressed for at least a week while reversible causes are addressed. Decompression allows some restoration of detrusor strength, which also facilitates urodynamic testing should it be necessary. α-Adrenergic blockers are effective for men with symptoms of prostatism, but clinical trials excluded patients with significant urinary retention. Bethanechol, although designed to improve bladder emptying in patients without obstruction, has not proved effective for this purpose. Decompression in some elderly patients can reduce but not eliminate residual urine; provided that it does not cause symptoms or renal compromise, subclinical retention need not necessarily be treated in all elderly patients, even if obstruction is present. [pp 1219–1222 and 1231]

9. **e. should be tailored to the individual.** The cost of pads is rarely covered by insurance and can easily exceed $1 per day. Menstrual pads, although often employed for incontinence, are usually inappropriate. They are designed to absorb small amounts of slowly leaking viscous fluid rather than rapid gushes of urine. From among the numerous types of pads and garments, selection should be tailored to the individual's needs and comorbidity; the type of incontinence matters less than the severity. [p 1229]

10. **e. None of the above.** The patient's altered pattern of fluid excretion may occur for a variety of reasons. The most common one is accumulation of peripheral edema due to venous insufficiency, peripheral vascular disease, low albumin states (malnutrition, hepatic disease), drugs (e.g., nonsteroidal anti-inflammatory drugs, dihydropyridine calcium channel blockers [e.g., nifedipine], or thiazolidinediones [e.g., rosiglitazone]), or congestive heart failure. Each can be readily addressed. Before doing so, however, it is important to realize that the multiple pathologic conditions so often found in the elderly may be causal, contributory, consequential, or unrelated to the condition for which the patient seeks help. In this individual, daytime leakage is the problem. Addressing the excess nocturnal excretion will not improve the daytime problem and, if it shifts the excess nocturnal excretion to the daytime (e.g., by use of pressure gradient stockings), it may actually exacerbate the daytime leakage. Thus, in this situation, the nocturnal overexcretion should not be treated. Daytime predominance of incontinence suggests that the patient has stress incontinence, or DO associated with bladder neck incompetence that is exacerbated when she is upright. Once the cause is sorted out, the appropriate intervention can be prescribed, but in this individual it should not include alteration of fluid intake or excretion. This case highlights the need to tailor the evaluation and treatment to the individual patient. [p 1225]

11. **False.** Cystometry provides information on the bladder only, not the outlet, and only during filling, not voiding. Thus, it is insufficient to adequately characterize urinary tract dysfunction. Rather than the primary cause of this patient's leakage, the detected DO may be incidental to aging and unrelated to his incontinence; in this instance, bladder relaxants will only lead to side effects. Alternatively, DO may be due to bladder neck incompetence following prostatic resection, or to urethral obstruction; a relaxant will likely exacerbate both. Further historical information is necessary, as is characterization of urethral function. Often, simply addressing issues outside the urinary tract—such as cognition, mobility, depression, manual dexterity, or fluid excretion and toileting—is sufficient to restore continence in an older adult. Such an approach is beneficial for other reasons: it avoids medication side effects and cost (drugs are often not covered by insurance), and it improves many of the patient's other symptoms and quality of life. [pp 1219–1222 and 1228]

12. **False.** Although anticholinergic agents can cause urinary incontinence, they do so by well-known mechanisms. In the absence of urinary retention, excess fluid intake engendered by xerostomia, or confusion, they should not be impugned as the cause of the leakage, and the search for a cause should continue. [pp 1220–1221]

SECTION VI

BENIGN PROSTATIC HYPERPLASIA

Chapter 37

The Molecular Biology, Endocrinology, and Physiology of the Prostate Gland and Seminal Vesicles

Alan W. Partin • Ronald Rodriguez

Questions

1. Which of the following is not considered a sex accessory tissue?

   a. Prostate gland
   b. Seminal vesicles
   c. Tunica albuginea
   d. Ampullae
   e. Bulbourethral gland

2. Which of the following biologic substances does not appear in the seminal plasma?

   a. Tyrosine kinase
   b. Fructose
   c. Citric acid
   d. Spermine
   e. Prostaglandins

3. Which fetal hormone stimulates the development of the wolffian ducts?

   a. Estradiol
   b. Dihydrotestosterone (DHT)
   c. Estrone
   d. Testosterone
   e. Inhibin

4. Which fetal hormone stimulates the growth of the prostate during development?

   a. Estradiol
   b. DHT
   c. Estrone
   d. Testosterone
   e. Inhibin

5. Which biologic substance is responsible for regression of the müllerian ductal system?

   a. Insulin
   b. Glucagon
   c. Cholesterol
   d. Müllerian-inhibiting substance
   e. Müllerian inhibition substance

6. At what point in neonatal development (time) does the neonatal surge of testosterone occur?

   a. 1 week
   b. 6 months
   c. 2 months
   d. 5 months
   e. 8 months

7. Which of the following is true regarding neuroendocrine cells found within the prostate?

   a. The major secretory product is somatostatin.
   b. A minor component of the secretory products is serotonin.
   c. Another name for neuroendocrine cells is AFUD.
   d. A major secretory product of the neuroendocrine cells is thyroid-stimulating hormone (TSH).
   e. Insulin is the major stimulator of secretion in the neuroendocrine cell system within the prostate.

8. Which α_1-adrenergic receptor subtype is linked to smooth muscle contraction in the prostate?

   a. α_{1d}
   b. α_{1a}
   c. α_{1b}
   d. α_2
   e. α_{2b}

9. Which of the following is true regarding testosterone?

   a. Testosterone is synthesized by the Sertoli cells of the testes.
   b. Testosterone is synthesized by the Leydig cells of the testes.
   c. Testosterone is a direct precursor of pregnenolone.
   d. 5α-Reductase is an enzyme that converts DHT into testosterone.
   e. Aromatase converts estrogens into testosterone.

10. The role of prolactin within the prostate is thought to:

    a. enhance the synthesis of fructose.
    b. enhance the uptake of androgens into the prostate through an effect on the synthesis of citric acid.
    c. enhance the conversion of testosterone to DHT.

d. enhance the conversion of estrogen to DHT.
e. stimulate secretion of the neuroendocrine cells through its effect on somatostatin.

11. The normal concentration of DHT in the plasma of normal males is:

    a. 100 ng/100 ml.
    b. 300 ng/100 ml.
    c. 400 ng/100 ml.
    d. 50 ng/100 ml.
    e. 20 ng/100 ml.

12. Dehydroepiandrosterone has been suggested as a major source of testosterone within the plasma. What percentage of total testosterone has been determined to be derived from dehydroepiandrosterone?

    a. 1%
    b. 2%
    c. 5%
    d. 15%
    e. 20%

13. To what is the majority of testosterone found in the plasma bound?

    a. Insulin
    b. Cholesterol
    c. Prostaglandins
    d. p53
    e. Testosterone-estradiol–binding globulin (TeBG)

14. Which of the following is not a well-recognized type of growth control regulating the prostate?

    a. Endocrine factors
    b. Neuroendocrine factors
    c. Anabolic factors
    d. Autocrine factors
    e. Extracellular matrix factors

15. Which of the following is true regarding androgen receptor intracellular event?

    a. DHT or testosterone binding to specific nucleotide receptors in the cytoplasm
    b. Dimerization and activation of the steroid receptor
    c. Endocytosis of native androgen
    d. Transport of the active receptor and androgen from the nucleus to the cell membrane
    e. Release of coactivators from the androgen receptor elements

16. How many isoenzymes of 5α-reductase exist?

    a. 1
    b. 4
    c. 2
    d. 7
    e. 3

17. Which 5α-reductase isoenzyme predominates in the prostate gland?

    a. Type I
    b. Type II
    c. Type III
    d. Type IV
    e. Type V

18. Which hormone has been determined to cause squamous cell metaplasia in prostatic growth?

    a. Androgen
    b. Insulin
    c. TSH
    d. Estrogen
    e. Inhibin

19. Which growth factor has been determined to play the most important role in maintaining the structure and functional integrity of prostatic growth?

    a. Fibroblast growth factor (FGF)
    b. Transforming growth factor (TGF)-β
    c. Epidermal growth factor (EGF)
    d. FGF-7
    e. FGF-1

20. Which biologic peptide has a profound effect on regulating the muscular tone of the prostate as well as constriction of blood vessels and elevation of blood pressure?

    a. Acetylcholine
    b. Epinephrine
    c. Insulin
    d. Endothelin
    e. Fructose

21. What percentage of the prostatic epithelial cells are lost after castration?

    a. 90%
    b. 50%
    c. 10%
    d. 3%
    e. 1%

22. The expression of which protein is thought to be induced after castration within the prostate and is directly associated with epithelial cell involution?

    a. p53
    b. PTEN
    c. TURP-7
    d. trpm-2
    e. PROS-1

23. What is the average volume of the normal human ejaculate?

    a. 7 ml
    b. 2 ml
    c. 20 ml
    d. 300 ml
    e. 3 ml

24. What proportion of the total human ejaculate comes from the prostate?

    a. 1/2
    b. 1/6
    c. 1/4
    d. 1/8
    e. 1/16

25. Seminal plasma has unusually high concentrations of all of the following except:

    a. citric acid.
    b. insulin.
    c. fructose.
    d. spermine.
    e. prostaglandins.

26. What is the source of fructose in human seminal plasma?

    a. Prostate gland
    b. Bulbourethral gland
    c. Vas deferens
    d. Seminal vesicles
    e. Tissue thromboplastin

27. All of the following are secretory products of the prostate except which one?

a. hK17
b. hK3
c. KLK-L1
d. prostatic acid phosphatase (PAP)
e. PSP-94

28. Which statement is false regarding prostate-specific antigen (PSA)?

a. PSA is a glycoprotein.
b. PSA is a chymotrypsin-like protease.
c. PSA's molecular weight is approximately 33,000.
d. Approximately 7% of the molecule consists of carbohydrates.
e. PSA is found exclusively within the epithelial cells of the prostate gland.

Answers

1. **c. Tunica albuginea.** Sex accessory tissues include the prostate gland, seminal vesicles, ampullae, and bulbourethral glands, and they are believed to play a major, but unknown, role in the reproductive process. [p 1238]

2. **a. Tyrosine kinase.** In the human, the sex accessory tissues produce extremely high concentrations of many important and potent biologic substances that appear in the seminal plasma, such as fructose (2 mg/ml), citric acid (4 mg/ml), spermine (3 mg/ml), and prostaglandins (200 μg/ml); extremely high concentrations of zinc (150 μg/ml); proteins (40 mg/ml); and specific proteins such as immunoglobulins, proteases, esterases, and phosphatases. [p 1238]

3. **d. Testosterone.** The wolffian ducts develop into the seminal vesicles, epididymis, vas deferens, ampulla, and ejaculatory duct, and the developmental growth of this group of glands is stimulated by fetal testosterone and not DHT. [p 1238]

4. **b. DHT.** In contrast, the prostate first appears and starts its development from the urogenital sinus during the third month of fetal growth, and development is directed primarily by DHT, not testosterone. [p 1238]

5. **d. Müllerian-inhibiting substance.** Growth factors will be discussed later, but it is important to note that the müllerian-inhibiting substance, which is expressed early in gonadal differentiation in the male, causes the regression of the müllerian duct as a prerequisite for virilization in the male. [p 1239]

6. **c. 2 months.** In the human male, neonatal surges in testosterone are observed to peak between 2 and 3 months of age. During this period, serum testosterone levels rise to 60 times that of normal prepubertal levels and often reach the adult serum testosterone range of about 400 ng/dl. [p 1240]

7. **d. A major secretory product of the neuroendocrine cells is thyroid-stimulating hormone (TSH).** There are three types of prostate neuroendocrine cells, with the major type containing both serotonin and TSH. The two minor cell types contain calcitonin and somatostatin. Neuroendocrine cells are also termed APUD, for amine precursor uptake decarboxylase cells, and bring about their regulatory activity by the secretion of hormonal polypeptides or biogenic amines such as serotonin (5-hydroxytryptamine), which is a common marker for these cells. [p 1242]

8. **b. α_{1a}** Research work has demonstrated three subtypes of the α_1-adrenergic receptor (α_{1a}, α_{1b}, and α_{1d}), of which the α_{1a} receptor appears to be linked to contraction. [p 1242]

9. **b. Testosterone is synthesized by the Leydig cells of the testes.** Foremost among the hormones and growth factors that stimulate the prostate is the prohormone testosterone, which must be converted within the prostate into the active androgen DHT. Testosterone is synthesized in the Leydig cells of the testes from pregnenolone by a series of reversible reactions; however, once testosterone is reduced by 5α-reductase into DHT or to estrogens by aromatase, the process is irreversible. In other words, whereas testosterone can be converted into DHT and into estrogens, estrogens and DHT cannot be converted into testosterone. [p 1245]

10. **b. enhance the uptake of androgens into the prostate through an effect on the synthesis of citric acid.** Prolactin is believed to enhance the uptake of androgens into the prostate and to affect the synthesis of citric acid. [p 1246]

11. **d. 50 ng/100 ml.** The concentration of DHT in the plasma of normal men is very low, 56 + 20 ng/100 ml, in comparison to testosterone. [pp 1247–1248]

12. **a. 1%.** Less than 1% of the total testosterone in the plasma is derived from dehydroepiandrosterone. [p 1248]

13. **e. testosterone-estradiol–binding globulin (TeBG).** The majority of testosterone bound to plasma protein is associated with TeBG. [p 1249]

14. **c. Anabolic factors.** These interactive types of growth control are usually accomplished by several generalized systems, as depicted in the schematic in Figure 37–5, and include (1) endocrine factors or long-range signals arriving at the prostate by serum transport of hormone originating from the secretions of distant organs (this would include serum hormone-like steroids such as testosterone, estrogens, and serum endocrine polypeptide hormones such as prolactin and gonadotropins); (2) neuroendocrine signals originating from neural stimulation such as 5-hydroxytryptamine, acetylcholine, and norepinephrine; (3) paracrine factors or soluble tissue growth factors that stimulate or inhibit growth and are elaborated over short ranges between neighboring cells within the prostate tissue compartment such as β-fibroblast growth factor and epidermal growth factor; (4) autocrine factors or growth factors such as autocrine motility factor, produced and released by a cell and then fed back on the same cell's external membrane receptors to regulate its own growth or function; (5) intracrine factors, factors that share structural and regulatory features with autocrine factors but that work inside the cell; (6) extracellular matrix factors, insoluble tissue matrix systems that make direct and coupled contact by being attached through integrins and adhesion molecules of the basal membrane to couple cytoskeleton organization with the extracellular matrix components that include the glycosaminoglycans such as heparin sulfate; and (7) cell-cell interactions. [p 1250]

15. **b. dimerization and activation of the steroid receptor.** A simplified schematic of the temporal sequence of intracellular events is depicted in Figures 37–9 and 37–10 and includes (1) cellular uptake of testosterone; (2) testosterone converted to DHT by metabolism of 5α-reductase; (3) DHT or testosterone binding to specific androgen receptors in the cytoplasm; (4) dimerization and activation of the steroid receptor by a variety of post-translational steps including, for instance, phosphorylation; (5) active nuclear transportation of the activated androgen receptor in an ATP-dependent man-

ner; (6) chromatin remodeling via interaction with coregulatory molecules; (7) transactivation or transrepression, via interactions with other coactivators or corepressors, in a histone acetyl transferase-dependent process; (8) binding of the activated receptor/coactivator complex to androgen receptor elements that are short, specific sequences of DNA recognized by androgen receptor dimers; (9) gene regulation, in which the receptor acts as a transcription factor and, when bound to the DNA and matrix in proximity to androgen target genes, increases the RNA polymerase (Pol II) transcription of the DNA into messenger RNA. [p 1250]

16. **c. 2.** In the human, rat, and monkey, there are two isozymes of 5α-reductase. [p 1252]

17. **b. Type II.** The type II enzyme is mutated in 5α-reductase deficiency and is the dominant isoform present in the prostate gland. [pp 1252–1253]

18. **d. Estrogen.** Estrogens can cause a florid squamous cell metaplasia in prostatic growth that can be offset by androgens. [p 1254]

19. **c. Epidermal growth factor (EGF).** A comparison of EGF and TGF-α concluded that EGF appears to be the predominant EGF-related growth factor in both normal prostate and benign prostatic hyperplasia (BPH). It is believed that these two growth factors are important for maintaining the structural and functional integrity of BPH. [p 1269]

20. **d. Endothelin.** There has been increased interest in the biologic properties of the peptide endothelins, of which there are three kinds: endothelin-1, -2, and -3. The most potent activity of these peptides is in constricting blood vessels and elevating blood pressure in mammals, and they may have profound effects on the muscular tone of the prostate as well as its growth. [p 1271]

21. **a. 90%.** Castration causes a 90% loss in the total number of prostatic epithelial cells and a slower, but less complete, reduction of approximately 40% in the number of stromal cells. [p 1272]

22. **d. trpm-2.** It has been reported that a temporal series of proteins is induced in the prostate gland after castration, and the most actively studied was trpm-2, in the work of Tenniswood and colleagues. This was followed by the cloning of the gene. This trpm-2 protein was dramatically increased 48 hours after castration and was associated with epithelial cell involution in the prostate gland. The trpm-2 protein now appears to be a secondary marker associated with, but not causing, involution. This protein has been shown to be similar to clusterin, a sulfated glycoprotein-2 normally found in Sertoli cells and present in human seminal plasma, and is suggested to be important in fertility. [p 1275]

23. **e. 3 ml.** The average volume of the normal human ejaculate is approximately 3 ml, ranging from 2 to 6 ml, and it has two components, spermatozoa and seminal plasma. [p 1276]

24. **b. 1/6.** The major contribution to the volume of seminal plasma (average 3 ml) comes from the seminal vesicles (1.5 to 2 ml); from the prostate (0.5 ml); and from Cowper's gland and glands of Littre (0.1 to 0.2 ml). [p 1276]

25. **b. insulin.** In relation to other body fluids, the seminal plasma is unusual because of its very high concentrations of potassium, zinc, citric acid, fructose, phosphorylcholine, spermine, free amino acids, prostaglandins, and enzymes, most notably acid phosphatase, diamine oxidase, β-glucuronidase, lactate dehydrogenase, α-amylase, prostate-specific antigen, and seminal proteinase. [pp 1276–1277]

26. **d. Seminal vesicles.** The source of fructose in human seminal plasma is the seminal vesicles. Patients with congenital absence of the seminal vesicles also have an associated absence of fructose in their ejaculates. [p 1277]

27. **a. hK17.** Major secretory protein markers that are found in abundance and have clinical significance include (1) prostate-specific antigen (human kallikrein 3 [hK3 (protein) or *KLK3* (gene)]; (2) human kallikrein 2 (hK2 or *KLK2*); (3) prostate KLK-L1; (4) prostatic acid phosphatase (PAP); and (5) prostate-specific protein (PSP-94), also termed β-microseminoprotein or β-MSP. [p 1279]

28. **b. PSA is a chymotrypsin-like protease.** PSA is a glycoprotein that acts as a serine protease, of 33,000 daltons, contains 7% carbohydrate, and is found almost exclusively in the epithelial cells of the prostate. [pp 1279–1280]

Chapter 38

Etiology, Pathophysiology, Epidemiology, and Natural History of Benign Prostatic Hyperplasia

Claus G. Roehrborn • John D. McConnell

Questions

1. Benign prostatic hyperplasia (BPH) is characterized by:
   a. a rapid proliferation of stromal cells.
   b. a rapid proliferation of epithelial cells.
   c. a rapid proliferation of prostatic stem cells.
   d. an imbalance between cell proliferation and cell death.

2. The role of androgens in the development of BPH is to:
   a. cause active proliferation of epithelial cells.
   b. cause active proliferation of stromal cells.
   c. prevent programmed cell death in epithelial cells.
   d. prevent programmed cell death in stromal cells.

3. The primary site of dihydrotestosterone (DHT) production in the prostate gland is the:

   a. stromal cell.
   b. vascular endothelial cell.
   c. epithelial cell.
   d. neuroendocrine cell.

4. New epithelial gland formation in the hyperplastic prostate most likely involves:

   a. overexpression of androgen receptors in the epithelium.
   b. reawakening of the embryonic process in which the underlying stroma induces epithelial development.
   c. excessive conversion of testosterone to estrogen by aromatase.
   d. atrophy of adjacent stromal cells.

5. Which of the following growth factors may mediate the stromal cell's androgen-dependent regulation of the epithelium?

   a. insulin-like growth factor.
   b. acidic fibroblastic growth factor (FGF), or FGF-1.
   c. basic FGF, or FGF-2.
   d. keratinocyte growth factor (KGF), or FGF-7.

6. Evidence that BPH has an inheritable genetic component is best demonstrated in families with multiple members who:

   a. also have a familial pattern of prostate cancer.
   b. have undergone prostatectomy for BPH at a young age.
   c. have 5α-reductase deficiency.
   d. have androgen receptor gene mutations.

7. The only other mammalian species known to develop BPH, the dog, does not develop lower urinary tract obstruction because the dog prostate:

   a. experiences only stromal hyperplasia.
   b. does not surround the urethra.
   c. does not have a prostatic capsule.
   d. lacks a middle lobe.

8. The majority of active smooth muscle tone in the prostate is mediated by the:

   a. α_{1A} receptor.
   b. ATP receptor.
   c. endothelin receptor.
   d. bradykinin receptor.

9. In aging men with BPH, lower urinary tract symptoms (LUTS) occur as a result of:

   a. obstruction-related changes in bladder function.
   b. age-related changes in bladder function.
   c. nocturnal polyuria.
   d. all of the above.

10. In aging men with BPH, bladder trabeculation represents:

    a. evidence of a neurogenic bladder.
    b. smooth muscle hypertrophy.
    c. smooth muscle hyperplasia.
    d. increased detrusor collagen.

11. The prevalence of a disease is defined as:

    a. number of diseased people per 100,000 population per year.
    b. number of existing cases per 100,000 population at a distinct target date.
    c. number of deaths per 100,000 population per year.
    d. number of deaths per number of diseased persons.

12. With regard to the autopsy prevalence of BPH or stromoglandular hyperplasia, which of the following statements is correct?

    a. It is commonly found in men of all ages.
    b. It is very uncommon in men younger than the age of 30 years.
    c. It is found in 100% of men starting at the age of 40 years.
    d. Because of the lack of a definition of stromoglandular hyperplasia, international comparisons are impossible.

13. Which of the following statements regarding the International Prostate Symptom Score (IPSS) is correct?

    a. Moderate symptom severity is defined as a score of 10 to 20 points.
    b. The IPSS score addresses irritative and obstructive symptoms and issues of incontinence.
    c. Quantitative symptom scores in BPH are not as important as objective measures are, such as a flow rate recording.
    d. The IPSS has been translated and validated in many languages.

14. Which statement is correct regarding prostate volume?

    a. International studies show significant similarity in prostate volume in white, age-stratified men.
    b. Prostate volume assessment by digital rectal examination is reproducible across examiners.
    c. Although there is a steady increase in total prostate volume with advancing age, the transition zone volume increases only marginally.
    d. MRI measurements are in general smaller compared with transrectal ultrasonographic measurements.

15. With regard to liver diseases and BPH, which of the following statements is true?

    a. Ethanol consumption increases circulating levels of estrogens.
    b. The risk of having surgery for BPH is increased in heavy drinkers.
    c. The intake of ethanol can decrease serum testosterone levels by a variety of mechanisms.
    d. Most autopsy studies find a higher prevalence of BPH in men with liver cirrhosis.

16. Which of the following statements about medications influencing symptoms and flow rate is true?

    a. There is no documented influence of any medication on symptoms or flow rate.
    b. Antihistamines and bronchodilators significantly decrease urinary flow rates.
    c. Calcium channel blockers and β blockers reduce urinary flow rates significantly.
    d. Antidepressants, antihistamines, and bronchodilators increase the symptom score by several points.

17. With regard to correlations between baseline parameters, which of the following statements is true?

    a. A clinically useful correlation exists between prostate volume and serum prostate-specific antigen (PSA).
    b. Many studies have shown a significant correlation between the transition zone volume and symptom severity.
    c. Correlations among symptoms, degree of bother, interference with activities of daily living, and quality of life are poor.
    d. Urinary flow rate and prostate volume correlate highly with serum PSA.

18. Which of the following statements is correct regarding the study of the natural history of BPH?

a. Placebo groups from treatment trials are useful because they are not affected by treatment biases.
b. A longitudinal population-based study has the fewest biases and is the most useful type of study.
c. Control groups from intervention or medical therapy trials reflect the natural history of the disease in unselected community-dwelling men.
d. Placebo groups have fewer selection biases compared with population-based studies.

19. With regard to the magnitude of the placebo response and its perception, which of the following statements is correct?

    a. The placebo response does not depend on the baseline severity score.
    b. Most patients report subjective improvement when the drop from baseline is greater than 30%.
    c. The higher the baseline score is, the greater the drop that is required for patients to subjectively feel improved.
    d. The perception of improvement is independent of the baseline score.

20. Descriptive studies of the incidence rates of acute urinary retention (AUR) have demonstrated that:

    a. depending on the population studied, incidence rates ranging from less than 5 to more than 130 cases per 1000 person-years have been reported.
    b. the incidence rates reported do not differ significantly between different studies and populations.
    c. AUR has been poorly defined and therefore no incidence rates can be calculated.
    d. incidence rates of less than 10 per 1000 person-years have been reported in all watchful waiting studies.

21. What is the most significant finding regarding analytical epidemiology of AUR?

    a. Serum PSA is a more powerful predictor of AUR than age.
    b. Serum PSA and prostate volume have limited ability to predict episodes of AUR.
    c. Urinary flow rates in placebo control groups are strong predictors of AUR episodes.
    d. Age has been found to be the most significant risk factor for AUR in population-based studies.

22. Which of the following statements regarding surgery for BPH is true?

    a. The incidence rates for surgery are similar across wide geographical regions and ethnic backgrounds.
    b. Compared with AUR, surgery is a softer end point.
    c. Surgery is a less common end point than AUR.
    d. Most patients with BPH eventually require surgery for their condition.

Answers

1. **d. an imbalance between cell proliferation and cell death.** In a given organ, the number of cells and thus the volume of the organ depend on the equilibrium between cell proliferation and cell death. The relative role of cell proliferation in human BPH is questioned because there is no clear evidence of an active proliferative process. Although it is possible that the early phases of BPH are associated with a rapid proliferation of cells, the established disease appears to be maintained in the presence of an equal or a reduced rate of cell replication. Once the proliferating cells mature through a process of terminal differentiation, they have a finite life span before undergoing programmed cell death. In this paradigm, the aging process induces a block in this maturation process so that the progression to terminally differentiated cells is reduced, reducing the overall rate of cell death. [p 1298]

2. **c. prevent programmed cell death in epithelial cells.** Not only are androgens required for normal cell proliferation and differentiation in the prostate gland, they also actively inhibit cell death. [p 1298]

3. **a. stromal cell.** Immunohistochemical studies with type 2 5α-reductase-specific antibodies show primarily stromal cell localization of the enzyme. [p 1299]

4. **b. reawakening of the embryonic process in which the underlying stroma induces epithelial development.** The process of new gland formation in the hyperplastic prostate suggests a "reawakening" of embryonic processes in which the underlying prostatic stroma induces epithelial cell development. [p 1301]

5. **d. keratinocyte growth factor (KGF), or FGF-7.** KGF, a member of the FGF family (FGF-7), is produced in prostatic stromal cells. However, cell surface receptors for stromal-derived KGF are expressed exclusively in epithelial cells. As a result, KGF (or a homologue) is the leading candidate for the factor mediating the stromal cell–based hormonal regulation of the prostatic epithelium. [p 1301]

6. **b. have undergone prostatectomy for BPH at a young age.** There is substantial evidence that BPH has an inheritable genetic component. In a retrospective case-control analysis of surgically treated patients and control subjects, the BPH patients had resected prostate weights that were in the highest quartile (>37 g) and whose age at prostatectomy was in the lowest quartile. The hazard-function ratio for surgically treated BPH among first-degree male relatives of the BPH cases as compared with the first-degree male relatives of the control subjects was 4.2 (95% CI, 1.7 to 10.2), demonstrating a very strong relationship. Results were most consistent with an autosomal dominant inheritance pattern. Utilizing this model, approximately 50% of cases of men undergoing prostatectomy for BPH at younger than 60 years of age could be attributable to an inheritable form of disease. [p 1302]

7. **c. does not have a prostatic capsule.** In the dog, the only other species known to develop naturally occurring BPH, symptoms of bladder outlet obstruction and urinary symptoms rarely develop because the canine prostate lacks a capsule. Presumably the capsule transmits the "pressure" of tissue expansion to the urethra and leads to an increase in urethral resistance. Thus, the clinical symptoms of BPH in the human may be due not only to age-related increases in prostatic size but also to the unique anatomic structure of the human gland. [p 1304]

8. **a. α_{1A} receptor.** Active smooth muscle tone in the human prostate gland is regulated by the adrenergic nervous system. Receptor binding studies clearly demonstrate that the α_{1A} receptor is the most abundant adrenoreceptor subtype present in the human prostate. Moreover, this receptor clearly mediates active tension in human prostatic smooth muscle. [p 1306]

9. **d. all of the above.** It is clear that many of the clinical symptoms of prostatism are related to obstruction-induced changes in bladder function rather than to outflow obstruction directly. Obstruction-induced changes in the bladder are of two basic types: first, those changes that lead to detrusor instability or decreased compliance, which are clinically associated with symptoms of frequency and urgency; and second, those changes associated with decreased detrusor contractility, which are associated with further deterioration in the force of the urinary stream, hesitancy, intermittency, increased residual urine, and (in a minority of cases) detrusor failure. [p 1306]

10. **d. increased detrusor collagen.** One study demonstrated that the major endoscopic detrusor change, trabeculation, is due to an increase in detrusor collagen. [p 1306]

11. **b. number of existing cases per 100,000 population at a distinct target date.** The following definitions of relevant rates apply: incidence, the number of diseased people per 100,000 population per year; prevalence, the number of existing cases per 100,000 population at a distinct target date; mortality, the number of deaths per 100,000 population per year; and fatality, the number of deaths due to the disease per number of diseased people. [p 1307]

12. **c. It is very uncommon in men younger than the age of 30 years.** The 1984 landmark study by Berry and colleagues summarized the data from five studies demonstrating that no men younger than age 30 had evidence of BPH, and that the prevalence rose with each age group to peak at 88% in men in their 80s. Several rigorously performed autopsy studies in the United States, England, Austria, Norway, Denmark, China, Japan, and India showed that the prevalence increases rapidly in the 4th decade of life, reaching nearly 100% in the 9th decade. It is striking that the age-specific autopsy prevalence is remarkably similar in all populations studied regardless of ethnic and geographic origin. [p 1307]

13. **d. The IPSS score has been translated and validated in many languages.** The IPSS score addresses irritative and obstructive symptoms but no incontinence symptoms. It is widely accepted that quantitative symptom scores are far more important than, for example, urinary flow rate recordings. The self-administered seven-item AUA Symptom Index (also known as the IPSS) has been a pivotal event in the research of LUTS and BPH. With the total score running from 0 to 35 points, patients scoring 0 to 7 points have been classified as mildly symptomatic, those scoring 8 to 19 points as moderately symptomatic, and those scoring 20 to 35 points as severely symptomatic. The instrument is an integral part of virtually every epidemiologic study as well as treatment studies in the field, and the availability of validated translations in many common languages allows cross-cultural comparisons of unprecedented scope. Socioeconomic factors do not seem to influence responses to the questionnaire, and fundamentally similar responses are obtained when the questionnaire is self-administered, read to the patient, mailed in, or administered in some other way. However, there is no question that subtle differences in comprehension of the translated questionnaire, as well as different perception of the symptoms, willingness to admit to the symptoms, and other factors are the cause for cross-cultural differences in symptom severity reported in the literature. Figure 38–9 shows the prevalence of at least moderate to severe symptoms stratified by decade of life as reported in 11 cross-sectional population-based studies from around the world. [pp 1309–1310]

14. **a. International studies show significant similarity in prostate volume in white, age-stratified men.** Prostate size can be estimated by digital rectal examination, although the reliability across observers is in general considered poor. For the purpose of epidemiologic studies, transrectal ultrasonography (TRUS) and MRI measurements are preferred, although MRI measurements are somewhat expensive when attempting cross-sectional examinations of populations and yield in general a larger volume compared with TRUS measurements. TRUS volume measurements using the prolate ellipsoid volume formula represent the most widely accepted measure of prostate volume with reasonable statistical performance characteristics, particularly when performed by a single or several well-trained examiners. In general, in all cross-sectional studies, prostate volume as assessed by TRUS has been found to increase slowly but steadily with advancing age. The slight differences in the absolute volume measures and the different slopes of increase with advancing age may be caused by differences in the population examined. Overall, total prostate volume increased in a number of international cross-sectional studies from approximately 25 ml for men in their 30s to 35 to 45 ml for men in their 70s, whereas transition zone volume increased from 15 to 25 ml for similarly aged men. In fact, the similarities between the transition zone volume measurements done in Spain, the United States (Dallas, Texas), and the Netherlands are striking (see Fig. 38–10). [pp 1310–1311]

15. **c. The intake of ethanol can decrease serum testosterone levels by a variety of mechanisms.** Alcohol may decrease plasma testosterone levels and production and increase the clearance of testosterone. Despite this hypothetical reason for a lower incidence of BPH, inverse relationships have been described. Two studies reported a multivariate-adjusted relative risk of 0.49 and an age-adjusted relative risk of 0.75, respectively, for the risk of having surgery for BPH among men who consumed more than three glasses of alcohol per day, lower than in age-matched control subjects. However, one might argue that the poorer health of heavy drinkers might bias physicians against surgery. One study, in fact, found no increased risk for either the clinical diagnosis or surgical rates. It is interesting to note, however, that of five studies examining the relationship between liver cirrhosis and BPH based on autopsy material, four found a lower prevalence of BPH in men with cirrhosis, whereas one study—admittedly with some design flaws—found a higher prevalence. Because most cirrhosis cases are alcohol induced, the separation of the effects of alcohol versus cirrhosis is virtually impossible. [p 1312]

16. **d. Antidepressants, antihistamines, and bronchodilators increase the symptom score by several points.** Very limited information is available. Cold medications containing α-sympathomimetic drugs exacerbate LUTS by the expected effect on the smooth muscles of the bladder outlet. A careful analysis of the data from the Olmsted County study demonstrated that daily use of antidepressants, antihistamines, or bronchodilators is associated with a 2- to 3-point increase in the IPSS compared with the IPSS in age-matched nonusers, and daily use of antidepressants is associated with a decrease in the age-adjusted flow rate. [p 1313]

17. **a. A clinically useful correlation exists between prostate volume and serum prostate-specific antigen (PSA).** All relevant parameters such as symptom severity and frequency, degree of bother, interference with activities of daily living, disease-specific health-related quality of life (HRQOL), maximum flow rate, and prostate volume tend to worsen with advancing age. However, reported correlations between these parameters as well as urodynamic pressure-flow studies are in general weak, with some exceptions. Strong correlations exist among measures of symptom severity and frequency (IPSS score), degree of bother, disease-specific HRQOL, and interference scores. The correlation between serum PSA and

prostate volume, both total and transition zone, has been described in greater detail. Although the variability is significant, precluding the accurate prediction of prostate volume by serum PSA in individual patients, there is a nearly linear relationship between these parameters, which can be shown in both population-based and clinical studies. The relationship is further influenced by patients' age, with older patients having a greater increase in prostate volume per unit of serum PSA (see Fig. 38–13). With the exception of age, correlations between various measures of LUTS and BPH are modest in community-based population studies and weak in BPH clinical and trial populations, not precluding, however, a clinically meaningful relationship. The relationship between serum PSA and prostate volume is moderate. Symptoms, flow rate, and prostate volume measures cannot predict the presence and degree of obstruction reliably. [pp 1313–1314]

18. **b. A longitudinal population-based study has the fewest biases and is the most useful type of study.** Control groups of men being randomized to receive no treatment, placebo, or sham treatment while being compared with a matched group of men receiving active therapeutic interventions also suffer from a variety of biases. As the watchful waiting cohorts, they have initial and constant contact with health care providers, they know from the design of the study that they are randomized to the perceived less effective or ineffective arm, and thus they may have a lower threshold than community-dwelling men to cross over to active therapy. However, because of a sense of obligation, they may elect to be followed until the trial is over, and then they choose an active treatment. They are also subject to a mean bias, because they were subjected to inclusion/exclusion criteria. Longitudinal population-based studies, although difficult and expensive to conduct, are likely the best vehicle to understand the natural history of the disease. [p 1316]

19. **c. The higher the baseline score is, the greater the drop that is required for patients to subjectively feel improved.** One study reported an important observation by assessing the relationship between changes in the AUA Symptom Index and patients' global rating of improvement in more than 1200 men treated in a medical treatment trial for BPH. The authors noted that a mean decrease in the Symptom Index of 3.1 points was associated with a slight improvement; however, this relationship was strictly dependent on the baseline AUA Symptom Index. For patients to perceive a slight, moderate, or marked improvement, increasing drops in AUA Symptom Index were required with increasing baseline symptom severity. For patients starting with a lower versus higher baseline score, the drop had to be −7.4 vs −15.3 points, respectively, to perceive a marked improvement, −4.0 vs −8.7 for a moderate improvement, −1.9 vs −6.1 for a slight improvement, −0.2 vs −2.0 for no improvement, and +3.3 vs +1.2 for worsening to be perceived. [pp 1319–1320]

20. **a. depending on the population studied, incidence rates ranging from less than 5 to more than 130 cases per 1000 person-years have been reported.** Older estimates of occurrence of AUR range from 4 to 15 to as high as 130 per 1000 person-years, which leads to 10-year cumulative incidence rates ranging from 4% to 73%. The self-reported rate of AUR in a cross-sectional study in 2002 Spanish men was 5.1%. More recent data from carefully controlled studies in better defined populations shed additional light on the incidence rates in community-dwelling men and clinical BPH populations. AUR occurred in the VA Cooperative study over 3 years in one man after transurethral prostatic resection and in 8 of 276 men in the watchful waiting arm for an incidence rate of 9.6 per 1000 person-years. Outcomes were reported for 500 men diagnosed by urologists with BPH who were candidates for prostatectomy by established criteria but elected to be followed conservatively. In 1574 person-years, 40 episodes of AUR occurred at a constant rate throughout the 4 years of follow-up, for an incidence rate of 25 per 1000 person-years. During 15,851 person-years of follow-up in the Physicians Health Study, 82 men reported an episode of AUR, for an incidence rate of 4.5 per 1000 person-years. Of the 2115 men aged 40 to 79 years in the Olmsted County Study, 57 had a first episode of AUR during 8344 person-years of follow-up (incidence 6.8 per 1000 person-years). The best data from men diagnosed with BPH stem from the Proscar Long Term Efficacy and Safety Study (PLESS). In PLESS, 1376 placebo-treated men with enlarged prostates and moderate symptoms had complete follow-up for 4 years; 99 experienced an episode of AUR for a calculated incidence rate of 18 per 1000 person-years. The placebo treatment groups from three 2-year studies with a similar patient population were meta-analyzed; of 2109 patients, 57 experienced AUR over the 2 years with a constant hazard ratio, for an incidence rate of 14 per 1000 person-years. [pp 1324–1325]

21. **d. Age has been found to be the most significant risk factor for AUR in population-based studies.** The Olmsted County Study analyses focused on age, symptom severity, maximum flow rate, and prostate volume (see Figs. 38–14 and 38–15). Incidence rates per 1000 person-years increased from 2.6 to 9.3 for men in their 40s to their 70s if they had mild symptoms, and from 3.0 to 34.7 if they had more than mild symptoms (see Fig. 38–18). The relative risk increased for older men, men with moderate to severe symptoms (3.2 times), those with a flow rate under 12 ml/second (3.9 times), and those with a prostate volume greater than 30 ml by TRUS (3.0 times). The highest relative risk by proportional hazard models exists for 60- to 69-year-old men with more than mild symptoms and a flow rate of less than 12 ml/second (10.3 times), and for 70- to 79-year-old men except if they had mild symptoms and a flow rate over 12 ml/second. All other men older than 70 years had a relative risk ranging from 12.9 to 14.8. Although age in community-dwelling men is an important risk factor, in BPH trial populations of men who already are diagnosed with BPH, other factors can be analyzed. In the placebo groups of three 2-year studies and a 4-year study (PLESS), prostate volume, serum PSA, and symptom severity all were predictors of AUR episodes. The risk for both types of AUR increases with increasing serum PSA as well as prostate volume stratified by tertiles (see Fig. 38–21). An analysis of more than 100 possible outcome predictors alone or in combination revealed a combination of serum PSA, urinating more than every 2 hours, symptom problem index, maximum urinary flow rate, and hesitancy as being only slightly superior to PSA alone in predicting AUR episodes. [pp 1324–1325]

22. **b. Compared with AUR, surgery is a softer end point.** Both surgery and AUR represent distinct end points in the disease progression of BPH. There are, however, distinct differences. AUR is an outcome mandating management, and surgery is one of the commonly employed management styles. AUR is probably one of the clearer indications for surgery, leaving the treating physician little choice in a patient in whom a trial without catheter failed. However, most patients undergo surgery not for AUR but for symptoms. Depending on local practice pattern, AUR accounts for 5% to more than 30% of the indications for surgery. AUR can be compared to a fracture. It is impossible for the physician in the interaction with the patient to increase or decrease the probability for that outcome to occur. Furthermore, once it has occurred, no interaction or consultation can undo it. In contrast, it is easy to see how patients can be influenced in their decision to undergo surgery by consultation with the

physician. The interaction style, the quoted probabilities of beneficial and harmful outcomes to occur, and many other factors cause considerable variability in the incidence rates of prostate-related surgery, an observation that caused the Agency for Health Care Policy and Research to develop guidelines for the treatment of BPH. From this brief discussion it becomes clear that surgery for BPH is a softer end point from an epidemiologic point of view than AUR, and data on rates of prostatectomy need to be interpreted in light of variation in its use, from provider to provider, region to region, health care plan to health care plan, and over time. [pp 1325–1326]

Chapter 39

Natural History, Evaluation, and Nonsurgical Management of Benign Prostatic Hyperplasia

Herbert Lepor • Franklin C. Lowe

Questions

1. Where does benign prostatic hyperplasia (BPH) originate?

   a. In the transition zone
   b. In the peripheral zone
   c. In the periurethral glands
   d. In the transition zone and periurethral zone

2. A strong correlation exists between prostate volume and:

   a. serum prostate-specific antigen (PSA).
   b. American Urological Association (AUA) symptom score.
   c. peak urinary flow rate.
   d. postvoid residual.

3. Medications that may exacerbate lower urinary tract symptoms (LUTS) include:

   a. α antagonists.
   b. α agonists.
   c. β agonists.
   d. muscarinic agonists.

4. What is the primary objective of the digital rectal examination (DRE) in evaluation of men with LUTS?

   a. To estimate prostate volume
   b. To obtain prostatic secretions
   c. To identify prostate nodules
   d. To determine rectal tone

5. In older men with LUTS, which test should be routinely performed to discriminate the differential diagnosis?

   a. Urinalysis
   b. Peak flow rate
   c. Serum creatinine assay
   d. Renal ultrasonography

6. It is advisable in a man with BPH and a slightly elevated creatinine level to perform a(an):

   a. transurethral resection of the prostate (TURP).
   b. intravenous pyelography.
   c. renal sonography.
   d. urodynamic study.

7. What percentage of men have histologically proven BPH with a serum PSA value of 4.0 ng/ml or greater?

   a. 5%
   b. 15%
   c. 30%
   d. 50%

8. An AUA symptom score of 20 indicates severe:

   a. LUTS.
   b. BPH.
   c. bladder outlet obstruction.
   d. bladder dysfunction.

9. An absolute indication for surgery (TURP or open prostatectomy) is:

   a. severe symptoms.
   b. postvoid residual (PVR) urine of 300 ml or more.
   c. single episodes of acute urinary retention.
   d. refractory gross hematuria secondary to BPH.

10. A low peak flow rate suggests:

    a. severe symptoms.
    b. bladder outlet obstruction.
    c. impaired detrusor contractility.
    d. b or c.

11. What is the next step for a man with a PVR of 300 ml?

    a. Repeat the PVR assay
    b. Upper urinary tract imaging.
    c. Urodynamic testing.
    d. TURP

12. The probability that a urodynamic study will decrease the failure rate of TURP in men with a peak flow rate of 15 ml/second is approximately:

    a. 10%.
    b. 25%.
    c. 50%.
    d. 75%.

13. What is the percentage of men with LUTS who have uninhibited contraction?

    a. 10%
    b. 30%

c. 60%
d. 80%

14. What is the probability that uninhibited detrusor contractions (UDCs) in men with BPH will resolve after TURP?

    a. Never
    b. Unlikely
    c. Likely
    d. Always

15. The finding of bladder trabeculation suggests:

    a. high-grade obstruction.
    b. high successful rate after TURP.
    c. high PVR.
    d. none of the above.

16. Imaging of the upper tract is indicated for:

    a. prostate glands weighing more than 50 g.
    b. a urinalysis demonstrating hematuria.
    c. bladder trabeculation.
    d. severe LUTS.

17. An improvement in the AUA symptom score of 5 units correlates with which level of symptoms improved?

    a. Marked.
    b. Moderate.
    c. Slight.
    d. None.

18. Urodynamic testing reliably predicts response after:

    a. TURP.
    b. α blockers.
    c. 5α-reductase inhibitors.
    d. none of the above.

19. There is compelling evidence that PVR is:

    a. related to symptom severity.
    b. associated with the risk for urinary tract infection (UTI).
    c. both a and b.
    d. neither a nor b.

20. The definition of detrusor instability is bladder pressure greater than which level at a bladder volume of 300 ml or less?

    a. 5 cm H_2O.
    b. 15 cm H_2O.
    c. 40 cm H_2O.
    d. 60 cm H_2O.

21. The likelihood that a man with acute urinary retention will develop a subsequent episode of urinary retention within 1 week is approximately:

    a. 20%.
    b. 40%.
    c. 60%.
    d. 80%.

22. The incidence of developing acute urinary retention is related to:

    a. prostate size.
    b. age.
    c. severity of symptoms.
    d. all of the above.

23. The best way to eliminate bias in a clinical study is to use:

    a. honest investigators.
    b. a placebo-controlled double-blind design.
    c. randomization.
    d. a large sample size.

24. The larger the sample size, the:

    a. less treatment effect required to achieve statistical significance.
    b. better the study.
    c. greater treatment effect required to achieve statistical significance.
    d. none of the above.

25. Which of the following is the attractive feature of medical therapy relative to TURP?

    a. Fewer side effects.
    b. Reversible side effects.
    c. Less serious side effects.
    d. All of the above.

26. During the past decade, the incidence of TURP in the United States has decreased by approximately:

    a. 10%.
    b. 50%.
    c. 100%.
    d. 200%.

27. Which of the following percentages of men older than 50 years of age have moderate or severe LUTS?

    a. 2%.
    b. 5%.
    c. 30%.
    d. 50%.

28. The ideal candidate for medical therapy should have:

    a. severe symptoms.
    b. moderate symptoms.
    c. minimal symptoms.
    d. bothersome symptoms.

29. Smooth muscle accounts for what percentage of the area density of the prostate?

    a. 5%.
    b. 10%.
    c. 20%.
    d. 40%.

30. The tension of prostate smooth muscle is mediated by the:

    a. α_1 receptor.
    b. α_2 receptor.
    c. β_2 receptor.
    d. muscarinic cholinergic receptor.

31. What is the advantage of terazosin over prazosin?

    a. Its longer half-life
    b. Its better absorption
    c. Its greater α_1-receptor selectivity
    d. None of the above

32. Which α_1 receptor subtype mediates prostate smooth muscle tension?

    a. α_{1a}
    b. α_{1b}
    c. α_{1c}
    d. α_{1d}

33. The improvement in AUA symptom score after terazosin administration depends on baseline:

    a. age.
    b. prostate size.
    c. PVR.
    d. none of the above.

34. The mean treatment-related improvement in response to terazosin is approximately:

a. 2 AUA symptom score units.
b. 4 AUA symptom score units.
c. 6 AUA symptom score units.
d. 8 AUA symptom score units.

35. The durability of the improvements in symptom scores and peak flow rate for α_1 blockers has been reported up to:

   a. 12 months.
   b. 42 months.
   c. 60 months.
   d. 92 months.

36. Which of the following α blockers does not lower blood pressure in men with uncontrolled hypertension?

   a. Terazosin.
   b. Doxazosin.
   c. Tamsulosin.
   d. Prazosin.

37. Retrograde ejaculation is most commonly seen with:

   a. terazosin.
   b. prazosin.
   c. finasteride.
   d. tamsulosin.

38. Approximately what percentage of men have both BPH and hypertension?

   a. 5%
   b. 15%
   c. 30%
   d. 50%

39. What is the likely mechanism for dizziness after α_1-blocker therapy?

   a. vascular.
   b. central nervous system.
   c. carotid baroreceptor.
   d. none of the above.

40. The major advantage of tamsulosin 0.4 mg over terazosin 10 mg is:

   a. greater efficiency.
   b. less retrograde ejaculation.
   c. no dose titration.
   d. greater lowering of blood pressure.

41. The embryologic development of the prostate is mediated primarily by:

   a. testosterone.
   b. dihydrotestosterone.
   c. androstenedione.
   d. estradiol.

42. Finasteride significantly decreases the long-term risk of:

   a. acute urinary retention.
   b. surgical intervention.
   c. all of the above.
   d. none of the above.

43. Finasteride is most effective at relieving hematuria in men:

   a. with prostatitis.
   b. with enlarged prostates.
   c. after transurethral prostatectomy.
   d. with obstructing prostates.

44. The adverse event that limits the use of flutamide as a primary treatment of BPH is:

   a. breast tenderness.
   b. diarrhea.
   c. erectile dysfunction.
   d. loss of libido.

45. The primary advantage of Cetrorelix, a gonadotropin-releasing hormone antagonist, for the treatment of BPH is:

   a. lower cost.
   b. ability to titrate the level of androgen suppression.
   c. ease of administration.
   d. rapid response.

46. A Veterans Administration study demonstrated that terazosin is more effective than finasteride at relieving symptoms in men with:

   a. small prostates.
   b. intermediate-size prostates.
   c. large prostates.
   d. all of the above.

47. In the Veterans Administration study, finasteride was no better than placebo at:

   a. improving symptoms.
   b. lowering micturition voiding pressure.
   c. decreasing prostate size.
   d. all of the above.

48. The amount spent on phytotherapy for the treatment of BPH is estimated to be:

   a. $10 million.
   b. $100 million.
   c. $1 billion.
   d. $10 billion.

49. The definitive mechanism of action for *Serenoa repens* is:

   a. inhibition of 5α-reductase.
   b. inhibition of cyclooxygenase.
   c. inhibition of lipoxygenase.
   d. inconclusive.

50. The next major step in the treatment of LUTS will require:

   a. unraveling the pathophysiology of LUTS.
   b. more selective α_1 blockers.
   c. duel inhibitors of dihydrotestosterone.
   d. new strategies for relaxing prostate smooth muscle.

Answers

1. **d. In the transition zone and periurethral zone.** The proliferative process originates in the transition zone and the periurethral glands. [p 1338]

2. **a. serum prostate-specific antigen (PSA).** A strong correlation exists between serum PSA levels and prostate volume. [p 1338]

3. **b. α agonists.** Current prescription and over-the-counter medications should be examined to determine whether the patient is taking drugs that impair bladder contractility (anticholinergics) or that increase outflow resistance (α-sympathomimetics). [pp 1338–1339]

4. **c. To identify prostate nodules.** The DRE and neurologic

examination are done to detect prostate or rectal malignancy, to evaluate anal sphincter tone, and to rule out any neurologic problems that may cause the presenting symptoms. [p 1339]

5. **a. Urinalysis.** In older men with BPH and a higher prevalence of serious urinary tract disorders, the benefits of an innocuous test such as urinalysis clearly outweigh the harm involved. [p 1339]

6. **c. renal sonography.** An elevated serum creatinine level in a patient with BPH is an indication for imaging studies (ultrasonography) to evaluate the upper urinary tract. [p 1339]

7. **c. 30%.** Twenty-eight percent of men with histologically proven BPH have a serum PSA level greater than 4.0 ng/ml. [p 1340]

8. **a. LUTS.** The International Prostate Symptom Score (IPSS), which is identical to the AUA Symptom Index, is recommended as the symptom scoring instrument to be used for the baseline assessment of symptom severity in men presenting with LUTS. When the IPSS system is used, symptoms can be classified as mild (0 to 7), moderate (8 to 19), or severe (20 to 35). The IPSS cannot be used to establish the diagnosis of BPH. [p 1340]

9. **d. refractory gross hematuria secondary to BPH.** Surgery is recommended if the patient has refractory urinary retention (at least one failed attempt at catheter removal) or any of the following conditions, clearly secondary to BPH: recurrent urinary tract infection, recurrent gross hematuria, bladder stones, renal insufficiency, or large bladder diverticula. [pp 1340–1341]

10. **d. b or c.** One study found that flow rate recording cannot distinguish between bladder outlet obstruction and impaired detrusor contractility as the cause for a low Qmax. [p 1341]

11. **a. Repeat the PVR assay.** Residual urine volume measurement has significant intraindividual variability that limits its clinical usefulness. [p 1342]

12. **a. 10%.** One study recommended invasive urodynamic testing for patients with a Qmax higher than 15 ml/second. For the population in their study, this would have resulted in an additional 9% of patients being excluded from surgery and a decrease in failure rate to 8.3%. [p 1343]

13. **c. 60%.** Uninhibited contractions are present in about 60% of men with LUTS and correlate strongly with irritative voiding symptoms. [p 1343]

14. **c. Likely.** UDCs resolve in most patients after surgery. [p 1343]

15. **d. none of the above.** Bladder trabeculation may predict a slightly higher failure rate in patients managed by watchful waiting but does not predict the success or failure of surgery. [p 1344]

16. **b. a urinalysis demonstrating hematuria.** Upper urinary tract imaging is not recommended for routine evaluation of men with LUTS unless they also have one or more of the following: hematuria; urinary tract infection; renal insufficiency (ultrasonography recommended); history of urolithiasis; history of urinary tract surgery. [p 1344]

17. **b. Moderate.** The group mean changes in American Urological Association Symptom Index for subjects rating their improvement as markedly, moderately, or slightly improved, unchanged, or worse was −8.8, −5.1, −3.0, −0.7, and +2.7, respectively. [p 1345]

18. **d. none of the above.** Urodynamic testing does not predict symptom improvement after α blockade, transurethral microwave thermotherapy, or prostatectomy. [p 1346]

19. **d. neither a nor b.** One study reported no correlation between the AUA symptom score and PVR volume. There are also no data documenting that the incidence of UTI is related to PVR volume. [p 1346]

20. **b. 15 cm H_2O.** The definition of detrusor instability is the development of a detrusor contraction exceeding 15 cm H_2O at a bladder volume less than or equal to 300 ml. [p 1346]

21. **d. 80%.** Of 59 Danish patients presenting to an emergency department with acute retention, 73% had recurrent urinary retention within 1 week after removal of the catheter. [p 1346]

22. **d. all of the above.** The incidence of acute urinary retention was related to age, severity of symptoms, and size of the prostate gland. [p 1346]

23. **b. a placebo-controlled double-blind design.** The only mechanism to ensure that the potential bias of the subject and the investigator does not influence the outcome is a randomized double-blind placebo-controlled design. [p 1347]

24. **a. less treatment effect required to achieve statistical significance.** The larger the number of subjects enrolled in a study, the smaller the change required to achieve statistical significance. [p 1347]

25. **d. All of the above.** The attractive features of medical therapy relative to prostatectomy is that clinically significant outcomes are obtained with fewer, less serious, and reversible side effects. [p 1348]

26. **b. 50%.** A 55% reduction in transurethral prostatectomy has occurred despite the progressively increasing number of men enrolled in the Medicare program. [p 1348]

27. **c. 30%.** Approximately 30% of American men older than 50 years of age have moderate to severe symptoms. [p 1348]

28. **d. bothersome symptoms.** The ideal candidate for medical therapy should have symptoms that are bothersome and have a negative impact on the quality of life. [p 1348]

29. **d. 40%.** Smooth muscle is one of the dominant cellular constituents of BPH, accounting for 40% of the area density of the hyperplastic prostate. [p 1349]

30. **a. α_1 receptor.** The tension of prostate smooth muscle is mediated by the α_1 adrenoceptors. [p 1349]

31. **a. Its longer half-life.** Terazosin and doxazosin are long-acting α blockers that have been shown to be safe and effective for the treatment of BPH. [p 1349]

32. **a. α_{1a}.** Prostate smooth muscle tension has been shown to be mediated by the α_{1a} adrenoceptors. [p 1350]

33. **d. none of the above.** The relationships between percent change in total symptom score and peak flow rate versus baseline age, prostate size, peak flow rate, PVR volume, and total symptom score were examined to identify clinical or urodynamic factors that predicted response to terazosin therapy. No significant association was observed between treatment effect and any of these baseline factors. [p 1352]

34. **b. 4 AUA symptom score units.** The treatment-related improvement (terazosin minus placebo) in the AUA symptom score and urinary peak flow rate was 1.4 ml/second and 3.9 symptom units, respectively. [p 1352]

35. **b. 42 months.** The initial improvements in symptom scores and peak flow rate in 450 subjects were maintained for up to 42 months. [pp 1352–1353]

36. **c. Tamsulosin.** The advantage of not lowering blood pressure in men who are hypertensive at baseline is controversial. [p 1355]

37. **d. tamsulosin.** The treatment-related incidences of asthenia, dizziness, rhinitis, and abnormal ejaculation observed for 0.4 mg of tamsulosin were 2%, 5%, 3%, and 11%, respectively, and for 0.8 mg of tamsulosin were 3%, 8%, 9%, and 18%, respectively. [p 1355]

38. **c. 30%.** Approximately 30% of men treated for BPH have coexisting hypertension. [p 1357]

39. **b. Central nervous system.** The α_1-mediated dizziness and asthenia are likely due to effects at the level of the central nervous system. [p 1358]

40. **c. no dose titration.** The major advantage of 0.4 mg tamsulosin and slow-release alfuzosin is the lack of requirement for dose titration. [p 1358]

41. **b. dihydrotestosterone.** The embryonic development of the prostate is dependent on the androgen dihydrotestosterone. [p 1359]

42. **c. all of the above.** The Proscar Long-Term Efficacy and Safety Study (PLESS) represents the longest duration multicenter randomized double-blind placebo-controlled study reported in the medical therapy of BPH literature. The unique findings of PLESS were related to incidences of both acute urinary retention and surgical intervention for BPH. The risk reduction of acute urinary retention and BPH-related surgery was clinically relevant, especially in men with very large prostates. [pp 1361–1362]

43. **c. after transurethral prostatectomy.** These preliminary observations have been confirmed by a randomized double-blind placebo-controlled study demonstrating that finasteride prevents recurrent gross hematuria secondary to BPH after prostatectomy. [p 1363]

44. **a. breast tenderness.** The incidences of breast tenderness and diarrhea in the flutamide group were 53% and 11%, respectively. [p 1364]

45. **b. ability to titrate the level of androgen suppression.** A potential advantage of a gonadotropin-releasing hormone antagonist over the luteinizing hormone–releasing hormone agonists in the treatment of BPH is the ability to titrate the level of androgen suppression. [p 1364]

46. **d. all of the above.** In the study, the mean group differences between terazosin vs placebo and terazosin vs finasteride for all of the outcome measures other than prostate volume were highly statistically significant. Terazosin was more effective than finasteride in those subjects with large prostates. [pp 1365–1366]

47. **a. improving symptoms.** The mean group differences between finasteride and placebo were not statistically significant for AUA symptom index, symptom problem index, BPH impact index, and peak flow rate. [p 1365]

48. **c. $1 billion.** Usage of these agents in the United States and throughout the world has escalated. It has been estimated that more than $1 billion was spent in the United States alone for these products. [p 1367]

49. **d. inconclusive.** Although experimental data have suggested numerous possible mechanisms of actions for the phytotherapeutic agents (see Table 39–13), it is uncertain which, if any, of these proposed mechanisms is responsible for the clinical responses. [p 1369]

50. **a. unraveling the pathophysiology of LUTS.** Our current understanding of the pathophysiology of clinical BPH is rudimentary. It is, therefore, imperative to develop a more comprehensive understanding of the pathophysiology of symptoms. [p 1372]

Chapter 40

Minimally Invasive and Endoscopic Management of Benign Prostatic Hyperplasia

John M. Fitzpatrick • Winston K. Mebust

Questions

1. Intraprostatic stents were developed after first being used to treat which of the following conditions?

    a. Peripheral vascular disease
    b. Coronary artery disease
    c. Urethral strictures
    d. Bronchial obstruction
    e. Lacrimal duct obstruction

2. The recognized role for the use of intraprostatic stents is:

    a. to replace transurethral resection of the prostate (TURP).
    b. in preoperative patients likely to develop retention.
    c. in patients unfit for TURP.
    d. in patients receiving anticoagulants.
    e. for temporary relief of obstruction.

3. The most common complication associated with temporary stents is:

    a. urinary retention.
    b. stent migration.
    c. clot retention.
    d. urinary incontinence.
    e. encrustation.

148 BENIGN PROSTATIC HYPERPLASIA

4. Which of the following statements is true of transurethral needle ablation (TUNA)?

   a. It causes necrosis at 15 days.
   b. It induces fibrosis at 7 days.
   c. It causes damage to α-adrenergic receptors at 1 week.
   d. It affects nitric oxide synthase receptors, which are least vulnerable to damage.
   e. It does not affect prostate-specific antigen (PSA) staining.

5. The complication most commonly reported after TUNA is:

   a. hemorrhage.
   b. urinary retention.
   c. irritative voiding symptoms.
   d. urinary tract infection.
   e. urethral strictures.

6. Transurethral microwave therapy (TUMT) has been shown to:

   a. damage nerve fibers, with necrosis possible.
   b. induce apoptosis of prostatic cells.
   c. be superior to TURP in terms of clinical efficacy.
   d. cause retrograde ejaculation.
   e. induce post-treatment voiding difficulties with low-energy treatment.

7. Treating symptomatic benign prostatic hyperplasia with the laser:

   a. causes the greatest degree of tissue vaporization with the holmium laser.
   b. is most appropriate for large prostates.
   c. is associated with a low incidence of postoperative urinary infection.
   d. has a hemorrhage rate of 8%.
   e. causes erectile dysfunction in 46% of patients.

8. An absolute indication for TURP is:

   a. postvoid residual urine volume of 250 ml.
   b. recurrent urinary infections.
   c. American Urological Association symptom score of 20 or greater.
   d. detrusor pressure at a maximum flow of 65 cm H_2O.
   e. inability to use medical treatment because of side effects.

9. Postoperative complications have been related to preoperative measurement of:

   a. urinary flow rate.
   b. detrusor pressure at maximum urinary flow rate.
   c. postvoid residual urine.
   d. prostatic size.
   e. serum creatinine value.

10. Outflow obstruction can be predicted by:

    a. serum creatinine level.
    b. urine culture results.
    c. maximum urinary flow rate.
    d. cystoscopy.
    e. pressure-flow studies.

11. TURP should commence with:

    a. incision of the bladder neck.
    b. resection of the middle lobe.
    c. resection of the bladder neck.
    d. resection of tissue at 12 o'clock.
    e. resection of tissue at 3 or 9 o'clock.

12. The most common complication after TURP is:

    a. failure to void.
    b. hemorrhage requiring transfusion.
    c. clot retention.
    d. urinary tract infection.
    e. transurethral resection syndrome.

13. Transurethral vaporization of the prostate (TUVP) results in:

    a. vaporization.
    b. coagulation.
    c. desiccation.
    d. vaporization and desiccation.
    e. cauterization.

14. In short-term studies, TUVP has been shown to be comparable to TURP in what area?

    a. Urinary flow rate improvement
    b. Incidence of postoperative hemorrhage
    c. Postoperative urinary infection
    d. Sexual complications
    e. Improvement in postvoid residual urine

15. Which of the following statements is true of transurethral incision of the prostate (TUIP)?

    a. It is appropriate for large prostates.
    b. It has a high complication rate.
    c. It causes retrograde ejaculation in up to 37% of cases.
    d. It commonly results in TURP syndrome.
    e. It was described by Bottim in 1900.

Answers

1. **b. Coronary artery disease.** Stents were first introduced as a method of treating certain cardiovascular conditions. [p 1380]

2. **c. in patients unfit for TURP.** Eventually it became clear that the major role for stents was likely to be found in the management of patients who were unfit for surgery, either in the short or in the long term, in whom the alternative would have been months or indeed a lifetime of indwelling urethral catheterization. [p 1381]

3. **d. urinary incontinence.** In the largest number of patients (318) reported from one center, complications were divided into none, moderate, and severe. In the patients who were described as having severe complications, stress or urge incontinence occurred in 63, emptying problems in 8, and frequency and/or nocturia (>3 episodes) in 57. [p 1381]

4. **c. It causes damage to α-adrenergic receptors at 1 week.** In studies with the TUNA system, necrosis was maximal at 7 days, with fibrosis developing by 15 days. In treated areas, there was an absence of staining for PSA, smooth muscle actin, and α-adrenergic neural tissue. Nitric oxide synthase receptors were found to be most vulnerable to thermal damage and occurred earliest, with damage to the α-adrenergic receptors maximal at 1 to 2 weeks. [p 1386]

5. **b. urinary retention.** By far the most common complication reported, however, is post-treatment urinary retention, occurring at a rate of 13.3% to 41.6%. It can be expected that

within the first 24 hours, about 40% of patients will experience urinary retention. [p 1388]

6. **b. induce apoptosis of prostatic cells.** In one study, apoptosis was verified by the terminal deoxynucleotidyl nick-end labeling (TUNEL) technique in sections showing histologic changes suggestive of apoptosis, such as pyknotic nuclei and chromatin segregation. Necrotic areas were frequently seen in the prostate to a depth of 4 to 5 cm. Outside these necrotic areas, normal and apoptotic areas were interspersed, the latter confirmed by TUNEL. The area of tissue damage seen after TUMT was relatively small compared with the volume of the prostates. The heat was implicated as the cause of the apoptosis, but there was no speculation as to the exact mechanism whereby heat brought about this effect. [p 1391]

7. **a. causes the greatest degree of tissue vaporization with the holmium laser.** The vaporization techniques using the neodymium:yttrium-aluminum-garnet (Nd:YAG) laser with high-energy density beams at high power (60 to 100 W) at a wavelength of 1064 nm have been effective for removing small amounts of tissue immediately during the procedure. However, this is a relatively inefficient technique because of the high power required. The holmium:yttrium-aluminum-garnet (Ho:YAG) laser energy is absorbed by water (unlike the Nd:YAG) at a wavelength of 2140 nm and causes considerable tissue vaporization. The methods of using the Ho:YAG laser have evolved because of several modifications in both the technology and the methodology. The technique has passed through simple vaporization to combined endoscopic laser ablation of the prostate and is now used to resect large pieces of prostatic tissue. [p 1398]

8. **b. recurrent urinary infections.** Although symptoms constitute the primary reason for recommending intervention, in patients with an obstructing prostate there are some absolute indications. These are acute urinary retention, recurrent infection, recurrent hematuria, and azotemia. [p 1404]

9. **e. serum creatinine value.** Patients with a serum creatinine level greater than 1.5% had a 25% incidence of postoperative complications, versus an incidence of 17% in those who had a normal creatinine level. [p 1405]

10. **e. pressure-flow studies.** Pressure-flow studies are recommended as an optional test. This is one of the best ways to evaluate a patient's degree of obstruction and detrusor function, particularly when the diagnosis is unclear. [p 1405]

11. **d. resection of tissue at 12 o'clock.** The resection begins at the bladder neck, starting at the 12-o'clock position and carried down to the 9-o'clock position, in a stepwise manner. [p 1406]

12. **a. failure to void.** The most common complications in the immediate postoperative period were, in one study, failing to void (6.5%), bleeding requiring transfusion (3.9%), and clot retention (3.3%). [p 1411]

13. **d. vaporization and desiccation.** With TUVP, two electrosurgical effects are combined: vaporization and desiccation. Vaporization steams tissue away using high heat, and coagulation uses lower heat to dry out tissue. [p 1412]

14. **a. Urinary flow rate improvement.** One study showed that in a relatively small number of cases, TUVP was as effective as TURP in relieving urodynamically proven outflow obstruction, but the overall complication rate for TUVP was 17.5%. [p 1413]

15. **c. It causes retrograde ejaculation in up to 37% of cases.** TUIP causes a decrease in retrograde ejaculation compared with TURP. The incidence of retrograde ejaculation after TURP ranges from 50% to 95%, but after TUIP it has been reported as occurring in 0% to 37% of cases. [p 1414]

Chapter 41

Retropubic and Suprapubic Open Prostatectomy

Misop Han • Harold J. Alfert • Alan W. Partin

Questions

1. Which of the following represents a major advantage of open prostatectomy over transurethral resection of prostate (TURP) in the management of prostatic adenoma?
   a. Removal of the prostatic adenoma under direct vision
   b. Decreased risk of hypernatremia
   c. Shortened convalescence period
   d. Decreased potential for perioperative hemorrhage
   e. Enhanced preservation of erectile function

2. The suprapubic prostatectomy, in comparison to the retropubic prostatectomy, allows:
   a. direct visualization of the prostatic adenoma during enucleation.
   b. better visualization of the prostatic fossa after enucleation to obtain hemostasis.
   c. easier management of a large median lobe and/or bladder calculi.
   d. an extraperitoneal approach.
   e. possible management of concomitant ureteral calculi.

3. The suprapubic approach to prostatectomy is ideal for the patient with a large prostatic adenoma and:
   a. multiple small bladder calculi.
   b. a total prostate-specific antigen value greater than 10.0 ng/ml.
   c. erectile dysfunction.

d. a symptomatic bladder diverticulum.
e. the presence of a dilated renal pelvis.

4. What are the most appropriate definitive treatment options for the patient with a 120 g prostatic adenoma and a symptomatic bladder diverticulum?

   a. retropubic open prostatectomy with fulguration of the bladder diverticulum.
   b. a long-acting α-adrenergic antagonist and prophylactic antibiotics.
   c. TURP followed by bladder diverticulectomy in 3 months.
   d. TURP and partial cystectomy.
   e. suprapubic prostatectomy with bladder diverticulectomy.

5. The contraindications to open prostatectomy include:

   a. biopsy-proven prostate cancer.
   b. a bladder diverticulum.
   c. large bladder calculi secondary to obstruction.
   d. recurrent urinary tract infection.
   e. acute urinary retention.

6. Which of the following statements is true of both retropubic prostatectomy and suprapubic prostatectomy?

   a. They are performed in the space of Retzius.
   b. They are ideal for patients with a large, obstructive prostatic adenoma and a concomitant, small bladder tumor.
   c. They allow direct visualization of prostatic adenoma during enucleation.
   d. They cause no trauma to the urinary bladder.
   e. They require the control of dorsal vein complex before enucleation of an obstructive prostatic adenoma.

7. What is the most common adverse event related to the open prostatectomy?

   a. Erectile dysfunction
   b. Bladder neck contracture
   c. Retrograde ejaculation
   d. Deep vein thrombosis
   e. Stress urinary incontinence

Answers

1. **a. Removal of the prostatic adenoma under direct vision.** When compared with TURP, open prostatectomy offers the advantages of lower retreatment rate and more complete removal of the prostatic adenoma under direct vision and avoids the risk of dilutional hyponatremia (the TURP syndrome) that occurs in approximately 2% of patients undergoing TURP. The disadvantages, as compared with TURP, include the need for a lower midline incision and a resultant longer hospitalization and convalescence period. In addition, there may be an increased potential for perioperative hemorrhage. [p 1423]

2. **c. easier management of a large median lobe and/or bladder calculi.** Because the suprapubic procedure allows direct visualization of the bladder neck and bladder mucosa, this operation is ideally suited for patients with a large median lobe protruding into the bladder or large bladder calculi. [p 1424]

3. **d. a symptomatic bladder diverticulum.** The suprapubic approach is also ideal for a patient with a large prostatic adenoma and a clinically significant bladder diverticulum. [p 1424]

4. **e. suprapubic prostatectomy with bladder diverticulectomy.** Open prostatectomy should be considered when the obstructive tissue is estimated to weigh more than 75 g. If sizable bladder diverticula justify removal, suprapubic prostatectomy and diverticulectomy should be performed concurrently. [p 1424]

5. **a. biopsy-proven prostate cancer.** Contraindications to open prostatectomy include a small fibrous gland, the presence of prostate cancer, previous prostatectomy, or pelvic surgery that may obliterate access to the prostate gland. [p 1424]

6. **a. They are performed in the space of Retzius.** For both the retropubic prostatectomy and the suprapubic prostatectomy, a mild Trendelenburg position is used to increase the distance between the umbilicus and the pubic symphysis and give optimal exposure to the retropubic space. In both procedures, a lower midline incision from the umbilicus to the pubic symphysis permits the linea alba to be incised, allowing the rectus abdominis muscles to be separated in the midline and the transversalis fascia to be incised sharply to expose the space of Retzius. [p 1425]

7. **c. Retrograde ejaculation.** Retrograde ejaculation occurs in approximately 80% to 90% of patients after open prostatectomy. [p 1433]

SECTION VII

REPRODUCTIVE FUNCTION AND DYSFUNCTION

Chapter 42

Male Reproductive Physiology

Peter N. Schlegel • Matthew Hardy

Questions

1. What is the proportion of testicular volume composed of seminiferous tubules in the human testis?

    a. 5%
    b. 10% to 20%
    c. 50% to 60%
    d. 70% to 80%
    e. 90% to 95%

2. Testicular blood supply is derived from all of the following sources except:

    a. internal spermatic artery.
    b. deferential artery.
    c. external spermatic artery.
    d. cremasteric artery.
    e. pudendal artery.

3. In what percentage of cases is more than one artery identifiable in the spermatic cord during inguinal dissection?

    a. 10%
    b. 20%
    c. 50%
    d. 80%
    e. 95%

4. What is the temperature differential between the temperature in the testes and rectal temperature in a normal man?

    a. 0°C
    b. 0–1°C
    c. 1–2°C
    d. 2–3°C
    e. 4–5°C

5. Primary, acute regulation of testosterone is dependent on which of the following hormones?

    a. Luteinizing hormone (LH)
    b. Steroid acute regulatory protein
    c. Follicle-stimulating hormone (FSH)
    d. Estradiol
    e. Inhibin

6. At what age does a testosterone peak occur during a human male's life?

    a. 2 months
    b. 6 to 9 months
    c. 30 to 40 years
    d. 50 to 60 years
    e. >70 years

7. Which hormones play a central role in the regulation of Sertoli cell function?

    a. LH, FSH
    b. FSH, estradiol
    c. Prolactin, LH
    d. FSH, testosterone
    e. Androgen-binding protein (ABP), testosterone

8. Structural components of the blood-testis barrier are seen at which of the following levels?

    a. Sertoli-Sertoli cell junctions
    b. Leydig cells
    c. Basement membrane
    d. Desmosomes between spermatocytes
    e. Spermatids

9. What is the normal developmental pattern of spermatogenic cells?

    a. Sertoli-spermatogonia-spermatocyte
    b. Spermatocyte-spermatogonia-spermatid
    c. Spermatid-Sertoli-spermatocyte
    d. Spermatogonia-spermatid-spermatocyte
    e. Spermatogonia-spermatocyte-spermatid

10. When does mitotic activity of gonocytes end?

    a. Week 36 of gestation
    b. 3 months of life
    c. 2 years of life
    d. 9 years of life
    e. 14 years of life

11. Development of type A spermatogonia to type B spermatogonia depends on:

    a. c-kit.
    b. Fas.
    c. DBY.
    d. SRY.
    e. ABP.

12. Spermiogenesis includes all of the following processes except:

    a. loss of cytoplasm.
    b. formation of the acrosome.

c. flagella formation.
d. migration of cytoplasmic organelles.
e. cell division.

13. The hormone needed for maintenance of spermatogenesis is:

   a. testosterone.
   b. dihydrotestosterone.
   c. estradiol.
   d. oxytocin.
   e. inhibin.

14. What proportion of men with nonobstructive azoospermia have microdeletions of the Y chromosome?

   a. <1%
   b. 2% to 5%
   c. 5% to 10%
   d. 20% to 30%
   e. 50%

15. Major components of the epididymis include:

   a. caput, corpus, cauda.
   b. globus minor, ductus deferens, cauda.
   c. rete testis, efferent ductules, caput.
   d. efferent ductules, caput, cauda.
   e. septa, efferent ductules, corpus.

16. The progenitors of basal cells in the epididymis are:

   a. goblet cells.
   b. pyramidal cells.
   c. neutrophils.
   d. macrophages.
   e. stromal cells.

17. With chronic obstruction, optimal sperm quality is found in what region of the epididymis?

   a. Rete testis
   b. Efferent ducts
   c. Proximal epididymis
   d. Middle epididymis
   e. Distal epididymis

18. Changes in sperm characteristics during epididymal transit include:

   a. increasingly positive charge.
   b. sulfhydryl reduction.
   c. decreased phospholipid content.
   d. reduced membrane rigidity.
   e. increased capacity for glycolysis.

19. Which spermatozoal region contains mitochondria?

   a. The tail
   b. The head
   c. The acrosome
   d. The mid-piece
   e. The dynein cross-arms

20. Human embryonic mitotic activity is controlled by sperm:

   a. DNA.
   b. RNA.
   c. acrosome.
   d. centrosome.
   e. mitochondria.

21. After ejaculation, what happens to the contents of the vas deferens?

   a. They are returned to the seminal vesicles.
   b. They are maintained in the ampulla.
   c. They are released into the ejaculatory ducts.
   d. They are propelled back into the epididymis.
   e. They are released into the bladder.

Answers

1. **d. 70% to 80%.** In humans, interstitial tissue takes up 20% to 30% of the total testicular volume. [p 1441]

2. **e. pudendal artery.** The arterial supply to the human testis and epididymis is derived from three sources: the internal spermatic artery, the deferential artery, and the external spermatic or cremasteric artery. [p 1442]

3. **c. 50%.** An intraoperative dissection study of more than 100 spermatic cords identified a single internal spermatic artery in 50% of cases, with two arteries in 30% of spermatic cords and three arteries in 20%. [pp 1442–1443]

4. **d. 2–3°C.** The countercurrent exchange of heat in the spermatic cord provides blood to the testis that is 2°C to 3°C cooler than the rectal temperature in the normal individual. [p 1442]

5. **a. Luteinizing hormone (LH).** LH stimulates Leydig cells to secrete testosterone. [p 1440]

6. **a. 2 months.** A testosterone peak occurs at approximately 2 months of age. [p 1447]

7. **d. FSH, testosterone.** The consensus is that FSH and testosterone play an important role in the regulation of Sertoli cell function, including ABP production. [p 1449]

8. **a. Sertoli-Sertoli cell junctions.** Sertoli-Sertoli tight junctions prevent the deep penetration of electron-opaque tracers into the seminiferous epithelium from the testicular interstitium. The blood-testis barrier appears to have three different levels within the testis. The primary level is formed by tight junctions between Sertoli cells and segregates premeiotic germ cells (spermatogonia) from other germ cells. [p 1449]

9. **e. Spermatogonia-spermatocyte-spermatid.** Proceeding from the least to the most differentiated, they were named dark type A spermatogonia (Ad); pale type A spermatogonia (Ap); type B spermatogonia (B); preleptotene primary spermatocytes (R); leptotene primary spermatocytes (L); zygotene primary spermatocytes (z); pachytene primary spermatocytes (p); secondary spermatocytes (II); and Sa, Sb1, Sb2, Sc, Sd1, and Sd2 spermatids. [p 1452]

10. **d. 9 years of life.** From 7 to 9 years of life, mitotic activity of gonocytes is detectable, with spermatogonia populating the base of the seminiferous tubule in numbers equal to those of the Sertoli cells. [p 1452]

11. **a. c-kit.** Evidence has suggested that a growth factor/receptor called the *kit* ligand/c-*kit* receptor system is involved in spermtagonial stem cell self-renewal. In fact, the c-*kit* receptor is a marker for type A cells in rats. The result of this process is that some type A_4 spermatogonia differentiate into intermediate and then type B spermatogonia that proceed through spermatogenesis, in a c-*kit*–dependent process, whereas other A_4 spermatogonia renew the stem cell population of type A_1 spermatogonia. [p 1453]

12. **e. cell division.** During spermiogenesis, the products of meiosis, the round Sa spermatids, metamorphose into mature spermatids (see Fig. 42–13). During this metamorphosis, extensive changes occur in both the spermatid cytoplasm and the nucleus, but cell division is not required. These changes have been described in detail and include loss of cytoplasm, formation of the acrosome, formation of the flagellum, and migration of cytoplasmic organelles to positions characteristic of the mature spermatozoon. [pp 1453–1454]

13. **a. testosterone.** Testosterone will initiate and qualitatively maintain spermatogenesis in humans. [p 1456]

14. **c. 5% to 10%.** The detection of microdeletions of a region of the Y chromosome referred to as interval 6 in 5% to 10% of azoospermic men has focused attention on this area as the site for a critical factor (azoospermic factor) important for spermatogenesis. [p 1456]

15. **a. caput, corpus, cauda.** Anatomically, the epididymis is divided into three regions: the caput, the corpus, and the cauda epididymis (see Fig. 42–16). On the basis of histologic criteria, each of these regions can be subdivided into distinct zones separated by transition segments. The human caput epididymis consists of 8 to 12 ductuli efferentes and the proximal segment of the ductus epididymis. The lumen of the ductuli efferentes is large and somewhat irregular in shape near the testis and becomes narrow and oval near the junction with the ductus epididymis. Distal to this junction, the diameter of the duct increases slightly and thereafter remains relatively constant throughout the corpus, or body, of the epididymis. In the bulky cauda epididymis, the diameter of the duct enlarges substantially, and the lumen acquires an irregular shape. [p 1457]

16. **d. macrophages.** Basal cells are thought to be derived from macrophages. [p 1460]

17. **c. Proximal epididymis.** Data from studies of patients with congenital absence of the vas deferens or with epididymal obstruction frequently report poor motility in spermatozoa aspirated from the distal epididymis, with optimal sperm quality in the proximal epididymis. [p 1462]

18. **e. increased capacity for glycolysis.** Spermatozoa undergo numerous metabolic changes during epididymal transit. Studies using experimental animals described the acquisition of an increased capacity for glycolysis, changes in intracellular pH and calcium content, modification of adenylate cyclase activity, and alterations in cellular phospholipid and phospholipid-like fatty acid content. [p 1463]

19. **d. The mid-piece.** The middle piece of the spermatozoon is a highly organized segment consisting of helically arranged mitochondria surrounding a set of outer dense fibers and the characteristic 9 + 2 microtubular structure of the sperm axoneme. [p 1464]

20. **d. centrosome.** In humans, the mitotic activity of embryos appears to be organized normally by the paternally derived centrosome. [p 1456]

21. **d. They are propelled back into the epididymis.** Studies have shown that after sexual stimulation and/or ejaculation, an interesting phenomenon occurred. The contents of the ductus deferens were propelled back toward the proximal epididymis and even into the cauda epididymis, because the distal portion of the ductus deferens contracted with greater amplitude, frequency, and duration than did the proximal portion of the ductus deferens. [p 1467]

Chapter **43**

Male Infertility

Mark Sigman • Jonathan P. Jarow

Questions

1. What are the baseline pregnancy rates by intercourse for fertile and infertile couples?

   a. 50% per month for fertile couples and 30% per month for infertile couples.
   b. The same for both fertile and infertile couples.
   c. 10% per month for fertile couples and 3% per month for infertile couples.
   d. 25% per month for fertile couples and 1% to 3% per month for infertile couples.
   e. 50% per month for fertile couples and 25% per month for infertile couples.

2. How many days does the average sperm remain viable within the normal female reproductive tract?

   a. 1
   b. 3
   c. 5
   d. 7
   e. 10

3. How many days does the average egg remain receptive to fertilization after ovulation?

   a. 1
   b. 2
   c. 4
   d. 6
   e. 10

4. Which of the following lubricants is least likely to adversely affect sperm motility?

   a. K-Y jelly
   b. Astroglide
   c. Saliva
   d. Surgilube
   e. Peanut oil

5. After an acute toxic event such as a febrile illness, how long would you expect sperm counts to be depressed?
   a. 1 week
   b. 3 weeks
   c. 3 months
   d. 6 months
   e. 1 year

6. Which of the following is true of couples in which the woman is approaching 40 years of age?
   a. Pregnancy rates are the same as when the woman is 25 years old.
   b. Treatment is often more aggressive than when the woman is younger.
   c. It is important to treat the infertility in a slow, stepwise manner.
   d. Treatment approaches never include in vitro fertilization (IVF).
   e. Insemination with donor sperm should be encouraged.

7. What percentage of testicular volume is directly involved in producing sperm?
   a. 20%
   b. 40%
   c. 50%
   d. 80%
   e. 100%

8. The evaluation of the infertile male:
   a. should always include at least two semen analyses.
   b. should include semen analysis only if results of the female evaluation are normal.
   c. includes semen analyses, the results of which will determine whether the patient is fertile or sterile.
   d. needs to be performed only if the couple does not conceive after IVF.
   e. should usually include the analysis of semen samples collected by coitus interruptus rather than by masturbation.

9. Low-volume ejaculates may be due to all of the following except:
   a. varicocele.
   b. ejaculatory duct obstruction.
   c. partial retrograde ejaculation.
   d. androgen deficiency.
   e. sympathetic denervation.

10. Couples from whom the semen demonstrates low (<14%) sperm morphology as measured by rigid criteria:
    a. rarely conceive by intercourse.
    b. have low fertilization rates during standard IVF.
    c. probably have infertility due to a varicocele in the male.
    d. have the same fertilization rate during IVF as do couples with normal morphology scores.
    e. cannot conceive by any method.

11. Which of the following statements regarding sperm density and fertility is true?
    a. Couples in which the man has a sperm density below 100 million sperm/ml are likely to be infertile.
    b. Couples in which the man has a sperm density of 70 to 100 million sperm/ml will always be fertile.
    c. Couples in which the man has a sperm density below 20 million sperm/ml are more likely to have a male infertility factor than couples in which the man has a sperm density greater than 20 million sperm/ml.
    d. Couples in which the man has a sperm density greater than 5 million sperm/ml have normal fertility as long as the sperm motility is normal.
    e. Couples in which the man has a sperm density below the average of the normal male population will likely be sterile.

12. Initial hormonal evaluation of an infertile man with a sperm count of 5 million sperm/ml should include assays of testosterone level and:
    a. prolactin.
    b. follicle-stimulating hormone (FSH).
    c. FSH, luteinizing hormone (LH), and prolactin.
    d. FSH and thyroid function.
    e. sex steroid hormone binding globulin (SHBG).

13. What is the next step in the management of an infertile man with low serum testosterone and LH levels associated with a normal prolactin level?
    a. Cranial MRI
    b. Testosterone therapy
    c. Thyroid function studies
    d. Gonadotropin-releasing hormone (GnRH) stimulation test
    e. Gonadotropin therapy

14. The most common cause of low ejaculate volume is:
    a. retrograde ejaculation.
    b. hypogonadism.
    c. incomplete collection.
    d. ejaculatory duct obstruction.
    e. failure of emission.

15. Patients with cystic fibrosis have infertility caused by:
    a. immotile sperm.
    b. obstruction secondary to inspissated secretions.
    c. obstruction due to absence of the vasa.
    d. abnormal spermatogenesis.
    e. hypogonadism.

16. Vasal agenesis is best diagnosed by:
    a. palpation.
    b. scrotal ultrasonography.
    c. vasography.
    d. surgical exploration.
    e. transrectal ultrasonography.

17. Fructose present in the semen is produced by which of the following organs?
    a. Prostate gland
    b. Seminal vesicles
    c. Epididymis
    d. Testis
    e. Glands of Littre

18. What is the best next step in the management of an azoospermic man with normal serum testosterone and FSH, normal testicular volume, and palpable vasa?
    a. Vasography
    b. Transrectal ultrasonography
    c. Testis biopsy
    d. Cranial MRI
    e. Donor insemination

19. What percentage of infertile men have endocrine disorders?
    a. 2%
    b. 10%
    c. 20%
    d. 40%
    e. 50%

20. Isolated asthenospermia may be due to all of the following except:

    a. antisperm antibodies.
    b. lack of dynein arms in the axoneme.
    c. genital tract infection.
    d. varicocele.
    e. prolactinoma.

21. Potential risk factors for the presence of antisperm antibodies include all of the following except:

    a. vasectomy.
    b. Kartagener's syndrome.
    c. cryptorchidism.
    d. genital trauma.
    e. sperm agglutination.

22. Which of the following statements is true regarding direct antisperm antibody assays?

    a. They detect antisperm antibodies in serum.
    b. They are performed only in females.
    c. They determine antibody titers.
    d. They detect antisperm antibodies on sperm.
    e. They are positive in 30% of infertile men.

23. Round cells in semen:

    a. may be white blood cells or immature germ cells.
    b. are most often white blood cells.
    c. always indicate the presence of a genital tract infection.
    d. are normally present in numbers greater than 5 million/ml.
    e. indicate the presence of antisperm antibodies.

24. Which of the following statements is true of semen cultures?

    a. They should be obtained in most men as part of the infertility evaluation.
    b. They often demonstrate distal urethral organisms.
    c. If positive for any bacteria, they indicate a need to treat the male with antibiotics.
    d. They are necessary only in the absence of pyospermia.
    e. They should be obtained for all patients with increased numbers of immature germ cells in the semen.

25. Color Doppler scrotal ultrasonography to detect varicoceles should be obtained in which of the following patient groups?

    a. All infertile men
    b. All infertile men with clinical varicoceles
    c. Infertile men with equivocal examinations
    d. Infertile men with low testosterone levels
    e. After varicocele repair

26. What percentage of patients with unilateral vasal agenesis have upper tract abnormalities?

    a. 10%
    b. 30%
    c. 50%
    d. 80%
    e. 95%

27. Which of the following statements is true regarding the postcoital test?

    a. It need not be performed in couples in which the man's sperm demonstrates poor motility.
    b. Abnormal results always indicate a significant infertility factor.
    c. Results are rarely abnormal because of poor timing relative to ovulation.
    d. Results are dependent on the sperm quality but independent of the cervical mucus quality.
    e. Normal results rule out the presence of a male factor.

28. Differentiation between late maturation arrest and normal spermatogenesis on a testicular biopsy sample is best accomplished by:

    a. spermatid count per tubule.
    b. Sertoli cell count per tubule.
    c. touch preparation.
    d. ratio of spermatids to Sertoli cells.
    e. absolute spermatid count.

29. An azoospermic patient has anosmia, bilateral atrophic testes, and low serum testosterone and LH levels. What is the best treatment for his infertility?

    a. Gonadotropins
    b. Testosterone
    c. Anti-estrogens
    d. Bromocriptine
    e. Cabergoline

30. An infertile man has low testosterone and LH levels and elevated prolactin levels. Cranial MRI reveals a 4 cm pituitary tumor. What is the best next step in management?

    a. Pituitary radiation
    b. Cabergoline
    c. Hypophysectomy
    d. Gonadotropins
    e. Testosterone

31. Which of the following hormone patterns suggests androgen insensitivity?

    a. High testosterone, high LH, normal FSH
    b. High testosterone, normal LH, normal FSH
    c. High testosterone, low LH, low FSH
    d. Low testosterone, high LH, high FSH
    e. Low testosterone, low LH, low FSH

32. Genetic causes of defects in spermatogenesis:

    a. occur with the same frequency in all infertile men regardless of the sperm count.
    b. are all detected by karyotype analysis.
    c. include karyotypic abnormalities and Y chromosome microdeletions.
    d. result in a strict correlation between the genetic findings and testicular histology.
    e. always result in azoospermia.

33. An extra X chromosome in the male:

    a. leads to a higher risk of testicular cancer.
    b. is the hallmark of Klinefelter's syndrome.
    c. means that sperm cannot be recovered from the testicles through attempts at testicular sperm retrieval.
    d. is found in sex reversal syndrome.
    e. has no effect on spermatogenesis.

34. Genes involved in spermatogenesis:

    a. are located on the short arm of the Y chromosome.
    b. when absent, result in intersex phenotypes.
    c. are rarely present in infertile men.
    d. include *DAZ*.
    e. are absent only when the karyotype is abnormal.

35. What percentage of patients with a history of unilateral cryptorchidism have abnormal semen analysis findings?

    a. 10%
    b. 25%

c. 50%
d. 75%
e. 100%

36. Which of the following statements is true regarding varicoceles?

    a. They should be looked for with the patient supine.
    b. They usually result in infertility.
    c. They may affect sperm motility and sperm count.
    d. They result in lower testicular temperatures.
    e. They should always be repaired if identified.

37. Which of the following statements is true regarding Sertoli-cell-only syndrome?

    a. It is diagnosed by examination of testicular histology.
    b. It is caused by a specific deletion on the X chromosome.
    c. It is associated with the absence of Leydig cells.
    d. It is found exclusively in patients with abnormal androgenization.
    e. If present, it precludes finding sperm in testicular tissue.

38. Which of the following situations applies after chemotherapy?

    a. Patients should immediately try to conceive.
    b. Spermatogenesis returns within one spermatogenic cycle.
    c. FSH levels are rarely elevated
    d. Patients who develop azoospermia never regain spermatogenesis.
    e. There is no increased risk of congenital abnormalities in children conceived by these patients.

39. What is the effect of radiation therapy directed at the retroperitoneum, as given to patients with testicular seminoma?

    a. It results in an increase in congenital abnormalities in children born to these patients.
    b. It results in erectile dysfunction in most patients.
    c. It has no effect on spermatogenesis if gonadal shielding is used.
    d. It should be delayed until after the patient desires no more children.
    e. It temporarily depresses spermatogenesis.

40. What is the background spontaneous pregnancy rate for couples with infertility caused by idiopathic oligospermia?

    a. 10%
    b. 25%
    c. 40%
    d. 60%
    e. 75%

41. What is the purported mechanism of action of anti-estrogenic improvement of male fertility?

    a. Reduction of estradiol in the testis
    b. Blocking of conversion of testosterone to estradiol
    c. Enhancement of gonadotropin action in the testis
    d. Blocking of feedback inhibition in the pituitary
    e. Blocking of inhibin

42. Exogenous testosterone administration has a contraceptive effect in the male by:

    a. lowering intratesticular testosterone concentration.
    b. inducing testosterone toxicity.
    c. increasing hepatic production of SHBG.
    d. altering the ratio of testosterone to estradiol.
    e. increasing the testicular production of androgen-binding protein.

43. What is the currently recommended management of a couple with infertility caused by bilateral absence of the vasa deferentia?

    a. Alloplastic spermatocele
    b. Vasal reconstruction
    c. Sperm harvesting and IVF
    d. Donor insemination
    e. Adoption

44. A patient with retrograde ejaculation secondary to prior bladder neck incision is best managed with:

    a. donor insemination.
    b. imipramine.
    c. epididymal sperm aspiration and IVF.
    d. bladder wash and intrauterine insemination.
    e. pseudoephedrine.

45. The initial management of aspermia in a man with a T6 spinal cord injury should be:

    a. vibratory stimulation.
    b. electroejaculation.
    c. seminal vesicle sperm aspiration and IVF.
    d. vasal sperm aspiration and IVF.
    e. epididymal sperm aspiration and IVF.

46. What is the best initial therapy of a patient with low serum testosterone and gonadotropin levels and an elevated 17-hydroxyprogesterone level?

    a. GnRH
    b. Gonadotropins
    c. Testosterone
    d. Cabergoline
    e. Corticosteroids

47. Which of the following management options is inappropriate for the couple in which the man has antisperm antibodies?

    a. IVF with intracytoplasmic sperm injection
    b. Clomiphene therapy for the man
    c. Intrauterine insemination
    d. Donor insemination
    e. Immunosuppressive therapy for the man

48. Which of the following statements is true regarding ultrastructural spermatozoal defects?

    a. They are best detected by 400× microscopic examination of live sperm.
    b. They improve with hormone therapy of the man.
    c. They may be associated with abnormalities of other organ systems.
    d. They result in total necrospermia (dead sperm).
    e. They should be suspected in patients with sperm counts of less than 10 million sperm/ml.

49. Which of the following statements is true regarding controlled ovarian hyperstimulation?

    a. It is commonly used in conjunction with intrauterine insemination and IVF.
    b. It is used only when the female is anovulatory.
    c. It does not increase the risk of multiple gestations with intrauterine insemination.
    d. It should routinely be employed with therapeutic donor insemination.
    e. When combined with intrauterine insemination, it does not increase pregnancy rates compared with intercourse alone for couples in which the man has sperm counts of less than 20 million/ml.

50. Which of the following is true regarding intracytoplasmic sperm injection?

    a. It is used in conjunction with intrauterine insemination.
    b. It involves the injection of spermatogonia into oocytes.

c. It is now the accepted treatment for all men who desire fertility after vasectomy.
d. It is an appropriate option for couples in which the man has idiopathic oligospermia.
e. It should be employed only after therapeutic donor insemination has failed.

51. Which of the following statements is true regarding epididymal sperm aspiration?

a. It is the retrieval technique of choice for patients with nonobstructive azoospermia.
b. It should be reserved for oligospermic patients.
c. It is usually combined with intrauterine insemination.
d. It is used for retrieving sperm from men with Klinefelter's syndrome.
e. It is an appropriate option for men with congenital bilateral absence of the vas deferens.

Answers

1. **d. 25% per month for fertile couples and 1% to 3% per month for infertile couples.** The chance of a fertile couple conceiving is estimated to be approximately 20% to 25% per month, 75% by 6 months, and 90% by 1 year. Of infertile couples without treatment, 25% to 35% will conceive at some time by intercourse alone. Within the first 2 years, 23% will conceive, whereas an additional 10% will do so within 2 more years. This baseline pregnancy rate of 1% to 3% per month (in nonazoospermic couples) must be kept in mind while managing infertile couples and evaluating the results of therapy. [pp 1475–1476]

2. **c. 5.** Studies have shown that conception may occur when sexual relations take place up to 5 days before ovulation but, owing to the short life span of oocytes, will not occur if intercourse is performed the day after ovulation. [p 1476]

3. **a. 1.** There is a 12- to 24-hour period in which the oocyte is within the fallopian tube and is capable of being fertilized. [p 1476]

4. **e. Peanut oil.** Most of the commonly used lubricants, such as Astroglide, Lubafax, K-Y jelly, Keri lotion, Surgilube, and saliva, adversely affect sperm motility. Lubricants that do not impair in vitro sperm motility include peanut oil, safflower oil, vegetable oil, and raw egg white. In general, a couple should be advised to use a lubricant only if necessary and to use a minimal amount of one that does not impair sperm function. [p 1477]

5. **c. 3 months.** After a febrile illness, spermatogenesis may be impaired for 1 to 3 months. [p 1477]

6. **b. Treatment is often more aggressive than when the woman is younger.** It is common to recommend more aggressive therapy in couples in which the woman is approaching 40 years old and to take a slower, stepwise approach in younger couples. [pp 1478–1479]

7. **d. 80%.** Because the majority of the testicular volume (~80%) consists of seminiferous tubules and germinal elements, a reduction in the number of these cells is typically manifested by a reduction in testicular volume or testicular atrophy. [p 1479]

8. **a. should always include at least two semen analyses.** All patients should have at least two semen analyses. [p 1480]

9. **a. varicocele.** Small-volume ejaculates may be produced in patients with obstruction of the ejaculatory ducts, androgen deficiency, retrograde ejaculation, sympathetic denervation, absence of the vas deferens and seminal vesicles, drug therapy, or bladder neck surgery. [p 1481]

10. **b. have low fertilization rates during standard IVF.** Using these criteria, Kruger and associates found that in a group of men with sperm densities greater than 20 million sperm/ml and motility greater than 30%, fertilization rates during IVF were 37% for those with less than 14% normal sperm by strict criteria and 91% for those with greater than 14% normal sperm. [pp 1482–1483]

11. **c. Couples in which the man has a sperm density below 20 million sperm/ml are more likely to have a male infertility factor than couples in which the man has a sperm density greater than 20 million sperm/ml.** The World Health Organization defines the following reference values: volume of 2.0 ml or more; pH of 7.2 or more; sperm concentration of 20×10^6 or more spermatozoa per milliliter; total sperm number of 40×10^6 or more spermatozoa per ejaculate; motility of 50% or more with grade "a+b" motility or 25% or more with grade "a" motility; morphology of 15% or more by strict criteria; viability of 75% or more; white blood cells of less than 1 million/ml. The finding of parameters below these levels is suggestive of infertility, whereas the finding of parameters of above these levels is suggestive of fertility. [p 1484]

12. **b. follicle-stimulating hormone (FSH).** We recommend that all men with an indication in the history or physical examination or a sperm density of less than 10 million/ml have serum FSH and testosterone levels measured because endocrine abnormalities are rarely present when the sperm concentration is greater than 10 million/ml. [p 1485]

13. **a. Cranial MRI.** If the testosterone level remains low, a serum prolactin assay and pituitary MRI should be performed. [p 1485]

14. **c. incomplete collection.** Low ejaculate volume in the nonazoospermic patient is most often due to collection problems, which warrants repeated collection. [p 1486]

15. **c. obstruction due to absence of the vasa.** Congenital bilateral absence of the vasa deferentia (CBAVD) is due to an abnormality in the cystic fibrosis transmembrane conductance regulator (*CFTR*) gene. [p 1477]

16. **a. palpation.** CBAVD is a clinical diagnosis based on physical examination, and further radiologic imaging is not routinely necessary, although a small percentage of these patients have upper tract abnormalities. An abdominal ultrasonographic scan may be obtained. [p 1487]

17. **b. Seminal vesicles.** The seminal vesicles produce fructose in an androgen-dependent process. [p 1483]

18. **c. Testis biopsy.** Patients with vasa present, normal testicular volume, and normal serum FSH levels require testicular biopsy to differentiate between spermatogenic abnormalities and ductal obstruction. [p 1487]

19. **a. 2%.** Although male reproductive function is critically dependent on endocrinologic control, less than 3% of infertile men have a primary hormonal cause. [p 1484]

20. **e. prolactinoma.** Spermatozoal structural defects, prolonged abstinence periods, genital tract infection, antisperm antibodies, partial ductal obstruction, varicoceles, and idiopathic causes may be responsible for cases of asthenospermia. [p 1488]

21. **b. Kartagener's syndrome.** Risk factors for the development of antisperm antibodies include conditions that may disrupt the blood-testis barrier. [p 1490]

22. **d. They detect antisperm antibodies on sperm.** Direct assays detect the presence of antisperm antibodies on the patient's sperm. [p 1490]

23. **a. may be white blood cells or immature germ cells.** Under wet mount microscopy, immature germ cells and leukocytes appear similar and are known as round cells. [p 1491]

24. **b. They often demonstrate distal urethral organisms.** Semen may be cultured for bacterial organisms; however, these cultures frequently yield low concentrations of multiple organisms because of distal urethral contamination. [p 1492]

25. **c. infertile men with equivocal examinations.** Color duplex scrotal ultrasonography should be reserved for those patients with an inadequate physical examination because of either obesity or testicular sensitivity. [p 1494]

26. **d. 80%.** Ipsilateral renal anomalies are present in up to 80% of men with unilateral absence of the vas deferens, with the most common anomaly being renal agenesis. [p 1495]

27. **a. It need not be performed in couples in which the man's sperm demonstrates poor motility.** Because patients with very poor quality semen invariably have poor postcoital test results, it is not necessary to perform this test in this group of patients. [p 1496]

28. **c. touch preparation.** Cases of late maturation arrest are often difficult to differentiate from normal spermatogenesis without the use of a testicular touch preparation. [p 1499]

29. **a. Gonadotropins.** Gonadotropin therapy is required for the initiation of spermatogenesis. [p 1501]

30. **b. Cabergoline.** Although surgery and radiation therapy were used in the past to treat patients with prolactin-secreting pituitary tumors, the vast majority of patients respond to medical therapy. The two most commonly used agents today are bromocriptine and cabergoline. Cabergoline has the advantages of fewer side effects and less frequent dosing required. [p 1503]

31. **a. High testosterone, high LH, normal FSH.** Patients with partial androgen insensitivity have elevated serum testosterone and LH levels. [p 1503]

32. **c. include karyotypic abnormalities and Y chromosome microdeletions.** Genetic causes for male infertility include karyotypic abnormalities (structural or numerical chromosomal abnormalities), Y chromosome microdeletions, and autosomal gene mutations. [p 1497]

33. **b. is the hallmark of Klinefelter's syndrome.** The presence of an extra X chromosome is the genetic hallmark of Klinefelter's syndrome. [p 1504]

34. **d. include DAZ** The gene deleted in azoospermia (*DAZ*) is one of the genes thought to be responsible for spermatogenic defects in patients with deletions in this interval. [p 1505]

35. **b. 25%.** Sperm concentrations below 12 to 20 million/ml are found in 50% of patients with bilateral cryptorchidism and in approximately 25% of patients with unilateral cryptorchidism. [p 1506]

36. **c. They may affect sperm motility and sperm count.** Semen samples from men with varicoceles have demonstrated decreased motility in 90% of patients and sperm concentrations of less than 20 million sperm/ml in 65% of patients. [p 1507]

37. **a. It is diagnosed by examination of testicular histology.** Sertoli-cell-only syndrome is a histologic diagnosis. [p 1508]

38. **e. There is no increased risk of congenital abnormalities in children conceived by these patients.** There appears to be no increased risk of birth defects in children born to patients who have received chemotherapy. [p 1509]

39. **e. It temporarily depresses spermatogenesis.** Semen quality will usually return to baseline within 2 years after radiation therapy for seminoma. [p 1509]

40. **b. 25%.** There is a significant background pregnancy rate (26%) for untreated couples with abnormal semen parameters. [p 1511]

41. **d. Blocking feedback inhibition in the pituitary.** They increase pituitary gonadotropin secretion by blocking feedback inhibition, thus increasing serum FSH and LH levels as well as the testicular production of testosterone. [p 1511]

42. **a. lowering intratesticular testosterone concentration.** Continuous androgen administration has a contraceptive effect on men by lowering intratesticular testosterone concentration and should never be used in the treatment of infertility. [p 1512]

43. **c. Sperm harvesting and IVF.** The currently recommended management of couples with infertility due to CBAVD is sperm retrieval combined with IVF using intracytoplasmic sperm injection after appropriate genetic testing and counseling of the couple regarding the risk of cystic fibrosis. [p 1512]

44. **d. bladder wash and intrauterine insemination.** Those patients with retrograde ejaculation unresponsive to medical therapy or due to ablation of the bladder neck may be treated by recovery of sperm from the bladder urine combined with intrauterine insemination. [p 1513]

45. **a. vibratory stimulation.** Penile vibratory stimulation results in ejaculation in approximately 70% of spinal cord–injured men. Although specially designed equipment with specific vibration frequency and amplitudes is available, many practitioners have had good results using readily available vibrators intended for general use. This approach should be used in patients with upper motor neuron lesions such as spinal cord injuries above T10. [p 1513]

46. **e. Corticosteroids.** Glucocorticoid therapy results in a reduction of adrenocorticotropic hormone levels, which induces a decrease in peripheral adrenal androgens, thus stimulating endogenous gonadotropin secretion and testicular steroidogenesis. [p 1502]

47. **b. Clomiphene therapy for the man.** Although we present the patient with the option of corticosteroid treatment, we encourage couples to consider intrauterine insemination or IVF with intracytoplasmic sperm injection if the semen is of adequate quality. For couples wishing to proceed with immunosuppressive therapy, we recommend an intermediate cyclic steroid regimen such as the one used by Hendry and coauthors. [p 1514]

48. **c. They may be associated with abnormalities of other organ systems.** When these clinical findings are combined with situs inversus, which is present in 50% of these cases, the patient has Kartagener's syndrome. [p 1514]

49. **a. It is commonly used in conjunction with intrauterine insemination and IVF.** Controlled ovarian hyperstimulation, hormonal stimulation of superovulation using gonadotropins, plays a crucial part in most forms of assisted reproductive techniques. [p 1515]

50. **d. It is an appropriate option for couples in which the man has idiopathic oligospermia.** IVF with intracytoplasmic sperm injection is indicated in cases of severe male factor infertility, in couples with prior failed or poor fertilization during regular IVF cycles, or in cases in which the sperm demonstrate significant fertilizing ability defects (such as with rounded-head sperm). [p 1517]

51. **e. It is an appropriate option for men with congenital bilateral absence of the vas deferens.** Microsurgical epididymal sperm aspiration is commonly employed to retrieve sperm out of the ductal system in cases with obstructive azoospermia such as congenital bilateral absence of the vasa deferentia. [p 1517]

Chapter 44

Surgery for Male Infertility and Other Scrotal Disorders

Marc Goldstein

Questions

1. Which of the following venous structures are intentionally preserved during varicocelectomy?

    a. External spermatic veins
    b. Internal spermatic veins
    c. Gubernacular veins
    d. Vasal veins
    e. Cremasteric veins

2. In the evaluation for vasectomy reversal, which of the following clinical findings is suggestive of epididymal obstruction?

    a. Varicocele
    b. Hydrocele
    c. Sperm granuloma
    d. Normal serum follicle-stimulating hormone (FSH) level
    e. Vasal gap larger than 2 cm

3. All of the following reduce the potential complications of vasography except:

    a. using water-soluble, low-ionic contrast medium.
    b. diluting the contrast medium.
    c. flushing with saline or lactated Ringer's solution after contrast medium infusion.
    d. performing vasography as an isolated diagnostic procedure.
    e. using low injection pressure.

4. Which of the following is not an indication for crossed vasovasostomy?

    a. Right: inguinal vas obstruction and normal testis; left: patent vas and atrophic testis
    b. Right: epididymal obstruction, patent vas, and normal testis; left: ejaculatory duct obstruction, patent vas, and normal testis
    c. Right: inguinal vas obstruction and normal testis; left: epididymal obstruction, patent vas, and normal testis
    d. Right: epididymal obstruction, and patent vas above vasectomy site; left: sperm in testicular end of vas and vasectomy site in convoluted vas
    e. Right: congenital absence of epididymis and normal patent vas; left: normal testis and partial absence of vas ending retroperitoneally.

5. A 25-year-old healthy man, presenting with primary infertility, was found to have azoospermia on two semen analyses and normal serum testosterone and FSH. Scrotal examination findings were normal. A subclinical varicocele was documented on the left side. Which of the following is the best option for management?

    a. Karyotype analysis
    b. Surgical repair of the varicocele
    c. Vasogram
    d. Surgical sperm retrieval for assisted reproduction
    e. Testis biopsy

6. Compared with the other surgical options for varicocelectomy, the advantages of performing a subinguinal microsurgical varicocelectomy include all of the following except:

    a. lower rate of arterial injury.
    b. lower rate of postoperative hydrocele.
    c. lower rate of varicocele recurrence.
    d. fewer number of veins to be ligated.
    e. lower overall complication rate.

7. Which of the following maneuvers should be avoided when bridging a large vasal gap during vasovasostomy?

    a. Mobilization of the vas deferens toward the external inguinal ring
    b. Dissection of the sheath of the convoluted vas deferens off the epididymis and allowing the testis to drop upside down
    c. Separation of the cauda and corpus epididymis from the testis
    d. Mobilization of the vas deferens toward the internal inguinal ring
    e. Unraveling of the convoluted vas deferens

8. During a vasovasostomy, difficulty with saline injection toward the abdominal vas was encountered. Which of the following is the least likely to provide evidence to confirm a vasal obstruction?

a. Testicular biopsy with touch preparation
b. Formal radiocontrast vasogram
c. Transrectal ultrasonographic scan
d. Indigo carmine vasogram and examination of the urine
e. Threading a suture into the abdominal vas

9. In which of the following scenarios is a testis biopsy least helpful?

a. Failure to retrieve motile sperm from the epididymis
b. Sperm retrieval for nonobstructive azoospermia
c. Diagnostic evaluation of men with congenital absence of vas and normal FSH levels
d. Diagnostic evaluation in azoospermic men with normal findings on scrotal examination and normal serum testosterone and FSH levels
e. Sperm retrieval for men diagnosed with a Sertoli-cell-only pattern in the testes

10. Which of the following scenarios has the lowest patency rate for vasectomy reversal?

a. Motile sperm in the vas and vasovasostomy
b. Nonmotile sperm in the vas and vasovasostomy
c. Motile sperm in the vas and unilateral crossed vasovasostomy
d. Thick, white vasal fluid devoid of sperm and vasovasostomy
e. Copious clear vasal fluid but no sperm and vasovasostomy

11. In the evaluation for azoospermia, all of the following tests should be considered to confirm a diagnosis of obstructive azoospermia except:

a. transrectal ultrasonography.
b. testicular biopsy.
c. antisperm antibody assay.
d. epididymal biopsy.
e. serum testosterone and FSH assay.

12. In discussing the management options for an adult with bilateral cryptorchidism, which of the following is correct?

a. The patient has no chance of fathering children biologically.
b. No further management is necessary.
c. Spermatogenic function is more likely than the endocrinogenic function of the testes to be preserved.
d. In adults with cryptorchidism the risk of testes tumor is similar to the risk in the general population.
e. Bilateral orchiopexy should be considered.

13. Which of the following is true regarding varicocele?

a. Treatment in infertile men rarely results in improved semen parameters.
b. Severity of testicular insult is related to the size of the varicoceles.
c. Severity of testicular insult from varicocele is duration independent.
d. Because of the severity of testicular insult, repair of large varicoceles is not warranted.
e. Surgical treatment of subclinical varicoceles results in greater improvement in semen quality than treatment of large varicoceles.

14. After a bilateral vasoepididymostomy, a patient remained azoospermic in two semen analyses until 6 months postoperatively, when the analysis revealed 8 million sperm/ml with 60% motility. What is the next management step?

a. A plan for intrauterine insemination with ejaculated sperm
b. A plan for assisted reproduction with intracytoplasmic sperm injection (ICSI) and ejaculated sperm
c. Cryopreservation of semen
d. No follow-up is necessary
e. Scrotal ultrasound

15. Which of the following vessels has the least direct contribution to the arterial supply of the vas deferens?

a. Deferential artery
b. Hypogastric artery
c. Inferior epididymal artery
d. External spermatic artery
e. Superior vesicle artery

16. Which of the following is a disadvantage of the intussusception vasoepididymostomy?

a. Inability to assess epididymal fluid for sperm before setting up for anastomosis
b. Lower patency rate than end-to-side and end-to-end techniques
c. Difficult hemostasis
d. Placement of sutures into a collapsed epididymal tubule
e. Transection of the epididymis required before anastomosis

17. Sperm retrieval by percutaneous testicular biopsy is most appropriate with which of the following types of patients?

a. Patients with congenital bilateral absence of vas
b. Patients with previous orchiopexy
c. Patients with severe hypospermatogenesis on previous biopsy
d. Patients with hydroceles
e. Patients with Klinefelter's syndrome

18. All of the following situations are appropriate for assisted reproduction with ICSI as a first line of treatment except:

a. obstruction with multiple failures of reconstruction.
b. mild oligoasthenospermia with varicoceles and a female partner of 29 years of age.
c. Klinefelter's syndrome.
d. only few viable sperm found in the ejaculate.
e. postchemotherapy azoospermia.

19. In which of the following settings are vasovasostomy and vasoepididymostomy contraindicated?

a. Previous vasectomy more than 20 years ago
b. Concomitant scrotal pain
c. Concomitant hydrocele
d. Concomitant varicoceles
e. Nonobstructive azoospermia

20. In the presence of epididymal obstruction, which of the following statements is false?

a. The quality of sperm is better in caput than caudal tubules
b. Vasoepididymostomy to the caudal tubules has a better patency rate than the caput tubules
c. Vasovasostomy can yield a satisfactory patency rate
d. A scrotal sonogram may demonstrate epididymal fullness and hydrocele
e. Intraoperative sperm cryopreservation is possible

21. Which of the following statements is true regarding microsurgical testicular sperm extraction?

a. Sertoli-cell-only pattern is a contraindication for the procedure.
b. Small seminiferous tubules typically give a higher sperm yield.
c. It can be performed percutaneously.
d. It can better preserve the blood supply to testis parenchyma than a nonmicrosurgical method.

e. It should not be used in men with nonobstructive azoospermia.

22. For managing chronic orchialgia, which of the following statements is true?

    a. Imaging studies are not indicated.
    b. Effective surgical treatment with epididymectomy should be considered early.
    c. A specific cause should be identified for effective treatment.
    d. If no specific cause is identified, surgical treatment such as epididymectomy or total denervation should be offered.
    e. Varicocele is never causative.

23. All of the following are expected outcomes of varicocele repair except:

    a. improved sperm motility.
    b. increased risk of multiple gestation.
    c. improved sperm counts.
    d. elevated serum testosterone levels.
    e. return of sperm to the ejaculate in azoospermic men.

24. A 30-year-old man presenting with primary infertility was found to be azoospermic on two semen analyses. Which of the following findings would contraindicate a testicular biopsy for diagnostic purposes?

    a. Ejaculate volume below 2.0 ml
    b. Semen pH less than 7.2
    c. Semen negative for fructose
    d. Serum FSH greater than 25 IU/l
    e. Absence of vasa deferentia and normal serum FSH level

25. Which of the following is true regarding percutaneous epididymal sperm aspiration (PESA) compared with microsurgical epididymal sperm aspiration (MESA)?

    a. PESA yields a better quantity of sperm.
    b. PESA can be performed with local anesthesia.
    c. MESA is the procedure of choice for nonobstructive azoospermia.
    d. PESA is associated with a higher pregnancy rate.
    e. PESA yields better sperm quality.

26. In which of the following scenarios is a vasogram indicated?

    a. Azoospermia, Sertoli-cell-only on testis biopsy
    b. Azoospermia, testicular volume of 10 ml, FSH value 25 IU/l
    c. Azoospermia, normal testicular volume and biopsy
    d. Azoospermia, no palpable vasa deferentia
    e. Sperm count 5.0×10^6/ml, 5% motility, grade II varicoceles bilaterally

27. All of the following diagnoses can be made from a radiocontrast vasogram except:

    a. inguinal vasal obstruction.
    b. ejaculatory duct obstruction.
    c. seminal vesicle agenesis.
    d. spermatogenic failure.
    e. partial agenesis of vasa deferentia.

28. Which of the following is true regarding hydrocelectomy?

    a. Hematoma is the most frequent complication.
    b. In repair of large hydrocele, epididymal injury rarely occurs.
    c. A window operation is the procedure of choice for large hydroceles.
    d. Sclerotherapy should be attempted before surgical treatment.
    e. Jaboulay's bottleneck operation is associated with a high recurrence rate.

29. Which of the following is true regarding varicocele in the pediatric population?

    a. There is a high rate of testicular atrophy after inadvertent ligation of testicular artery.
    b. The rate of recurrence after nonmicrosurgical repair is higher than in the adult population.
    c. Subclinical varicoceles should be treated.
    d. Treatment of varicocele should be offered only after the age of 18 years when there is interest in fertility.
    e. Surgical repair in this age group is best performed scrotally.

30. Which of the following is the best diagnostic study to determine whether an azoospermic man has ejaculatory duct obstruction?

    a. Semen fructose test
    b. Complete semen analysis
    c. Antisperm antibody assay
    d. Transrectal ultrasonography
    e. Cystoscopy

31. All of the following are potential complications of transurethral resection of the ejaculatory ducts except:

    a. urinary incontinence.
    b. retrograde ejaculation.
    c. recurrent epididymitis.
    d. testicular atrophy.
    e. urethral stricture.

32. Which of the following treatments for hydrocele is contraindicated in a younger man interested in fertility?

    a. Jaboulay's hydrocele excision
    b. Lord's plication
    c. Window operation
    d. Dartos pouch technique
    e. Sclerotherapy

33. What is the pathogenesis of postvaricocelectomy hydrocele?

    a. Increased testicular venous pressure
    b. Lymphatic obstruction
    c. Soft tissue fibrosis
    d. Arterial injury
    e. Catch-up growth of testes

34. In which of the following scenarios is a subinguinal incision for varicocelectomy contraindicated?

    a. Obese patients
    b. Previous ipsilateral inguinal hernia repair
    c. Prepubertal varicocele
    d. Large varicocele
    e. Prior orchiopexy

35. Which of the following is correct regarding the ejaculatory duct?

    a. It is a single midline duct formed by the confluence of the seminal vesicle ducts.
    b. It enters into the middle of the verumontanum.
    c. It joins with the prostatic ducts.
    d. It is a paired duct formed by the confluence of each seminal vesicle duct and vasa deferentia.
    e. It enters directly into the vesicle trigone.

36. A nontransilluminating, nontender mass is noted in the epididymis on physical examination and confirmed to be solid by sonography. What is the most likely diagnosis?

a. Epididymal cyst
b. Spermatocele
c. Hydrocele
d. Lymphoma
e. Adenomatoid tumor

37. All of the following are potential complications of vasography except:

    a. vasal obstruction at the site of vasography.
    b. perivasal hematoma.
    c. sperm granuloma at the site of vasography.
    d. injury to the vasal artery.
    e. retrograde ejaculation.

38. What is the estimated percentage of men who develop antisperm antibodies after vasectomy?

    a. 0% to 20%
    b. 20% to 40%
    c. 40% to 60%
    d. 60% to 80%
    e. >80%

39. Intraoperatively during a vasectomy reversal, a sperm granuloma is found on the left side. What does this indicate?

    a. Concomitant epididymal obstruction that requires a vasoepididymostomy
    b. Infection requiring postoperative antibiotics for 5 to 7 days
    c. The need for genetic counseling
    d. That sperm will be found at the testicular end of the vas
    e. That the procedure should be abandoned and the patient should undergo re-exploration in 3 months

40. When is the best time to perform vasography?

    a. At the time of diagnostic testis biopsy
    b. At the time of reconstruction if a prior testis biopsy result was normal
    c. At the time of scrotal ultrasonography with color flow Doppler
    d. At the time of transrectal ultrasonography revealing normal seminal vesicles
    e. At the time of electroejaculation

41. Twelve years after vasectomy, a man was found on routine examination to have asymptomatic sperm granulomas bilaterally. All of the following scenarios are true except which one?

    a. Microrecanalization is possible with the appearance of rare sperm in the ejaculate.
    b. If vasectomy reversal is performed, only bilateral vasovasostomy is likely to be necessary.
    c. The epididymides are unlikely to be indurated.
    d. The epididymides are likely to be obstructed.
    e. No treatment is necessary for asymptomatic sperm granuloma.

42. What is the most common complication of nonmicrosurgical varicocelectomy?

    a. Vasal obstruction
    b. Testicular atrophy
    c. Varicocele recurrence
    d. Epididymal injury
    e. Hydrocele

43. Which of the following techniques of varicocele repair has the highest recurrence rate?

    a. Retroperitoneal ligation
    b. Laparoscopic ligation
    c. Microsurgical ligation
    d. Nonmicrosurgical ligation
    e. Radiographic embolization

44. A midline cyst compressing the ejaculatory duct is found on a transrectal ultrasonographic scan. What does the presence of sperm in the cyst aspirate suggest?

    a. Congenital absence of vas on at least one side
    b. Nonobstructive azoospermia
    c. Bilateral epididymal obstruction
    d. The possibility of XXY karyotype
    e. Patency of a vas deferens and epididymis on at least one side

45. Six months after transurethral resection of the ejaculatory ducts, the patient develops retrograde ejaculation. What is the next step of management?

    a. Watchful waiting
    b. Intrauterine insemination
    c. ICSI
    d. A trial of pseudoephedrine
    e. Electroejaculation

46. Which of the following is an indication for repeated vasectomy?

    a. Painless sperm granuloma
    b. Tender epididymitis
    c. Rare nonmotile sperm found in spun semen analysis 12 weeks after vasectomy
    d. Rare motile sperm found in semen analysis 6 weeks after vasectomy
    e. Motile sperm found in semen analysis 3 months after vasectomy

47. After vasectomy, where in the reproductive tract does most of the pressure-induced injury occur?

    a. Testis
    b. Epididymis
    c. Convoluted portion of the vas
    d. Straight portion of the vas
    e. Ejaculatory duct

48. Simultaneous vasectomy reversal and microsurgical varicocelectomy should be approached with caution because of:

    a. testicular ischemia from arterial insufficiency.
    b. higher risk of testicular venous congestion.
    c. higher risk of lymphatic obstruction.
    d. prolonged anesthesia time.
    e. high likelihood of epididymal injury requiring a vasoepididymostomy.

49. One year after vasovasostomy, a progressive decline in sperm motility and sperm counts is noted. What does this indicate?

    a. Progressive spermatogenic failure
    b. Infection
    c. Arterial injury to the testis and epididymis
    d. Ejaculatory duct obstruction
    e. Stricture of the vasovasostomy

50. In which of the following scenarios would a diagnostic testicular biopsy provide valuable clinical information?

    a. Men with azoospermia and an FSH level of 25 IU/L
    b. Men with a 47,XXY karyotype
    c. Men with a fecundity history who seek vasectomy reversal
    d. Men with primary infertility, azoospermia, normal physical examination findings, and normal serum FSH level
    e. Men with anejaculation caused by high spinal cord injury

51. Which of the following is true regarding retractile testes in adults?

    a. As in the pediatric population, surgical repair is never indicated.
    b. A dartos pouch operation is the treatment of choice.
    c. Simple three-stitch orchiopexy of the tunica albuginea to the dartos, as for torsion prophylaxis, is effective in preventing retraction.
    d. Bilateral orchiopexy is necessary for unilateral retractile testis.
    e. Coexisting varicocele is common.

52. Which of the following is true regarding vasoepididymostomy?

    a. End-to-side anastomosis currently has the highest patency rate.
    b. Microsurgical technique does not significantly improve the surgical outcome.
    c. Assisted reproduction with ICSI is a more cost-effective option.
    d. It should be reserved for azoospermic patients with spermatogenic arrest.
    e. It should be performed only to an epididymal tubule containing sperm.

53. When a vasoepididymostomy is performed for fertility reasons, which of the following should be routinely done in the same setting?

    a. Intraoperative epididymal sperm aspiration for sperm cryopreservation
    b. Testicular biopsy for sperm cryopreservation
    c. A touch preparation of testicular tissue
    d. A squash preparation of testicular tissue
    e. A radiocontrast vasogram

54. Which of the following statements is true regarding chronic intermittent testicular torsion?

    a. The torsion episodes are similar to acute torsion episodes but are less severe.
    b. Physical examination of the scrotum is reliable in making the diagnosis.
    c. Ipsilateral orchiopexy is the treatment of choice.
    d. Dartos pouch orchiopexy is not effective.
    e. The torsion is always associated with congenital absence of the vas.

55. Regarding the management of chronic orchialgia of undetermined origin, all of the following statements are true except which one?

    a. Denervation is an effective surgical treatment.
    b. Orchiectomy is the primary surgical treatment of choice.
    c. Various forms of conservative management should be attempted initially.
    d. Epididymectomy is an effective treatment for postvasectomy orchialgia.
    e. Psychosocial stress factors should be considered potential causes.

56. Which of the following is the most important factor in ensuring a high patency rate after a vasovasostomy?

    a. Age of the patient
    b. Time since vasectomy
    c. Surgeon's technique and experience
    d. Presence of motile sperm in the vasal fluid
    e. Presence of a sperm granuloma at the vasectomy site

57. Which of the following surgical sperm retrieval techniques is inappropriate for the clinical situation indicated?

    a. PESA for congenital absence of vas
    b. Percutaneous testicular sperm aspiration (TESA) after failed vasoepididymostomy
    c. Electroejaculation in a man with post-retroperitoneal lymph node dissection for left testicular embryonal carcinoma
    d. MESA for spermatogenic maturation arrest
    e. Testicular sperm extraction (TESE) in a man with azoospermia from chemotherapy

58. In recent years, the use of microsurgery in the treatment of male infertility has expanded to all of the following procedures except which one?

    a. Varicocelectomy
    b. Surgical sperm retrieval
    c. Vasectomy reversal
    d. Diagnostic testis biopsy
    e. Orchiopexy for retractile testis

59. Which of the following is true for end-to-side open tubule vasoepididymostomy?

    a. It permits easy placement of microsutures to a distended epididymal tubule.
    b. It requires tedious hemostasis.
    c. It causes disruption of blood supply to the caudal epididymis.
    d. It is the procedure of choice in the presence of ejaculatory duct obstruction.
    e. It allows examination of epididymal fluid before microanastomosis is performed.

60. All of the following conditions can lead to orchialgia except which one?

    a. Sperm granuloma
    b. Varicocele
    c. Hernia repair
    d. Congenital absence of vas
    e. Vasectomy

Answers

1. **d. Vasal veins.** All veins within the cord, with the exception of the vasal veins, are doubly ligated. Scrotal or gubernacular collateral veins have been demonstrated radiographically to be the cause of 10% of recurrent varicoceles. All external spermatic veins are identified and doubly ligated with hemoclips and divided (see Fig. 44–59). The gubernaculum is inspected for the presence of veins exiting from the tunica vaginalis. These are either cauterized or doubly clipped and divided. [pp 1574–1575]

2. **b. Hydrocele.** The presence of a hydrocele in the face of excurrent ductal system obstruction is often associated with secondary epididymal obstruction. Surgeons attempting reconstruction should be aware of the possibility of the need for a vasoepididymostomy. [p 1547]

3. **d. performing vasography as an isolated diagnostic procedure.** All other options can reduce the complications of vasography. Vasography should not be performed as an iso-

4. **d. Right: epididymal obstruction, patent vas above vasectomy site, and normal testis; left: sperm in testicular end vas and vasectomy site in convoluted vas.** Crossover is indicated in the following circumstances: (1) unilateral inguinal obstruction of the vas deferens associated with an atrophic testis on the contralateral side. A crossover vasovasostomy should be performed to connect a healthy testicle to the contralateral unobstructed vas. (2) Obstruction or aplasia of the inguinal vas or ejaculatory duct on one side and epididymal obstruction on the contralateral side. It is preferable to perform one anastomosis with a high probability of success (vasovasostomy) than two operations with a much lower chance of success, such as unilateral vasovasoepididymostomy and contralateral transurethral resection of the ejaculatory ducts. [p 1554]

5. **e. Testis biopsy.** Testis biopsy is indicated in azoospermic men with testis of normal size and consistency, palpable vasa deferentia, and normal serum FSH levels. Varicoceles that are impalpable on a good physical examination are considered subclinical and probably do not warrant treatment. [pp 1534 and 1571]

6. **d. fewer number of veins to be ligated.** At the subinguinal level, significantly more veins are encountered, the artery is more often surrounded by a network of tiny veins that must be ligated, and the testicular artery has often divided into two or three branches, making arterial identification and preservation more difficult without using a microscope for the procedure. [p 1573]

7. **e. Unraveling of the convoluted vas deferens.** When large vasal gaps are present, a gauze-wrapped index finger is used to bluntly separate the cord structures from the vas. Blunt finger dissection through the external ring will free the vas to the internal inguinal ring if additional abdominal side length is necessary. These maneuvers will leave all the vasal vessels intact. When the vasal gap is extremely large, additional length can be achieved by dissecting the entire convoluted vas free of its attachments to the epididymal tunica (see Fig. 44–24), allowing the testis to drop upside down. If the amount of vas removed is so large that even these measures fail to allow a tension-free anastomosis, the incision can be extended to the internal inguinal ring, the floor of the inguinal canal cut, and the vas rerouted under the floor, as in a difficult orchiopexy. An additional 4 to 6 cm of length can be obtained by dissecting the epididymis off of the testis from the vasoepididymal junction to the caput epididymis (see Fig. 44–25). The superior epididymal vessels are left intact and provide adequate blood supply to the testicular end of the vas. With this combination of maneuvers, gaps up to 10 cm wide can be bridged. The convoluted vas should not be unraveled. This disturbs the blood supply at the anastomotic line. [pp 1548–1549 and 1554]

8. **a. Testicular biopsy with touch preparation.** If further proof of patency of the vas deferens is desired, 1 ml of 50% dilute indigo carmine dye can be injected and the bladder catheterized. The presence of blue-green dye in the urine confirms patency of the vas. Indigo carmine diluted 50/50 with Ringer's solution is preferred over methylene blue because, even at low concentrations, methylene blue kills sperm and renders them useless for cryopreservation or immediate in vitro fertilization (IVF) or intracytoplasmic sperm injection (ICSI). If a large amount of fluid is found in the vasal lumen and microscopic examination reveals the presence of sperm, the obstruction is toward the seminal vesicle end of the vas. In these cases, the vas is usually markedly dilated. A 2-0 proline suture can be passed toward the seminal vesicle end of the vas and a clamp placed on the proline when the suture passes no further. This is particularly useful for delineating the site of inguinal obstruction from prior groin surgery. Formal vasography is then performed. After the vasa have been cannulated, vasograms are performed with the injection of 0.5 ml of water-soluble contrast media (see Fig. 44–6). If vasography reveals obstruction at the site of the ejaculatory ducts (see Fig. 44–7), indigo carmine dye is injected in both vasa to facilitate a transurethral resection of the ejaculatory ducts. If both vasa are visualized after injection of contrast material into only one vas (see Fig. 44–8), both vasa empty into a single cavity, usually a midline ejaculatory duct cyst. If transrectal ultrasonography reveals dilated seminal vesicles and/or a midline (müllerian duct) cyst, transrectal fine-needle aspiration followed by instillation of contrast material and indigo carmine dye should be performed. If motile sperm are found, they should be cryopreserved. [p 1534]

9. **c. Diagnostic evaluation of men with congenital absence of vas.** Testis biopsy is indicated in azoospermic men with testes of normal size and consistency, palpable vasa deferentia, and normal serum FSH levels. Under these circumstances, biopsy will distinguish obstructive azoospermia from primary seminiferous tubular failure. In the testes of men with congenital absence of vasa, biopsy always reveals normal or at least some spermatogenesis, and biopsy is not necessary before definitive sperm aspiration and IVF with ICSI. [p 1534]

10. **d. thick, white vasal fluid devoid of sperm and vasovasostomy.** If the fluid expressed from the vas is found to be thick, white, water insoluble, and toothpaste-like in quality, microscopic examination rarely reveals sperm. Under these circumstances, the tunica vaginalis is opened and the epididymis inspected. If clear evidence of obstruction is found—for example, an epididymal sperm granuloma with dilated tubules above and collapsed tubules below—vasoepididymostomy is performed. When the surgeon is in doubt or is not very experienced with vasoepididymostomy, vasovasostomy should be performed. However, only 15% of men with bilateral absence of sperm in the vasal fluid after barbotage and an intensive search will have sperm return to the ejaculate after vasovasostomy. [p 1550]

11. **d. epididymal biopsy.** Before attempted surgical reconstruction of the reproductive tract, spermatogenesis in the patient should be evident. A testicular biopsy may be indicated to confirm the presence of spermatogenesis. Men with a low semen volume should have a transrectal ultrasonographic scan to alert one to the possibility of an additional ejaculatory duct obstruction. For serum and antisperm antibody studies, the presence of serum antisperm antibodies corroborates the diagnosis of obstruction and the presence of active spermatogenesis. At present, this test is of unknown prognostic value and is optional. For serum FSH assay, men with small soft testes should have serum FSH measured. An elevated FSH level suggests impaired spermatogenesis and potentially a poorer prognosis. [p 1547]

12. **e. Bilateral orchiopexy should be considered.** If the contralateral testis is normal, the patient may be fertile. If both testes are truly undescended, azoospermia is certain. In the past, bilateral orchiectomy was usually recommended in adults with undescended testes because of the substantially increased risk of testes tumor. Orchiectomy, however, condemns these men to absolute sterility and a lifetime of hormone replacement therapy. Bilateral orchiopexy in adults can result in induction of spermatogenesis and pregnancy. It will also preserve testicular hormonal function. [p 1581]

13. **b. Severity of testicular insult is related to the size of the varicoceles.** Larger varicoceles appear to cause more damage

than small varicoceles; large varicoceles are associated with greater preoperative impairment in semen quality than are small varicoceles. [p 1578]

14. **c. Cryopreservation of semen.** With the older end-to-end or end-to-side vasoepididymostomy method, at 14 months after surgery 25% of initially patent anastomoses have shut down. For this reason, we recommend banking sperm both intraoperatively and as soon as sperm appear in the ejaculate postoperatively. [p 1564]

15. **d. External spermatic artery.** The blood supply of major scrotal organs is summarized in Table 44–1: blood supply to the vas deferens includes the deferential artery at the seminal vesicle end and the deferential artery and inferior epididymal artery at the testicular end. [p 1534]

16. **a. Inability to assess epididymal fluid for sperm before setting up for anastomosis.** This method, also known as the triangulation technique, was introduced by Berger. There are several advantages of this method over previous techniques (see Table 44–3): two or three sutures placed in the epididymal tubule provide four and six points of fixation, and the anastomosis is virtually bloodless. However, one cannot assess tubular fluid for sperm before the anastomosis set-up. [pp 1558 and 1560]

17. **a. Patients with congenital bilateral absence of vas.** The percutaneous methods are most appropriate in men with normal spermatogenesis and obstructive azoospermia, when adequate numbers of sperm can be retrieved in a small amount of tissue. [p 1568]

18. **b. mild oligoasthenospermia with varicoceles and a female partner of 29 years of age.** Assisted reproduction can be offered to men with surgically unreconstructable obstruction such as congenital absence of the vas deferens; men with few viable sperm in the ejaculate; azoospermic men with varicoceles (half of these men will respond to varicocelectomy with return of enough sperm to ejaculate to achieve pregnancy using IVF with ICSI); and men with nonobstructive azoospermia. [p 1570]

19. **e. Nonobstructive azoospermia.** Before attempted surgical reconstruction of the reproductive tract, spermatogenesis in the patient should be evident. A prior history of natural fertility prevasectomy is usually adequate. In other cases, a testicular biopsy may be indicated to confirm the presence of spermatogenesis. [p 1547]

20. **c. Vasovasostomy can yield a satisfactory patency rate.** If clear evidence of obstruction is found, vasoepididymostomy is performed. When there is doubt or the physician is not very experienced with vasoepididymostomy, vasovasostomy should be performed. However, only 15% of men with bilateral absence of sperm in the vasal fluid after barbotage and an intensive search will have sperm return to the ejaculate after vasovasostomy. [p 1550]

21. **d. It can better preserve the blood supply to testis parenchyma than a nonmicrosurgical method.** The use of an operating microscope for standard open diagnostic testes biopsy allows identification of an area in the tunica albuginea free of blood vessels (see Fig. 44–54A), minimizing the risk of injury to the testicular blood supply and allowing a relatively blood-free biopsy specimen. [pp 1568–1569]

22. **c. A specific cause should be identified for effective treatment.** Chronic orchialgia is defined as intermittent or constant scrotal pain, which may be unilateral, bilateral, or bilaterally alternating, lasting longer than 3 months. Chronic testicular pain has a variety of potential causes. All men with chronic orchialgia should undergo a high-resolution scrotal ultrasonographic study with color flow Doppler to completely evaluate the scrotal contents and rule out any underlying pathologic condition such as of testis tumor. Successful treatment requires identification of the cause so that specific therapy can be instituted. [p 1581]

23. **b. increased risk of multiple gestation.** Varicocelectomy results in significant improvement in the findings of semen analysis in 60% to 80% of men. Reported pregnancy rates after varicocelectomy vary from 20% to 60%. A randomized controlled trial of surgery versus no surgery in infertile men with varicoceles revealed a pregnancy rate of 44% at 1 year in the surgery group versus 10% in the control group. In our series of 1500 microsurgical operations, 43% of couples were pregnant at 1 year and 69% at 2 years when couples with female factors were excluded. Microsurgical varicocelectomy results in return of sperm to the ejaculate in 50% of azoospermic men with palpable varicoceles. Repair of large varicoceles results in a significantly greater improvement in semen quality than repair of small varicoceles (see Fig. 44–66). In addition, large varicoceles are associated with greater preoperative impairment in semen quality than are small varicoceles, and consequently overall pregnancy rates are similar regardless of varicocele size. Some evidence suggests that the younger the patient is at the time of varicocele repair, the greater the improvement after repair and the more likely the testis is to recover from varicocele-induced injury. Varicocele recurrence, testicular artery ligation, and postvaricocelectomy hydrocele formation are often associated with poor postoperative results. In infertile men with low serum testosterone levels, microsurgical varicocelectomy alone results in substantial improvement in serum testosterone levels. [p 1578]

24. **e. Absence of vasa deferentia and normal serum FSH level.** In the testes of men with congenital absence of vasa and normal serum FSH level, biopsy always reveals normal or at least some spermatogenesis, and biopsy is not necessary before definitive sperm aspiration and IVF with ICSI. [p 1534]

25. **b. PESA can be performed with local anesthesia.** Percutaneous puncture of the epididymis with a fine needle (see Fig. 44–52) has been successfully employed to obtain sperm and achieve pregnancies. The technique is less reliable than the open retrieval method, and the small quantities of sperm obtained are sometimes inadequate for cryopreservation. Reported pregnancy rates are half those achieved with open microsurgical techniques. [pp 1567–1568]

26. **c. Azoospermia, normal testicular volume and biopsy.** The absolute indications for vasography are azoospermia, plus complete spermatogenesis with many mature spermatids on testis biopsy, plus at least one palpable vas. Relative indications for vasography are severe oligospermia with normal testis biopsy; a high level of sperm-bound antibodies that may be due to obstruction; low semen volume and very poor sperm motility (partial ejaculatory duct obstruction). [p 1537]

27. **d. spermatogenic failure.** Vasography should answer the questions: Are there sperm in the vasal fluid? Is the vas obstructed? If the testis biopsy reveals many sperm, then the absence of sperm in vasal fluid indicates obstruction proximal to the vasal site examined, most likely an epididymal obstruction. Vasography is done in this case with saline or indigo carmine to confirm the patency of the seminal vesicle end of the vas before vasoepididymostomy. Copious vasal fluid containing many sperm indicates vasal or ejaculatory duct obstruction, and formal contrast vasography is performed to document the exact location of the obstruction. Copious thick, white fluid without sperm in a dilated vas indicates secondary epididymal obstruction in addition to a potential vasal or ejaculatory duct obstruction. [p 1537]

28. **a. Hematoma is the most frequent complication.** Hematoma is the most common complication of hydrocelectomy. When excision techniques are employed, the incidence of hematoma can be minimized by meticulously oversewing all raw edges of the sac and draining the scrotum when necessary. [p 1580]

29. **b. The rate of recurrence after nonmicrosurgical repair is higher than in the adult population.** The incidence of varicocele recurrence after surgical repair varies from 0.6% to 45%. Recurrence is more common after repair of pediatric varicoceles than of adult varicoceles. [p 1577]

30. **d. Transrectal ultrasonography.** Transrectal sonography has revolutionized the diagnosis and treatment of ejaculatory duct obstruction. A midline cystic lesion or dilated ejaculatory ducts and seminal vesicles can be visualized sonographically. [p 1564]

31. **d. testicular atrophy.** Reflux of urine into the ejaculatory ducts, vas, and seminal vesicles occurs after a majority of resections. This can be documented by voiding cystourethrography or by measuring semen creatinine levels. Reflux can lead to acute and chronic epididymitis. Recurrent epididymitis often results in epididymal obstruction. The incidence of epididymitis after transurethral resection is probably underestimated. Symptomatic chemical epididymitis may occur from refluxing urine. If epididymitis is chronic and recurrent, vasectomy or even epididymectomy may be necessary. Even when care has been taken to spare the bladder neck, retrograde ejaculation is common after transurethral resection. Transurethral instrumentation can increase the risk of urethral stricture. [p 1565]

32. **e. Sclerotherapy.** Sclerotherapy has been used with some success in the treatment of hydrocele. Sclerotherapy with tetracycline derivatives or other irritating agents may result in epididymal obstruction. It can be associated with substantial postoperative pain, and recurrence is not uncommon. When hydrocele recurs after sclerotherapy, it is usually multiloculated and more difficult to repair. Sclerotherapy is most useful in older men in whom fertility is no longer an issue. [p 1580]

33. **b. Lymphatic obstruction.** Analysis of the protein concentration of hydrocele fluid indicates that hydrocele formation after varicocelectomy is due to lymphatic obstruction. [p 1577]

34. **c. Prepubertal varicocele.** The external oblique aponeurosis should always be opened in children or prepubertal adolescents without prior inguinal surgery. In children, the testicular artery is very small and systemic blood pressure is low, making identification of the artery very difficult in a subinguinal approach. The fascia should also be opened in men with a solitary testis in whom preservation of the artery is crucial. Exposure of the cord more proximally (at the inguinal level) allows identification of the artery before it has branched, where clear pulsations are more readily observed. [p 1573]

35. **d. It is a paired duct formed by the confluence of each seminal vesicle duct and vasa deferentia.** The ejaculatory ducts course between the bladder neck and the verumontanum and exit at the level of and along the lateral aspect of the verumontanum (see Fig. 44–50). [pp 1564–1565]

36. **e. Adenomatoid tumor.** Most nontransilluminable epididymal masses are benign adenomatoid tumors. Malignant epididymal tumors are exceedingly rare. Like any potentially malignant testicular mass, they should be managed by inguinal exploration, clamping of the cord, and delivery of the testis and biopsy by frozen section. [p 1557]

37. **e. Retrograde ejaculation.** Complications of vasography include stricture, injury to the vasal blood supply, hematoma, and sperm granuloma. Multiple attempts at percutaneous vasography using sharp needles can result in stricture or obstruction at the vasography site. Careless or crude closure of a vasotomy can also result in stricture and obstruction. Non–water-soluble contrast agents may also result in stricture and should not be employed for vasography. If the vasal blood supply is injured at the site of vasography, vasovasostomy proximal to the vasography site may result in ischemia, necrosis, and obstruction of the intervening segment of vas. A bipolar cautery should be used for meticulous hemostasis at the time of vasotomy to prevent hematoma in the perivasal sheath. Leaky closure of a vasography site may lead to the development of a sperm granuloma, which can result in stricture or obstruction of the vas. [p 1540]

38. **d. 60% to 80%.** Systemic effects of vasectomy have been postulated. Vasectomy disrupts the blood-testis barrier, resulting in detectable levels of serum antisperm antibodies in 60% to 80% of men. Some studies suggest that the antibody titers diminish 2 or more years after vasectomy. Others suggest that these antibody titers persist. However, neither circulating immune complexes nor deposits are increased after vasectomy. [p 1546]

39. **d. That sperm will be found at the testicular end of the vas.** A sperm granuloma at the testicular end of the vas suggests that sperm have been leaking at the vasectomy site. This vents the high pressures away from the epididymis and is associated with a better prognosis for restored fertility regardless of the time interval since vasectomy. [p 1547]

40. **b. At the time of reconstruction if a prior testis biopsy result was normal.** There is no need to perform vasography at the time of testis biopsy for azoospermia unless immediate reconstruction is planned and the touch or wet preparation biopsy reveals mature sperm with tails. If performed carelessly, vasography can cause stricture or even obstruction at the vasography site, which can complicate subsequent reconstruction. [p 1537]

41. **d. The epididymides are likely to be obstructed.** Sperm granulomas form when sperm leak from the testicular end of the vas. Sperm are highly antigenic, and an intense inflammatory reaction occurs when sperm escape outside the reproductive epithelium. Sperm granulomas are rarely symptomatic. The presence or absence of a sperm granuloma at the vasectomy site seems to be of importance in modulating the local effects of chronic obstruction on the male reproductive tract. The sperm granuloma's complex network of epithelialized channels provides an additional absorptive surface that helps vent the high intraluminal pressure in the obstructed excurrent ducts. Numerous animal studies have correlated the presence or absence of sperm granuloma at the vasectomy site with the degree of epididymal and testicular damage. Species that always develop granulomas after vasectomy have minimal damage to the seminiferous tubules. Some studies of men undergoing vasectomy reversal have revealed somewhat higher success rates in men who have a sperm granuloma at the vasectomy site, whereas another large study has not. Although sperm granulomas at the vasectomy site are present microscopically in 10% to 30% of men undergoing reversal, it is likely that, given enough time, virtually all men develop sperm granulomas at the vasectomy site, the epididymis, or the rete testis. When chronic postvasectomy pain is localized to the granuloma, excision and occlusion of the vasa with intraluminal cautery usually relieve the pain and prevent recurrence. Men with postvasectomy congestive epididymitis may be relieved of

pain by open-ended vasectomy designed to purposefully produce pressure, relieving sperm granuloma. [p 1546]

42. **e. Hydrocele.** Hydrocele formation is the most common complication reported after nonmicroscopic varicocelectomy. The incidence of this complication varies from 3% to 33%, with an average incidence of about 7%. [p 1577]

43. **a. Retroperitoneal ligation.** A disadvantage of a retroperitoneal approach is the high incidence of varicocele recurrence, especially in children and adolescents, when the testicular artery is intentionally preserved. Recurrence rates after retroperitoneal varicocelectomy are about 15%. Failure is usually due to preservation of the periarterial plexus of fine veins (venae comitantes) along with the artery. These veins have been shown to communicate with larger internal spermatic veins. If left intact, they may dilate with time and cause recurrence. [p 1572]

44. **e. Patency of a vas deferens and epididymis on at least one side.** The fine-needle aspirate is examined for sperm. If sperm are present, it means at least one vas and epididymis are patent. [pp 1540–1541]

45. **d. A trial of pseudoephedrine.** Pseudoephedrine (Sudafed), 120 mg orally 90 minutes before ejaculation may prevent retrograde ejaculation. If this is not successful, sperm can be retrieved from alkalinized urine and used for either intrauterine insemination or IVF with ICSI. [p 1565]

46. **e. Motile sperm found in semen analysis 3 months after vasectomy.** No technique of vasal occlusion, short of removing the entire scrotal vas, is 100% effective. Follow-up semen analysis with the goal of obtaining at least one and preferably two absolutely azoospermic specimens 4 to 6 weeks apart is recommended. If any motile sperm are found in the ejaculate 3 months after vasectomy, the procedure should be repeated. If rare nonmotile sperm are found, contraception may be cautiously discontinued and repeated semen analysis done every 3 months. Rare complete sperm in a spun semen analysis pellet are found in 10% of semen specimens at a mean of 10 years after vasectomy. [p 1545]

47. **b. Epididymis.** Micropuncture studies have revealed that in humans, the markedly increased pressures that occur on the testicular side of the vas as well as the epididymis after vasectomy are not transmitted to the seminiferous tubules. Therefore, little disruption of spermatogenesis is expected in humans. The brunt of pressure-induced damage after vasectomy falls on the epididymis and efferent ductules. These structures become markedly distended and then adapt to reabsorb large volumes of testicular fluid and sperm products. [p 1546]

48. **b. higher risk of testicular venous congestion.** When varicocelectomy is properly performed, all spermatic veins are ligated and the only remaining avenues for testicular venous return are the vasal veins. In men who have had vasectomy and are presenting for reversal, the vasal veins are likely to be compromised from either the original vasectomy or the reversal itself. Furthermore, the integrity of the vasal artery in those men is also likely to be compromised. Varicocelectomy in such men requires preservation of the testicular artery as the primary remaining testicular blood supply as well as preservation of some avenue for venous return. Microscopic varicocelectomy can ensure preservation of the testicular artery in most cases. [p 1550]

49. **e. Stricture of vasovasostomy.** Late stricture and obstruction are disappointingly common. Progressive loss of sperm motility followed by decreasing counts indicates stricture. [pp 1555–1556]

50. **d. Men with primary infertility, azoospermia, normal physical examination findings, and normal serum FSH level.** Testis biopsy is indicated in azoospermic men with testis of normal size and consistency, palpable vasa deferentia, and normal serum FSH levels. [p 1534]

51. **b. A dartos pouch operation is the treatment of choice.** When scrotal orchiopexy is performed for retractile testis, a dartos pouch operation should be performed. Simple suture orchiopexy of the tunica albuginea of the testis to the dartos, such as is performed sometimes to prevent torsion, will not prevent retraction of these testes into the groin. Creation of a dartos pouch will keep the testis well down into the scrotum and permanently prevent retraction. This is also the most reliable and safest technique for the prevention of testicular torsion. [p 1581]

52. **e. It should be performed only to an epididymal tubule containing sperm.** Specific treatments for male factor infertility, such as microsurgical reconstruction for obstructive azoospermia and varicocelectomy for impaired testes, remain the safest and most cost-effective ways of managing infertile men. Microsurgical approaches allow accurate approximation of the vasal mucosa to that of a single epididymal tubule, resulting in marked improvement in the patency and pregnancy rates. If the level of obstruction is not clearly delineated, after the buttonhole opening is made in the tunica, a 70 μm diameter tapered needle from the 10-0 nylon microsuture is used to puncture the epididymal tubule, beginning as distal as possible, and fluid is sampled from the puncture site. When sperm are found, the puncture sites are sealed with microbipolar forceps, a new buttonhole is made in the epididymal tunica just proximally, and the tubule is prepared as described previously. Patency rates with the intussusception technique can exceed 80%. With the classic end-to-side or older end-to-end method, the patency rate is about 70%, and 43% of men with sperm will impregnate their wives after a minimum follow-up of 2 years. [pp 1533, 1557, 1558, and 1564]

53. **a. Intraoperative epididymal sperm aspiration for sperm cryopreservation.** Once sperm are identified, they are aspirated into glass capillary tubes and flushed into media for cryopreservation. [p 1559]

54. **a. The torsion episodes are similar to acute torsion episodes but are less severe.** Men with chronic intermittent torsion often have a history of intermittent episodes of sudden-onset testicular pain, as in acute testicular torsion. However, the pain with intermittent torsion spontaneously disappears after anywhere from a few minutes to a few hours. [p 1582]

55. **b. Orchiectomy is the primary surgical treatment of choice.** The underlying cause of chronic orchialgia may not always be obvious. Lower urinary tract symptoms, distal ureteral stone, occult hernia, irritable bowel syndrome, and referred pain are some of the possible causes of the symptoms. Even when no specific cause can be found, conservative therapy, including nonsteroidal anti-inflammatory drugs, sitz baths, and scrotal support for a period of 3 to 6 months, is indicated. Not infrequently, these patients fail to respond to conservative management, including pharmacologic, local anesthesia, and even psychological or behavioral therapy. Microsurgical total denervation of the spermatic cord is a measure with reported success in 80% of cases in recent small series. [p 1583]

56. **c. Surgeon's technique and experience.** The responsibilities assumed by the surgeon demand the utmost in judgment and

skill. Many of the procedures described in this chapter are among the most technically demanding in all of urology. Acquisition of the skills required to perform them demands intensive laboratory training in microsurgery and a thorough knowledge of the anatomy and physiology of the male reproductive system. Attempting such surgery only occasionally and without proper training is a terrible disservice to the patient, the couple, and future humanity. [p 1534]

57. **d. MESA for spermatogenic maturation arrest.** MESA is indicated for men with normal spermatogenesis and unreconstructable obstruction such as congenital bilateral absence of the vas deferens. [p 1568]

58. **e. Orchiopexy for retractile testis.** The use of the operating microscope to identify individual seminiferous tubules that are more likely to contain sperm has improved the success rates of testicular sperm extraction and minimized morbidity significantly. The use of microsurgical techniques has also extended to varicocelectomy. [p 1533]

59. **e. It allows examination of vasal fluid before microanastomosis is performed.** End-to-side techniques of vasoepididymostomy have the advantage of being minimally traumatic to the epididymis and relatively bloodless (see Table 44–3). The end-to-side technique does not disturb the epididymal blood supply. When the level of epididymal obstruction is clearly demarcated by the presence of markedly dilated tubules proximally and collapsed tubules distally, the site at which the anastomosis should be performed is readily apparent. The end-to-side approach has the advantage of allowing accurate approximation of the muscularis and adventitia of the vas deferens to a precisely tailored opening in the tunica of the epididymis. This is the preferred technique when vasoepididymostomy is performed simultaneously with inguinal vasovasostomy, because it is possible to preserve the vasal blood supply deriving from epididymal branches of the testicular artery (see Fig. 44–43). This provides blood supply to the segment of vas intervening between the two anastomoses. Maintenance of the deferential artery's contribution to the testicular blood supply is also important in situations in which the integrity of the testicular artery is in doubt because of prior surgery such as orchiopexy, nonmicroscopic varicocelectomy, or hernia repair. [pp 1557–1558]

60. **d. Congenital absence of vas.** Large varicoceles can cause a persistent, aching discomfort often described by patients as a heavy sensation or a sensation of increased heat in the scrotum. Chronic testicular pain after hernia repair may be associated with nerve entrapment injuries. Postvasectomy chronic orchialgia is disappointingly common and difficult to treat. Although early pain lasting a few weeks is fairly common after vasectomy, present in up to 30% of men, long-term pain requiring some kind of interventional or surgical therapy probably occurs in approximately 1 in 1000 vasectomized men. Sperm granulomas are easily palpable on the testicular end of the vas after vasectomy. If they are exquisitely tender and palpation duplicates the pain that the patient feels, removal of the granuloma with intraluminal cautery of the vas will usually relieve the pain. [pp 1582–1583]

SECTION VIII

SEXUAL FUNCTION AND DYSFUNCTION

Chapter 45

Physiology of Penile Erection and Pathophysiology of Erectile Dysfunction and Priapism

Tom F. Lue

Questions

1. Which of the following statements is true regarding the tunica albuginea of the human penis?
   a. It consists of a single layer of strong fibrous tissue, enclosing both the corpora cavernosa and the corpus spongiosum.
   b. It is a bilayered structure in the corpora cavernosa but a single-layered structure in the corpus spongiosum.
   c. It is commonly called Buck's fascia of the penis.
   d. It consists of collagen fibers, smooth muscle fibers, and elastic fibers.
   e. It extends all the way to the glans penis to give the glans penis a strong covering.

2. Which of the following statements is true regarding the thickness of the tunica albuginea?
   a. It is the same throughout the entire penis.
   b. It is less in the pendulous portion of the penis.
   c. It is less at the ventral groove of the penis.
   d. It is the same between the flaccid and the erect phases of the penis.
   e. It determines the girth of the penis.

3. All of the following statements about the accessory pudendal artery are true except which one?
   a. It may arise from the obturator artery.
   b. It may travel anterior to the prostate.
   c. It may be damaged during radical prostatectomy.
   d. It may be the dominant blood supply to the corpus cavernosum.
   e. It may occur in up to 80% of men.

4. The arterial supply of the corpus cavernosum is usually from which artery?
   a. The external pudendal artery
   b. The accessory pudendal artery
   c. The cavernous artery
   d. The dorsal artery
   e. The inferior epigastric artery

5. Which of the following statements is true regarding the venous channels draining the corpus cavernosum?
   a. They originate in the center of the corpus cavernosum.
   b. They originate in the emissary veins.
   c. They originate in the subtunical venules.
   d. They drain exclusively via the dorsal vein of the penis.
   e. They drain exclusively via the cavernous vein.

6. What causes venous flow reduction during erection?
   a. Active constriction of the superficial and deep dorsal veins
   b. Opening of a penile arteriovenous shunt
   c. Compression of the subtunical venules and emissary veins by the tunica albuginea
   d. Active contraction of emissary veins
   e. Relaxation of the ischiocavernous muscle

7. What actions are involved in penile erection?
   a. Arterial dilatation and venous constriction
   b. Relaxation of the ischiocavernous muscle
   c. Arterial dilatation, venous compression, and sinusoidal relaxation
   d. Contraction of the smooth muscles within the corpus cavernosum
   e. Filling and expansion of the sinusoidal spaces by nitric oxide (NO)

8. Where does the innervation of the penis come from?
   a. Sacral S2, S3, and S4 spinal segments
   b. T10–T12 and S2–S4 spinal segments
   c. The dorsal nerve
   d. The cavernous nerve
   e. All of the above

9. Which of the following statements is true regarding the ischiocavernous and bulbocavernous muscles?
   a. They are innervated by the pudendal nerve.
   b. They are responsible for the rigid phase of erection.
   c. They are important in the expulsion of semen during ejaculation.
   d. They are striated muscles.
   e. All of the above.

169

10. Stimulation of which of the following areas of the brain has been reported to induce penile erection?

    a. Paraventricular area of the hypothalamus
    b. Midbrain raphe
    c. Substantia nigra
    d. Nucleus paragigantocellularis
    e. A5 catecholamine cell group and locus ceruleus

11. What is the most likely neurotransmitter for penile erection?

    a. Prostaglandin E_1
    b. NO
    c. Norepinephrine
    d. Acetylcholine
    e. Neuropeptide P

12. Of the ion channels identified on penile smooth muscle, which of the following have been shown to be involved in penile erection?

    a. Sodium and chloride channels
    b. Calcium and potassium channels
    c. Titanium and potassium channels
    d. Chloride and calcium channels
    e. Gold and silver channels

13. The action of NO within the penile smooth muscle cell involves:

    a. activation of adenylyl cyclase and elevation of the cyclic AMP level.
    b. activation of phosphodiesterase type 4.
    c. opening of calcium channels, which results in elevation of the cytosolic calcium level.
    d. activation of guanylyl cyclase and elevation of the cyclic GMP level.
    e. closure of potassium channels.

14. Which of the following is involved in detumescence of the penis?

    a. NO
    b. Phosphodiesterase type 5
    c. Phosphodiesterase type 3
    d. Acetylcholine
    e. Neuropeptide P

15. Which of the following accurately describes the gap junction?

    a. It is a communication between the tunica albuginea and the sinusoid spaces.
    b. It is a communication between the glans penis and the corpora cavernosa.
    c. It is a communication between the corpus cavernosum and corpus spongiosum.
    d. It is a communication among the intracavernous muscle cells.
    e. It is a junction of the presynaptic neurons and the receptors.

16. Neurotransmitters involved in modulating sexual function in the brain include:

    a. epinephrine, testosterone, and prolactin.
    b. dopamine, norepinephrine, serotonin, and oxytocin.
    c. endothelin and calcitonin gene-related peptide (CGRP).
    d. vasoactive intestinal polypeptide (VIP) and acetylcholine.
    e. all of the above.

17. Which of the following statements is true regarding apomorphine?

    a. It has a strong analgesic action but is not a narcotic.
    b. It is a central-acting dopamine receptor agonist.
    c. It produces penile erection when injected into the corpus cavernosum.
    d. It is an inhibitor of phosphodiesterase type 5, similar to sildenafil.
    e. It is often used as an antiemetic.

18. Central norepinephrine transmission seems to enhance sexual function, as evidenced by which of the following?

    a. Clonidine, an α_2-adrenergic agonist, enhances sexual function.
    b. Yohimbine, an α_2-adrenergic antagonist, enhances sexual function.
    c. Intracavernous injection of phenylephrine produces penile erection.
    d. Oral phentolamine enhances penile erection.
    e. Intracavernous injection of papaverine produces penile erection.

19. Which of the following statements is true, as reported by the Massachusetts Male Aging Study (MMAS)?

    a. The prevalence of erectile dysfunction (ED) in the United States is about 50% at 50 years of age, 60% at 60 years, and 70% at 70 years (including mild, moderate, and severe ED).
    b. The prevalence rate of severe ED remains the same but the prevalence rate of mild ED increases with age.
    c. The MMAS is a hospital-based, cross-sectional survey of sexual function in men and women in the United States.
    d. The MMAS surveyed more than 1700 hospitalized patients between 1995 and 1997.
    e. The MMAS study estimated that the incidence rate of ED is about 20 million new cases per year in the United States.

20. A 25-year-old healthy student complained of an inability to maintain an erection since meeting his new girlfriend. He did not have a problem with his previous sexual partners. A nocturnal penile tumescence study revealed that 70% of the erections recorded were of full rigidity. What is the most likely diagnosis?

    a. Psychogenic ED.
    b. Testosterone deficiency.
    c. Penile vascular insufficiency.
    d. Penile venous leakage.
    e. Primary ED.

21. A 58-year-old man complained of impotence after radical prostatectomy for cancer of the prostate. Impotence after radical prostatectomy is frequently a result of injury to which of the following?

    a. The dorsal nerve of the penis
    b. The cavernous nerve
    c. The genitofemoral nerve
    d. The sympathetic ganglion
    e. The ilioinguinal nerve

22. The function of testosterone includes all of the following except which one?

    a. It enhances sexual interest.
    b. It increases the frequency of sexual acts.
    c. It increases the frequency of nocturnal erections but has little or no effect on fantasy or visually induced erections.
    d. It maintains nitric oxide synthase activity in the penis (in rats).
    e. It prevents hair loss in men.

23. What is cavernosal (venogenic) ED?

    a. A disease of the deep dorsal vein
    b. A disease of the emissary vein

c. A disease of the preprostatic venous plexus
d. A disease of the tunica albuginea or cavernous smooth muscles
e. A disease of the internal pudendal vein

24. Which of the following is not part of the normal aging process?

    a. Greater latency to erection and loss of forceful ejaculation
    b. Decreased ejaculatory volume and a longer refractory period
    c. Decreased frequency and duration of nocturnal erection
    d. Decrease in penile tactile sensitivity
    e. Complete ED

25. Erectile dysfunction associated with diabetes can be a result of which of the following?

    a. Psychological impact
    b. Neurologic deficit
    c. Arterial insufficiency
    d. Endothelial cell dysfunction
    e. All of the above

26. All of the following are proposed molecular mechanisms of diabetic ED except:

    a. impaired NO synthesis.
    b. increased levels of oxygen free radicals.
    c. elevated levels of advanced glycosylation end products, which quench NO.
    d. selective degeneration of NO synthase-containing nerves.
    e. decreased level of phosphodiesterase type 5.

27. The causes of ED in an animal model of hyperlipidemia and hypercholesterolemia include all of the following except:

    a. increased production of contractile thromboxane and prostaglandin.
    b. increased production of oxytocin.
    c. the contractile effect of oxidized low-density lipoprotein.
    d. release of superoxide radicals.
    e. increased production of NO synthase inhibitors.

28. A 60-year-old hypertensive man complained of ED after taking a calcium channel blocker to lower his blood pressure. What is the most likely cause of his ED?

    a. The direct effect of the calcium channel blocker on penile smooth muscle.
    b. Arrhythmia caused by the calcium channel blocker.
    c. Decreased penile perfusion caused by a decline in blood pressure in the pudendal artery.
    d. Anxiety from taking new medication.
    e. A decreased level of testosterone resulting from the calcium channel blocker.

29. A 16-year-old African-American teenager suffers from a persistent painful erection for 6 hours. What is the most likely diagnosis?

    a. High flow (arterial) priapism
    b. Ischemic priapism from sickle cell anemia
    c. Sexual trauma
    d. Intracavernous injection of papaverine
    e. Cavernositis

30. A 36-year-old man sustained a straddle injury after falling off a ladder and landing on a concrete divider. The next morning he woke up with a 75% partial erection that persisted for 2 weeks. The erection was not painful. What is the most likely cause?

    a. Injury of the cavernous nerve
    b. Rupture of the cavernous artery
    c. Persistent fistula between the corpus cavernosum and the corpus spongiosum
    d. Autonomic dysfunction
    e. Malingering to get workers' compensation benefits

Answers

1. **b. It is a bilayered structure in the corpora cavernosa but a single-layered structure in the corpus spongiosum.** The tunical covering of the corpora cavernosa is a bilayered structure with multiple sublayers: (1) Inner layer bundles support and contain the cavernous tissue and are oriented circularly. Radiating from this inner layer are intracavernosal pillars, acting as struts, augmenting the septum that provides essential support to the erectile tissue. (2) Outer layer bundles are oriented longitudinally, extending from the glans penis to the proximal crura; they insert into the inferior pubic rami but are absent between the 5- and 7-o'clock positions. In contrast, the corpus spongiosum lacks an outer layer or intracorporeal struts, ensuring a low-pressure structure during erection. [pp 1592–1593]

2. **c. It is less at the ventral groove of the penis.** The outer tunical layer appears to play an additional role in compression of the emissary veins during erection. It also determines, to a large extent, the variability in tunical thickness and strength. At the 7-o'clock position, the tunical thickness is 0.8 ± 0.1 mm, at 9 o'clock 1.2 ± 0.2 mm, and at 11 o'clock 2.2 ± 0.4 mm. At 3, 5, and 1 o'clock, the measurements are nearly identical in mirror-image manner. (Differences at specific locations have been found to be statistically significant.) The stress on the tunica before penetration has been measured as $1.6 \pm 0.2 \times 10^7$ N/m² at the 7-o'clock position, $3.0 \pm 0.3 \times 10^7$ N/m² at 9 o'clock, and $4.5 \pm 0.5 \times 10^7$ N/m² at 11 o'clock. The strength and thickness of the tunica correlate in a statistically significant manner with location. The most vulnerable area is located on the ventral groove (between 5 and 7 o'clock), which lacks the longitudinally directed outer layer bundles; most prostheses tend to extrude here. [p 1593]

3. **e. It may occur in up to 80% of men.** The main source of blood supply to the penis is usually via the internal pudendal artery, a branch of the internal iliac artery. In many instances, however, accessory arteries exist, arising from the external iliac, obturator, vesical, and femoral arteries, and may occasionally become the dominant or only arterial supply to the corpus cavernosum. Damage to these accessory arteries during radical prostatectomy or cystectomy may result in vasculogenic erectile dysfunction (ED) after surgery. [p 1593]

4. **c. The cavernous artery.** The cavernous artery is responsible for tumescence of the corpus cavernosum and the dorsal artery for engorgement of the glans penis during erection. The bulbourethral artery supplies the bulb and corpus spongiosum. The cavernous artery enters the corpus cavernosum at the hilum of the penis, where the two crura merge. [p 1593]

5. **c. They originate in the subtunical venules.** The venous drainage from the three corpora originates in tiny venules

leading from the peripheral sinusoids immediately beneath the tunica albuginea. These venules travel in the trabeculae between the tunica and the peripheral sinusoids to form the subtunical venular plexus before exiting as the emissary veins. [p 1595]

6. **c. Compression of the subtunical venules and emissary veins by the tunica albuginea.** Sexual stimulation triggers release of neurotransmitters from the cavernous nerve terminals. This results in relaxation of these smooth muscles and the following events (see Fig. 45–3): (1) dilatation of the arterioles and arteries by increased blood flow in both the diastolic and the systolic phases; (2) trapping of the incoming blood by the expanding sinusoids; (3) compression of the subtunical venular plexuses between the tunica albuginea and the peripheral sinusoids, reducing the venous outflow; (4) stretching of the tunica to its capacity, which encloses the emissary veins between the inner circular and the outer longitudinal layers and further decreases the venous outflow to a minimum; (5) an increase in intracavernous pressure (maintained at about 100 mm Hg), which raises the penis from the dependent position to the erect state (the full erection phase); and (6) a further pressure increase (to several hundred mm Hg) with contraction of the ischiocavernous muscles (rigid erection phase). [p 1595]

7. **c. Arterial dilatation, venous compression, and sinusoidal relaxation.** Erection involves sinusoidal relaxation, arterial dilatation, and venous compression. The importance of smooth muscle relaxation has been demonstrated in animal and human studies. To summarize the hemodynamic events of erection and detumescence, seven phases can be observed in animal experiments. The changes in and the relationship between penile arterial flow and intracavernous pressure are shown in Figure 45–4. [p 1595]

8. **e. All of the above.** The sympathetic pathway originates from the 11th thoracic to the 2nd lumbar spinal segments and passes via the white rami to the sympathetic chain ganglia. Some fibers then travel via the lumbar splanchnic nerves to the inferior mesenteric and superior hypogastric plexuses, from which fibers travel in the hypogastric nerves to the pelvic plexus. In humans, the T10–T12 segments are most often the origin of the sympathetic fibers, and the chain ganglia cells projecting to the penis are located in the sacral and caudal ganglia. The parasympathetic pathway arises from neurons in the intermediolateral cell columns of the second, third, and fourth sacral spinal cord segments. The preganglionic fibers pass in the pelvic nerves to the pelvic plexus, where they are joined by the sympathetic nerves from the superior hypogastric plexus. The cavernous nerves are branches of the pelvic plexus that innervate the penis. Other branches of the pelvic plexus innervate the rectum, bladder, prostate, and sphincters. The cavernous nerves are easily damaged during radical excision of the rectum, bladder, and prostate. A clear understanding of the course of these nerves is essential to the prevention of iatrogenic ED. Recent human cadaveric dissection revealed medial and lateral branches of the cavernous nerves (the former accompany the urethra and the latter pierce the urogenital diaphragm 4 to 7 mm lateral to the sphincter) and multiple communications between the cavernous and dorsal nerves (see Fig. 45–6). [p 1597]

9. **e. All of the above.** Onuf's nucleus in the second to fourth sacral spinal segments is the center of somatomotor penile innervation. These nerves travel in the sacral nerves to the pudendal nerve to innervate the ischiocavernous and bulbocavernous muscles. Contraction of the ischiocavernous muscles produces the rigid erection phase. Rhythmic contraction of the bulbocavernous muscle is necessary for ejaculation. [p 1598]

10. **a. Paraventricular area of the hypothalamus.** Studies with animals have identified the medial preoptic area and the paraventricular nucleus of the hypothalamus and the hippocampus as important integration centers for sexual function and penile erection. Electrostimulation of this area induces erection, and lesions at this site limit copulation. [p 1598]

11. **b. NO.** Most researchers now agree that NO released from nonadrenergic/noncholinergic neurotransmission and from the endothelium is the principal neurotransmitter mediating penile erection. NO increases the production of cyclic GMP (cGMP), which in turn relaxes the cavernous smooth muscle. [p 1599]

12. **b. Calcium and potassium channels.** In the penis, the NO that is released from nerve endings or endothelial cells diffuses into smooth muscle cells, where it activates soluble guanylyl cyclase, producing cGMP. The mechanism by which intracellular cGMP promotes smooth muscle relaxation has not been settled. The most likely mechanism is the activation of cGMP-specific protein kinase, resulting in the phosphorylation and inactivation of myosin light chain kinase, thereby causing dissociation of myosin and actin and smooth muscle relaxation. Both cGMP and cGMP-specific protein kinase may also activate potassium channels, causing hyperpolarization and closure of voltage-dependent calcium channels and a decrease in intracellular calcium. [p 1601]

13. **d. activation of guanylyl cyclase and elevation of the cyclic GMP level.** Cyclic AMP (cAMP) and cGMP are the second messengers involved in smooth muscle relaxation. They activate cAMP- and cGMP-dependent protein kinases, which in turn phosphorylate certain proteins and ion channels, resulting in (1) opening of the potassium channels and hyperpolarization; (2) sequestration of intracellular calcium by the endoplasmic reticulum; and (3) inhibition of voltage-dependent calcium channels, blocking calcium influx. The consequence is a drop in cytosolic free calcium and smooth muscle relaxation. [p 1600]

14. **b. Phosphodiesterase type 5.** During the return to the flaccid state, cGMP is hydrolyzed to GMP by the highly specific cGMP-binding phosphodiesterase type 5. [p 1601]

15. **d. It is a communication among the intracavernous muscle cells.** Several studies have demonstrated the presence of gap junctions in the membrane of adjacent muscle cells. These intercellular channels allow exchange of ions such as calcium and second-messenger molecules. The major component of gap junctions is connexin43, a membrane-sparing protein of less than 0.25 μm that has been identified between smooth muscle cells of human corpus cavernosum. Cell-to-cell communication through these gap junctions most likely explains the synchronized erectile response, although their pathophysiologic impact is still unclear. [pp 1601–1602]

16. **b. dopamine, norepinephrine, serotonin, and oxytocin.** A variety of neurotransmitters (dopamine, norepinephrine, serotonin, and oxytocin) and neural hormones (oxytocin and prolactin) have been implicated in the regulation of sexual function. It is suggested that dopaminergic and adrenergic receptors may promote sexual function and that serotonin receptors inhibit it. [p 1602]

17. **b. It is a central-acting dopamine receptor agonist.** In men, apomorphine, which stimulates both D1 and D2 receptors, induces penile erection that is unaccompanied by sexual arousal. [p 1602]

18. **b. Yohimbine, an α_2-adrenergic antagonist, enhances sexual function.** Central norepinephrine transmission seems to have a positive effect on sexual function. In both humans and rats, inhibition of norepinephrine release by clonidine, an α_2-adrenergic agonist, is associated with a decrease in

sexual behavior, and yohimbine, an α_2-receptor antagonist, has been shown to increase sexual activity. [p 1604]

19. **a. The prevalence of erectile dysfunction (ED) in the United States is about 50% at 50 years of age, 60% at 60 years, and 70% at 70 years (including mild, moderate, and severe ED).** As reported in the MMAS study, between the ages of 40 and 70 years the probability of complete ED increased from 5.1% to 15%, the probability of moderate ED increased from 17% to 34%, and the probability of mild ED remained constant at about 17%. [p 1605]

20. **a. Psychogenic ED.** A classification recommended by the International Society of Impotence Research is shown in Table 45–4: organic, which includes vasculogenic (arteriogenic, cavernosal, and mixed), neurogenic, anatomic, and endocrinologic; and psychogenic, which includes the generalized type (generalized unresponsiveness and generalized inhibition) and the situational type (partner related; performance related; and psychological distress or adjustment related). [pp 1605 and 1606]

21. **b. The cavernous nerve.** Because of the close relationship between the cavernous nerves and the pelvic organs, surgery on these organs is a frequent cause of impotence. The incidence of iatrogenic impotence from various procedures has been reported as follows: radical prostatectomy, 43% to 100%; perineal prostatectomy for benign disease, 29%; abdominal perineal resection, 15% to 100%; and external sphincterotomy at the 3- and 9-o'clock positions, 2% to 49%. [p 1606]

22. **e. It prevents hair loss in men.** Mulligan and Schmitt in 1993 concluded the following: (1) testosterone enhances sexual interest; (2) testosterone increases the frequency of sexual acts; and (3) testosterone increases the frequency of nocturnal erections but has little or no effect on fantasy- or visually induced erections. [p 1607]

23. **d. A disease of the tunica albuginea or cavernous smooth muscles.** Veno-occlusive dysfunction may result from the following pathophysiologic processes: (1) The presence or development of large venous channels draining the corpora cavernosa. (2) Degenerative changes (Peyronie's disease, aging, and diabetes) or traumatic injury to the tunica albuginea (penile fracture), resulting in inadequate compression of the subtunical and emissary veins. In Peyronie's disease, the inelastic tunica albuginea may prevent the emissary veins from closing. Iacono and colleagues postulated that a decrease in elastic fibers in the tunica albuginea and an alteration of microarchitecture may contribute to impotence in some men. Changes in the subtunical areolar layer may impair the veno-occlusive mechanism as occasionally seen in patients after surgery for Peyronie's disease. (3) Structural alterations in the fibroelastic components of the trabeculae, cavernous smooth muscle, and endothelium may result in a venous leak. (4) Insufficient trabecular smooth muscle relaxation, causing inadequate sinusoidal expansion and insufficient compression of the subtunical venules, may occur in an anxious individual with excessive adrenergic tone or in a patient with inadequate neurotransmitter release. It has been shown that alteration of α-adrenoceptor or decrease in NO release may heighten the smooth muscle tone and impair the relaxation in response to endogenous muscle relaxant. (5) Acquired venous shunts—the result of operative correction of priapism—may cause persistent glans/cavernosum or cavernosum/spongiosum shunting. [p 1608]

24. **e. Complete ED.** A number of studies have indicated a progressive decline in sexual function in "healthy" aging men. Masters and Johnson in 1977 noted a number of changes in older men, including greater latency to erection, less turgid erection, loss of forceful ejaculation, decreased ejaculatory volume, and a longer refractory period. Decreased frequency and duration of nocturnal erection with increasing age were reported in a group of men who had regular intercourse. Other research has also indicated a decrease in penile tactile sensitivity with age. [pp 1609–1610]

25. **e. All of the above.** ED has been estimated to occur in 35% to 75% of men with diabetes mellitus, with onset occurring at an earlier age than in men without diabetes. Deterioration of sexual function was the first symptom in 12% of diabetic men. The incidence of ED in diabetes has been found to be age dependent: 15% at 30 years of age and 55% at 34 to 60 years. Diabetes may cause ED through its effects on central nervous system and peripheral nerve function, androgen production, psychological factors, vascular integrity, and endothelial and smooth muscle function. [p 1610]

26. **e. decreased level of phosphodiesterase type 5.** The following summarizes the proposed mechanisms of ED in diabetic animals: (1) impaired NO synthesis; (2) increase in endothelin B receptor binding sites and ultrastructural changes; (3) increased levels of oxygen free radicals and oxidative stress injury; and (4) NO-dependent selective nitrergic nerve degeneration. [p 1610]

27. **b. increased production of oxytocin.** In a rabbit model of atherosclerosis and hypercholesterolemia, decreased NO synthase activity and increased production of contractile thromboxane and prostaglandin are thought to be the causes of impaired smooth muscle relaxation in response to electrical stimulation. Others have proposed that the impaired NO-mediated smooth muscle relaxation in hypercholesterolemia may be due to the contractile effect of oxidized low-density lipoprotein, the release of superoxide radicals, and the increased production of NO synthase inhibitors. In addition, ultrastructural studies of cholesterol-fed rabbits have revealed early atherosclerotic changes in the corpus cavernosum. [p 1610]

28. **c. Decreased penile perfusion caused by a decline in blood pressure in the pudendal artery.** In hypertension, the increased blood pressure itself does not impair erectile function; rather, the associated arterial stenotic lesions are thought to be the cause. One study has demonstrated that NO availability is impaired because of the production of cyclooxygenase-derived vasoconstrictor substances and reduced endothelin B receptor-mediated NO activation. In addition to increased peripheral vascular resistance, alteration in the vessel architecture, resulting in an increased wall-to-lumen ratio and reduced dilatory capacity, may contribute to impotence in hypertensive patients. [p 1610]

29. **b. Ischemic priapism from sickle-cell anemia.** Sickle-cell disease affects 8% of African Americans. In a review of 321 pediatric patients, Tarry and colleagues in 1987 found a 6.4% incidence of priapism among their sickle-cell clinic patients. Red cell sickling and later sludging of blood occur within the corpora cavernosa, perhaps as a result of abnormal endothelial adherence, the mild acidosis accompanying hypoventilation during sleep, or mild trauma with masturbation and intercourse. When the venous channels are maximally compressed during nocturnal penile tumescence, the sludged red blood cells can then block the microscopic subtunical venules and trigger diffuse veno-occlusion. In one study of adults with homozygous sickle-cell disease in a Jamaican clinic, stuttering nocturnal attacks of priapism lasting 2 to 6 hours reportedly affected 42% of patients. These attacks, which begin soon after puberty and are not related to other vaso-occlusive crises, may occur over weeks to culminate in a major episode lasting 3 to 5 days. Anecdotally, pediatric patients are known subsequently to achieve erectile capability, but adults often do not recover it. The natural

history of sickle-cell priapism is one of recurrence. Although almost all cases are of the ischemic type, two cases of nonischemic priapism in patients with sickle-cell disease have been reported. [p 1611]

30. **b. Rupture of the cavernous artery.** Laceration of the cavernous artery or its branches within the corpora cavernosa, from trauma or intracavernous injection, can result in unregulated pooling of the blood into the sinusoidal spaces with consequent priapism. Nonischemic priapism after blunt perineal trauma typically has a delayed onset. Injury to the erectile tissue and the cavernous artery or its branches does not produce priapism until the patient has nocturnal erections, at which time vasodilatation causes rupture of the damaged artery and results in unregulated high flow into the corpora cavernosa. [p 1612]

Chapter 46

Evaluation and Nonsurgical Management of Erectile Dysfunction and Priapism

Gregory A. Broderick • Tom E. Lue

Questions

1. The urologist's role in the era of effective oral pharmacotherapy for treatment of erectile dysfunction (ED) includes specialized diagnostic testing. ED diagnostic evaluations may be of benefit to each of the following selected patients except which group?

   a. Patients with perineal trauma
   b. Patients who are refractory to phosphodiesterase inhibitor
   c. Patients with Peyronie's disease
   d. Men 50 years of age and older with one to three risk factors for organic ED
   e. Patients complaining of ED present since the onset of sexual maturity

2. In 1992, the National Institutes of Health (NIH) sponsored a consensus conference on impotence. The conference defined ED as the inability to achieve and/or maintain erection of sufficient rigidity and duration to permit satisfactory sexual performance and recognized clinical conditions that have come to be regarded as organic risk factors for ED, including which of the following?

   a. Increasing age
   b. Hypertension
   c. Atherosclerotic heart disease
   d. Diabetes mellitus
   e. All of the above

3. The Process of Care Model, which has been developed to assist physicians in the diagnosis and treatment of ED:

   a. is an algorithm.
   b. is a guide for urologists interested in diagnostic testing.
   c. deemphasizes the medical history.
   d. is a stepwise management approach that ranks treatment options.
   e. was designed before the introduction of oral pharmacotherapies.

4. The First International Consultation of ED was convened in Paris in 1999 and was cosponsored by the World Health Organization. ED was defined as the consistent or recurrent inability to attain and or maintain penile erection sufficient for sexual performance. Which of the following was also defined at the meeting?

   a. The term ED requires a 3-month duration.
   b. The term ED may also describe penile curvatures.
   c. The term ED may also describe anorgasmia and lack of desire.
   d. The term ED may also describe lack of desire.
   e. The diagnosis of ED should not be based solely on the patient's complaint.

5. The International Index of Erectile Function (IIEF) is the most widely used self-administered questionnaire (SAQ). The IIEF quantifies several domains of sexual function, except:

   a. erectile function.
   b. partner satisfaction.
   c. sexual desire.
   d. orgasmic function.
   e. overall satisfaction.

6. Which of the following statements is true regarding self-administered sex questionnaires?

   a. They distinguish psychogenic ED from organic ED.
   b. They correlate patient-perceived severity with the physiologic severity of ED.
   c. They are a good way to structure the male sexual history for physicians lacking expertise in ED.
   d. They predict therapeutic responses to different pharmacologic treatments.
   e. They are of no use in clinical trials.

7. When correlated with results of penile pharmacotesting and penile duplex Doppler study, which of the following risk factors is not associated with likelihood of abnormal penile blood flows?

   a. Smoking
   b. Diabetes mellitus
   c. Hypertension

d. Testosterone level
e. Age

8. The First International Consultation on ED in Paris in 1999 divided laboratory testing into three categories: recommended, optional, and specialized. What does recommended laboratory testing include?

   a. Fasting glucose or glycosylated hemoglobin, lipid profile, and testosterone
   b. Prolactin and luteinizing hormone
   c. Complete blood count
   d. Thyroid-stimulating hormone
   e. Prostate-specific antigen and urinalysis

9. How can nocturnal penile tumescence (NPT) be measured?

   a. The stamp test
   b. Snap gauges
   c. RigiScan
   d. NEVA
   e. All of the above

10. Karacan, in 1966, was the first to use NPT in the clinical evaluation of impotence. His observations included which of the following?

    a. Only 20% of NPT occurs during rapid eye movement sleep.
    b. NPT shows age-specific variation.
    c. NPT peaks during the third decade of life.
    d. The average adult has one NPT episode each night.
    e. The average duration of an NPT episode is 90 minutes.

11. According to the criteria of Levine and Lenting, each of the following statements describes NPTR as measured by RigiScan except which one?

    a. Normal radial rigidity is reflected by a value greater than 70%.
    b. Radial rigidity less than 40% represents a flaccid penis.
    c. The RigiScan measures axial buckling forces.
    d. Three to six erectile events is normal per 8-hour sleep recording.
    e. The average NPTR event lasts 10 to 15 minutes.

12. Udelson and Goldstein, in 1998, described the physics of ED in engineering terms. What are the factors that regulate penile axial rigidity?

    a. Intracavernous pressure
    b. Penile diameter to length ratio
    c. Penile flaccid diameter
    d. Cavernous smooth muscle mechanical properties
    e. All of the above

13. When ED testing is employed, no single test is likely to reveal the cause in all cases. Heaton and Morales suggested that RigiScan testing may be of value in all of the following situations except which one?

    a. Suspected venous leakage
    b. Suspected sleep disorder
    c. Legally sensitive case
    d. Suspected psychogenic dysfunction
    e. Measurement and comparison of drug effects in placebo-controlled trials

14. Audiovisual sexual stimulation (AVSS) has been noted to increase erectile responses to specific sexual stimuli during clinical testing with:

    a. vibration.
    b. intracavernous agents.
    c. topical agents.
    d. oral agents.
    e. all of the above.

15. The complex ED patient seen in referral from the primary caregiver may be a man with a significant psychological component to his ED. Certain authors have suggested that which significant percentage of patients will not sustain initial success with sildenafil citrate because of confounding psychological factors?

    a. 10%
    b. 25%
    c. 30%
    d. 55%
    e. 75%

16. Current neurologic testing in the evaluation of ED is of limited value for which of the following reasons?

    a. There is a lack of specificity in differentiating somatic from autonomic deficits.
    b. There are no clinical tests to assess neurotransmitter release in the penis.
    c. Neurologic disease is rarely reversible.
    d. ED in diabetes mellitus is multifactorial.
    e. All of the above.

17. Routine endocrine testing for ED is controversial; in contemporary series, the incidence of endocrinopathy in ED patients varies from a low of 1.7% to a high of 35%. After screening 300 patients with total serum testosterone, Johnson and Jarow made which of the following suggestions to increase cost-effectiveness?

    a. Testosterone assays should be restricted to men with decreased libido or bilateral testicular atrophy.
    b. Testosterone assays should be restricted to men with decreased libido.
    c. Testosterone assays should be restricted to men with testicular atrophy.
    d. Testosterone assays should be restricted to men older than 50 years of age.
    e. Testosterone assays should be abandoned in favor of assessing bioavailable testosterone.

18. There is mounting contemporary evidence from cross-sectional aging studies that androgens decline with age and are associated with a variety of clinical consequences. All of the following associations have been documented except which one?

    a. Decreased libido
    b. Venous leakage
    c. Osteoporosis
    d. Insulin resistance
    e. Depression

19. The urologist should be aware of drugs that directly alter androgen levels and bioavailability. Each of the following exerts adverse effects on male sexual function by direct interference with testosterone production at the level of the testes or by bioavailability except which one?

    a. Cimetidine
    b. Ketoconazole
    c. Cocaine
    d. Bicalutamide
    e. Flutamide

20. Which of the following statements about dehydroepiandrosterone (DHEA), an adrenal steroid, is correct?

    a. DHEA is secreted by the adrenal gland in response to luteinizing hormone stimulation.
    b. DHEA has direct androgenic activity.

c. Maximal DHEA levels are reached in the sixth decade of life for men.
d. Many human tissues, including adipose tissue, bone, muscle, skin, and prostate, contain dihydrotestosterone (DHT), by which DHEA is converted to testosterone.
e. DHEA sulfate (DHEAS) and free testosterone are the only hormones statistically correlated with the complaint of impotence in the original Massachusetts Male Aging Study.

21. Office intracavernous injection (ICI) pharmacotesting consists of a penile injection of a vasoactive agent followed by visual rating of the subsequent erection. Each of the following statements about office pharmacotesting with ICI is true except which one?
    a. It is the most commonly performed diagnostic procedure in the evaluation of ED.
    b. To produce an erection, arterial vasodilatation, sinusoidal relaxation, and decreased venous outflow must each occur in response to a vasodilating agent.
    c. It is minimally invasive and requires no monitoring equipment.
    d. A normal erection rules out veno-occlusive dysfunction, although some men with borderline arterial insufficiency will also achieve a rigid erection.
    e. Self-stimulation and audiovisual stimulation are of no additional benefit in ICI pharmacotesting.

22. Which of the following statements about penile blood flow studies (PBFSs) utilizing ICI pharmacotesting and duplex Doppler ultrasonography is true?
    a. The average patient with several vascular risk factors for ED should have PBFS before a trial of oral pharmacotherapy to ensure that adequate penile blood flow exists.
    b. Detection and quantification of flow in the flaccid penis are highly predictive of erectile responses to ICI.
    c. Color duplex Doppler study is helpful in the diagnosis of high-flow priapism and localization of cavernous arterial injury.
    d. The finding of echodense areas (acoustic shadows) within the tunica albuginea suggests that corporeal fibrosis has replaced the normal vascular sinusoids.
    e. Penile Doppler study, like pudendal arteriography, is an invasive third-line diagnostic test that should be reserved for patients who are candidates for arterial bypass.

23. The most common agent(s) used for ICI for the purposes of office pharmacotesting or initial home dosing is(are):
    a. alprostadil.
    b. papaverine.
    c. papaverine plus phentolamine (Regitine).
    d. alprostadil plus papaverine plus phentolamine.
    e. sildenafil.

24. When penile pharmacoangiography is compared with duplex Doppler penile ultrasonography in the same patients, which of the following Doppler parameters is consistently associated with severe arterial disease?
    a. End-diastolic velocity greater than 5 cm/second
    b. Peak systolic velocity less than 25 cm/second
    c. Peak systolic velocity greater than 25 cm/second but less than 35 cm/second and end-diastolic velocity greater than 5 cm/second
    d. Peak systolic velocity greater than 35 cm/second
    e. Resistive index greater than 0.9

25. Which of the following statements about cavernous veno-occlusive dysfunction (CVOD), defined as the inability to achieve and maintain erection despite adequate arterial flows, is true?
    a. With increasing intracorporeal pressures, full erection is associated with cessation of diastolic flows in the dorsal arteries.
    b. Deep dorsal vein flows should be interpreted as evidence of CVOD.
    c. The parameters of end-diastolic velocity and resistive index are used to document CVOD.
    d. Cavernous arterial Doppler waveforms do not change with progress from tumescence to rigidity in the normal patient.
    e. CVOD should be suspected if an erection lasts 30 or more minutes after the injection of 10 μg of alprostadil.

26. Dynamic infusion cavernosometry and cavernosography (DICC) was introduced by Goldstein and colleagues in 1989. Each of the following statements about DICC is true except which one?
    a. It involves infusing saline solution into the corpora at a rate sufficient to raise penile pressures above systolic blood pressure.
    b. Like the Doppler penile blood flow study, it is minimally invasive and permits the patient a period of privacy and self-stimulation.
    c. The pressure at which the cavernous arterial flows become detectable is defined as the cavernous artery systolic occlusion pressure (CASOP).
    d. CASOP correlates with peak systolic velocity measurements obtained by penile Doppler ultrasonography.
    e. Cavernosography involves the infusion of contrast solution into the corpora cavernosa during artificial erection to visualize sites of venous leakage.

27. In older patients with adequate arterial inflows but poorly sustained erections, venous leakage is likely secondary to:
    a. large veins.
    b. anomalous course of penile veins.
    c. congenitally excessive number of veins.
    d. corporeal smooth muscle pathology.
    e. trauma.

28. Wespes and colleagues used cavernous smooth muscle biopsies to show the relationship between corporeal smooth muscle content and ED. Each of the following has been suggested by this line of research except which one?
    a. The corporeal smooth muscle content in young hemodynamically normal men is 40% to 52%.
    b. Veno-occlusive dysfunction was associated with 19% to 36% smooth muscle content.
    c. Arterial dysfunction was associated with normal smooth muscle content but atherosclerotic blockage of one or both cavernous arteries.
    d. Smooth muscle is replaced by extracellular matrix, such as collagen, to varying degrees in vascular ED.
    e. Corporeal biopsy samples are retrieved at the time of penile prosthesis implantation and are not a standard technique in the diagnosis of ED.

29. In the patient with documented hypogonadism and ED, it is reasonable to initiate androgen therapy. Which of the following is true?
    a. Intramuscular preparations of testosterone are the cheapest form of treatment and mimic normal circadian levels of testosterone.
    b. Transdermal scrotal testosterone patches result in significant levels of DHT, because of a high content of 5α-reductase in scrotal skin.

c. The most common reaction to testosterone patches is contact dermatitis secondary to development of testosterone allergy.
d. Testosterone gel is rapidly absorbed by men and cannot alter female partners' testosterone levels.
e. Oral testosterone preparations are the safest, most effective means of delivering therapy.

30. Testosterone therapy has potential adverse effects. All of the following have been documented except which one?

   a. Suppression of luteinizing hormone and follicle-stimulating hormone, resulting in infertility
   b. Erythrocytosis
   c. Increased cardiovascular risks
   d. Osteoporosis
   e. Exacerbation of occult prostate cancer

31. Yohimbine is an α_2-adrenergic antagonist that historically has been used to treat ED. Which of the following statements is true?

   a. It is administered intramuscularly.
   b. In addition to activity on adrenergic receptors, it alters serotonin and dopamine transmission.
   c. It was recommended as first-line therapy in the 1996 American Urological Association guidelines on ED.
   d. It has demonstrated efficacy over placebo in patients with vascular ED.
   e. A principal side effect is hypotension.

32. Apomorphine has well-documented effects on sexual arousal. Which of the following statements is true?

   a. Apomorphine is an opiate.
   b. The main site of action for apomorphine is the penile vascular tissues.
   c. Apomorphine is a dopaminergic agonist, activating D1 and D2 receptors in the paraventricular nucleus.
   d. Clinical trials suggest that in human subjects apomorphine induces erection without sexual stimulation.
   e. The main side effect is penile pain.

33. Sildenafil is orally active and facilitates erectile responses to sexual stimulation. Which of the following statements is true?

   a. It enhances proerectile signaling in the brain.
   b. It prevents the breakdown of cyclic guanosine monophosphate (cGMP).
   c. It stimulates the production of nitric oxide, a gaseous neurotransmitter.
   d. Dosing needs to be reduced in men taking nitrates.
   e. It is a nonspecific inhibitor of phosphodiesterase, like papaverine.

34. Each of the following statements describes findings of the sildenafil clinical trials published in 1998 except which one?

   a. Erectile responses are dosage related over a range of 25 to 100 mg, with little benefit and considerably more side effects beyond 100 mg.
   b. Improved erections were seen in hypertensive patients.
   c. Improved erections were seen in patients with lower motor neuron spinal cord lesions.
   d. Improved erections were seen in diabetic patients.
   e. Cimetidine, ketoconazole, and erythromycin may impair hepatic metabolism of sildenafil.

35. Post-release product labeling was required by the Food and Drug Administration (FDA) cautioning the use of sildenafil in several patient populations. Each of the following represents a precautionary population except which group?

   a. Men with unstable angina
   b. Men with a history of life-threatening arrhythmia in the preceding 6 months
   c. Men with resting blood pressure less than 90/50 or higher than 170/110 mm Hg
   d. Men with diabetic neuropathy
   e. Men with retinitis pigmentosa

36. MUSE (medicated urethral system for erection) is a small semisolid pellet 3 × 1 mm composed of:

   a. papaverine.
   b. papaverine plus phentolamine.
   c. alprostadil.
   d. L-arginine.
   e. cyclic GMP–specific phosphodiesterase inhibitor.

37. Each of the following statements about papaverine therapy is true except which one?

   a. It is a nonspecific phosphodiesterase inhibitor increasing cyclic AMP (cAMP) and cyclic GMP (cGMP) in cavernous tissues.
   b. It is very stable at room temperature.
   c. It has a higher incidence of fibrosis than does alprostadil.
   d. Papaverine-induced erection is associated with idiopathic penile pain in 30% of men.
   e. Systemic side effects include dizziness.

38. Alprostadil is the synthetic form of a naturally occurring unsaturated 20-carbon fatty acid, prostaglandin E_1 (PGE_1). Which of the following statements is true?

   a. It causes corporeal smooth muscle relaxation through elevation of intracellular cGMP.
   b. Up to 90% is metabolized on the first passage through the lungs.
   c. Prolonged erection and priapism have been noted in up to 30% of men at dosages from 10 to 20 μg.
   d. Penile pain is reported in 5% or fewer patients at clinically effective dosages.
   e. Only one formulation is available in the United States: Caverject.

39. Bennett and colleagues, in 1991, introduced and popularized a three-drug mixture (papaverine, phentolamine, alprostadil) for ICI pharmacotherapy. Which of the following statements is true regarding Trimix?

   a. Trimix is the only FDA-approved combination ICI pharmacotherapy for ED.
   b. Trimix proved to be not as effective as alprostadil alone.
   c. The incidence of prolonged erection, fibrosis, and injection plaques is higher with Trimix than with papaverine plus phentolamine therapy.
   d. Vasoactive intestinal polypeptide (VIP) and phentolamine have the same pharmacologic activity and may be equally substituted as the third ingredient in Trimix.
   e. Trimix is more effective than papaverine plus phentolamine in patients with severe arteriogenic or veno-occlusive ED.

40. Patient acceptance of ICI therapy ranges from 49% to 84%. Which of the following statements is true?

   a. Reasons for declining to use ICI include penile pain, inadequate responses, fear of needles, unnaturalness.
   b. Dropout rates from ICI programs are reported to be up to 60%.
   c. Common reasons for dropouts from ICI programs include drug costs and insufficient erections.
   d. The incidence of prolonged erections for alprostadil monotherapy ICI is five times lower than that in ICI programs using papaverine or papaverine plus phentolamine.
   e. All of the above.

41. Vacuum erection devices (VEDs) became popular before the

introduction of oral pharmacotherapies for ED. Which of the following statements is true?

a. VEDs require physician prescription.
b. VEDs may be effective in the patient with a malfunctioning penile implant and after explantation.
c. Dropout rates for long-term VED are low compared with dropout rates for ICI.
d. VEDs induce and maintain erection without a constriction band in men with arterial insufficiency but not in men with venous leakage.
e. Combining ICI with VED does not enhance VED responses.

42. The Process of Care Model and the First World Consultation on ED in Paris recommended specialist referral and possible evidence-based assessments for complex ED patients. Specialist review is recommended for each of the following patients except which group?

a. Those with penile, pelvic, or perineal trauma
b. Men with Peyronie's disease
c. Men failing to respond to phosphodiesterase inhibitor therapy
d. Those with suspected psychological or psychiatric disease
e. Men 50 years of age or older with vascular risk factors

43. There are distinct clinical and physiologic differences between high-flow and low-flow priapism. Which of the following statements is true?

a. Priapism of 12 or more hours after intracavernous pharmacotherapy is generally high flow.
b. High-flow priapism is generally painful after 6 hours.
c. A corporeal aspirate of dark blood that is hypercarbic and acidotic is classic for low-flow priapism.
d. Trauma after penile or straddle injury more often leads to ischemic rather than arterial priapism.
e. The least invasive way of diagnosing low-flow priapism is with phalloarteriography.

44. Treatment of low-flow priapism has two goals: (1) to immediately reverse the painful erection and (2) to prevent permanent corporeal smooth muscle damage. Which of the following statements is true?

a. Priapism is a true urologic emergency and is best managed with immediate operative intervention: shunting.
b. Aspiration of the corpora and intracorporeal injection of an α-adrenergic agent is the treatment of choice in low-flow priapism.
c. Aspiration and intracorporeal injection of an α-adrenergic agent is contraindicated in patients taking sildenafil.
d. α-Adrenergic blockers may be effective in the management of low-flow priapism.

e. Applying ice to the penis usually avoids the need to aspirate and inject.

45. Sickle-cell priapism has some unique clinical and physiologic features. Each of the following statements is correct except which one?

a. Both adults and prepubertal children with sickle-cell disease may develop priapism.
b. Stuttering priapism with a series of prolonged nocturnal erections may occur with sickle-cell disease and sickle-cell trait and in patients without sickle-cell disease who have had a previous episode of true low-flow priapism.
c. Antiandrogens, luteinizing hormone–releasing hormone agonists, and estrogens have been described in the management of recurring priapism in sickle-cell patients.
d. Treatment of the man with sickle cell priapism should be by immediate operative shunting.
e. Sickle-cell priapism may or may not be accompanied by other signs of sickle-cell crisis. Systemic intervention is usually part of the management strategy with hydration, oxygenation, alkalinization, and transfusion to reduce the hemoglobin S level.

46. The long-term complication of conservatively managed low-flow priapism is ED secondary to fibrosis. The urologist should be prepared for complications of well-intentioned interventions with α-adrenergic agents, including all of the following except:

a. hypertension, headache, cardiac arrhythmia.
b. skin necrosis.
c. penile hematoma.
d. cellulitis.
e. temporary stress incontinence.

47. High-flow priapism has a different physiologic mechanism and a different clinical presentation and may merit an intervention different from that of low-flow priapism. Which of the following statements is false?

a. High-flow priapism is secondary to "dysregulation" of cavernous arterial inflows.
b. Sexual trauma, straddle injury, and laceration by needle have all been reported as culprits.
c. Shunting, although most invasive, has the highest degree of success in reversing high-flow priapism.
d. Arteriography with autologous clot embolization or coils may abort the high-flow erection but may also lead to permanent vascular ED.
e. Conservative management with follow-up color duplex Doppler sonography is recommended because of the likelihood of resolution of small cavernous-sinusoidal fistulas and preservation of potency in most cases of high-flow priapism.

Answers

1. **d. Men 50 years of age and older with one to three risk factors for organic ED.** Vascular, hormonal, and neurologic testing will not be needed by the typical ED patient who seeks help from his primary care provider but will be needed to manage complex cases. Whether or not ED testing can predict which drug or combination of drugs will work for a particular patient remains to be determined. For now, ED evaluations are of defined benefit in patients with complex conditions: oral agent–resistant ED, multiple medical disorders, high-risk cardiac conditions, pelvic or perineal trauma, primary ED in young patients (present since the age of sexual maturity), neurologic disease, endocrinopathy, and Peyronie's disease and to identify patients with a significant psychological component to ED (depression, anxiety). [p 1620]

2. **e. All of the above.** At the NIH Consensus Conference on Impotence, a multidisciplinary group reviewed the various

aspects of male sexual function (interest, performance, and satisfaction) and suggested refinement in terminology as a first step to increasing public and physician awareness. ED was defined as the inability to achieve and/or maintain erection of sufficient rigidity and duration to permit satisfactory sexual performance. The participants looked at multiple strategies for identifying and evaluating ED; they were compelled to acknowledge the statistical associations with increasing age, and the concurrence of distinct medical illnesses: diabetes, atherosclerotic peripheral and coronary disease, hypertension, cigarette smoking, and chronic renal insufficiency. [p 1620]

3. **d. is a stepwise management approach that ranks treatment options.** The Process of Care Model for the Evaluation and Treatment of Erectile Dysfunction was developed to coincide with the introduction of sildenafil in 1998. The model has as its goal to advance guidelines for the diagnosis and management of ED; it targets the primary care provider (PCP). Rather than an algorithm, it is a stepwise linear model. Central to its purpose is the identification and potential modification of ED risk factors. The model segregates therapies as first line (oral agents, vacuum erection devices, and couple/sexual therapy) to be administered by the PCP, and second- and third-line therapies, which are presumably to be administered by a specialist (intraurethral alprostadil and intracavernosal injection/surgical prosthesis). Referral is based on failure of first-line therapy and/or need for diagnostic testing or management. Common referral indications include treatment failures, penile curvature, young patients, pelvic/perineal trauma, cases requiring vascular or neurosurgical intervention, complicated endocrinopathy, complicated psychiatric or psychosexual disorders, and patient request. [pp 1620–1621]

4. **a. The term ED requires a 3-month duration.** ED was redefined as the consistent or recurrent inability to attain and or maintain penile erection sufficient for sexual performance. A 3-month duration of ED is required to meet the criteria of consistency; the exceptions are cases of trauma or surgically induced ED. The term ED should not be used to describe penile curvatures, prolonged erection, painful erection, premature ejaculation, anorgasmia, or lack of desire. [p 1621]

5. **b. partner satisfaction.** The IIEF is the most widely used SAQ, and it is statistically validated in at least seven languages. It was employed as the primary efficacy end point in the sildenafil citrate trials. The IIEF is a 15-item SAQ; it addresses and quantifies five domains: erectile function, orgasmic function, sexual desire, intercourse satisfaction, and overall satisfaction. [p 1623]

6. **c. They are a good way to structure the male sexual history for physicians lacking expertise in ED.** Sex questionnaires are a good way of structuring the male history, especially for nonurologists. Several important roles for erectile function SAQs remain to be clarified: (1) Do they accurately distinguish psychogenic from organic ED? (2) Does perceived severity match physiologic severity of ED? (3) Will SAQs be useful in predicting therapeutic responses to different pharmacologic treatments? [pp 1623–1624]

7. **d. Testosterone level.** One study of the correlation of three risk factors—smoking, diabetes mellitus, and hypertension— with results of penile duplex ultrasonography found that the incidence of abnormal findings increased significantly as the number of risk factors increased. [p 1624]

8. **a. Fasting glucose or glycosylated hemoglobin, lipid profile, and testosterone.** The First International Consultation on ED divided testing into three categories: recommended, optional, and specialized. Among the recommended laboratory assays was some combination of tests to identify the pathologies of diabetes mellitus, hyperlipidemia, and the hypothalamic-pituitary-gonadal axis (fasting glucose or glycosylated hemoglobin, lipid profile, and testosterone). [p 1626]

9. **e. All of the above.** NPT has been measured by the following methods: the stamp test, snap gauges, strain gauges, NPTR (RigiScan; originally from Dacomed Corp. and currently from Timm Medical Systems, Minneapolis, MN), sleep laboratory NPTR, and most recently NPT electrobioimpedance (NEVA, Timm Medical Technologies). [p 1627]

10. **b. NPT shows age-specific variation.** Karacan was the first to demonstrate that 80% of NPT occurs during rapid eye movement sleep. The average man has three to five episodes of NPT each night, with each episode potentially yielding 30 to 60 minutes of erection time. NPT shows age-specific variations. Total tumescence time during sleep peaks at the age of puberty, when as much of 20% of total sleep time may be spent with an erection. In the second decade of life, the average duration of a nocturnal erection is 38 minutes; for adult males, the average duration is 27 minutes. [p 1627]

11. **c. The RigiScan measures axial buckling forces.** Radial rigidity greater than 70% represents a nonbuckling erection, and a rigidity of less than 40% represents a flaccid penis. Measurements between 40% and 70% represent varying degrees of penile stiffness; number of erections considered normal is three to six per 8-hour session and lasting an average of 10 to 15 minutes. [p 1629]

12. **e. All of the above.** Udelson and Goldstein attempted to describe the physics of ED. ED in engineering terms is inadequate penile rigidity, which allows bending, leading to deformation (buckling) of an otherwise straight column (the erect penile shaft). The physical factors regulating penile axial rigidity are intracavernous pressure, penile geometry (penile diameter to length ratio and flaccid penile diameter), and penile tissue mechanical properties (cavernosal expandability). These physical principles explain why a thick short penis is more resistant to buckling than a long thin penis with the same intracavernous pressure. [p 1630]

13. **a. Suspected venous leakage.** Because of problems associated with various NPT tests, findings need to be confirmed independently by other studies. For these reasons, we have abandoned NPTR testing as a routine part of ED evaluation. We concur with Heaton and Morales, who described in 1997 the complex cases in which NPTR may be indicated: (1) suspected sleep disorder; (2) an obscure origin; (3) patient unresponsive to therapy; (4) planned invasive treatment; (5) a legally sensitive case; (6) measurement and comparison of drug effects in placebo-controlled drug trials; (7) suspected psychogenic cause. [p 1631]

14. **e. all of the above.** AVSS appears to enhance penile responses to a variety of test stimulants: vibratory, intracavernous, and topical and oral pharmacologic agents. AVSS likely decreases central inhibitory stimuli and activates central proerectile stimuli. All urologists interested in the management of complex ED patients need to appreciate the specific insights to be gained from this type of evidence-based testing. [p 1631]

15. **b. 25%.** The complex ED patient referred to the urologist may be a man with mixed ED, a patient in whom pharmacologic treatment has failed because only one component of his problem has been identified. Some studies have suggested that as many as 25% of patients will not sustain initial success with sildenafil citrate because of confounding (or unaddressed) psychological factors: anxiety, low desire, relationship problems, sexual apathy, and avoidance. [p 1632]

16. **e. All of the above.** It is clear that the effect of neurologic deficit on penile erection is a complicated phenomenon and, with a few exceptions, neurologic testing will rarely change management. Moreover, there is no reliable test to assess neurotransmitter release, which leaves a major gap in the current assessment of overall neurologic function associated with penile erection. Therefore, for practical reasons, one study suggested that neurologic evaluation of impotence in patients with neurologic pathology should differ from that in other subjects; in particular, the aim is to identify or exclude a hidden or underestimated neurologic lesion. In our opinion, the aim of neurourologic testing is to (1) uncover reversible neurologic disease such as dorsal nerve neuropathy secondary to long-distance bicycling; (2) assess the extent of neurologic deficit from a known neurologic disease such as diabetes mellitus or pelvic injury; and (3) determine whether a referral to a neurologist is necessary (e.g., work-up for possible compression lesion of the spinal cord). [p 1633]

17. **a. Testosterone assays should be restricted to men with decreased libido or bilateral testicular atrophy.** The value of routine endocrinologic testing among patients complaining of ED is controversial. In a large series, the overall incidence of endocrinopathy in impotent patients was 17.5%. In contemporary series, reported incidences of endocrinopathy among ED patients vary from a low of 1.7% to a high of 35%, with most large series closer to the former figure. These differences are likely attributable to the population being screened: patients presenting to urologists versus those presenting to endocrinologists. Johnson and Jarow attempted to determine whether specific historical or physical findings could identify a subgroup of patients at risk for hypogonadal ED and avoid screening of the overall population. They screened 330 men referred to a urologic practice by drawing a total testosterone and found 10 to have low total testosterone (240 to 950 ng/dl). In these patients, repeated hormone studies, including total testosterone, bioavailable (free) testosterone (9 to 30 mg/dl), and pituitary hormones (luteinizing hormone, follicle-stimulating hormone, prolactin) led to the discovery of seven patients (2.1%) with true hypogonadism. When the history and physical findings in these patients were reviewed, testicular atrophy was observed in five patients; six reported decreased libido. All of their patients with hypogonadism had either decreased libido or bilateral testicular atrophy. Routine endocrine screening of ED patients, with its high cost, may add little information beyond a complete history and physical examination. Other investigators have also suggested that only men with clinical evidence of hypogonadism (decreased libido and/or bilateral testicular atrophy) need to be evaluated. [p 1635]

18. **b. Venous leakage.** There is mounting contemporary evidence from cross-sectional studies that testosterone or one of its metabolites decreases with aging. In the geriatric literature, multiple clinical consequences are associated with age-related decline in androgens: decreased libido, impotence, osteoporosis, insulin resistance, decreased lean muscle mass, increased body fat, and depression. Similarly, the health benefits of androgen replacement therapy are being promoted: increased bone density, increased muscle mass, improved sense of well-being, and improved metabolic profile (glucose and lipids). [p 1636]

19. **c. Cocaine.** Patients experiencing treatment failures of first-line therapy (sildenafil failure, vacuum erection device failures) are likely to have undergone little if any evaluation by the primary care provider directed at identifying an underlying endocrinopathy. In these men and certainly all patients presenting with a complaint of decreased libido, the urologist should be aware of drugs that can adversely alter androgen levels and bioavailability. Those that inhibit testosterone production include spironolactone, common chemotherapy agents such as methotrexate, alkylating agents, ketoconazole, metronidazole, flutamide, cimetidine, and cyproterone. Those that inhibit gonadotropin releasing-hormone (GnRH) release or production include progesterone, estrogen, and GnRH agonists (leuprolide, goserelin). Those that elevate prolactin levels include estrogen, phenothiazines, tricyclic antidepressants, reserpine, opioid analgesics, and cocaine. [p 1637]

20. **d. Many human tissues, including adipose tissue, bone, muscle, skin, and prostate, contain dihydrotestosterone (DHT), by which DHEA is converted to testosterone.** DHEA is an adrenal steroid, which is converted to more active androgens. DHEA is secreted by the adrenal gland in response to adrenocorticotropic hormone stimulation. DHEA does not have any direct androgenic activity. Human tissues contain numerous sites where enzymes can convert DHEA to testosterone via DHT: adipose tissue, bone, muscle, breast, prostate, skin, and brain. Maximal levels of DHEA are reached in the third decade of life for men. Thereafter, it is estimated that a slow, steady decline of 2% per year occurs. DHEA, but not testosterone, correlated with the complaint of impotence in the original MMAS. [p 1637]

21. **e. Self-stimulation and audiovisual stimulation are of no additional benefit in ICI pharmacotesting.** Office pharmacotesting consists of an intracavernous injection and a visual rating of the subsequent erection. This test is the most commonly performed diagnostic procedure for ED. It is simple, is minimally invasive, and requires no monitoring equipment. This screening test allows the clinician to bypass neurogenic and hormonal influences and to evaluate the vascular status of the penis directly and objectively. The pharmacologic test yields important information regarding penile vascular status. A positive response (normal erectile rigidity of sustained duration) implies psychogenic impotence, presumably excluding significant venous or arterial pathology. More contemporary studies suggest that a normal response rules out the possibility of venous leakage, although some patients (about 20%) with arterial insufficiency will also achieve a rigid erection. Generally, a normal office pharmacotest with ICI and stimulation suggests that neurogenic, psychogenic, or hormonal factors may be primarily responsible for ED, although pharmacotesting is unable to distinguish among them. Regardless, further evaluation for veno-occlusive dysfunction is rendered unnecessary. The patient's fear of injection often produces a heightened sympathetic response, which inhibits the response of the cavernous smooth muscle to the intracavernous agent. This may produce a false-positive result. To avoid this error, we have found it helpful to give patients as much privacy as possible during this study. They are also instructed to perform self-stimulation if a rigid erection does not result within 15 minutes. This technique is known as the combined injection and stimulation test. [pp 1638–1639]

22. **c. Color duplex Doppler study is helpful in the diagnosis of high-flow priapism and localization of cavernous arterial injury.** When diagnostic testing is indicated in the evaluation of the complex patient, the PBFS, which consists of an intracavernous pharmacotest with ICI and measurement by duplex Doppler ultrasonography, is the most reliable and least invasive evidence-based assessment of ED. Duplex sonography is more accurate than continuous wave sonography because the examiner can see a real-time image of the central cavernous arteries, avoiding the pitfall of erroneously measuring the dorsal vessels. Color duplex Doppler ultrasonography is a further advance in sonography; it aids in visualizing vessels with the Doppler computer assigning color to

flowing blood. Current color duplex Doppler ultrasonography probes consist of linear arrays with frequency ranges from 7 to 10 MHz. The higher the frequency, the better the near field resolution; some investigators have reported adequate high-resolution penile imaging with (noncolor) gray scale 13.5-MHz probes. Ultrasonography provides clear advantages over previous techniques: first, in contrast to pudendal arteriography, duplex sonography is noninvasive and can be performed in the office; second, high-resolution color duplex Doppler ultrasonography allows the ultrasonographer to image the individual cavernous arteries selectively and to perform dynamic blood flow analysis simultaneously. The color duplex Doppler ultrasonography device provides an additional advantage of rapid acquisition of vessels and collateral flows among the cavernous, dorsal, and spongiosal arteries, which may be crucial in planning penile vascular and reconstructive surgeries. It is the best tool available for the diagnosis of high-flow priapism and localization of arterial rupture. In most centers, it has replaced cavernosometry and cavernosography for diagnosing venous leakage. With color duplex Doppler ultrasonography, slow cavernous blood flows are visible, but detection of flow in the flaccid penis (before injection of vasodilator) depends on the patient's level of sympathetic tone and anxiety and on ambient room temperature. Flaccid cavernous arterial flow measurements are of no predictive value. High-resolution ultrasonography is used to image the corpora cavernosa, the corpus spongiosum, and the tunica albuginea. The corpus cavernosum and corpus spongiosum have a homogeneous echogenicity, which is distinguished from the hyperechoic tunica albuginea and septum. The tunica albuginea should have uniform thickness and echogenicity; the subcutaneous tissues and Buck's fascia are not identifiable sonographically except by the location of the dorsal vascular bundle: paired dorsal arteries and deep dorsal vein complex. The finding of echodense areas or calcification (acoustic shadows) within the corporeal bodies or the tunica albuginea may represent intrinsic sinusoidal disease, fibrosis, or Peyronie's plaques. The cavernous arteries are usually identified near the septum at the base and centrally located in the middle and distal shaft. [pp 1639–1640]

23. **a. alprostadil.** Alprostadil is an effective agent and should be considered the drug of first choice for the diagnosis and management of ED in the oral agent failure/contraindication group of patients. In 1996, prostaglandin E_1 (PGE_1) became the first and remains the only penile injectable approved by the Food and Drug Administration (FDA) for the management of ED. It is available in the United States in two proprietary forms: Caverject (Pharmacia and Upjohn) and Edex (Schwarz Pharma). Its advantages are a lower incidence of prolonged erection, systemic side effects, and fibrosis (presumably because of its local metabolism by prostaglandin hydroxydehydrogenase present in the penile tissue). The disadvantages include a higher incidence of painful erection and higher cost, and once reconstituted into liquid from powder it has a shortened half-life if not refrigerated. [p 1658]

24. **b. Peak systolic velocity less than 25 cm/second.** When penile angiographic findings are compared with duplex Doppler examination findings from the same patients, peak systolic velocity less than 25 cm/second is consistently associated with severe arterial disease. In the Mayo Clinic series, peak systolic velocity less than 25 cm/second had a sensitivity of 100% and specificity of 95% in selected patients with abnormal pudendal arteriographic findings. The Mayo Clinic recommends that if a patient has a good clinical response to vasodilating injection and bilateral peak systolic velocities are greater than 30 cm/second, arteriography is not necessary. When peak systolic velocity is compared with cavernous arterial systolic occlusion pressures (CASOP) generated during dynamic infusion cavernosometry, a peak systolic velocity of 25 cm/second or more predicts a normal CASOP with a sensitivity of 95% and specificity of 95%. Severe unilateral cavernous arterial insufficiency results in asymmetry of peak systolic velocity greater than 10 cm/second. [p 1642]

25. **c. The parameters of end-diastolic velocity and resistive index are used to document CVOD.** CVOD is defined as the inability to achieve and maintain erection despite adequate arterial inflow. When the Doppler spectral waveform continues to exhibit forward diastolic flow despite peak systolic velocity greater than 35 cm/second, a low-resistance state persists in the sinusoids and the patient may have venogenic impotence. Unlike the cavernous arteries, the dorsal arteries are not subjected to changing intracorporeal pressure, whereas full erection is associated with reduction or cessation of intracorporeal diastolic flow (measured by end-diastolic velocities). Dorsal arterial flows in the full or rigid erection phase are associated with high end-diastolic velocity. Deep dorsal vein flow also persists during rigid erection; these flows are a function of rate of dorsal arterial inflow to the glans and should not be interpreted as evidence of corporeal venous leakage. The suspicion of venous leakage is raised when the patient has an excellent arterial response to injected vasodilator (>30 to 35 cm/second peak systolic velocity), with well-maintained end-diastolic velocity (>5 to 7 cm/second), accompanied by transient rigidity after self-stimulation. One study described progressive changes in Doppler spectral waveform pattern with increasing intracorporeal pressure in potent volunteers stimulated by injection (papaverine/phentolamine). Rigid erection was associated with intracorporeal pressures ranging from 83 to 106 mm Hg. [pp 1643–1644]

26. **b. Like the Doppler penile blood flow study, it is minimally invasive and permits the patient a period of privacy and self-stimulation.** This variation of penile blood pressure determination was introduced by Padma-Nathan and Goldstein in 1989. It involves infusing saline solution into the corpora at a rate sufficient to raise the intracavernous pressure above the systolic blood pressure. A pencil Doppler transducer is then applied to the side of the penile base. The saline infusion is stopped, and the intracavernous pressure is allowed to fall. The pressure at which the cavernous arterial flow becomes detectable is defined as the CASOP. Results have been shown to correlate well with those of arteriography and peak systolic velocity obtained by high-resolution duplex Doppler ultrasonography. However, despite these advantages, dynamic infusion cavernosometry is nonetheless a more invasive procedure and more prone to psychological inhibition and is not feasible if the intracavernous pressure cannot be raised above the systolic blood pressure (e.g., in patients with severe venous leakage). Cavernosography involves the infusion of radiocontrast solution into the corpora cavernosa during an artificial erection to visualize the site of venous leakage. It should always be performed after activation of the veno-occlusive mechanism by intracavernous injection of a vasodilator. Leakage sites to the glans, corpus spongiosum, superficial and deep dorsal veins, and cavernous and crural veins can then be detected. [pp 1644, 1645, 1647]

27. **d. corporal smooth muscle pathology.** It has become increasingly evident that, in older men with secondary ED, venous leakage is the consequence of corporal smooth muscle pathology and not congenitally large, anomalous, or excessive penile veins. [p 1647]

28. **c. Arterial dysfunction was associated with normal smooth muscle content but atherosclerotic blockage of**

one or both cavernous arteries. Wespes and colleagues have advocated corporeal biopsy with light microscopy and computerized morphometric analysis as an adjunctive technique in the diagnosis of vascular impotence. In patients receiving penile implants and in cadaveric specimens, researchers have observed an age-related decrease in smooth muscle content within the corpora cavernosa. When computerized morphometry was used to compare young patients with penile curvature but hemodynamically adequate erection with elderly patients with ED, the corpora cavernosa in the young were composed of 40% to 52% smooth muscle; in the elderly with corporeal veno-occlusive dysfunction, 19% to 36% smooth muscle; and in those with arterial impotence, 10% to 25% smooth muscle (collagen was correspondingly increased). In another study in which penile biopsies were performed in 50 patients, the biopsy gun specimens were as representative as the open biopsy specimens. The most severe lesions were observed in the erectile tissue, in particular in the smooth muscle of the trabeculae and the helicine arteries, which had been reduced and replaced by connective tissue. [p 1647]

29. **b. Transdermal scrotal testosterone patches result in significant levels of DHT, because of a high content of 5α-reductase in scrotal skin.** Parenteral depot preparations of testosterone, like testosterone cypionate and enanthate, have been available for years, are the cheapest form of androgen supplementation, and are effective in restoring serum levels of testosterone to normal. They are administered through deep intramuscular injection and result in supraphysiologic levels of testosterone for 72 hours with gradual steady decline over 2 to 3 weeks. Depot preparations of testosterone do not replicate normal circadian levels; the initial supraphysiologic testosterone "rush" may be perceived as disconcerting to some patients, but others enjoy an improved sense of well-being, aggression, and libido. The most common preparations are the 17β-hydroxyl esters. Enanthate and cypionate are generally administered every 2 to 4 weeks at dosages of 200 to 400 mg. Testosterone propionate has a shorter half-life, requiring dosing every other day. Scrotal skin patches required shaving and were difficult to keep in place; also, because of high levels of 5α-reductase activity in scrotal skin, significantly high levels of DHT are produced. Daily endogenous testosterone production is approximately 7 mg. When taken orally, testosterone preparations are largely rendered metabolically inactive during the first-pass circulation through the liver. Metabolic inactivation requires oral dosing to exceed 200 mg/day to maintain normal serum levels. Large dosages of testosterone are toxic to the liver and can lead to hepatitis, cholestatic jaundice, hepatomas, hemorrhagic liver cysts, and hepatocarcinoma. [pp 1649–1650]

30. **d. Osteoporosis.** In a young hypogonadal man, testosterone replacement is clearly the treatment of choice. However, the risks may outweigh the benefits in some patients. Supraphysiologic levels of testosterone will suppress luteinizing hormone and follicle-stimulating hormone production and result in infertility. Breast tenderness or gynecomastia is not uncommon with parenteral testosterone dosing. Long-term androgen therapy requires a commitment from the patient and specialist for follow-up. Testosterone and its metabolite DHT are growth factors. Erythrocytosis is the most common laboratory alteration noted with long-term therapy. One study noted that the mean hematocrit increased from 42 to 49 after 3 months of treatment. Androgens may induce or worsen sleep apnea. Cardiovascular risks are increased in some patients by increases in red cell mass; in addition, in young patients abusing testosterone therapy, moderate elevations of low-density lipoprotein and decreases in high-density lipoprotein have been noted. Increases in thromboxane A_2 and platelet aggregation have also been attributed to testosterone therapy. A number of studies in the literature suggest that androgen replacement does not induce prostate cancer in men with normal prostates, and placebo-controlled studies show little difference in prostate volume, prostate-specific antigen, and obstructive symptoms. The possibility of exacerbating an occult cancer of the prostate in men undergoing testosterone replacement remains a urologist's nightmare. [pp 1650–1651]

31. **b. In addition to activity on adrenergic receptors, it alters serotonin and dopamine transmission.** Yohimbine, an α_2-adrenergic antagonist, is obtained from the bark of the yohimbe tree. It acts centrally, to promote sexual behavior by blocking presynaptic autoreceptors and increasing adrenergic receptor activity, which also alters serotonin and dopamine transmission. Documented experimental effects from either systemically or intracranially administered yohimbine on the male sexual response are behavioral. As an initial treatment, 5.4 mg three times daily has been recommended; other investigators have reported efficacy by doubling that dosage or using the drug on an as-needed basis (two tablets 1 to 2 hours before anticipated sexual activity). The American Urological Association, in its guidelines for the management of organic ED published in 1996, advised that there was no efficacy of yohimbine over placebo in patients with organic ED. Side effects of yohimbine include gastrointestinal intolerance, palpitations, headache, agitation, anxiety, and increase in blood pressure (precautions are advised in men with cardiovascular disease). [p 1652]

32. **c. Apomorphine is a dopaminergic agonist, activating D1 and D2 receptors in the paraventricular nucleus.** Apomorphine is chemically unrelated to morphine; it is not an opiate. It acts in the brain within the paraventricular nucleus. The paraventricular nucleus functions as the sexual drive center in mammals. Apomorphine is a dopaminergic agonist, activating D1 and D2 receptors. Dopaminergic stimulation is proerectile; early reports of patients treated for Parkinson's disease showed increased spontaneous erections, without increased libido. Apomorphine is a D1/D2 dopaminergic agonist that stimulates proerectile signaling; in human subjects sexual arousal is necessary. The proprietary agent acts sublingually by buccal absorption and erection efficacy is lost if the tablet is swallowed. The drug has a rapid onset of action with mean time to erection of 12 minutes; the pharmacology permits a window of sexual opportunity of approximately 2 hours from ingestion. [pp 1652–1653]

33. **b. It prevents the breakdown of cyclic GMP.** Sildenafil citrate (Viagra, Pfizer Pharmaceuticals) is a selective inhibitor of phosphodiesterase-5 (PDE5), the enzyme that breaks down the intracellular second messenger of erection, cGMP. When nitric oxide enters a vascular smooth muscle cell, it stimulates the enzyme guanylate cyclase to convert cGTP in cGMP. This intracellular second messenger cGMP triggers the mobilization of intracellular calcium by causing it to be pumped out of the cell or sequestered in the sarcoplasmic reticulum; the result is smooth muscle relaxation. PGE_1 works via a similar second messenger cAMP to decrease intracellular calcium. The breakdown of these second messengers (cAMP and cGMP) is regulated by the set of enzymes known as phosphodiesterases. Sildenafil enhances the natural effects of nitric oxide on corporeal arterial and sinusoidal smooth muscle by inhibiting catabolism of cGMP by PDE5. Sildenafil is a peripheral conditioner that is orally active and facilitates the natural responses to sexual stimulation by its activity in the end organ, the penis. [pp 1653–1654]

34. **c. Improved erections were seen in patients with lower**

motor neuron spinal cord lesions. Improvements in erections were reported in 56%, 77%, and 84% of subjects taking 25, 50, and 100 mg, respectively, of sildenafil, and in 25% in the placebo group. At the end of the U.S. flexible-dose study (6 months), 75% of subjects were taking 100 mg, 23% of subjects were taking 50 mg, and 2% preferred the 25-mg dosage. At the end of a 12-week dosage escalation study in U.S. trials, 74% of subjects responding to a global efficacy SAQ reported improved erections, compared with 19% taking a placebo. Treatment effect was principally assessed by SAQs and was largely based on items 3 and 4 of the IIEF-15 (ability to initiate and maintain erection). Overall responses to sildenafil appear to be dosage related over the range 25 to 100 mg, with little benefit and considerably more side effects above 100 mg. Sildenafil is metabolized in the liver by the cytochrome P450 isoenzymes. Age greater than 65 years, hepatic impairment, drugs that inhibit the microsomal cytochrome P450 isoenzymes 3A4 and 2C9 (cimetidine, ketoconazole, erythromycin), and severe renal insufficiency are associated with increased plasma levels of sildenafil. [p 1654]

35. **d. Men with diabetic neuropathy.** The American Heart Association and American College of Cardiology guidelines caution that sildenafil dosing is potentially hazardous in men with coronary ischemia (positive exercise test) who are not taking nitrates, in men with congestive heart failure and borderline low blood pressure and low blood volume, and in men taking complicated multidrug antihypertensives. A postrelease product labeling update from the FDA also cautions use in several populations of patients who were not part of the original clinical trials: men suffering a myocardial infarction, stroke, or life-threatening arrhythmia in the prior 6 months; men with resting blood pressure less than 90/50 or higher than 170/110 mm Hg; men with cardiac failure; men with unstable angina; and men with retinitis pigmentosa. One study demonstrated that patients taking antihypertensive medications do show considerable decreases in blood pressure during sleep, after taking sildenafil. [pp 1654–1655]

36. **c. alprostadil.** Alprostadil, the synthetic formulation of PGE_1, is the only pharmacologic agent approved by the FDA for the management of ED via intracavernous and intraurethral routes. Alprostadil stimulates adenylate cyclase to increase intracellular levels of cAMP, lowering intracellular concentrations of calcium and thus relaxing arterial and trabecular smooth muscle. Drug is transferred from the urethra to the corpus spongiosum to the corpus cavernosum via venous channels (via circumflex and emissary veins perforating the tunica albuginea). MUSE consists of very small semi-solid pellets (3 × 1 mm) administered into the distal urethra (3 cm) by a proprietary applicator (MUSE VIVUS, Menlo Park, CA). [p 1655]

37. **d. Papaverine-induced erection is associated with idiopathic penile pain in 30% of men.** Papaverine is an alkaloid isolated from the opium poppy. Its molecular mechanism of action is through its inhibitory effect on phosphodiesterase, leading to increased cAMP and cGMP in penile erectile tissue. Papaverine also blocks voltage-dependent calcium channels, thus impairing calcium influx, and it may also impair calcium-activated potassium and chloride currents. All of these actions relax cavernous smooth muscle and penile vessels. Papaverine is metabolized in the liver, and the plasma half-life is about 1 to 2 hours. The advantages are its low cost and stability at room temperature. The major disadvantages are the higher incidence of priapism (0% to 35%) and corporeal fibrosis (1% to 33%), thought to be a result of low acidity (pH 3 to 4), and occasional elevation of liver enzymes. Systemic side effects include dizziness, pallor, and cold sweats, which may be the result of vasovagal reflex or hypotension from its vasodilatory effect in patients with veno-occlusive dysfunction. [pp 1656–1657]

38. **b. Up to 90% is metabolized on the first passage through the lungs.** Alprostadil is the synthetic form of a naturally occurring unsaturated 20-carbon fatty acid (i.e., alprostadil refers to the exogenous form, PGE_1 to the endogenous compound). It causes smooth muscle relaxation, vasodilatation, and inhibition of platelet aggregation through elevation of intracellular cAMP. After intracavernous injection, 96% of alprostadil is locally metabolized within 60 minutes, and no change in peripheral blood levels has been observed. In patients with veno-occlusive dysfunction, alprostadil may rise to 10 times baseline, but up to 90% is metabolized on the first pass through the lungs. A review of the published literature found that, in doses of 10 to 20 μg, alprostadil produced full erections in 70% to 80% of patients with ED. The most frequent side effects were pain at the injection site or during erection (occurring in 16.8% of patients), hematoma/ecchymosis (1.5%), and prolonged erection/priapism (1.3%). [pp 1657–1658]

39. **e. Trimix is more effective than papaverine plus phentolamine in patients with severe arteriogenic or veno-occlusive ED.** Phentolamine is a nonspecific α-adrenergic antagonist with equal affinity for blocking both α_1- and α_2-adrenoreceptors. VIP, originally isolated from the small intestine, is a potent smooth muscle relaxant. One study proposed that VIP may be a neurotransmitter for penile erection. VIP receptors are present in the cavernous smooth muscle cells. Intracorporeal injection of VIP alone does not produce rigid erection. Its efficacy appears to be in combination therapies with phentolamine (VIP 25 μg, phentolamine 0.5 mg/ml). Statistically, the triple-drug combination was more effective in patients with severe arteriogenic or mild veno-occlusive dysfunction. The incidence of prolonged erection was lower when compared with papaverine plus phentolamine but not significantly different from alprostadil alone. In summary, the triple-drug combination has been shown to be as effective as alprostadil alone but has a much lower incidence of painful erection. Generally, Trimix is reserved for men in whom PGE_1 monotherapy has failed or who have significant penile pain at higher concentrations of PGE_1. [p 1659]

40. **e. All of the above.** In several studies, the percentage of patients accepting injection therapy when it was offered in the office ranged from 49% to 84%. The reasons for declining included penile pain, inadequate response, fear of the needle, unnaturalness, and loss of sex drive. In long-term studies, 13% to 60% of patients dropped out for a number of reasons. These include loss of interest, loss of the partner, poor erectile response, penile pain, concomitant illness, recovery of spontaneous erection, and ultimate choice of other therapy. One study segregated dropouts into short and long term. They found that of patients who were instructed in self-injection therapy and never initiated home treatment, dissatisfaction and unnaturalness of the process was most commonly cited. Among dropouts from home therapy (63%), most common complaints were drug costs and insufficient erection for penetration. Another group calculated that priapism occurred in 1.3% of 8090 patients in 48 studies with alprostadil. The incidence was found to be about five times lower with alprostadil than with papaverine or the combination of papaverine and phentolamine (1.5% vs 10% vs 7%). The use of ICI therapy is contraindicated in patients with sickle cell anemia, schizophrenia or a severe psychiatric disorder, severe venous incompetence, or severe systemic disease. In patients taking an anticoagulant or aspirin, com-

pressing the injection site for 7 to 10 minutes after injection is recommended. In patients with poor manual dexterity, the sexual partner can be instructed to perform the injection. [p 1660]

41. **b. VEDs may be effective in the patient with a malfunctioning penile implant and after explantation.** The vacuum constriction device has become more popular in the last decade as an effective and safe treatment for ED. It consists of a plastic cylinder connected directly or by tubing to a vacuum-generating source (manual or battery-operated pump). After the penis is engorged by the negative pressure, a constricting ring is applied to the base to maintain the erection. To avoid injury, the ring should not be left in place for longer than 30 minutes. Combining ICI with the vacuum constriction device may enhance the erection. The device can also be used successfully by men with a malfunctioning penile prosthesis in place and has been used after explantation. A retrospective review of patients found that 20% rejected the device primarily and 30.9% rejected it after a period ranging to 16 weeks. The primary dropout rate was 50.9%, and the secondary dropout rate was 7.3% after 10 months. Long-term users (41.8%) reported 98% satisfaction; partner satisfaction was 85%. [pp 1660–1661]

42. **e. Men 50 years of age or older with vascular risk factors.** We have defined complex ED patients as (1) those with penile, pelvic, or perineal trauma; (2) young men with primary ED (present since age of sexual maturity); (3) men with Peyronie's disease; (4) men who fail to respond to oral phosphodiesterase inhibitors or for whom PDE5 inhibitors are contraindicated; and (5) men with a significant psychological or psychiatric component. Currently, patients who undergo diagnostic testing in our practice are men with complex ED. [p 1661]

43. **c. A corporeal aspirate of dark blood that is hypercarbic and acidotic is classic for low-flow priapism.** The diagnosis of priapism is usually based on history and physical examination. Priapism associated with intracavernous pharmacotherapy occurs more often in patients with neurogenic and psychogenic impotence, and the diagnosis is evident. Sickle-cell priapism often occurs in teenagers, and recurrence is very common. Acute low-flow (veno-occlusive) priapism, if lasting more than several hours, is usually painful because of changes associated with tissue ischemia. In contrast, most cases of high-flow (arterial) priapism are painless and usually follow perineal injury or direct injury to the penis. We prefer blood gas determination and, if doubt exists, a color-coded duplex ultrasonographic scan of the cavernous arteries and the corpora cavernosa. Minimal arterial flow with distended corpora cavernosa is seen in low-flow priapism, whereas a ruptured artery with unregulated blood pooling in the area of injury can often be seen in trauma-induced high-flow priapism. [pp 1661–1662]

44. **b. Aspiration of the corpora and intracorporeal injection of an α-adrenergic agent is the treatment of choice in low-flow priapism.** Treatment is aimed at the primary cause of priapism if it can be identified. The goal is to abort the erection, thereby preventing permanent damage to the corpora (which would lead to impotence), and to relieve pain. Medical management should always be tried before resorting to surgery. There is ample evidence that the risk of fibrosis and impotence increases with time. Generally, the incidence of impotence is less if erection is aborted in less than 24 hours. Medical treatment is aimed at decreasing arterial inflow and increasing venous outflow. The first line of treatment involves aspiration of the corpora and intracavernous injection with an α-adrenergic agonist. Intracavernous injection of an α-adrenergic agonist remains the most effective treatment for low-flow priapism and is almost 100% effective if the priapism is treated within 12 hours of onset. [p 1662]

45. **d. Treatment of the man with sickle-cell priapism should be by immediate operative shunting.** Sickle-cell disorder accounts for approximately 28% of all cases of priapism; 42% of adults and 64% of children with sickle-cell disease will eventually develop it. Although high-flow priapism in patients with sickle-cell disease has been reported, the majority of cases are of the low-flow type. Treatment should be prompt and conservative, as priapism often recurs in these patients. Having ruled out other causative factors, one should treat the patient by aggressive hydration, oxygenation, and metabolic alkalinization to reduce further sickling. Supertransfusion and erythrocytapheresis should be used as second-line therapy. Irrigation and injection, as above, should be performed as soon as possible. [p 1662]

46. **e. temporary stress incontinence.** Untreated veno-occlusive priapism leads to corporeal fibrosis and impotence. Complications of treatment can be classified as early and late. Early complications include acute hypertension, headache, palpitation, and cardiac arrhythmia from α-adrenergic agents and bleeding, infection, and urethral injury from needle puncture. Two deaths and one case of skin necrosis were reported after injection of undiluted metaraminol (2 to 4 mg). Hematoma of the shaft after corporeal aspiration and irrigation is also common. Infections are usually in the form of cellulitis. Therefore, strict asepsis in carrying out penile irrigation and use of antibiotics are both mandatory to avoid this potentially disastrous complication. If undiagnosed, it may lead to abscess formation. Urethral injury is a rare complication of treatment that may lead to stricture or urethrocutaneous fistula. Injury to the urethra can occur during needle aspiration and irrigation, when one of the distal shunts is performed, or during the cavernosospongiosal shunt procedure. [p 1663]

47. **c. Shunting, although most invasive, has the highest degree of success in reversing high-flow priapism.** Priapism after intracavernous pharmacotherapy is generally low-flow ischemic priapism. Ischemic priapism is a urologic emergency, and the first task at hand is distinguishing high-flow arterial priapism from low-flow ischemic priapism. Ischemic priapism most commonly occurs after excessive dosing of a vasoactive agent. Ischemic priapism is generally quite painful after 6 hours. Almost all cases can be successfully aborted with injection of a dilute α-adrenergic agonist, provided that treatment begins within 12 hours of onset. Tissue damage can thus be prevented and potency preserved. High-flow priapism itself does not cause erectile tissue damage, but injury to the erectile tissue and nerves may be associated with delayed recovery of potency after treatment. The best diagnostic tool is a color-coded duplex ultrasonogram. Angiographic embolization with autologous clot or coils is generally considered the treatment of choice for high-flow priapism. Embolization must be highly selective to occlude only the lesion. Consideration should be given to conservative treatment and follow-up observation with color Doppler study in cases of high-flow priapism. [p 1663]

Chapter 47

Surgery for Erectile Dysfunction

Ronald W. Lewis • Gerald H. Jordan

Questions

1. What are three essential elements of informed consent for patients considering penile prosthesis surgery?

    a. Other options for treatment, results expected from the surgery, and possible complications of the surgery
    b. The high cost of prosthetic surgery compared with the cost of other therapy, the length of penile erection after surgery, and the infection rate associated with prosthetic surgery
    c. The role of the partner in the use of the device, the high infection rate associated with prosthesis surgery, and the nature of the incision for this surgery
    d. The cosmetic defect associated with all prosthetic surgery, complications associated with the device, and the low cost of the device
    e. That penile prosthesis surgery is never a first-line therapy for erectile dysfunction, the high cost of the devices, and risks of the surgery

2. Choice of incision for erectile dysfunction involves which of the following factors?

    a. It is primarily a one-incision choice.
    b. The choice is never a subcoronal circumferential incision.
    c. It also depends on the choice of the surgeon.
    d. There is easier access to the urethra with the infrapubic incision.
    e. A paramedian abdominal incision is the only incision for exposure of the inferior epigastric artery in penile revascularization surgery.

3. The two broad categories for penile prostheses are:

    a. semirigid and malleable.
    b. two- and three-piece inflatable devices.
    c. rods and cylinders.
    d. semirigid and inflatable devices.
    e. mechanical and malleable devices.

4. Selection of a penile prosthesis for an individual is based on which three considerations?

    a. Height of the patient, penile size, and mechanical aptitude of the patient.
    b. Patient preference, cost of the device, and surgeon preference.
    c. Penile length, presence of diabetes mellitus in the patient, and infection potential.
    d. Girth of the penis, presence of penile scarring, and blood type of the patient.
    e. Immune competence of the patient, cost of the device, and penile size.

5. What are two disadvantages of the semirigid devices compared with the inflatable devices?

    a. Less concealability and greater chance of pressure erosion.
    b. More difficult surgical placement and less concealability.
    c. Higher infection rates and greater chance of erosion.
    d. More mechanical problems and higher cost of the device.
    e. Lack of penile length and lower cost.

6. What is the most important fact that the patient considering a penile prosthesis should know?

    a. Restoration of girth of erection is usually disappointing.
    b. Rigidity of erection obtained from the penile prosthesis is usually suboptimal.
    c. No device will restore the full length previously achieved by the patient with his natural erection.
    d. The infection rate associated with penile prostheses is high.
    e. Moderate pain is usually associated with a penile prosthesis.

7. The advantage of placement of a Foley catheter at the time of surgical placement of a three-piece inflatable device is:

    a. a decrease in the infection rate.
    b. protection of the urethra from injury.
    c. facilitated dilatation of the corporeal bodies.
    d. help in avoidance of bladder perforation during placement of the reservoir.
    e. help in accurately sizing intracorporeal length.

8. The corporotomy incision for placement of the prosthetic cylinders may be placed on any of the following positions of the corporeal bodies except which one?

    a. Basal lateral surface
    b. Distal lateral surface
    c. Dorsal surface
    d. Ventral surface

9. Corporeal perforation is most likely to occur in which part of the corpora during dilatation?

    a. The crural end of the corpora
    b. The lateral middle portion of the corpora
    c. The subglandular portion of the corpora
    d. The dorsal surface of the corpora

10. What is the unique feature for cylinder sizing of the American Medical Systems (AMS) Ultrex cylinder?

    a. The cylinder selection should be 2 cm shorter than the total measured length.
    b. The cylinder length used should be exactly the measured length.
    c. The cylinder diameter selection is markedly different compared with that for other devices.
    d. The cylinder selected must be 1 cm longer than the total measured length.
    e. The cylinder selected must be 1 cm shorter than the total measured length.

11. Two potential complications of failure to make an adequate

space for the reservoir of the three-piece inflatable devices are which of the following?

   a. Bowel perforation and infection
   b. Encapsulation of the reservoir and perforation of the reservoir
   c. Entrapment of the reservoir and infection of the space
   d. Autoinflation and failure to obtain optimal deflation of the cylinders
   e. Kinking of the Mentor new reservoir lockout valve and autoinflation

12. What is the incidence of infection in the placement of a primary penile prosthesis?

    a. 10% to 20%
    b. 1% to 9%
    c. 5% to 15%
    d. <0.5%
    e. >30%

13. What is the most prudent course of action in the face of frank purulent pus in association with a penile prosthesis?

    a. Placement of drains
    b. Removal of only those grossly infected elements
    c. Removal with antibiotic irrigation and immediate replacement
    d. Immediate replacement
    e. Removal of the entire device

14. All of the following are steps for prevention of infection in genitourinary prosthetics except:

    a. short hospital stay.
    b. elimination of other sites of infection preoperatively.
    c. antiseptic soap shower or bath 2 or 3 nights preoperatively.
    d. prophylactic perioperative antibiotics.
    e. shaving of the operative site the night before surgery.

15. The three most common position problems with penile prosthetic surgery are:

    a. poor cylinder placement, superficial placement of tubing, and poor reservoir placement.
    b. inadequate cylinder length, high-riding pump, and kinked reservoir neck.
    c. poor seating of the crural cylinder, superficial placement of tubing, and crossover placement of cylinders.
    d. malposition of the reservoir, too low a position of the pump, and cylinder placement outside the corpora.

16. How long can the patient expect to have mild to moderate pain after penile prosthesis placement?

    a. 4 to 6 weeks
    b. 3 months
    c. 6 months
    d. Only a few days
    e. 9 months

17. With placement of the modern inflatable penile prosthesis, the patient can expect mechanical failure in what percentages of cases?

    a. 10%
    b. 5%
    c. Less than 1%
    d. 50%
    e. 20%

18. In three-piece penile prosthesis reoperation, what is the most likely source of fluid leak?

    a. The reservoir
    b. The cylinder
    c. The pump
    d. The tubing at the connector site
    e. The rear tip extender site

19. All of the following statements are true regarding the condition of reoperation of penile prosthesis except which one?

    a. If a reoperation is done for mechanical failure and the device has been present for 5 years, replacement of all of the device is recommended.
    b. The most difficult problem in reoperation is intracorporeal fibrosis, and it may often be necessary to make more than one corporeal incision.
    c. Corporeal reconstruction is never indicated.
    d. Infection rate may be 10 to 20 times higher in reoperation cases than for the initial operation.
    e. Special cavernotomes may be necessary to treat the fibrosis.

20. What is the percentage rate of satisfaction with a penile prosthesis for patient and partners?

    a. 10% to 20%
    b. 20% to 30%
    c. 30% to 50%
    d. Over 100%
    e. 60% to 80%

21. Among patients who have erectile dysfunction, who are the best candidates for penile revascularization surgery?

    a. Patients older than 70 years of age.
    b. Patients with generalized arterial sclerosis.
    c. Young, healthy male patients who have a history of perineal or pelvic trauma.
    d. Patients with vascular disease who smoke.
    e. Patients with veno-occlusive disorders.

22. The arterial inflow source most commonly used for penile revascularization surgery is:

    a. the inferior epigastric artery.
    b. the superficial perineal artery.
    c. the obturator artery.
    d. the superior epigastric artery.
    e. the epididymal artery.

23. Which of the following statements regarding Peyronie's disease is correct?

    a. Most patients with Peyronie's disease understand the effects of their disease and thus require little counseling.
    b. The majority of patients with Peyronie's disease will eventually require surgery.
    c. Surgery, when required, can be viewed as palliation for the effects of the Peyronie disease process.
    d. In many patients with Peyronie's disease, medical therapy has proved curative.

24. All of the following agents are associated, in the literature, with the development of Peyronie's disease except which one?

    a. Methyldopa antihypertensives
    b. β Blockers
    c. Paget's disease of the bone
    d. Diabetes mellitus

25. Which of the following statements regarding Peyronie's disease is incorrect?

    a. Smith, using an autopsy study, found the asymptomatic incidence of Peyronie's disease to be 22%.

b. The symptomatic incidence of Peyronie's disease has been estimated to be 10%.
c. The average age at onset of Peyronie's disease is in the middle 50s.
d. The asymptomatic prevalence of Peyronie's disease is established to be approximately 0.4% to 1.0%.

26. With regard to the anatomy of the penis pertinent to Peyronie's disease:

    a. the linear longitudinal layer attenuates at the 12-o'clock position (dorsal midline).
    b. the circular lamina of the tunica albuginea attenuates at the 6-o'clock position (ventral midline).
    c. the septal fibers interweave with the circular fiber lamina of the tunica albuginea.
    d. the longitudinal lamina of the tunica albuginea is thickest at the ventral midline.

27. Current theory involving the etiology of Peyronie's includes all of the following assumptions except which one?

    a. The inciting event leading to Peyronie's disease seems to be buckling trauma during erection.
    b. Transforming growth factor-β1 (TGF-β1) has been implicated as a cause of the abnormal disordered healing.
    c. TGF-β1, -β2, and -β3, if not cleared from an area of injury, lead to accumulation of further TGF-βs.
    d. The accumulation of plaque has been associated with other disorders governed by increased cholesterol and lipid levels.

28. Series that observe the natural history of Peyronie's disease document which of the following?

    a. The majority of patients present with sudden onset of stable deformity.
    b. Many patients require surgery to resolve their painful erections.
    c. All patients eventually develop stable deformity.
    d. Total resolution of the Peyronie disease process occurs relatively frequently.

29. With regard to the relationship of erectile dysfunction and Peyronie's disease, select the correct response:

    a. In most published series, the stratification of erectile problems, functional versus organic, is not clear.
    b. The highly emotional aspects of Peyronie's disease are expressed in many men via disordered erectile function.
    c. Many patients tend to abandon their sexual activities in response to the emotional trauma of Peyronie's disease.
    d. All of the above.

30. With regard to the presenting complaints of patients with Peyronie's disease, select the incorrect response:

    a. Distal flaccidity occurs because of vascular blockage due to the plaque.
    b. Painful erections virtually always resolve as the disease becomes quiescent.
    c. Penile deformity can be migratory or present stable.
    d. Foreshortening of the penis is a frequent complaint of patients with Peyronie's disease.

31. With regard to medical management of Peyronie's disease, select the correct response:

    a. Vitamin E has proved efficacious for the treatment of Peyronie's disease.
    b. The use of aminobenzoate potassium (Potaba) is not strongly advocated, as it has not proved definitively to be efficacious and it has a significant side effect profile.
    c. Nonsteroidal anti-inflammatory agents are useful in some patients.
    d. Colchicine is thought to be useful by virtue of effects on purine metabolism.
    e. Tamoxifen, by virtue of its action on tubulin, has proved to be highly effective.

32. With regard to intralesional injection protocols for Peyronie's disease, select the incorrect response:

    a. The use of intralesional steroids is not recommended.
    b. Verapamil injection protocols are logistically laborious, but the injections are well tolerated.
    c. Collagenase injection protocols are available only as a part of study protocols.
    d. Interferon injections are proposed to work by mechanisms similar to those of verapamil but are better tolerated.

33. Surgery is absolutely indicated in patients with Peyronie's disease for which of the following reasons?

    a. Persistent pain with erection
    b. Severe foreshortening of the penis
    c. Erectile dysfunction or curvature that precludes intercourse
    d. All of the above

Answers

1. **a. Other options for treatment, results expected from the surgery, and possible complications of the surgery.** The three essential elements of informed consent are other options for therapy, an explanation of what the prosthesis will do for the patient, and possible complications of such surgery (see Table 47–1). [p 1674]

2. **c. It also depends on the choice of the surgeon.** For placement of a two- or three-piece inflatable penile prosthesis, a penile scrotal or infrapubic incision (in either case vertical or horizontal) is optimal, depending on the preference of the surgeon. [p 1674]

3. **d. semirigid and inflatable devices.** Penile prostheses are basically of two broad categories: the malleable or semirigid devices, and the inflatable devices. [p 1674]

4. **b. Patient preference, cost of the device, and surgeon preference.** Selection of the appropriate device for the individual patient is largely based on three considerations: the patient's preference, the cost of the device, and the surgeon's preference. [p 1675]

5. **a. Less concealability and greater chance of pressure erosion.** Patients who use condom catheters are more likely to have neurologic disease and lack of penile sensation and are therefore more prone to cylinder erosion with the semirigid or malleable devices. Besides this drawback of the semirigid devices, other disadvantages include less concealability and inability to change in girth. [p 1675]

6. **c. No device will restore the full length previously achieved by the patient with his natural erection.** No pe-

nile prosthesis will restore the full length previously achieved by the patient with his natural erection. [p 1676]

7. **d. help in avoidance of bladder perforation during placement of the reservoir.** Placement of a Foley urinary catheter is recommended, especially in patients with corporeal fibrosis and in patients who will have placement of a suprapubic reservoir, because an empty bladder facilitates creation of the reservoir pouch and avoids injury to the bladder. [p 1677]

8. **c. Dorsal surface.** The tunica albuginea surface is exposed on the lateral surface of the corpus cavernosum, a corporotomy incision. The corporotomy incision should not be placed on the dorsal surface because of potential nerve and blood vessel injury there. [p 1677]

9. **a. The crural end of the corpora.** This should be carefully done by placement of the dilatation tool of choice toward the crura or the glans, with care taken to abut against the ischial tuberosity in the crural direction, because this is where intraoperative perforation is most likely to occur. [pp 1677–1678]

10. **e. The cylinder selected must be 1 cm shorter than the total measured length.** The appropriate-length individual cylinders with or without rear-tip extenders (total length 1 cm less with the AMS Ultrex cylinder) are then placed into their respective intracorporeal spaces, directly for the semirigid devices and with a cylinder placement tool for inflatable devices. [p 1678]

11. **d. Autoinflation and failure to obtain optimal deflation of the cylinders.** Placing the pump into the peritoneum has been advocated by some surgeons to eliminate the risk of entrapment of the reservoir, which might lead to autoinflation. This can be avoided by carefully creating an adequate space initially, which can be ascertained when filling the reservoir after placement. Complications of failure to make an adequate space for the reservoir are spontaneous transfer of fluid and inability to fully deflate the cylinders, therefore producing poor flaccidity. [p 1681]

12. **b. 1% to 9%.** One of the most dreaded complications associated with penile prostheses is infection. In excellent reviews by Carson in 1989 and 1993, the reported incidence was 0.6% to 8.9%. [p 1683]

13. **d. Immediate replacement.** It is advisable, in the face of frank purulent material, for the entire device to be removed. [p 1683]

14. **e. shaving of the operative site the night before surgery.** Steps to prevent infection include a short hospital stay preoperatively and postoperatively; elimination of other sites of infection preoperatively; antiseptic soap shower or bath 2 or 3 nights before and the morning of surgery; and prophylactic perioperative antibiotics. Shaving should be done immediately before preparation of the skin incision site. [p 1683]

15. **b. inadequate cylinder length, high-riding pump, and kinked reservoir neck.** The three most common position problems are inadequate cylinder length, resulting in an SST deformity; a high-riding pump or pump/reservoir combination; and a kinked reservoir neck. [p 1684]

16. **a. 4 to 6 weeks.** It is not unusual for the patient to experience some degree of discomfort or minor penile pain 4 to 6 weeks postoperatively. [p 1684]

17. **b. 5%.** For patients who have primary placement of a modern penile prosthesis, reoperation for mechanical failure can be expected in 5% of the cases when the device has been in place for 5 to 10 years. The chance of mechanical failure is greater in patients who have experienced previous prosthetic problems. Those patients requiring secondary placement also have a more significant risk for infection, as do those with other predisposing infection risk factors. [p 1687]

18. **d. The tubing at the connector site.** In operating for leakage of fluid from an inflatable penile prosthesis with tubing connectors, exploration of the connector sites first is recommended, because this is the area most frequently associated with pressure-induced failure. [p 1687]

19. **c. Corporeal reconstruction is never indicated.** When replacing a failed part of a multicomponent device, it is recommended that, if the device has been present for 5 years or longer, all of the device be replaced. The patient needs to be informed that reoperation, particularly the reoperation involving corporeal reconstruction, may have 10 to 20 times higher infection rates than the initial operation. The most difficult problem in reoperation is intracorporeal fibrosis. It is often necessary to make more than one corporeal incision to prepare a space for placement of a new cylinder. Special tools such as the Carrion-Rossello cavernotomes may be helpful. Even with optimal corporeal dilatation, the standard penile prosthesis cylinder will be unable to be placed in the majority of cases of severe fibrosis without corporeal reconstruction. [p 1687]

20. **e. 60% to 80%.** In general, patient and partner satisfaction with penile prostheses ranges from 60% to 80%. [p 1688]

21. **c. Young, healthy male patients who have a history of perineal or pelvic trauma.** It is a rare patient with erectile dysfunction who should be offered the choice of vascular surgery. Those patients with discrete focal arterial lesions found on pudendal arteriography, particularly younger patients who have a history of trauma, who do not have insulin-dependent diabetes, who are not currently users of tobacco, and who do not have neurologic disease are the best candidates for penile revascularization procedures. [p 1689]

22. **a. the inferior epigastric artery.** It is preferable to connect the donor arterial vessel, usually the inferior epigastric artery (occasionally in the absence of a suitable epigastric artery, a saphenous vein connected to the femoral artery may serve as the input arterial supply), to a branch of the dorsal penile artery in an end-to-side fashion, or, when able, with an end-to-end anastomosis, which allows the most efficient runoff. [pp 1690–1691]

23. **c. Surgery, when required, can be viewed as palliation for the effects of the Peyronie disease process.** For most patients, reassurance is sufficient and a necessity. For others, medical therapy is useful. Fortunately, only a minority of patients will have deformity that precludes their having intercourse. The vast majority of patients with Peyronie's disease do not require surgery. [p 1696]

24. **a. Methyldopa antihypertensives.** Peyronie's disease was associated with Dupuytren's contracture. Approximately 30% to 40% of men with Peyronie's disease will also have Dupuytren's contracture. Other associated conditions are plantar fascial contracture (Ledderhose's disease) and tympanosclerosis. Peyronie's disease is also reported as seen in patients with external trauma to the penis, diabetes mellitus, gout, Paget's disease, use of β blockers, use of phenytoin, and urethral instrumentation. An association that has not stood the test of time is that with phenytoin. [p 1696]

25. **b. The symptomatic incidence of Peyronie's disease has been estimated to be 10%.** The symptomatic incidence of Peyronie's disease has been estimated at 10%. In white men, the average age at onset of Peyronie's disease is 53 years. The asymptomatic prevalence is estimated at 0.4% to 1%.

An autopsy study of 100 men without known Peyronie's disease found 22 of the 100 men to have lesions compatible with the disease. [p 1696]

26. **c. the septal fibers interweave with the circular fiber lamina of the tunica albuginea.** The tunica albuginea is bilaminar throughout most of its circumference. It is composed of an outer longitudinal layer and an inner circular layer. The tunica albuginea varies in thickness from 1.5 to 3 mm depending on the position on the circumference. The outer longitudinal layer attenuates in the ventral midline, and thus the tunica is monolaminar at that point. The outer longitudinal layer is thickest on the ventrum adjacent to the corpus spongiosum and on the dorsum, and thinnest on the lateral aspect. [pp 1696–1697]

27. **d. The accumulation of plaque has been associated with other disorders governed by increased cholesterol and lipid levels.** Somers and Dawson have shown that Peyronie's disease most likely begins with buckling trauma causing injury to the septal insertion of the tunica albuginea. It has been proposed that the avascular nature of the tunica albuginea may impede clearance of many of these growth factors. The TGFs, particularly TGF-β1, are capable of autoinducement. Thus, the accumulation of TGF-β1 is capable of inducement of further accumulation. The presence of TGF-β stimulating further release of TGF-β1 could lead to an ongoing, smoldering, inflammatory process, ending with disordered healing. There is good reason to suspect TGF-β1 as possibly involved with the formation of Peyronie's plaque, as it has been implicated in a number of soft tissue fibroses as well as with erectile dysfunction. [pp 1697–1698]

28. **c. All patients eventually develop stable deformity.** In most cases of Peyronie's disease, there are two phases: an active phase that is often associated with painful erections and with changing deformity of the penis, followed by a quiescent secondary phase, which is characterized by stabilizing of the deformity, with disappearance of painful erections, if they were present; and, in general, stability of the process. Up to one third of patients, however, present with what appears to be sudden development of painless deformity. [p 1698]

29. **d. All of the above.** In articles concerning the natural history of the disease, erectile dysfunction is prominently mentioned. A major failure of the literature is that patients are not stratified with regard to functional issues versus organic issues as they relate to erectile dysfunction. Jones, in 1997, dealt best with the counseling issues of men with sexual dysfunction. He described counseling a man with Peyronie's disease as being much the same as counseling a person who has suffered a death and is grieving. A major point made by Jones in dealing with Peyronie's disease patients is that to avoid or limit emotional factors, patients and their partners need to hear the suggestion that they must "keep sexual expression alive." [pp 1698–1699]

30. **a. Distal flaccidity occurs because of vascular blockage due to the plaque.** The presenting symptoms of Peyronie's disease include (1) in many patients, penile pain with erection, (2) penile deformity, (3) shortening with and without an erection, (4) notice of a plaque or indurated area in the penis, and (5) in many patients, erectile dysfunction. Some patients also complain of being awakened in the morning with pain during their erection. Spontaneous improvement in pain virtually always occurs as the inflammation resolves. A small group of patients with extensive disease will have "circumferential plaques" and, because of the resulting hinge effect, an unstable penis. Most patients, however, complain of distal flaccidity. [p 1699]

31. **b. The use of aminobenzoate potassium (Potaba) is not strongly advocated, as it has not proved definitively to be efficacious and it has a significant side effect profile.** Any section on the medical management of Peyronie's disease must begin with the disclaimer that few medical management regimens have been subjected to double-blind drug testing. There are no blinded or controlled studies that have examined the use of vitamin E, but vitamin E is cheap, safe, and possibly effective. Aminobenzoate potassium has been looked at in a small blinded study that showed it to be efficacious. It is poorly tolerated by some patients and is relatively costly. Its use is not strongly advocated. Four actions are attributed to colchicine. Colchicine binds tubulin and causes it to depolymerize and thus inhibits mobility and adhesion of leukocytes. It inhibits cell mitosis by disrupting spindle cell fibers and thus functions as a potent anti-inflammatory. It blocks the lipoxygenase pathway of arachidonic acid metabolism, furthering its anti-inflammatory effect. It interferes with the transcellular movement of protocollagen. Nonsteroidal anti-inflammatory drugs and steroids have been used anecdotally, but no studies support an indication for the use of these drugs. Tamoxifen, it is thought, facilitates the release of TGF-β from fibroblasts. [p 1700]

32. **d. Interferon injections are proposed to work by mechanisms similar to those of verapamil but are better tolerated.** A number of intralesional injection protocols have been examined. It is the recommendation of the consensus committee on penile curvatures that the use of intralesional steroids be eliminated or at least initiated with extreme caution because of the rather significant local side effects, the inconsistent pattern of improvement in well-established curvature, the lack of studies showing proven efficacy, and reports of patients who felt their condition deteriorated after the injections. A number of nonblinded studies have suggested efficacy with the use of intralesional verapamil, but no blinded studies suggest that the use of verapamil as an intralesional agent is efficacious. Collagenase has been subjected to two double-blind studies, but intralesional collagenase is currently available only on study protocol. The use of interferons as intralesional therapy for Peyronie's disease was reported in 1991. The mechanism of action of interferon is very similar to that proposed for verapamil. Verapamil is well tolerated. Complications are associated only with the injection procedure per se and are minimal. However, almost all patients injected with interferon develop a "flu-like syndrome." Interferon is expensive, and, given the lack of blinded studies, its use cannot be recommended. [p 1700]

33. **c. Erectile dysfunction or curvature that precludes intercourse.** For a patient to be a surgical candidate, the patients must have stable and mature disease. Indications for surgery include deformity that precludes intercourse and/or erectile dysfunction that precludes intercourse. [p 1700]

Chapter 48

Female Sexual Function and Dysfunction

Ridwan Shabsigh

Questions

1. Which of the following statements is NOT true regarding the bulb of the vestibule?

   a. Deep to the labia are two masses of erectile tissue called the bulb of the vestibule.
   b. The bulb of the vestibule is part of the crura of the clitoris.
   c. Each bulb is attached to the inferior surface of the perineal membrane and is covered by bulbocavernosus muscle.
   d. These muscles aid in constricting the venous supply to the erectile vestibular bulbs.
   e. The bulb runs on either side of the vaginal orifice and becomes engorged with blood during sexual arousal, which causes narrowing of the opening into the vagina and squeezes against the penis during sexual intercourse.

2. Which of the following statements is true about the bulbocavernosus reflex?

   a. The efferent pathway is through the pelvic nerve.
   b. The center of the reflex arch is in the brain stem.
   c. It exists only in males.
   d. It is speculated that through this reflex, tonic stimulation of the clitoris may lead to development of the orgasmic platform.
   e. It is a polysynaptic response seen in males and females and elicited by sympathetic afferents.

3. Which of the following statements is NOT true about the effects of androgens on female sexual functioning?

   a. Among women after adrenalectomy and/or oophorectomy, androgens but not estrogens appear to be responsible for sexual desire; testosterone replacement restores sexual desire after adrenalectomy and oophorectomy.
   b. In premenopausal women, studies have shown a positive correlation between midcycle androgen level and sexual function, including intercourse frequency, masturbation frequency, and genital response.
   c. In postmenopausal women, free testosterone was the only hormone correlated with sexual desire.
   d. In postmenopausal women not receiving hormone replacement therapy, sexual activity correlated with androgen level.
   e. In postmenopausal women, testosterone is efficacious for treating atrophic vaginitis.

4. Which of the following statements is NOT true about the effects of androgens on female sexual functioning?

   a. Testosterone is contraindicated in combination with estrogen.
   b. Testosterone is converted to two active metabolites: dihydrotestosterone and estradiol.
   c. Age is associated with a decline in androgens, a blunting of the midcycle testosterone surge, and an increase in hypoactive sexual desire.
   d. Testosterone levels among premenopausal women in their middle 40s are about half those of women in their 20s.
   e. Postmenopausal women report fewer sexual fantasies, reduced vaginal lubrication, and less sexual satisfaction compared with premenopausal women.

5. Which of the following is NOT a change associated with menopause?

   a. Reduced sexual responsiveness
   b. Dyspareunia
   c. Increased vaginal wall congestion during arousal
   d. Decreased sexual activity
   e. Diminished sexual desire

6. Which of the following statements is true about the relationship between diabetes and female sexual dysfunction (FSD)?

   a. There is a strong correlation between depression and sexual dysfunction in diabetic patients with neuropathy.
   b. Diabetes has no effect on female sexual function.
   c. Diabetic neuropathy is frequently reversible.
   d. Peripheral vascular disease does not contribute to FSD in diabetic patients.
   e. FSD in patients with diabetes is caused by hormonal imbalance.

7. Which of the following statements is NOT true regarding the effects of spinal cord injury on female sexual functioning?

   a. About 50% of women with spinal cord injury are able to achieve arousal and orgasm regardless of severity or completeness of the injury.
   b. Among women with spinal cord injury, 7% to 23% are unable to achieve orgasm.
   c. Psychogenic stimulation may result in cognitive subjective arousal.
   d. Genital arousal in response to psychogenic stimulation is related to the degree of preservation of the sympathetic innervation at T11–L2.
   e. Women with complete lower motor neuron lesions at S3–S4 are more likely to achieve orgasm.

8. Which of the following statements is NOT true about the effects of selective serotonin reuptake inhibitors (SSRIs) on female sexual functioning?

   a. Up to 50% of males and females taking antidepressants experience some degree of sexual dysfunction.
   b. Sexual side effects of SSRIs occur only when depression is not adequately treated.

c. Decreased desire, impaired physiologic arousal (i.e., vaginal lubrication), dyspareunia, and difficulty achieving orgasm are among the most common complaints in women.
d. Sexual dysfunction can be a cause of patient noncompliance with antidepressant treatment.
e. The recent introduction of oral sildenafil citrate presents a possible new opportunity for managing this significant side effect.

9. The multivariate analysis of the National Health and Social Life Survey identified all of the following independent predictors associated with the presence of FSD except which one?

    a. Nonmarried women were slightly more likely to experience difficulty with orgasm and sexual anxiety than were married women.
    b. Highly educated women were half as likely to report low sexual desire, problems achieving orgasm, sexual pain, and sexual anxiety as women who did not graduate from high school.
    c. Negative experiences such as forced sex or adult-child sexual contact were highly associated with arousal disorder.
    d. Lubrication difficulty decreased with age.
    e. All types of FSD were associated with emotional or stress-related problems, or low happiness and low physical satisfaction.

10. Which of the following statements is NOT true about dyspareunia?

    a. The first step in treatment of dyspareunia is to address potential reversible causes.
    b. Nonsteroidal anti-inflammatory drugs are the treatment of first choice.
    c. Atrophic vaginitis, decreased elasticity, thinning and fragility of vaginal tissue, and poor lubrication are readily amenable to treatment with estrogen.
    d. Systemic or topical applications of estrogens may help in alleviating dyspareunia in the elderly.
    e. Lubricants are effective in the treatment of idiopathic dyspareunia.

Answers

1. **b. The bulb of the vestibule is part of the crura of the clitoris.** Deep to the labia are two masses of erectile tissue called the bulb of the vestibule. Each bulb is attached to the inferior surface of the perineal membrane and is covered by bulbocavernosus muscle. These muscles aid in constricting the venous supply to the erectile vestibular bulbs. The bulb runs on either side of the vaginal orifice and becomes engorged with blood during sexual arousal. Bulb engorgement narrows the opening into the vagina and squeezes against the penis during sexual intercourse. [p 1711]

2. **d. It is speculated that through this reflex, tonic stimulation of the clitoris may lead to development of the orgasmic platform.** The best-studied reflex is the bulbocavernosus reflex, a polysynaptic response seen in males and females and elicited by pudendal sensory fibers. Although its sexual significance is unclear, it is speculated that through this reflex, tonic stimulation of the clitoris may lead to development of the orgasmic platform. [p 1713]

3. **e. In postmenopausal women, testosterone is efficacious for treating atrophic vaginitis.** Among women after adrenalectomy and/or oophorectomy, androgens and not estrogens appeared to be responsible for sexual desire. Testosterone replacement restores sexual desire after adrenalectomy and oophorectomy. In premenopausal women, studies have shown a positive correlation between midcycle androgen level and sexual function, including intercourse frequency, masturbation frequency, and genital response. In a group of 59 healthy, postmenopausal women, free testosterone was the only hormone correlated with sexual desire. In postmenopausal women not receiving hormone replacement therapy, sexual activity correlated with androgen level. [p 1715]

4. **a. Testosterone is contraindicated in combination with estrogen.** Circulating free testosterone diffuses into the target cells where testosterone is converted to two active metabolites: dihydrotestosterone and estradiol. Age is associated with a decline in androgens, a blunting of the midcycle testosterone surge, and an increase in hypoactive sexual desire. Testosterone levels among premenopausal women in their middle 40s are about half those of women in their 20s. This decline in testosterone continues into the postmenopausal years and appears more related to age than to menopause. Postmenopausal women report fewer sexual fantasies, reduced vaginal lubrication, and less sexual satisfaction compared with premenopausal women. [pp 1714, 1715]

5. **c. Increased vaginal wall congestion during arousal.** General menopause-related changes in sexual function have been described in the medical literature: reduced sexual responsiveness, dyspareunia, decreased sexual activity, and diminished sexual desire. [p 1716]

6. **a. There is a strong correlation between depression and sexual dysfunction in diabetic patients with neuropathy.** There is a strong correlation between depression and sexual dysfunction in diabetic patients with neuropathy. Sexual dysfunction parameters included difficulty achieving orgasm, problems with arousal, painful orgasm, lubrication problems, lack of desire, and inability to masturbate or have intercourse. Diabetic patients with neuropathy had significantly more problems in each category. Among these diabetic women with neuropathy, there was a significant positive correlation between the severity of the reported sexual dysfunction and the severity of the depression. [p 1719]

7. **e. Women with complete lower motor neuron lesions at S3–S4 are more likely to achieve orgasm.** About 50% of women with spinal cord injury are able to achieve arousal and orgasm regardless of severity or completeness of the injury. Psychogenic stimulation may result in cognitive subjective arousal. However, genital arousal in response to psychogenic stimulation is related to the degree of preservation of the sympathetic innervation at T11–L2. Among women with spinal cord injury, 7% to 23% are unable to achieve orgasm. Women with complete lower motor neuron lesions at S3–S4 are less likely to achieve orgasm. [pp 1721, 1722]

8. **b. Sexual side effects of SSRIs occur only when depression is not adequately treated.** Sexual dysfunction is one of the most common side effects associated with SSRIs. Although estimates of its prevalence vary, largely based on the method of investigation, up to 50% of males and females taking antidepressants experience some degree of sexual dysfunction. Decreased desire, impaired physiologic arousal (i.e., vaginal lubrication), dyspareunia, and difficulty achiev-

ing orgasm are among the most common complaints in women. Given the widespread use of antidepressants and the need to take antidepressant medications for prolonged periods, sexual dysfunction can be a cause of patient noncompliance with antidepressant treatment. Many antidotes have been proposed, but none have demonstrated efficacy in randomized placebo-controlled clinical studies. The recent introduction of oral sildenafil citrate presents a possible new opportunity for managing this significant side effect. [p 1721]

9. **d. Lubrication difficulty decreased with age.** A multivariate analysis of these data identified several independent predictors associated with the presence of FSD, which may eventually prove to have a causal role. Nonmarried women were slightly more likely to experience difficulty with orgasm and sexual anxiety than married women. Highly educated women were half as likely to report low sexual desire, problems achieving orgasm, sexual pain, and sexual anxiety as women who did not graduate from high school. Negative experiences such as forced sex or adult-child sexual contact were highly associated with arousal disorder. One of the most interesting results of this predictor analysis was the association of emotional or stress-related problems, or low happiness and low physical satisfaction, with all categories of sexual dysfunction. [p 1723]

10. **b. Nonsteroidal anti-inflammatory drugs are the treatment of first choice.** The first step in the treatment of dyspareunia is to address potential reversible causes such as vaginitis, endometriosis, and anatomic abnormalities. Estrogens and lubricants can be used to treat dyspareunia in patients with poor lubrication. Hormone replacement therapy is the major form of therapy for these elderly patients. Estrogen therapy alleviates symptoms such as vasomotor instability, minor psychological disturbance, and sexual difficulties. Atrophic vaginitis, decreased elasticity, thinning and fragility of vaginal tissue, and poor lubrication are readily amenable to treatment with estrogen. There is some evidence that hormone replacement therapy will increase lubrication during intercourse and may increase sexual enjoyment, desire, and orgasmic frequency. Systemic or topical applications of estrogens may help alleviate dyspareunia in the elderly. [p 1729]

SECTION IX

PEDIATRIC UROLOGY

Chapter 49

Normal and Anomalous Development of the Urogenital System

John M. Park

Questions

1. The fetal kidneys develop from which of the following embryonic structures?

   a. Paraxial (somite) mesoderm
   b. Intermediate mesoderm
   c. Neural tube
   d. Lateral mesoderm

2. Which of the following statements is NOT true of the mesonephros?

   a. It serves as a transient excretory organ during the development of definitive kidneys, the metanephros.
   b. Certain elements of the mesonephros persist as part of the reproductive tract.
   c. The excretory portion of the mesonephros begins to degenerate during the first year of life.
   d. Development of the mesonephric ducts precedes that of the mesonephric tubules.

3. At what gestational time point does the metanephros development begin?

   a. 20th day
   b. 24th day
   c. 28th day
   d. 32nd day

4. Which of the following statements is true of the metanephric development?

   a. It requires the reciprocal inductive interaction between müllerian duct and metanephric mesenchyme.
   b. The calyces, pelvis, and ureter derive from the differentiation of the metanephric mesenchyme.
   c. Older, more differentiated nephrons are located at the periphery of the developing kidney, whereas newer, less differentiated nephrons are found near the juxtamedullary region.
   d. In humans, although renal maturation continues postnatally, nephrogenesis is completed by birth.

5. The fused lower pole of the horseshoe kidney is trapped by which of the following structures during the ascent?

   a. Inferior mesenteric artery
   b. Superior mesenteric artery
   c. Celiac artery
   d. Common iliac artery

6. The homozygous gene disruption (gene knock-out) in which of the following molecules does not lead to a significant renal maldevelopment in mice?

   a. WT-1
   b. Pax-2
   c. GDNF
   d. p53

7. Which of the following statements is NOT true of the GDNF?

   a. It is a ligand for the c-*ret* receptor tyrosine kinase.
   b. GDNF gene knock-out mice demonstrate an abnormal renal development.
   c. It is expressed in the metanephric mesenchyme but not in the ureteric bud.
   d. GDNF arrests the ureteric bud growth in vitro.

8. Which of the following statements is NOT true of the renin-angiotensin system (RAS) during renal and ureteral development?

   a. The embryonic kidney is able to produce all components of the RAS.
   b. Both subtypes of angiotensin II receptor, AT_1 and AT_2, are expressed in the developing metanephros.
   c. AT_1 gene knock-out mice demonstrate a spectrum of congenital urinary tract abnormalities including ureteropelvic junction obstruction and vesicoureteral reflux.
   d. Infants born to mothers treated with angiotensin-converting enzyme inhibitors during pregnancy have increased rates of oligohydramnios, hypotension, and anuria.

9. The bladder trigone develops from which of the following structures?

   a. Mesonephric ducts
   b. Müllerian ducts
   c. Urogenital sinus
   d. Metanephric mesenchyme

10. The urachus involutes to become:

a. the verumontanum.
b. the median umbilical ligament.
c. appendix testes.
d. the epoophoron.

11. Which of the following statements is NOT true of bladder development?

    a. The bladder body is derived from the urogenital sinus while the trigone develops from the terminal portion of the mesonephric ducts.
    b. Bladder compliance seems to be low during early gestation, and it gradually increases thereafter.
    c. Epithelial-mesenchymal inductive interactions appear to be necessary for proper bladder development.
    d. Histologic evidence of smooth muscle differentiation begins near the bladder neck and proceeds toward the bladder dome.

12. The primordial germ cell migration and the formation of the genital ridges begin at which time point during gestation?

    a. Third week
    b. Fifth week
    c. Seventh week
    d. Ninth week

13. Which of the following statements is NOT true of the paramesonephric (müllerian) ducts?

    a. Both male and female embryos form paramesonephric (müllerian) ducts.
    b. In male embryos, the paramesonephric ducts degenerate under the influence of the MIS (müllerian-inhibiting substance) produced by the Leydig cells.
    c. In male embryos, the paramesonephric ducts become the appendix testis and the prostatic utricle.
    d. In female embryos, the paramesonephric ducts form the female reproductive tract, including fallopian tubes, uterus, and upper vagina.

14. Which of the following structures in the male reproductive tract develops from the urogenital sinus?

    a. Vas deferens
    b. Seminal vesicles
    c. Prostate
    d. Appendix epididymis

15. Which of the following statements is NOT true of human prostate development?

    a. It requires the conversion of testosterone into dihydrotestosterone by 5α-reductase.
    b. It is dependent on epithelial-mesenchymal interactions under the influence of androgens.
    c. It is first seen at the 10th week of gestation.
    d. It requires the hormonal effects of MIS.

16. In female embryos, the remnants of the mesonephric ducts persist as the following structures except:

    a. epoophoron.
    b. paroophoron.
    c. hymen.
    d. Gartner's duct cysts.

17. Which of the following statements is NOT true of the external genitalia development?

    a. The appearance of the external genitalia is similar in male and female embryos until the 12th week.
    b. The external genital appearance of males who are deficient in 5α-reductase is similar to that of females.
    c. In males, the formation of distal glandular urethra may occur by the fusion of urethral folds proximally and the ingrowth of ectodermal cells distally.
    d. In females, the urethral folds become the labia majora, and the labioscrotal folds become the labia minora.

18. The testicles descend to the level of internal inguinal ring by which time point during gestation?

    a. Sixth week
    b. Third month
    c. Sixth month
    d. Ninth month

19. Which of the following statements is NOT true of the SRY (the sex-determining region of the Y chromosome)?

    a. Its expression triggers the primitive sex cord cells to differentiate into the Sertoli cells.
    b. Approximately 25% of sex reversal conditions in humans are attributable to SRY mutations.
    c. It is located on the short arm of the Y chromosome.
    d. It causes the regression of mesonephric ducts.

Answers

1. **b. Intermediate mesoderm.** Mammals develop three kidneys in the course of intrauterine life. The embryonic kidneys are, in order of their appearance, the pronephros, the mesonephros, and the metanephros. The first two kidneys regress in utero, and the third becomes the permanent kidney. In terms of embryology, all three kidneys develop from the intermediate mesoderm. [p 1737]

2. **c. The excretory portion of the mesonephros begins to degenerate during the first year of life.** The second kidney, the mesonephros (plural, mesonephroi), is also transient, but in mammals it serves as an excretory organ for the embryo while the definitive kidney, the metanephros, begins its development. Development of the mesonephric ducts (also called wolffian ducts) precedes the development of the mesonephric tubules. Soon after the appearance of the mesonephric ducts during the fourth week, mesonephric vesicles begin to form. Initially, several spherical masses of cells are found along the medial side of the nephrogenic cords at the cranial end. This differentiation progresses caudally and results in the formation of 40 to 42 pairs of mesonephric tubules, but only about 30 pairs are seen at any one time, because the cranially located tubules start to degenerate starting at about the fifth week. By the fourth month, the human mesonephroi have almost completely disappeared, except for a few elements that persist into maturity. Certain elements of the mesonephroi are retained in the mature urogenital system as part of the reproductive tract. [p 1740]

3. **c. 28th day.** The definitive kidney, or the metanephros (plural, metanephroi), forms in the sacral region as a pair of new structures, called the ureteric buds, sprouts from the distal portion of the mesonephric duct and comes in contact with the blastema of metanephric mesenchyme at about the 28th day. [p 1740]

4. **d. In humans, although renal maturation continues postnatally, nephrogenesis is completed by birth.** It requires the inductive interaction between the ureteric bud and metanephric mesenchyme. The calyces, pelvis, and ureter derive from the ureteric bud. Older, more differentiated nephrons are located in the inner part of the kidney near the juxtamedullary region. In humans, although renal maturation continues to take place postnatally, nephrogenesis is completed before birth. [pp 1741–1742]

5. **a. Inferior mesenteric artery.** The inferior poles of the kidneys may also fuse, forming a horseshoe kidney that crosses over the ventral side of the aorta. During ascent, the fused lower pole becomes trapped under the inferior mesenteric artery and thus does not reach its normal site. [p 1743]

6. **d. p53.** Mutant WT-1 mice do not form ureteric buds, and in *Pax*-2 gene knock-out mice, no mesonephric ducts, müllerian ducts, ureteric buds, or metanephric mesenchyme form, and the animals die within 1 day of birth because of renal failure. Ureteric bud formation is impaired in GDNF (glial cell line-derived neurotrophic factor) knock-out mice, but *p53* gene knock-out mice do not demonstrate significant renal developmental anomaly. [pp 1746–1748]

7. **d. GDNF arrests the ureteric bud growth in vitro.** GDNF promotes ureteric bud growth in vitro. Although the importance of c-*ret* in kidney development was clearly demonstrated, it is only recently that its ligand, GDNF, has been identified. GDNF is a secreted glycoprotein that possesses a cystine-knot motif. GDNF is expressed within the metanephric mesenchyme prior to ureteric bud invasion, and ureteric bud formation is impaired in GDNF knock-out mice. [pp 1746–1747]

8. **c. AT_1 gene knock-out mice demonstrate a spectrum of congenital urinary tract abnormalities, including ureteropelvic junction obstruction and vesicoureteral reflux.** AT_2 gene knock-out mice demonstrate a spectrum of congenital urinary tract abnormalities, including ureteropelvic junction obstruction, multicystic dysplastic kidney, megaureter, vesicoureteral reflux, and renal hypoplasia. [p 1748]

9. **a. Mesonephric ducts.** The terminal portion of the mesonephric duct, called the common excretory ducts, becomes incorporated into the developing bladder and forms the trigone. [p 1749]

10. **b. The median umbilical ligament.** By the 12th week, the urachus involutes to become a fibrous cord, which becomes the median umbilical ligament. [p 1752]

11. **d. Histologic evidence of smooth muscle differentiation begins near the bladder neck and proceeds toward the bladder dome.** Between the 7th and 12th weeks, the surrounding connective tissues condense and smooth muscle fibers begin to appear, first at the region of the bladder dome and later proceeding toward the bladder neck. [pp 1752–1753]

12. **b. Fifth week.** During the fifth week, primordial germ cells migrate from the yolk sac along the dorsal mesentery to populate the mesenchyme of the posterior body wall near the 10th thoracic level. In both sexes, the arrival of primordial germ cells in the area of future gonads serves as the signal for the existing cells of the mesonephros and the adjacent coelomic epithelium to proliferate and form a pair of genital ridges just medial to the developing mesonephros. [p 1753]

13. **b. In male embryos, the paramesonephric ducts degenerate under the influence of the MIS (müllerian-inhibiting substance) produced by the Leydig cells.** A new pair of ducts, called the paramesonephric (müllerian) ducts, begins to form just lateral to the mesonephric ducts in both male and female embryos. These ducts arise by the craniocaudal invagination of thickened coelomic epithelium, extending all the way from the third thoracic segment to the posterior wall of the developing urogenital sinus. The caudal tips of the paramesonephric ducts adhere to each other as they connect with the urogenital sinus between the openings of the right and left mesonephric ducts. The cranial ends of the paramesonephric ducts form funnel-shaped openings into the coelomic cavity (the future peritoneum). As developing Sertoli cells begin their differentiation in response to the SRY (sex-determining region of the Y chromosome), they begin to secrete MIS, which causes the paramesonephric (müllerian) ducts to regress rapidly between the 8th and 10th weeks. Small müllerian duct remnants can be detected in the developed male as a small tissue protrusion at the superior pole of the testicle, called the appendix testis, and as a posterior expansion of the prostatic urethra, called the prostatic utricle. In female embryos, MIS is absent, so the müllerian ducts do not regress and instead give rise to fallopian tubes, uterus, and vagina. [pp 1753–1754]

14. **c. Prostate.** Vas deferens, seminal vesicles, and appendix epididymis all develop from the mesonephric ducts. The prostate and bulbourethral glands develop from the urethra. [p 1754]

15. **d. It requires the hormonal effects of MIS.** The prostate gland begins to develop during the 10th week as a cluster of endodermal evaginations budding from the pelvic urethra. These presumptive prostatic outgrowths are induced by the surrounding mesenchyme, and this process depends on the conversion of testosterone into dihydrotestosterone by 5α-reductase. Similar to renal and bladder development, prostatic development depends on mesenchymal-epithelial interactions but under the influence of androgens. There is no evidence that MIS plays a direct role in prostate development. [pp 1755–1756]

16. **c. Hymen.** In the absence of MIS, the mesonephric (wolffian) ducts degenerate and the paramesonephric (müllerian) ducts give rise to the fallopian tubes, uterus, and upper two thirds of the vagina. The remnants of mesonephric ducts are found in the mesentery of the ovary as the epoophoron and paroophoron, and near the vaginal introitus and anterolateral vaginal wall as Gartner's duct cysts. The hymen develops from the endodermal membrane located at the junction between the vaginal plate and the definitive urogenital sinus, which is the future vestibule of the vagina. [p 1756]

17. **d. In females, the urethral folds become the labia majora, and the labioscrotal folds become the labia minora.** The early development of the external genital organ is similar in both sexes. Early in the fifth week, a pair of swellings called cloacal folds develops on either side of the cloacal membrane. These folds meet just anterior to the cloacal membrane to form a midline swelling called the genital tubercle. During the cloacal division into the anterior urogenital sinus and the posterior anorectal canal, the portion of the cloacal folds flanking the opening of the urogenital sinus becomes the urogenital folds, and the portion flanking the opening of the anorectal canal becomes the anal folds. A new pair of swellings, called the labioscrotal folds, then appears on either side of the urogenital folds. In the absence of dihydrotestosterone, the primitive perineum does not lengthen, and the labioscrotal and urethral folds do not fuse across the midline in the female embryos. The phallus bends inferiorly, becoming the clitoris, and the definitive urogenital

sinus becomes the vestibule of the vagina. The urethral folds become the labia minora, and the labioscrotal folds become the labia majora. The external genital organ develops in a similar manner in genetic males who are deficient in 5α-reductase and therefore lack dihydrotestosterone. [pp 1757–1758]

18. **b. Third month.** The testicle reaches the level of internal inguinal ring by the third month and passes through the inguinal canal to reach the scrotum between the seventh and ninth months. [p 1758]

19. **d. It causes the regression of mesonephric ducts.** When the Y-linked master regulatory gene, called *SRY*, is expressed in the male, the epithelial cells of the primitive sex cords differentiate into Sertoli cells, and this critical morphogenetic event triggers subsequent testicular development. Analysis of DNA narrowed the location of the *SRY* to a relatively small region within the short arm of the chromosome. It is now clear that only about 25% of sex reversals in humans can be attributed to disabling mutations of the *SRY*. [pp 1761–1762]

Chapter 50

Renal Function in the Fetus, Neonate, and Child

Robert L. Chevalier • Stuart S. Howards

Questions

1. The pronephros, mesonephros, and metanephros have the following significance in human embryogenesis, respectively:
   a. none, none, none.
   b. none, none, gives rise to the ureteric bud.
   c. none, gives rise to the gonad, gives rise to the ureteric bud.
   d. none, gives rise to the ureteric bud, induces nephrogenesis.
   e. gives rise to the gonad, gives rise to the ureteric bud, induces nephrogenesis.

2. When does urine production begin in the human fetus?
   a. At 2 to 3 weeks
   b. At 4 to 6 weeks
   c. At 10 to 12 weeks
   d. At 14 to 16 weeks
   e. At 20 to 22 weeks

3. During the first 24 hours of life:
   a. 100% of infants void.
   b. 80% of infants void.
   c. 60% of infants void.
   d. 80% of term infants void, whereas 50% of premature infants void.
   e. 60% of term infants void, whereas 40% of premature infants void.

4. During the first 2 weeks of life, the glomerular filtration rate (GFR):
   a. is stable.
   b. increases 2% to 3% per day.
   c. varies based primarily on hydration.
   d. is stable in term infants but increases 50% in premature infants.
   e. increases 100% in term infants.

5. At 1 week of age, the serum creatinine level of term and premature infants is usually:
   a. less than 1.0 mg/dl in both.
   b. less than 1.0 mg/dl for term infants but up to 1.5 mg/dl for premature infants.
   c. less than 0.7 mg/dl in both.
   d. less than 0.7 mg/dl for term infants but greater than 2.0 mg/dl for premature infants.
   e. greatly variable depending on the mother's serum creatinine concentration.

6. The sequelae of renal tubular acidosis in the infant include:
   a. growth retardation.
   b. growth retardation, osteodystrophy.
   c. growth retardation, osteodystrophy, polyuria.
   d. growth retardation, osteodystrophy, polyuria, nephrocalcinosis.
   e. growth retardation, osteodystrophy, polyuria, nephrocalcinosis, nephrolithiasis.

7. Sonographic evaluation of the urinary tract should be done in children with renal tubular acidosis to rule out what?
   a. Renal atrophy
   b. Obstruction
   c. Nephrolithiasis
   d. Obstruction and nephrolithiasis
   e. Renal atrophy, obstruction, and nephrolithiasis

8. What are the normal values for the ratio of calcium to creatinine in the urine of term infants and older children?
   a. Less than 0.4 and 0.2, respectively
   b. Less than 0.2 and 0.4, respectively
   c. Less than 0.2 and 0.2, respectively
   d. Less than 0.8 and 0.4, respectively
   e. Less than 0.4 and 0.8, respectively

9. After the postnatal diuresis begins, what are the appropriate values of "maintenance" intravenous administration of sodium and potassium, respectively, in an infant with normal renal function?
   a. 10 to 15 mEq/kg/day and 5 to 10 mEq/kg/day
   b. 10 to 15 mEq/kg/day and 2 to 3 mEq/kg/day

c. 2 to 3 mEq/kg/day and 5 to 10 mEq/kg/day
d. 2 to 3 mEq/kg/day and 0 mEq/kg/day
e. 2 to 3 mEq/kg/day and 2 to 3 mEq/kg/day

10. What effect does the maternal administration of nonsteroidal anti-inflammatory drugs (NSAIDs) such as indomethacin have?

   a. It has no effect on neonatal renal function.
   b. It has no effect on neonatal renal function in the term infant but can cause renal insufficiency in the premature infant.
   c. It can cause renal insufficiency and oliguria in the neonate.
   d. It causes a concentrating deficit in the neonate.
   e. It causes a concentrating defect in the premature neonate but not in the term infant.

11. When does compensatory renal growth in the child with a solitary kidney begin?

   a. In utero
   b. At birth
   c. At 2 weeks of age
   d. At 1 month of age
   e. At 3 months of age

Answers

1. **d. None, gives rise to the ureteric bud, induces nephrogenesis.** The pronephros appears at 3 weeks, never progresses beyond a rudimentary stage, and involutes by 5 weeks. The mesonephros is seen at 5 weeks of gestation, appears to have transitory function, and degenerates by 11 to 12 weeks. Its major role in renal development is related to the fact that its ductal system gives rise to the ureteric bud. The metanephros begins its inductive phase after 5 weeks of gestation, and, in the human, nephrogenesis is completed by 34 to 36 weeks. [pp 1765–1766]

2. **c. At 10 to 12 weeks.** Urine production in the human kidney is known to begin at about 10 to 12 weeks. Throughout gestation, however, the placenta primarily handles salt and water homeostasis. [p 1766]

3. **a. 100% of infants void.** In a study of 500 normal neonates, Clark found that every infant voided within the first 24 hours of life regardless of gestational age. [p 1767]

4. **e. Increases 100% in term infants.** The GFR doubles during the first week in term infants. Because of the dependence of the GFR on gestational age, for infants born before 34 weeks, the GFR rises slowly. After a postconceptual age of 34 weeks is reached, a rapid rise is observed. [p 1767]

5. **b. Less than 1.0 mg/dl for term infants but up to 1.5 mg/dl for premature infants.** By 7 days in the term infant, the plasma creatinine concentration is normally less than 1 mg/dl, whereas in preterm infants levels can remain as high as 1.5 mg/dl for the first month of life. [p 1768]

6. **e. Growth retardation, osteodystrophy, polyuria, nephrocalcinosis, nephrolithiasis.** Appropriate evaluation and treatment are important to prevent the sequelae of renal tubular acidosis. These sequelae include growth retardation, osteodystrophy, nephrocalcinosis or nephrolithiasis, and polyuria. [p 1769]

7. **d. Obstruction and nephrolithiasis.** Sonographic examination of the urinary tract should be performed not only to identify hydronephrosis but also to reveal nephrocalcinosis or nephrolithiasis that can develop in children with type I renal tubular acidosis. [p 1771]

8. **a. Less than 0.4 and 0.2, respectively.** Urinary calcium excretion in the neonate is most easily assessed by determination of the calcium/creatinine ratio (mg/mg) in a random urine sample. In contrast to the older child, in whom a ratio exceeding 0.2 should be considered abnormal, the ratio in the infant receiving breast milk can rise to 0.4 in the term infant and to 0.8 in the preterm neonate. [p 1771]

9. **e. 2 to 3 mEq/kg/day and 2 to 3 mEq/kg/day.** Once the physiologic postnatal diuresis has begun, 2 to 3 mEq/kg/day sodium can be prescribed. Potassium chloride, 2 mEq/kg/day, can be added to the fluid prescription once urine output is established. [p 1772]

10. **c. It can cause renal insufficiency and oliguria in the neonate.** Maternal administration of NSAIDs such as indomethacin can result in prolonged renal insufficiency and oliguria in the neonate. Prolonged intrauterine exposure can also impair fetal renal development. Administration of indomethacin to neonates with patent ductus arteriosus frequently results in decreased GFR and oliguria. Caution should be exercised in the administration of NSAIDs to any infant or child with a single functioning kidney or with renal impairment, because such patients are at increased risk for additional nephron injury and deterioration of GFR. [p 1774]

11. **a. In utero.** Studies demonstrate unequivocally that compensatory renal growth can begin prenatally. Because the placenta provides the excretory function for the fetus, an increased excretory burden on the kidney is not required to initiate compensatory growth. Rather, alterations in growth factors or inhibitors presumably modulate the prenatal changes. [p 1774]

Chapter 51

Perinatal Urology

Craig A. Peters

Questions

1. A neonate is reported to have a single cyst on the upper pole of the left kidney. What does this most likely represent?

   a. A benign simple cyst
   b. Cystic neuroblastoma
   c. Duplication anomaly with upper pole dilatation
   d. Upper pole dilatation caused by reflux
   e. Neurenteric cyst

2. During gestation, the makeup of the amniotic fluid (AF) becomes increasingly:

   a. like fetal plasma.
   b. the product of fetal urine output.
   c. an ultrafiltrate from the placenta.
   d. hyperosmotic to fetal plasma.
   e. a product of gastrointestinal secretions.

3. What is the most reliable predictor of vesicoureteral reflux in the fetus?

   a. Pelvic dilatation greater than 7 mm at 30 weeks
   b. Intermittent ureteral dilatation
   c. Calyceal dilatation
   d. Echogenic renal parenchyma
   e. There are no reliable predictors of reflux.

4. A 24-week fetus is found to have evidence of a ureterocele and has bilateral moderately severe hydronephrosis of all renal units. What is the likely cause?

   a. Concomitant posterior urethral valves
   b. Bilateral ectopic ureters
   c. Obstruction of the ureteral orifices by the ureterocele
   d. Bladder outlet obstruction by the ureterocele
   e. Associated neurogenic bladder dysfunction

5. The characteristic ultrasonographic appearance of a multicystic dysplastic kidney (MCDK) in utero is multiple noncommunicating cysts and:

   a. absence of a large central cyst with minimal parenchyma.
   b. presence of a large central cyst with echogenic parenchyma.
   c. presence of a large central cyst without parenchyma.
   d. absence of a large central cyst with thick echogenic parenchyma.
   e. a peripheral array around a large central cyst.

6. A 34-week fetus has bilateral large echogenic kidneys without recognizable cysts. There is little amniotic fluid. What is the likely diagnosis?

   a. Bilateral MCDK
   b. Bilateral congenital mesoblastic nephromas
   c. Congenital medullary nephronophthisis
   d. Bilateral fetal renal vein thrombosis
   e. Autosomal recessive polycystic kidneys

7. A fetus with intracardiac masses consistent with rhabdomyosarcomas should be screened for:

   a. Down syndrome.
   b. Beckwith-Wiedemann syndrome.
   c. trisomy 14.
   d. tuberous sclerosis.
   e. Denys-Drash syndrome.

8. A characteristic feature of congenital obstructive nephropathy is:

   a. increased glomerulogenesis.
   b. decreased renin-angiotensin activation.
   c. interstitial fibrosis.
   d. medullary hyperplasia.
   e. relative loss of smooth muscle α-actin expression.

9. A fetus with apparent obstructive uropathy has had adequate amniotic fluid until about 32 weeks' gestation. The kidneys are dilated and nonechogenic. What is the likely outcome in this child?

   a. Early neonatal respiratory death
   b. Pulmonary insufficiency with death by 4 months of age
   c. Early neonatal death because of renal failure
   d. Moderate renal insufficiency
   e. Normal renal and pulmonary function

10. What is the most compelling reason for in utero urinary tract shunting for obstructive uropathy?

    a. Severe bilateral hydronephrosis
    b. Echogenic kidneys at 24 weeks' gestation
    c. Decreasing amniotic fluid volume after 28 weeks
    d. Absence of bladder refilling on percutaneous aspiration
    e. Oligohydramnios at 21 weeks associated with severe hydronephrosis

11. A neonatal boy with prenatal hydronephrosis is found to have bilateral grade 5 reflux and a bladder capacity of 200 ml. There is no trabeculation. What is the best explanation for his large bladder capacity?

    a. Recycling of refluxed urine
    b. Bladder outlet obstruction from valves
    c. Neurogenic bladder
    d. Prune-belly variant
    e. Impaired bladder emptying

12. A neonatal boy with bilateral grade 4 reflux may be expected to have which pattern on urodynamic studies?

    a. Normal bladder dynamics
    b. Impaired contractility
    c. Bladder outlet obstruction
    d. Small capacity, high pressure
    e. Hypertonicity and instability

13. A 7-day-old boy with hypospadias and undescended testes is

seen in the emergency room with hypotension, hyponatremia, hyperkalemia, and dehydration. The most appropriate management is intravenous fluid resuscitation and:

   a. intravenous antibiotics.
   b. hypertonic saline.
   c. parenteral corticosteroids.
   d. abdominal CT.
   e. voiding cystourethrogram.

14. A newborn boy has a penile abnormality. The surface of the penis closest to the abdomen appears to be a mucosal surface, with the defect extending from the pubis to the glans. The foreskin is dangling from the opposite side of the glans. The scrotum is normal. The pubic bones feel more widely spaced than normal. What is this condition, most likely?

    a. Penoscrotal hypospadias
    b. Superior vesical fissure
    c. Classic bladder exstrophy
    d. Congenital urethrocutaneous fistula
    e. Epispadias

15. In cloacal exstrophy, what is the principal goal for early management?

    a. Bladder closure with delayed hindgut functionalization
    b. Early hindgut functionalization
    c. Removal of the atretic hindgut and early ileal functionalization
    d. Total bladder reconstruction with delayed hindgut functionalization
    e. Omphalocele closure, mucous fistula for hindgut, and ileostomy

16. A 5-month-old child undergoes a KUB (kidney, ureter, bladder) study for abdominal distention. There are calcifications in the left upper quadrant in a peripheral, eggshell pattern. What is the most likely cause?

    a. Neuroblastoma
    b. Renal vein thrombosis
    c. Renal artery stenosis
    d. Adrenal hemorrhage
    e. Wilms' tumor

Answers

1. **c. Duplication anomaly with upper pole dilatation.** A single upper pole cyst is likely not a cyst but a dilated upper pole, probably a duplication anomaly with upper pole hydronephrosis. A dilated ureter is likely to be found as well, and this may be associated with an ectopic ureterocele or an ectopic ureter causing obstruction. The other entities can be distinguished by the fact that they do not usually appear as elements of the functional renal units. [p 1783]

2. **b. The product of fetal urine output.** The time of onset of changes in the AF is crucial and reflects a normal shift from the point at which most of the AF is a placental transudate to the point at which it becomes predominantly a product of fetal urine. This occurs after 16 weeks, and by 20 or 22 weeks most AF is fetal urine. Oligohydramnios, the condition of reduced AF, may therefore be due to urinary tract obstruction and may become evident only after 18 or 20 weeks' gestation. [p 1785]

3. **e. There are no reliable predictors of reflux.** Vesicoureteral reflux may be evident by a variable degree of collecting system dilatation; however, there is no reliable way to predict the presence of reflux or its grade based on fetal ultrasonographic findings. Although any of the characteristics given may suggest the possibility of reflux and would prompt the performance of a voiding cystourethrogram, they are neither specific nor sensitive. [p 1785]

4. **d. Bladder outlet obstruction by the ureterocele.** Bilateral hydronephrosis may imply bilateral reflux but may also indicate an element of bladder outlet obstruction caused by prolapse of the ureterocele into the bladder neck. It would be unusual for the other causes to occur in a child with a ureterocele. [p 1786]

5. **a. Absence of a large central cyst with minimal parenchyma.** The classic ultrasonographic appearance of an MCDK was initially defined by Saunders as being a nonreniform structure, with multiple, randomly arrayed, noncommunicating, fluid-filled cystic spaces; no central large cyst; and minimal to no recognizable renal parenchyma. There are examples of MCDKs that have a more substantial amount of parenchyma visible, which is invariably echogenic. [p 1787]

6. **e. Autosomal recessive polycystic kidneys.** Autosomal recessive polycystic kidney disease is characterized by markedly enlarged, brightly echogenic kidneys without recognizable cysts. The cysts are too small to be resolved individually by ultrasonography. As the condition progresses, oligohydramnios will develop. [p 1787]

7. **d. Tuberous sclerosis.** The finding of a cardiac mass (rhabdomyosarcoma) is associated with tuberous sclerosis, and possible renal masses. Therefore, screening for this condition and the possibility of renal masses, including angiomyolipomas and Wilms' tumor, should be done. [p 1789]

8. **c. Interstitial fibrosis.** Congenital obstructive uropathy is characterized by increased interstitial fibrosis that leads to functional abnormalities. The obstructed kidney will show patterns that may be characterized as injury responses. These include fibrosis, inflammation, and altered growth. This condition is probably induced in part by overexpression of the renin-angiotensin system mediated through transforming growth factor-β. There is usually a loss of medullary structures and decreased glomerulogenesis. [p 1791]

9. **d. Moderate renal insufficiency.** The timing of the onset of oligohydramnios is important in assessing its potential consequences. As would be predicted from an understanding of the pathophysiology, late-onset oligohydramnios is not associated with pulmonary insufficiency, with a threshold of about 30 weeks. There may be some degree of renal insufficiency, but with nonechogenic kidneys, this is unlikely to result in end-stage failure early in life; similarly, it would be unlikely for this child to have completely normal renal function. [p 1792]

10. **e. Oligohydramnios at 21 weeks associated with severe hydronephrosis.** At present, fetal intervention for obstructive uropathy is indicated when the life of the fetus is at risk. This is only when oligohydramnios is present in the setting of presumed bladder outlet obstruction. Bilateral hydronephrosis alone may not require intervention, and bilateral renal echogenicity may indicate dysplasia. In the absence of oligohydramnios, renal echogenicity is not necessarily associated with an adverse outcome. The absence of bladder re-

filling indicates nonsalvageable renal functional impairment. [p 1793]

11. **a. Recycling of refluxed urine.** This is a description of the megacystis-megaureter association in which there is massive bilateral reflux. The bladder empties, but the refluxed urine immediately refills the bladder, effectively causing retention. The constant recycling of bladder urine into the upper tracts prevents true bladder emptying. In the absence of trabeculation, this case is unlikely to be valve obstruction or a neurogenic bladder. Prune belly syndrome variants with massive reflux have been described but are quite rare and less likely to be the cause of this condition than the megacystis-megaureter association. [p 1797]

12. **e. Hypertonicity and instability.** Several studies have demonstrated markedly abnormal urodynamic patterns in boys with dilating reflux. These have generally shown a high incidence of bladder hypertonicity and instability. This raises the question of whether the high grades of reflux are a product of bladder dysfunction or just associated with it. [p 1799]

13. **c. Parenteral corticosteroids.** The most likely cause of this condition is congenital virilizing adrenal hyperplasia with salt wasting, which may produce life-threatening adrenal crisis at 7 to 10 days of life. With hypospadias and bilateral undescended testes, this condition should be presumed and immediate treatment initiated with resuscitation and steroid treatment. In addition, urinalysis for possible infection and electrolyte assays can be performed, as well as a pelvic ultrasonographic scan to look for the presence of a uterine structure, which will confirm the diagnosis. [p 1800]

14. **e. Epispadias.** In contrast to hypospadias, the urethral opening in epispadias is on the dorsal aspect of the penis and may be proximal (penopubic) or more distal (glanular). This condition is also characterized by a widened symphysis pubis. Penoscrotal hypospadias would be a defect on the opposite side, closest to the scrotum. Bladder exstrophy would have the defect extending up to the umbilicus, with the mucosal surface of the bladder visible. Superior vesical fissure is a defect in the bladder wall near the umbilicus with an intact penis. Congenital urethrocutaneous fistulas are ventral. [p 1802]

15. **b. Early hindgut functionalization.** The most crucial element of the early management of these children rests in preserving all aspects of the gastrointestinal and urinary tracts. Separation of the gastrointestinal and genitourinary tracts with the creation of an end-colostomy (not ileostomy) will permit the most efficient use of all levels of the gastrointestinal tract. Preservation of the hindgut not only will be crucial for nutrition and growth but may be needed later for urinary tract reconstruction. This is best accomplished by functional anastomosis of the ileum and hindgut with separation from the bladder plate. Bladder closure can be delayed if the bladder's condition or the child's health is not optimal. The hindgut should never be discarded and will often grow remarkably once it is functionalized. [p 1803]

16. **d. Adrenal hemorrhage.** The late appearance of an adrenal hemorrhage is that of peripheral eggshell calcifications, in contrast to diffuse stippled calcifications of neuroblastoma. The other conditions can unusually lead to calcifications, but they are not typically peripheral and thin. Ultrasonography would confirm the site of origin and appearance. [p 1806]

Chapter 52

Evaluation of the Pediatric Urologic Patient

Douglas A. Canning

Questions

1. When should newborn boys with bilateral hydronephrosis be evaluated?

   a. Within a week after referral
   b. Immediately after delivery
   c. At the time of discharge from the newborn nursery
   d. At the first well-child visit
   e. At the family's convenience

2. When should an infant with ambiguous genitalia undergo testing for congenital adrenal hyperplasia?

   a. At the family's convenience
   b. At the first well-child visit
   c. Before discharge from the newborn nursery
   d. At 6 weeks of age
   e. At 12 weeks of age

3. The peak incidence for gonorrhea in females in North America is at what age?

   a. 12 to 14 years
   b. 15 to 19 years
   c. 20 to 25 years
   d. 26 to 30 years
   e. 31 to 35 years

4. When should surgery for boys with undescended testes be performed?

   a. At birth
   b. At 3 months of age
   c. At 6 months of age
   d. At 1 year of age
   e. At 2 years of age

5. Common urologic sources of failure to thrive include which of the following?

   a. Urinary tract infection
   b. Renal tubular acidosis

c. Diabetes insipidus
  d. Chronic renal insufficiency
  e. All of the above

6. Neurofibromatosis type 1 (von Recklinghausen's disease) should be suspected if:

  a. three café-au-lait spots are present.
  b. five or more café-au-lait spots, each more than 5 mm in diameter, are present in prepubertal patients.
  c. six or more café-au-lait spots, each more than 15 mm in diameter, are present in postpubertal children.
  d. four café-au-lait spots, each more than 15 mm in diameter, are present in postpubertal children.
  e. b and c.

7. The Beckwith-Wiedemann syndrome includes which of the following findings?

  a. Macroglossia, hepatosplenomegaly, nephromegaly, and hypoglycemia
  b. Neuroblastoma, hepatosplenomegaly, nephromegaly, and hypoglycemia
  c. Preauricular sinus, hepatosplenomegaly, nephromegaly, and hypoglycemia
  d. Supernumerary digits, macroglossia, hepatosplenomegaly, and hypoglycemia
  e. Macroglossia, hepatosplenomegaly, nephromegaly, and hypospadias

8. In newborns with ambiguous genitalia, what does a symmetrical gonadal examination suggest?

  a. Congenital adrenal hyperplasia or true hermaphroditism
  b. Mixed gonadal dysgenesis or androgen insensitivity syndrome
  c. Congenital adrenal hyperplasia or mixed gonadal dysgenesis
  d. Congenital adrenal hyperplasia or androgen insensitivity syndrome
  e. True hermaphroditism or mixed gonadal dysgenesis

9. A newborn should have a hydrocele surgically corrected in the newborn period if:

  a. it is large.
  b. it is changing in volume.
  c. it accompanies a symptomatic hernia.
  d. a, b, and c.
  e. b and c.

10. The most commonly reported form of sexual abuse in children involves which of the following?

  a. Abuse of daughters by fathers
  b. Abuse of sons by fathers
  c. Abuse of sons by mothers
  d. Abuse of sisters by brothers
  e. Abuse of daughters by mothers

11. A presacral dimple in a newborn may indicate spina bifida if:

  a. it is deeper than 0.5 cm.
  b. it is on the midline.
  c. it is more than 2.5 cm from the anal verge.
  d. a and c.
  e. a, b, and c

12. What is genitourinary sinography used for?

  a. To identify the presence of a cervix in a patient with ambiguous genitalia
  b. To provide detail about the relative positions of the urethra, vagina, and distal hindgut in a patient with a cloaca
  c. To assess the distance between the perineum and the point of confluence between the vagina and the urethra
  d. a and c.
  e. a, b, and c.

13. Urethral meatal stenosis occurs in the newborn:

  a. as a result of birth trauma.
  b. after urinary tract infection.
  c. after a newborn physical examination.
  d. after healing of the inflamed, denuded glans after circumcision.
  e. from undergarment irritation.

Answers

1. **b. Immediately after delivery.** Infants with severe bilateral hydronephrosis should be evaluated immediately after delivery. Many will develop compromised renal function. A few will need a direct admission to the newborn intensive care unit or to a similar inpatient step-down unit. [pp 1812–1813]

2. **c. Before discharge from the newborn nursery.** Infants with ambiguous genitalia require immediate evaluation. Because congenital adrenal hyperplasia may result in salt wasting, which may be life-threatening in the infant, infants with ambiguous genitalia must be evaluated quickly and stabilized. If congenital adrenal hyperplasia is suspected, the infant should not be discharged from the nursery before appropriate testing is complete. [p 1813]

3. **b. 15 to 19 years.** The incidence of sexually transmitted diseases is declining but remains relatively high, with peak ages for women with gonorrhea in the United States between 15 and 19 years. [p 1817]

4. **c. At 6 months of age.** We operate on patients with undescended or absent testes when the patient is about 6 months of age. [p 1818]

5. **e. All of the above.** As urologists, we must be alert to common urologic sources of failure to thrive such as urinary tract infection, renal tubular acidosis, diabetes insipidus, and chronic renal insufficiency. [p 1819]

6. **e. b and c.** If there are five or more spots, each more than 5 mm in diameter in prepubertal patients, or six or more spots more than 15 mm in diameter in postpubertal children, neurofibromatosis type 1 (von Recklinghausen's disease) should be suspected. [p 1822]

7. **a. Macroglossia, hepatosplenomegaly, nephromegaly, and hypoglycemia.** Macroglossia can be associated with the Beckwith-Wiedemann syndrome, which also includes hepatosplenomegaly, nephromegaly, and hypoglycemia secondary to pancreatic β-cell hyperplasia in an infant that is large for gestational age. [p 1822]

8. **d. Congenital adrenal hyperplasia or androgen insensitivity syndrome.** Particular attention to the symmetry of the examination is important if intersex conditions are thought to exist. A symmetrical gonadal examination (gonads palpable on each side or impalpable on both sides) suggests a

global disorder such as congenital adrenal hyperplasia or androgen insensitivity. [p 1823]

9. **c. It accompanies a symptomatic hernia.** A hydrocele that changes in volume suggests a patent processus vaginalis. These infants are at risk for inguinal hernia. The processus vaginalis is not likely to close after birth. If a hernia has been symptomatic, the processus vaginalis should be corrected in the newborn period. [p 1823]

10. **a. Abuse of daughters by fathers.** The abuse of daughters by fathers and stepfathers is the most common form of reported incest, although brother-sister incest is considered to be the most common type. [p 1824]

11. **d. a and c.** A presacral dimple may indicate spina bifida or cord tethering if the dimple is off center, more than 2.5 cm from the anal verge at birth, or deeper than 0.5 cm. [p 1825]

12. **e. a, b, and c.** The genitourinary sinogram will help to differentiate a cervix from a prostatic utricle. If a cloaca is present, the sinogram will provide detail about the position of the rectum, vagina, and urethra and about the point of confluence and the distance to the perineum. [p 1828]

13. **d. After healing of the inflamed, denuded glans after circumcision.** Meatal stenosis is common after circumcision. It may result from contraction of the meatus after healing of the inflamed, denuded glans tissue that occurs after retraction of the foreskin or from damage to the frenular artery at the time of circumcision. [p 1829]

Chapter 53

Renal Disease in Childhood

Shane Roy III • H. Norman Noe

Questions

1. Which one of the following is considered to be the hallmark of glomerular bleeding?

    a. Gross hematuria
    b. Cola-colored urine
    c. Red blood cell (RBC) casts
    d. Proteinuria
    e. Painless hematuria

2. Which of the following findings on urinalysis enhances the diagnosis of a glomerular source of bleeding?

    a. Eumorphic RBC
    b. Greater than 10% dysmorphic RBC
    c. Proteinuria
    d. Granular casts
    e. Oval fat bodies

3. In the absence of urinary infection or glomerular disease, what is the most common cause of hematuria in children?

    a. Wilms' tumor
    b. Ureteropelvic junction obstruction
    c. Renal calculi
    d. Posterior urethral valves
    e. Hypercalciuria

4. Which one of the following forms of glomerulonephritis is associated with a low serum complement C3 concentration?

    a. Poststreptococcal acute glomerulonephritis
    b. IgA nephropathy
    c. Alport's syndrome
    d. Henoch-Schönlein purpura
    e. Hemolytic-uremic syndrome

5. What percentage of patients with immunoglobulin A nephropathy can be expected to have progressive renal failure after 10 to 20 years of follow-up?

    a. Less than 5%
    b. 20% to 25%
    c. 30% to 50%
    d. 75%
    e. 80% to 90%

6. Which of the following is the first step in evaluating a child with persistent proteinuria?

    a. Measuring the serum albumin concentration
    b. Obtaining a renal ultrasonographic scan
    c. Examining the urine for RBC casts
    d. Quantitating the proteinuria with a timed urine collection
    e. Measuring the serum complement level

7. Which of the following sets of values favors a diagnosis of minimal change nephrotic syndrome?

    a. Normal C3 value, proteinuria greater than 40 mg/m^2 per hour, and high serum cholesterol level
    b. Low C3 value, RBC casts on urinalysis, and elevated serum creatinine concentration
    c. Normal C3 value, hypertension, and serum albumin concentration less than 2.5 g/dl
    d. Normal C3 value, normal serum albumin concentration, and normal cholesterol level
    e. RBC casts, low C3 value, and hypertension

8. Which of the following diagnoses is most likely in a child with hypertension and a past history of urinary tract infections?

    a. Ureteropelvic junction obstruction
    b. Reflux nephropathy
    c. Wilms' tumor
    d. Renal artery stenosis
    e. Posterior urethral valves

9. Which of the following may not be associated with the diagnosis of the Fanconi's syndrome?

    a. Heavy metal exposure
    b. Ifosfamide therapy
    c. Exposure to outdated tetracycline
    d. Cyclophosphamide therapy
    e. Cystinosis

Answers

1. **c. Red blood cell (RBC) casts.** The hallmark of glomerular bleeding has been the presence of RBC casts with or without proteinuria. [p 1835]

2. **b. Greater than 10% dysmorphic RBC.** Although no rigid criteria have been established for correlating RBC dysmorphism with a specific diagnosis, it can be a reliable tool in distinguishing glomerular bleeding. One study indicated that a rate of 10% dysmorphism was diagnostic of glomerulonephritis and found a diagnostic specificity of 94% and a sensitivity of 92% in such cases. Although RBC morphology has proved to be a valuable adjunct to urine microscopy, the presence or absence of dysmorphic cells is not an absolute diagnostic finding. [p 1835]

3. **e. Hypercalciuria.** Hypercalciuria is a common condition and a frequent cause of hematuria in otherwise healthy children. Hypercalciuria is present in approximately 5% of healthy white children and is the most frequent cause of isolated hematuria in this group. Approximately 30% of children in whom hematuria is isolated (i.e., the urine is noninfected and the hematuria is nonglomerular) are found to be hypercalciuric. [p 1838]

4. **a. Poststreptococcal acute glomerulonephritis.** Hematuria with symptoms and signs of acute glomerulonephritis including edema, hypertension, oliguria, and the presence of dysmorphic RBCs and RBC casts on urine microscopy requires an investigation to determine the cause. A positive antistreptolysin-O or streptozyme titer and a decreased serum complement C3 concentration are usually present. [p 1838]

5. **c. 30% to 50%.** A poor prognosis in patients with IgA nephropathy is indicated by the presence of renal histologic findings of glomerulosclerosis, severe mesangial proliferation, glomerular crescents, and significant interstitial fibrosis associated with renal function impairment, hypertension, male gender, older age at the time of biopsy, and proteinuria of more than 2 g/day. Progressive renal failure may be expected in 30% to 50% of patients after 10 to 20 years of follow-up. No treatment has proved to be of benefit. [p 1839]

6. **d. Quantitating the proteinuria with a timed urine collection.** Persistent proteinuria exists when at least 80% of urine specimens contain excessive amounts of protein. The first step in evaluating a child with persistent proteinuria is to quantitate the urinary protein excretion by means of a timed urine sample (12- or 24-hour collection) or with a random Upr/Ucr ratio. Urinary protein excretion of more than 4 mg/m^2 per hour is abnormal, and a level above 40 mg/m^2 per hour is in the nephrotic range. A Upr/Ucr ratio (mg/mg) in a random urine sample of above 0.18 is abnormal, and above 1.0 it is in the nephrotic range. [p 1842]

7. **a. Normal C3 value, proteinuria greater than 40 mg/m$_2$ per hour, and high serum cholesterol level.** Children with the nephrotic syndrome present with edema or with proteinuria (40 mg/m^2 per hour) discovered during a routine office visit. Children with minimal change nephrotic syndrome almost always have a normal C3 value. A renal biopsy is necessary in children with the nephrotic syndrome who are younger than 1 year or older than 10 years of age, children with a low C3 level or a positive antinuclear antibody test, and those in whom the disease has a major "nephritic" component. [p 1842]

8. **b. Reflux nephropathy.** Proteinuria in the presence of a history of a past urinary tract infection or unexplained febrile illness treated with antibiotics should alert the physician to the fact that reflux nephropathy may exist. These children are usually hypertensive. [p 1843]

9. **d. Cyclophosphamide therapy.** In the past, the most common cause of Fanconi's syndrome in children was infantile nephropathic cystinosis. Acquired forms of Fanconi's syndrome may occur after exposure to heavy metals (lead, cadmium, mercury), antibiotics (gentamicin, outdated tetracycline, cephalosporin), or ifosfamide, and during the final stages of the nephrotic syndrome secondary to focal segmental glomerulosclerosis. [p 1844]

Chapter 54
Urinary Tract Infections in Children

Linda M. Dairiki Shortliffe

Questions

1. Boys have more urinary tract infections (UTIs) than girls:
   a. during the first year of life.
   b. when they become sexually active.
   c. during elementary school years.
   d. if they are uncircumcised toddlers.
   e. at puberty.

2. The best urinary indicators of infection on urinalysis are positive findings for which of the following?

   a. Pyuria, leukocyte esterase, and catalase
   b. Nitrite and microscopic red blood cell and white blood cell casts
   c. Glitter cells in spun urine
   d. Microscopic bacteria, leukocyte esterase, and nitrite
   e. Gram stain and nitrite

3. Bacteria that are more likely to infect the kidney do which of the following?

a. Show growth in mannose
b. Produce hemolysis
c. Contain P fimbriae
d. Show KOH staining
e. Produce urease

4. Which of the following is a source of bacterial persistence?

   a. Sexual activity
   b. The prepuce
   c. A struvite calculus
   d. Fecal colonization
   e. An increased postvoid residual

5. Cystitis can be differentiated from pyelonephritis by which sign or technique?

   a. Fever
   b. Presence of interleukin 6
   c. Flank pain
   d. The Fairley washout method
   e. Homans's sign

6. What is a typical radiologic finding of pyelonephritis?

   a. A hot spot on a technetium 99m dimercaptosuccinic acid (DMSA) nuclear renogram
   b. A focal renal wedge lesion on an intravenous pyelogram
   c. Parenchymal hyperechogenicity on a renal ultrasonogram
   d. Ureteral dilatation
   e. Renal pelvic debris levels

7. What causes renal scarring in association with pyelonephritis?

   a. A "water hammer" effect of vesicoureteral reflux on the kidney
   b. Intrarenal reflux with pyelotubular backflow
   c. Bacteriuria and vesicoureteral reflux
   d. Compound calyces
   e. Elevated bladder pressure

8. In children, the likelihood of renal scarring correlates:

   a. directly with the number of occurrences of UTI.
   b. with the severity of fever.
   c. directly with intrapelvic pressure.
   d. with renal dysplasia.
   e. with the duration of vesicoureteral reflux.

9. Which of the following is true when nocturnal enuresis accompanies recurrent UTIs in children?

   a. Treatment of nocturnal enuresis is associated with decreased numbers of UTIs.
   b. These are independent findings.
   c. Vesicoureteral reflux may be involved.
   d. Both findings are likely to resolve spontaneously by puberty.
   e. Dysfunctional voiding is likely.

10. Increased periurethral bacterial colonization is present:

    a. in children who get recurrent UTIs.
    b. on the foreskin of boys 5 years of age and older.
    c. when children are constipated.
    d. during antimicrobial therapy.
    e. in children with vesicoureteral reflux.

11. Compared with nonpregnant women, during pregnancy:

    a. women have a higher likelihood of getting a UTI.
    b. women are more likely to get renal scarring.
    c. the likelihood of bacteriuria progressing to pyelonephritis is increased.
    d. the likelihood of vesicoureteral reflux occurring is increased.
    e. asymptomatic bacteriuria is common.

12. During pregnancy, young female patients who have had surgically corrected vesicoureteral reflux for breakthrough UTIs:

    a. will be protected from UTI.
    b. do not need urinary tract antimicrobial prophylaxis.
    c. will not have accelerated renal insufficiency.
    d. should have their urine screened for bacteriuria.
    e. risk increased fetal complications.

13. Evaluation and management of the first UTI in a 2-year-old child should include:

    a. a DMSA scan.
    b. parenteral antimicrobial agents.
    c. a white blood cell count and nitrite test.
    d. erythrocyte sedimentation rate and creatinine assays.
    e. prophylactic antimicrobial agents until imaging.

14. When a child does not appear to improve after 2 to 4 days of appropriate antimicrobial therapy for the first UTI, what should the next step be?

    a. Perform a DMSA scan
    b. Obtain a complete blood count and blood cultures
    c. Perform renal and bladder ultrasonography
    d. Perform voiding cystourethrography
    e. Change antimicrobial therapy

15. What is a characteristic sign of mature renal scarring on a DMSA renogram?

    a. A focal circular area of diminished uptake
    b. Diffuse renal enlargement
    c. Wedge-shaped areas of increased uptake
    d. Polar areas of diminished uptake
    e. Areas of increased focal cortical activity

16. Which of the following is true when an asymptomatic UTI is diagnosed?

    a. It should be treated to prevent recurrence.
    b. In about one third of cases, the infection will clear spontaneously.
    c. The infecting bacterial species is commonly P piliated.
    d. The child does not need imaging evaluation unless it is the second UTI.
    e. The child should have monthly assays of urinary specimens to check for UTI.

17. In a 6-year-old girl with recurrent UTIs, slight diurnal incontinence, and normal genitourinary tract (by renal and bladder ultrasonography, and voiding cystourethrogram):

    a. monthly screening cultures should be performed.
    b. annual renal and bladder ultrasonography is warranted.
    c. urodynamics should be performed.
    d. constipation should be suspected.
    e. daily perineal hygiene should be initiated.

18. An 8-year-old boy recovering from a bone marrow transplantation has frequency, urgency, and dysuria with hematuria and is treated for a UTI. The cultures return in 48 hours showing no growth, so the antimicrobial treatment is stopped, but his symptoms continue. What should the next step be?

    a. Renal arteriography
    b. Cystoscopy
    c. Interferon and acyclovir
    d. Reculture urine
    e. Renal and bladder ultrasonography and voiding cystourethrography

19. A 12-year-old boy undergoes exploration for possible testicular torsion, but epididymitis is found. What should the next step be?

a. Antimicrobial treatment, renal and bladder ultrasonography, and voiding cystourethrogram
b. Antimicrobial treatment and testicular color flow Doppler ultrasonography in 3 months
c. No further treatment
d. Intravenous pyelogram
e. Testicular biopsy, special cultures, and testes ultrasonography

20. After 10 days of urethral catheter drainage, the urine from a 5-year-old child with multiple traumatic injuries grows 20,000 CFU/ml of *Candida glabrata* on several cultures. What is the next step?

a. Administer parenteral amphotericin before catheter removal
b. Change the catheter
c. Give intravesical amphotericin irrigation before catheter removal
d. Change the indwelling catheter and alkalinize the urine
e. Perform renal and bladder ultrasonography

21. After an acute UTI, when a drug is selected for low-dose urinary tract antimicrobial prophylaxis:

a. the same drug that was used for treatment is optimal.
b. serum concentrations of drug should be high.
c. urinary excretion should be rapid.
d. there should be minimal effect on the fecal flora.
e. the drug dosage should be higher for the first few weeks.

22. Nitrofurantoin is effective in treating recurrent bacteriuria for what reason?

a. It has high serum and tissue concentrating levels.
b. It has a hemolytic effect.
c. It affects the bacterial biofilm.
d. It diffuses into the vagina and decreases bacterial colonization.
e. It has low systemic absorption with high urinary drug concentrations, so it may generate less microbial resistance.

Answers

1. **a. During the first year of life.** More boys than girls get UTIs during the first year of life. [p 1847]

2. **d. Microscopic bacteria, leukocyte esterase, and nitrite.** The combination of positive leukocyte esterase and nitrite testing and microscopic confirmation of bacteria has almost 100% sensitivity for detection of UTIs, and when all three (or leukocyte esterase and nitrite tests) are negative, the negative predictive value approaches 100%. [p 1848]

3. **c. Contain P fimbriae.** A bacterial trait that may increase virulence for the urinary tract is a surface structure called pilus or fimbria (plural, pili or fimbriae). Two important markers for *Escherichia coli* virulence are mannose-resistant hemagglutination characteristics and the P blood group-specific adhesins. [p 1850]

4. **c. A struvite calculus.** Surgically correctable causes of bacterial persistence include infected stones, infected nonfunctioning or poorly functioning kidneys or renal segments, infected ureteral stumps after nephrectomy, vesicointestinal or urethrorectal fistula, vesicovaginal fistula, infected necrotic papillae in papillary necrosis, unilateral medullary sponge kidney, infected urachal cyst, and infected urethral diverticulum or periurethral gland. [p 1850]

5. **d. The Fairley washout method.** Although ureteral catheterization has been the gold standard for localizing upper and lower tract bacteriuria, this requires invasive cystoscopy and is an impractical way of following the course of infection. It cannot, moreover, reveal the extent of renal inflammation. The Fairley bladder washout localization technique requires urethral catheterization during acute infection and washing the bladder with sterile water to determine whether the source of bacteria is the bladder or is supravesical. [p 1851]

6. **d. Ureteral dilatation.** Other radiologic findings are thickening of the renal pelvis, hypoechogenicity and focal or diffuse hyperechogenicity, ureteral dilatation, DMSA cold spots, and renal swelling or nonexcretion of IVP. [p 1852]

7. **c. Bacteriuria and vesicoureteral reflux.** Renal scarring occurs only when both vesicoureteral reflux and bacteriuria are present. [p 1853]

8. **a. Directly with the number of occurrences of UTI.** The likelihood of renal scarring correlates directly with the number of occurrences of UTI. [p 1854]

9. **b. These are independent findings.** Epidemiologic studies have shown that nocturnal enuresis alone is unassociated with UTIs, but diurnal enuresis or a combination of diurnal and nocturnal enuresis is associated with pediatric UTIs, even when the enuretic episodes are as infrequent as once a week. [p 1858]

10. **a. In children who get recurrent UTIs.** The periurethral area of healthy girls and boys is massively colonized with aerobic bacteria during the first few weeks to months of life. After 5 years of age, only those women and children who suffer repeated UTIs remain more colonized by periurethral gram-negative bacteria than those who do not get infections. Times and conditions of increased periurethral colonization are, therefore, associated with increased risk of UTI. [p 1860]

11. **c. The likelihood of bacteriuria progressing to pyelonephritis is increased.** During pregnancy, 13.5% to 65% of women who are bacteriuric on a screening urinary culture will develop pyelonephritis if left untreated, whereas uncomplicated cystitis in a nonpregnant woman rarely progresses to pyelonephritis. The reason for this increased risk of pyelonephritis may be related to the hydronephrosis of pregnancy that occurs from hormonal and mechanical changes. [p 1862]

12. **d. Should have their urine screened for bacteriuria.** Postpubertal female patients who have vesicoureteral reflux and a predisposition for frequent UTIs will continue to have this predisposition for infections into adulthood and pregnancy. Moreover, those women who were prone to UTIs before pregnancy will continue to be more likely to develop UTI during and after pregnancy, whether or not they have vesicoureteral reflux. If vesicoureteral reflux is surgically corrected, these girls should not be assured that pyelonephritis during pregnancy is impossible or even unlikely, because most episodes of pyelonephritis occurring during pregnancy are seen in patients with nonrefluxing kidneys. The urine of these women should be screened routinely for bacteriuria during pregnancy. [pp 1862–1863]

13. **e. Prophylactic antimicrobial agents until imaging.** Nitro-

furantoin attains high urinary concentrations and low serum concentrations and as such may be a poor choice to treat any severe systemic and renal infection, but it is ideal for treating a bladder UTI when there is a normal urinary tract. Resistance rates to nitrofurantoin have changed little in the past decade. After the therapeutic regimen for acute UTI, the child should be started on a daily prophylactic antimicrobial agent until full radiologic evaluation of the urinary tract may be conveniently performed in the next days to weeks. [p 1865]

14. **c. Perform renal and bladder ultrasonography.** Circumstances such as newly diagnosed azotemia, a poor response to appropriate antimicrobial drugs after 3 to 4 days, an unusual infecting organism (tuberculosis or urea-splitting organisms such as *Proteus*), known partial obstruction such as a ureterocele, ureteropelvic junction obstruction, megaureters, nonfunctioning or poorly functioning renal units, or history of diabetes, papillary necrosis, or a neuropathic bladder may warrant acute or early upper and lower urinary tract imaging. [p 1868]

15. **d. Polar areas of diminished uptake.** Later, after the acute episode is healed, the scans will show (1) a normal pattern; (2) a generally diminished uptake and small kidney volume; (3) diminished uptake in the medial kidney; or (4) polar defects with diminished uptake in the renal poles. [p 1870]

16. **b. In about one third of cases, the infection will clear spontaneously.** Some investigators have found that in only about 30% of school-aged girls will infections clear spontaneously without treatment. Whether treated when diagnosed or not, the majority of these girls have or will get persistent infections or reinfections. [p 1870]

17. **d. Constipation should be suspected.** If constipation is found or even suspected, there may be an improvement in voiding and reduction in UTIs when it is treated. [p 1872]

18. **e. Renal and bladder ultrasonography and voiding cystourethrography.** BK, a DNA virus of the polyomavirus genus, has been found in the urine of patients who had bone marrow transplantation and other immunosuppressed patients with hemorrhagic cystitis. Although no antimicrobial treatment is indicated in healthy individuals with viral cystitis, radiologic evaluation should still be performed to eliminate other causes for hematuria as well. [p 1872]

19. **a. Antimicrobial treatment, renal and bladder ultrasonography, and voiding cystourethrogram.** Once the culture results and antimicrobial sensitivities are available, the most specific, most cost-effective agent with fewest side effects that achieves good tissue and urinary levels should be selected. During or after treatment of the acute urinary and epididymal infections, radiologic evaluation of the urinary tract should be performed as with any UTI. [p 1873]

20. **c. Give intravesical amphotericin irrigation before catheter removal.** Recent prospective studies with intravesical amphotericin B bladder irrigation and oral fluconazole appear to show that both may clear funguria, although fungal recurrences are common. Optimal dosages, length of treatment, and, for amphotericin, delivery (intermittent versus continuous) are indeterminate and controversial, but amphotericin B (50 mg/L) infused continuously at 42 ml/hour for 72 hours is effective. [p 1874]

21. **d. There should be minimal effect on the fecal flora.** The ideal prophylactic agent should have low serum levels, high urinary levels, and minimal effects on the normal fecal flora; should be well tolerated; and should be cheap. [p 1866]

22. **e. It has low systemic absorption with high urinary drug concentrations, so it may generate less microbial resistance.** Nitrofurantoin is an effective urinary prophylactic agent because its serum levels are low, its urinary levels are high, and it produces a minimal effect on the fecal flora. Although there is some evidence that agents that lack systemic absorption may result in less overall bacterial resistance and change to human microbial ecology than systemic agents, long-term studies are lacking. [p 1866]

Chapter 55

Anomalies of the Upper Urinary Tract

Stuart B. Bauer

Questions

1. Potter facies is a typical appearance for which of the following kidney abnormalities?
   a. Bilateral renal agenesis
   b. Unilateral renal agenesis
   c. Bilateral renal ectopia
   d. Horseshoe kidney
   e. Megacalycosis

2. Pulmonary development during gestation requires which of the following factors for maturation of the lungs?
   a. Surfactant
   b. Amniotic fluid
   c. Proline
   d. Acetylcholine
   e. Epinephrine

3. The absence of a kidney probably occurred during which week of development?
   a. Third week
   b. Fourth week
   c. Fifth week
   d. Seventh week
   e. Eighth week

4. In girls with unilateral renal agenesis, which of the follow-

ing conditions is likely to be seen after the onset of puberty?

   a. Hydrocolpos
   b. Gartner's duct cyst
   c. Contralateral reflux
   d. Cystocele
   e. Ectopic pregnancy

5. Which of the following findings on a physical examination suggests unilateral renal agenesis?

   a. Absent testis
   b. Communicating hydrocele
   c. Undescended testis
   d. Absent vas
   e. Hypospadias

6. Renal ectopia is the result of abnormal migration of the metanephric tissue during which week of gestation?

   a. Fourth week
   b. Sixth week
   c. Eighth week
   d. 10th week
   e. 12th week

7. Which of the following statements is true regarding renal ectopia?

   a. Boys are more likely than girls to have an associated genital abnormality.
   b. The arterial tree to the ectopic kidney derives from its normal location.
   c. The ectopic kidney is more prone to disease than is the normally positioned organ.
   d. Despite the ectopic kidney, the adrenal gland is usually in the normal location.
   e. The left colonic flexure does not reside in the renal fossa with a left ectopic kidney.

8. Which of the following statements is true about a horseshoe kidney?

   a. The two kidneys usually join at their superior poles.
   b. The isthmus functions almost as well as the remainder of the kidneys.
   c. The horseshoe kidneys are usually in their normal location.
   d. The majority of patients with Turner's syndrome have a horseshoe kidney.
   e. Patients with horseshoe kidneys rarely have other anomalies.

9. What is the most common tumor associated with a horseshoe kidney?

   a. Renal pelvic tumor
   b. Wilms' tumor
   c. Renal cell carcinoma
   d. Neuroblastoma
   e. Transitional cell carcinoma of the bladder

10. The posterior branch of the main renal artery supplies which of the following segments of the kidney?

    a. Upper
    b. Middle
    c. Anterior
    d. Posterior
    e. Renal pelvis

11. A renal artery aneurysm should be excised if it exhibits each of the following characteristics except which one?

    a. It has an incomplete ring-like calcification.
    b. The aneurysm is larger than 2.5 cm.
    c. The aneurysm increases in size with time.
    d. The patient is postmenopausal.
    e. The patient is hypertensive.

12. Which of the following statements is true with regard to calyceal diverticula?

    a. The diagnosis is best made by renal ultrasonography.
    b. Diverticula tend to collect milk-of-calcium stones.
    c. The diverticula communicate with the renal pelvis.
    d. Reflux is rarely associated with these diverticula.
    e. Calyceal diverticula begin as cysts and then rupture into the collecting system.

13. Megacalycosis has which of the following characteristics?

    a. It is more likely to occur in female patients.
    b. It is associated with an increased number of calyces that are dilated.
    c. The ureter is usually dilated as well.
    d. It has an autosomal recessive pattern of inheritance.
    e. The renal scan reveals an obstructive pattern.

Answers

1. **a. Bilateral renal agenesis.** Infants with bilateral renal agenesis generally look prematurely senile and have "a prominent fold of skin that begins over each eye, swings down in a semi-circle over the inner canthus and extends onto the cheek." [p 1887]

2. **c. Proline.** Hislop and colleagues in 1979 suggested that the anephric fetus fails to produce proline, which is needed for collagen formation in the bronchiolar tree. The kidney is the primary source of proline. Thus, pulmonary hypoplasia may result from absence of renal parenchyma and not from diminished amniotic fluid. [p 1888]

3. **b. Fourth week.** The abnormality most likely occurs no later than the fourth or fifth week of gestation. [p 1889]

4. **a. Hydrocolpos.** Obstruction of one side of a duplicated system is not uncommon, and unilateral hematocolpos or hydrocolpos has been described. [p 1890]

5. **d. Absent vas.** The diagnosis should be suspected during a physical examination when the vas deferens or body and tail of the epididymis are missing, or when an absent, septate, or hypoplastic vagina is associated with a unicornuate or bicornuate uterus. [p 1892]

6. **c. Eighth week.** This process of migration and rotation is completed by the end of the eighth week of gestation. [p 1895]

7. **d. Despite the ectopic kidney, the adrenal gland is usually in the normal location.** Rarely, the adrenal gland is absent or is abnormally positioned. [p 1896]

8. **d. The majority of patients with Turner's syndrome have a horseshoe kidney.** Horseshoe kidney may also be seen in as many as 60% of female patients with Turner's syndrome. [p 1905]

9. **c. Renal cell carcinoma.** One hundred fourteen cases of re-

nal carcinoma within a horseshoe kidney have been reported; more than half of these cancers were hypernephromas. [p 1906]

10. **d. Posterior.** The main renal artery divides initially into an anterior and a posterior branch. The anterior branch almost always supplies the upper, middle, and lower segments of the kidney. The posterior branch invariably nourishes the posterior and lower segments. [p 1909]

11. **d. The patient is postmenopausal.** Excision is recommended if (1) the hypertension cannot be easily controlled; (2) an incomplete ring-like calcification is present; (3) the aneurysm is larger than 2.5 cm; (4) the patient is female and likely to become pregnant because rupture during pregnancy is a likely possibility; (5) the aneurysm increases in size on serial angiograms; or (6) an arteriovenous fistula is present. [p 1912]

12. **b. Diverticula tend to collect milk-of-calcium stones.** Over time, these diverticula tend to progressively distend with trapped urine. Infection, milk-of-calcium stones, and true stone formation are complications of stasis or obstruction that can produce symptoms. [p 1913]

13. **b. It is associated with an increased number of calyces that are dilated.** Megacalycosis is best defined as nonobstructive enlargement of calyces because of malformation of the renal papillae. The calyces that are generally dilated may be increased in number. The ureteropelvic junction is normally funneled, without evidence of obstruction. [p 1914]

Chapter 56

Renal Dysgenesis and Cystic Disease of the Kidney

Kenneth I. Glassberg

Questions

1. Which of the following is a correct match?
   a. Von Hippel-Lindau disease—adenoma sebaceum
   b. Tuberous sclerosis—angiomyolipoma
   c. Autosomal dominant polycystic kidney disease (ADPKD)—salt-losing nephropathy
   d. Congenital nephrosis (Finnish type)—medullary cysts
   e. Autosomal recessive polycystic kidney disease—colonic diverticulosis

2. What is the most likely event to precede the development of renal cell carcinoma in von Hippel–Lindau disease?
   a. Hypertension of the *VHL* gene
   b. Development of chronic renal failure
   c. Development of angiomyolipoma
   d. Loss of *VHL* gene heterozygosity
   e. Development of adenoma sebaceum

3. The development of acquired renal cystic disease (ARCD) is most related to which factor?
   a. Age of the patient
   b. Duration of renal failure
   c. Recent initiation of hemodialysis
   d. *Escherichia coli* infection
   e. A genetic defect on chromosome 16

4. Which of the following statements regarding ADPKD is most correct?
   a. ADPKD will manifest with clinical symptoms in almost all patients possessing the genetic defect by age 40 years.
   b. Approximately 50% of patients with ADPKD will have cysts by 30 years of age.
   c. Approximately 25% of offspring of a patient with ADPKD will have the disease.
   d. ADPKD is associated with a high incidence of diverticulosis and mitral valve prolapse.
   e. ADPKD is associated with a high incidence of portal hypertension.

5. What is the characteristic ultrasonographic appearance of the kidneys in a newborn with autosomal recessive polycystic kidney disease?
   a. Bilateral large kidneys with large cysts
   b. Bilateral large, homogeneous, hyperechogenic kidneys
   c. Bilateral large, homogeneous, hypoechoic kidneys
   d. Bilateral small kidneys with large cysts
   e. Bilateral small kidneys with absent pyramids

6. Which of the following statements is most correct about ADPKD?
   a. The genetic defect is located on chromosome 6.
   b. Most affected infants have congenital hepatic fibrosis.
   c. Renal cysts will be present on ultrasonographic scans in almost 100% of affected patients by 15 years of age.
   d. Glomerular cysts are sometimes found in the kidneys of newborns diagnosed with ADPKD.
   e. The incidence of renal cell carcinoma in ADPKD is twice that in the normal population.

7. All of the following conditions frequently have cysts with epithelial hyperplasia except which one?
   a. Tuberous sclerosis
   b. Acquired renal cystic disease
   c. Simple cysts
   d. von Hippel–Lindau disease
   e. ADPKD

8. Which of the following statements is NOT true regarding unilateral multicystic dysplastic kidneys?

a. The majority of multicystic dysplastic kidneys get smaller or become sonographically undetectable with time.
b. There is an absence of communications between cysts on ultrasonographic scans.
c. Cysts are usually found to communicate with each other when injected intracystically with contrast material.
d. The sine qua non for diagnosis of a multicystic dysplastic kidney is the presence of primitive ducts.
e. Multicystic dysplastic kidneys appear more often in females and more often on the right side.

9. Which signaling molecule is most likely responsible for inducing renal epithelial cells to align into simple tubules?

    a. p Wnt-11
    b. p Wnt-4
    c. p VHL
    d. GDNF (glial cell line-derived neurotrophic factor)
    e. PAX-2

10. Which gene is associated with a multiple malformation syndrome and clear cell renal cell carcinoma?

    a. *PDK1*
    b. *PDK2*
    c. *TG737*
    d. *Wnt-2*
    e. *VHL*

11. A benign multilocular cyst is seen most often:

    a. in males younger than 4 years of age and in females older than 30 years of age.
    b. in females younger than 4 years of age and in males older than 30 years of age.
    c. in males between 4 and 30 years of age.
    d. equally in both sexes before 4 years of age and in females after 30 years of age.
    e. equally in both sexes before 4 years of age and in males after 30 years of age.

12. Which of the following pairs of genes is a possible example of those in a contiguous gene syndrome?

    a. *TSC1* and *VHL*
    b. *TSC2* and *PKD1*
    c. *PKD2* and *TSC1*
    d. *VHL* and *PKD1*
    e. *TSC2* and *PKD2*

13. Unilateral renal cystic disease is:

    a. the name given to a unilateral presentation of autosomal polycystic kidney disease.
    b. an inherited disease.
    c. a condition associated with hemodialysis.
    d. a unilateral condition in which multiple simple cysts are clustered together.
    e. most often diagnosed in children.

14. A high-density lesion is recognized with a postcontrast CT scan. No precontrast record was obtained. To help diagnose this high-density lesion as a possible neoplasm versus a benign cyst, what should first be considered?

    a. Evaluating for further enhancement on a CT image 15 to 30 minutes later
    b. Repeating the study without contrast enhancement at another visit
    c. Obtaining a renal angiogram
    d. Injecting a second bolus of contrast material
    e. Looking for de-enhancement on a CT image approximately 15 to 30 minutes later

15. What does GDNF most likely play a significant role in?

    a. Mesenchymal cell conversion to epithelial cell
    b. Epithelial cell alignment
    c. Ureteric branching
    d. Kidney migration
    e. Cyst formation

16. What does PAX-2 most likely play a significant role in?

    a. Ureteric budding
    b. Tubule formation
    c. Cyst formation
    d. Development of renal cell carcinoma
    e. Conversion of mesenchymal cells to epithelial cells

17. Which of the following entities has the highest likelihood of having a renal cell carcinoma develop?

    a. ADPKD
    b. Tuberous sclerosis
    c. von Hippel–Lindau disease
    d. Acquired renal cystic disease
    e. Medullary sponge kidney

18. What is the best study to help determine renal function when trying to differentiate severe hydronephrosis from a multicystic renal dysplastic kidney?

    a. Dimercaptosuccinic acid (DMSA) renal scan
    b. Intravenous urogram
    c. Mercaptoacetyltriglycine (MAG3) renal scan
    d. Diethylenetriaminepentaacetic acid (DTPA) renal scan
    e. Furosemide (Lasix) washout renal scan

19. Which one of the following criteria helps confirm the diagnosis of unilateral renal cystic disease?

    a. Absence of contralateral renal cysts; siblings with similar findings.
    b. Absence of cysts in the contralateral kidney; absence of cysts in family members.
    c. Absence of cysts in the contralateral kidney; diffuse, noncontiguous unilateral renal cysts.
    d. Genetic linkage studies; gross hematuria.
    e. Hypertension; absence of contralateral renal cysts.

20. Renal sinus cysts are most likely derived from:

    a. vascular elements.
    b. renal parenchyma.
    c. the renal pelvis.
    d. the lymphatic system.
    e. nephrogenic rests.

21. Most simple renal cysts identified in utero:

    a. represent the first sign of a multicystic kidney.
    b. represent the first sign of autosomal recessive polycystic kidney disease.
    c. represent the first sign of ADPKD.
    d. represent a calyceal diverticulum.
    e. resolve before birth.

22. Approximately what percentage of individuals older than 60 years will have an identifiable renal cyst by CT?

    a. 1% to 5%
    b. 10%
    c. 33%
    d. 75%
    e. 90%

23. Which term best describes an entity that presents with renal agenesis, renal dysplasia, or multicystic dysplasia and is seen in multiple family members?

    a. Oligomeganephronia
    b. Familial hypodysplasia

c. Renal aplasia
d. Familial adysplasia
e. Mayer-Rokitansky-Küster-Hauser syndrome

24. Which of the following group of antibiotics includes the best choice of antibiotics for treating an infected renal cyst in a patient with ADPKD?

    a. Trimethoprim-sulfamethoxazole, chloramphenicol, fluoroquinolones
    b. Cephalosporins, trimethoprim-sulfamethoxazole, doxycycline
    c. Gentamicin, cephalosporins, vancomycin
    d. Fluoroquinolones, metronidazole (Flagyl), vancomycin
    e. Doxycycline, amoxicillin, gentamicin

25. What is laparoscopic unrooting of renal cysts in patients with ADPKD most useful for?

    a. Managing hypertension
    b. Improving renal function
    c. Relieving pain
    d. Treating an infected cyst
    e. Diagnosis

26. In neonates with a unilateral multicystic kidney, what is the incidence of contralateral vesicoureteral reflux?

    a. 0% to 7%
    b. 18% to 43%
    c. 50% to 67%
    d. 75%
    e. 7% to 15%

27. What consequence does the identification of the defective *VHL* gene have?

    a. One only has to screen all siblings with an ophthalmologic examination.
    b. One has to obtain renal sonographic monitoring of those with a defect in both VHL genes.
    c. Follow-up of siblings has not changed.
    d. The incidence of angiomyolipoma can more readily be determined.
    e. Only those siblings identified with the gene defect require routine screening and follow-up.

28. What is the most likely cause of loin pain and hematuria in a 50-year-old patient with end-stage renal disease who has been undergoing dialysis for 5 years?

    a. Acute renal vein thrombosis
    b. Acute renal artery thrombosis
    c. Renal cell carcinoma
    d. ARCD
    e. Uric acid stones

29. What does the bud theory state?

    a. That growth receptors are located at the tips of the ureteric bud
    b. That the developing metanephric kidney induces the ureteric bud to form from the wolffian duct
    c. That a ureter that buds too early, or too late, or from the wrong site on the wolffian duct can lead to an abnormal ureteric orifice and renal dysplasia
    d. That GDNF stimulates Wnt-ll activity, which then is followed by a cascade of signaling events leading to ureteric bud formation and subsequent ureteric branching
    e. That cephalad ureteric budding leads to a lateral ureteral orifice

30. When patients with ARCD undergo renal transplantation, what happens?

    a. The cysts usually continue to grow.
    b. The cysts usually get smaller, and the risk of renal cell carcinoma dramatically falls.
    c. The cysts usually get smaller, but a significant risk for renal cell carcinoma persists.
    d. There is a significantly increased incidence of hematuria.
    e. The cysts calcify.

31. Major theories on the etiology of cyst development in ADPKD include which of the following?

    a. Calcification of tubular basement membrane
    b. Increased number of epidermal growth factor receptors at the base (i.e., nonluminal side) of renal tubular epithelial cells
    c. Increased apoptosis of renal tubular cells
    d. Apical (i.e., luminal side) location of Na^+,K^+-ATPase and epidermal growth factor receptors in renal tubular epithelial cells
    e. Fusion of podocytes

32. What is the main difference between a newborn with ADPKD with glomerular cysts and a newborn with sporadic glomerulocystic kidney disease?

    a. Absence of biliary dysgenesis in ADPKD.
    b. Retinal angiomas in sporadic glomerulocystic disease
    c. The presence of liver cysts in ADPKD
    d. More severely compromised kidneys in ADPKD
    e. Absence of affected family members in sporadic glomerulocystic disease

33. Which group of three findings best describes the typical ultrasonographic image of a multicystic dysplastic kidney?

    a. The cysts are organized around a central large cyst; there is no identifiable renal sinus; there are communications between the cysts
    b. The cysts have a haphazard distribution; there is absence of a central or medial large cyst; there are no obvious communications between the cysts.
    c. The cysts have a haphazard distribution; there is no obvious renal sinus; there is a large central cyst
    d. Connections exist between the cysts; a medial cyst is present; a renal sinus is usually present.
    e. The cysts are organized at the periphery; the largest is the central one; there is an identifiable renal sinus

34. The Mayer-Rokitansky-Küster-Hauser syndrome refers to which group of associated findings?

    a. Wilms' tumor, nephrotic syndrome, ambiguous genitalia
    b. Caudad ureteric budding, lateral orifice position, lower pole dysplasia
    c. Hypertension, vesicoureteral reflux, deep cortical depression over an area of the kidney with "thyroidization" of tubules
    d. Bilateral renal agenesis, respiratory failure, oligohydramnios
    e. Unilateral renal agenesis or renal ectopia, ipsilateral müllerian defects, vaginal agenesis

35. Which one of the following conditions is most representative of a neoplastic growth?

    a. Benign multilocular cyst
    b. Oligomeganephronia
    c. Multicystic dysplastic kidney
    d. Calyceal diverticulum
    e. Ask-Upmark kidney

36. Which of the following is the best match?

    a. Autosomal recessive polycystic kidney disease—congenital hepatic fibrosis

b. Medullary sponge kidney—predominance of glomerular cysts
   c. Juvenile nephronophthisis—cortical cysts
   d. Ask-Upmark kidney—hypotension
   e. von-Hippel–Lindau disease—adenoma sebaceum
37. Which of the following matches is correct?
   a. Autosomal recessive polycystic kidney disease—chromosome 2
   b. ADPKD—chromosomes 4, 16
   c. Tuberous sclerosis—chromosomes 9, 15
   d. von Hippel–Lindau disease—chromosome 4
   e. Juvenile nephronophthisis—chromosome 6

Answers

1. **b. Tuberous sclerosis—angiomyolipoma.** Angiomyolipomas occur in 40% to 80% of patients. [p 1956]

2. **d. Loss of *VHL* gene heterozygosity.** In kidney cells of individuals with von Hippel–Lindau disease, for example, once the wild-type allele mutates, heterozygosity is lost and there is a propensity to develop a clear cell renal cell carcinoma. [p 1927]

3. **b. Duration of renal failure.** At first, ARCD was thought to be confined to patients receiving hemodialysis. However, it shortly became apparent that the disorder is almost as common in patients receiving peritoneal dialysis and that it may develop in patients with chronic renal failure who are being managed medically without any type of dialysis. Thus, ARCD appears to be a feature of end-stage kidney disease rather than a response to dialysis. [p 1976]

4. **d. ADPKD is associated with a high incidence of diverticulosis and mitral valve prolapse.** A number of associated anomalies are common: cysts of the liver, pancreas, spleen, and lungs; aneurysms of the circle of Willis (berry aneurysms); colonic diverticula; and mitral valve prolapse. [p 1944]

5. **b. Bilateral large, homogeneous, hyperechogenic kidneys.** Sonography identifies very enlarged, homogeneously hyperechogenic kidneys, especially compared with the echogenicity of the liver. The increased echogenicity is a result of the return of sound waves from the enormous number of interfaces created by tightly compacted, dilated collecting ducts. [pp 1941–1942]

6. **d. Glomerular cysts are sometimes found in the kidneys of newborns diagnosed with ADPKD.** A variant form of ADPKD probably exists in which the renal cysts are located primarily in Bowman's space. One cytogenetic study provided evidence that such a condition is a form of ADPKD. The authors found that a fetus with cystic disease predominantly of the glomeruli had the same genetic linkages on chromosome 16 as did its ADPKD-affected mother. Another study suggested that glomerulocystic kidneys in members of families with ADPKD are variants; the glomerular cysts may be an early stage of polycystic kidney disease gene expression. [p 1947]

7. **c. Simple cysts.** That the incidence of renal cell carcinoma is not increased in ADPKD is also surprising in view of the frequent finding of epithelial hyperplasia. For example, two other conditions, tuberous sclerosis and von Hippel–Lindau disease, are associated with epithelial hyperplasia. The cyst lining is a single layer of flattened or cuboidal epithelium. The hyperplastic lining in the cyst is thought by some workers to be a precursor of renal tumors. [pp 1948, 1969, 1979]

8. **e. Multicystic dysplastic kidneys appear more often in females and more often on the right side.** At any age, the condition is more likely to be found on the left. Males are more likely to have unilateral multicystic dysplastic kidneys (2.4:1). [p 1961]

9. **b. p Wnt-4.** Wnt-4 stimulates transcription processes within epithelial cells as well as the development of cell adhesion molecules, which allow the kidney epithelial cells to adhere to one another in such a manner as to take on the shape of a tubule. [p 1927]

10. **e. *VHL*.** The gene associated with the transmission of von Hippel–Lindau disease is located on chromosome 3. In non–von Hippel–Lindau patients with sporadic clear cell renal cell carcinoma, 50% of cell lines are associated with a mutational form of the *VHL* gene. [p 1958]

11. **a. in males younger than 4 years of age and in females older than 30 years of age.** The great majority of patients present before the age of 4 years or after the age of 30 years. Five percent present between 4 and 30 years of age. The patient is twice as likely to be male if younger than 4 years and eight times as likely to be female if older than 30 years of age. [p 1966]

12. **b. *TSC2* and *PKD1*.** When severe polycystic kidneys are present in patients, particularly infants with tuberous sclerosis, they likely represent a contiguous gene syndrome, that is, defects in both *TSC2* and *PKD1*. [p 1955]

13. **d. a unilateral condition in which multiple simple cysts are clustered together.** Large renal cysts of varying size appearing side by side, often more numerous at one pole, have been referred to as unilateral renal cystic disease. Because the entity seems to represent nothing more than multiple simple cysts lying side by side within a kidney, for the present the author prefers to include it as a variation of the presentation of simple cysts. [p 1972]

14. **e. Looking for de-enhancement on a CT image approximately 15 to 30 minutes later.** Occasionally, a high-density (>30 HU), well-marginated lesion may be noticed on a postcontrast CT scan when no record of density of the previously unrecognized lesion was obtained. In such situations, one can look for "de-enhancement," a finding that occurs following the initial flow of contrast material to an organ and that offers proof of vascularity—that is, neoplasm. One study found 15 minutes to be a sufficient period of delay to detect de-enhancement. If there is still a question of de-enhancement, the patient can be taken off the table and returned 30 or more minutes later. [p 1970]

15. **c. Ureteric branching.** The presence of a signaling agent produced by the mesenchyme, GDNF, precedes the branching process. The receptor for GDNF is called tyrosine kinase c-*ret*, and it is located at the tip of the ureteric bud and later at the branching ureteric tips. In mice, either a deficiency in GDNF or an abnormality of c-*ret* can occasionally result in renal agenesis or, in some cases, severe dysgenesis. Once GDNF binds to its receptor, Wnt-11 becomes activated and its protein product induces ureteric branching. [pp 1927–1928]

16. **e. Conversion of mesenchymal cells to epithelial cells.** The tips of the branches induce the adjacent mesenchymal cells to condense around them and convert into pretubular clusters of epithelial cells. This conversion process is facilitated and modulated by PAX-2. When PAX-2 protein levels are reduced, mesenchymal cells fail to cluster and fail to change into epithelial cells. [p 1928]

17. **c. von Hippel–Lindau disease.** Tuberous sclerosis and von Hippel–Lindau disease are associated with epithelial hyperplasia (and adenomas as well) and have an increased incidence of renal cell carcinoma (tuberous sclerosis, 2%, and von Hippel–Lindau disease, 35% to 38%). [p 1948]

18. **a. Dimercaptosuccinic acid (DMSA) renal scan.** In these difficult cases, radioisotope studies may be helpful. Hydronephrotic kidneys generally show some function on a DMSA scan, whereas renal concentration is seldom seen with multicystic kidneys. [p 1962]

19. **b. Absence of cysts in the contralateral kidney; absence of cysts in family members.** Such a diagnosis requires long-term follow-up demonstrating absence of cyst development in the contralateral kidney and no family members with cystic disease. [p 1972]

20. **d. The lymphatic system.** The predominant type of renal sinus cyst appears to be one derived from the lymphatics. [p 1983]

21. **e. resolve before birth.** In 28 of 11,000 fetuses with renal cysts, 25 fetuses had the cysts resolve before birth. Of two cysts that remained postnatally, in one it was the first sign of a multicystic kidney. [p 1969]

22. **c. 33%.** In adults, the frequency of renal cyst occurrence increases with age. Using CT, one group demonstrated a 20% incidence of cysts by 40 years of age and approximately 33% incidence of cysts after 60 years of age. [p 1969]

23. **d. Familial adysplasia.** Renal agenesis, renal dysplasia, multicystic dysplasia, and renal aplasia usually appear as isolated sporadic occurrences. On rare occasions, this group of anomalies may appear in many family members, but heterogeneously. In other words, one family member may have renal agenesis whereas another has renal dysplasia and still another has a multicystic dysplastic or aplastic kidney. When all or part of this group of anomalies is seen in one family, an encompassing term for these four entities is used: familial renal adysplasia. [p 1931]

24. **a. Trimethoprim-sulfamethoxazole, chloramphenicol, fluoroquinolones.** In the experience of one group of researchers, the only dependable antibiotics were those that were lipid soluble, namely, trimethoprim-sulfamethoxazole and chloramphenicol. Chloramphenicol produced better results. The fluoroquinolones, which are also lipid soluble, are proving useful. If a patient with suspected pyelonephritis does not respond to an antibiotic and if the antibiotic used is not lipid soluble, one must consider whether the infection may be present in a noncommunicating cyst. [p 1951]

25. **c. Relieving pain.** At a mean follow-up of 2.2 years, subjective pain was reduced by 62% in 11 of 15 patients, and those who had bilateral unroofing faired better. The remaining 4 had less impressive results. Unfortunately, the effect of laparoscopic unroofing in those with hypertension was quite variable. [p 1951]

26. **b. 18% to 43%.** Contralateral vesicoureteral reflux is seen even more often than contralateral ureteropelvic junction obstruction, being identified in 18% to 43% of infants. [p 1961]

27. **e. Only those siblings identified with the gene defect require routine screening and follow-up.** Recommendations by Levine and colleagues published in 1990 for all asymptomatic relatives now applies only to those with genetic evidence of the disease. [p 1958]

28. **d. ARCD.** The most common presentation of ARCD is loin pain, hematuria, or both. Bleeding occurs in as many as 50% of patients. [p 1978]

29. **c. That a ureter that buds too early, or too late, or from the wrong site on the wolffian duct can lead to an abnormal ureteric orifice and renal dysplasia.** According to the Mackie and Stephens "bud" theory, abnormal ureteric budding can lead not only to an ectopic orifice but also to inappropriate penetration of the blastema, causing renal dysplasia. According to this theory, an ectopic orifice is a sign of abnormal ureteric budding and metanephric development (i.e., dysplasia). [p 1931]

30. **c. The cysts usually get smaller, but a significant risk for renal cell carcinoma persists.** A number of investigators have found that the cysts of ARCD regress after renal transplantation (see Fig. 56–30). One study found improvement in the number and size of cysts in 16 of 25 (64%) ARCD patients 1 year after transplantation. Therefore, it was considered that the incidence of renal cell carcinoma might fall after transplantation as well. However, another group found that although the majority of cysts either disappear or become smaller, 18% of patients develop new cysts after transplantation, and a more recent report of four cases of renal carcinoma occurring in the native kidney 3 to 8 years after transplantation suggested that the risk of carcinoma does not lessen after transplantation. In a different series of 96 transplant patients, renal cell carcinoma had developed in 6 patients and 5 of the 6 had associated ARCD. The authors suggested that the malignant potential of ARCD persists for many years after transplantation. They also found a higher incidence of renal cell carcinoma in older transplant patients and in men. We must keep in mind that although the native kidneys may become smaller after transplantation and although the cysts may disappear from view on ultrasonographic follow-up, it does not necessarily mean that the cells that previously surrounded these cysts have disappeared. [p 1982]

31. **d. Apical (i.e., luminal side) location of Na^+,K^+-ATPase and epidermal growth factor receptors in renal tubular epithelial cells.** The receptors for epidermal growth factor have been identified ectopically on the apical side of cells adjacent to the cyst fluid. Na^+,K^+-ATPase in polycystic epithelial cells was located in the apical position in cells lining the cyst rather than in the usual basolateral position. If this is the case, fluid would preferably enter the cyst lumen rather than leave it. [pp 1944–1945]

32. **e. Absence of affected family members in sporadic glomerulocystic disease.** ADPKD should not be referred to as glomerulocystic kidney disease to avoid confusing it with sporadic glomerulocystic kidney disease, a condition that seems to be histologically identical to ADPKD in infants except for the absence of affected family members. [p 1947]

33. **b. The cysts have a haphazard distribution; there is absence of a central or medial large cyst; there are no obvious communications between the cysts.** Renal masses in infants most often represent either multicystic kidney disease or hydronephrosis, and it is important to distinguish the two, especially if the surgeon wishes to remove a nonfunctioning hydronephrotic kidney or repair a ureteropelvic junction obstruction while leaving a multicystic organ in situ. In newborns, ultrasonography is generally the first study performed.

In a few cases, it is difficult to distinguish multicystic kidney disease from severe hydronephrosis. In general, however, the multicystic kidney has a haphazard distribution of cysts of various sizes without a larger central or medial cyst and without visible communications between the cysts. Frequently, very small cysts appear in between the large cysts. In comparison, in ureteropelvic junction obstruction, the cysts or calyces are organized around the periphery of the kidney, connections can usually be demonstrated between the peripheral cysts and a central or medial cyst that represents the renal pelvis, and there is absence of small cysts between the larger cysts (see Fig. 56–19). When there is an identifiable renal sinus, the diagnosis is more likely to be hydronephrosis than multicystic kidney. [p 1962]

34. **e. Unilateral renal agenesis or renal ectopia, ipsilateral müllerian defects, vaginal agenesis.** The term Mayer-Rokitansky-Küster-Hauser syndrome refers to a group of associated findings that include unilateral renal agenesis or renal ectopia, ipsilateral müllerian defects, and vaginal agenesis. Drash syndrome includes Wilms' tumor, nephrotic syndrome, and ambiguous genitalia; the findings of caudad ureteric budding, lateral orifice position, and lower pole dysplasia follow the bud theory; the grouping of hypertension, vesicoureteral reflux, and deep cortical depression over an area of the kidney with "thyroidization" of tubules defines the Ask-Upmark kidney; and the grouping of bilateral renal agenesis, respiratory failure, and oligohydramnios can lead the fetus to be born with Potter's syndrome and Potter facies. [pp 1930–1954]

35. **a. Benign multilocular cyst.** For the benign multilocular cystic lesion, certain authors prefer the term cystic nephroma because this term implies a benign but neoplastic lesion. [p 1966]

36. **a. Autosomal recessive polycystic kidney disease—congenital hepatic fibrosis.** All patients with autosomal recessive polycystic kidney disease have varying degrees of congenital hepatic fibrosis. [p 1938]

37. **b. ADPKD—chromosomes 4, 16.** For the genetic cystic disease ADPKD, the chromosomal defect is on chromosome 16 for PKD1 and 4 for PKD2; PKD3 has not been mapped. Autosomal recessive polycystic kidney disease involves chromosome 6; tuberous sclerosis involves chromosomes 9 and 16; von Hippel–Lindau disease involves chromosome 3; and juvenile nephronophthisis involves chromosome 2. [pp 1939–1940]

Chapter 57

Anomalies and Surgery of the Ureteropelvic Junction in Children

Michael C. Carr

Questions

1. Obstruction at the ureteropelvic junction can be due to all of the following except:
   a. interruption in development of circular musculature of the ureteropelvic junction.
   b. persistent fetal convolutions.
   c. Ostling's folds.
   d. upper ureteral polyps.
   e. lower pole crossing vessel.

2. Congenital malformations seen in association with ureteropelvic junction obstruction include all of the following except:
   a. contralateral ureteropelvic junction obstruction.
   b. multicystic dysplastic kidney.
   c. renal agenesis.
   d. renal dysplasia.
   e. autosomal dominant polycystic kidney disease.

3. Which radiographic modality provides the most useful information to assess whether a ureteropelvic junction obstruction exists?
   a. Renal ultrasonography
   b. Intravenous urography
   c. Mercaptoacetyltriglycine (MAG3)-furosemide (Lasix) renography
   d. Nuclear voiding cystourethrography
   e. Doppler ultrasonography

4. Which surgical repair for ureteropelvic junction obstruction would yield the greatest likelihood of success if there is a long segment of ureteral stenosis?
   a. Dismembered pyeloplasty
   b. Endopyelotomy
   c. Laparoscopic Anderson-Hynes pyeloplasty
   d. Spiral flap (Culp-DeWeerd) pyeloplasty
   e. Davis intubated ureterotomy

5. The key steps in performing a dismembered pyeloplasty include all the following except:
   a. spatulating the ureter on the lateral margin an adequate distance.
   b. excising as much redundant renal pelvis as possible.
   c. ensuring that a tension-free anastomosis exists.
   d. placing a feeding tube into the ureter during the suturing of the anastomosis.
   e. placing a Penrose drain adjacent to the repair.

6. Surgical options in the repair of a failed pyeloplasty include all the following except:
   a. endopyelotomy.
   b. ureterocalicostomy.
   c. redo pyeloplasty.
   d. transureteroureterostomy.
   e. nephrectomy.

Answers

1. **c. Ostling's folds.** Ostling's folds are now considered folds that are not obstructive and disappear with a person's linear growth. They are rarely seen in an older child or adult. [p 1997]

2. **e. autosomal dominant polycystic kidney disease.** Ureteropelvic junction obstruction is the most common anomaly encountered in the opposite kidney; it occurs in 10% to 40% of cases. Renal dysplasia and multicystic dysplastic kidney are the next most frequently observed contralateral lesions. In addition, unilateral renal agenesis has been noted in almost 5% of children. [p 1998]

3. **c. Mercaptoacetyltriglycine (MAG3)-furosemide (Lasix) renography.** Intravenous urography was previously the primary radiographic study used to define ureteropelvic junction obstruction. In most institutions, this has been supplanted with radionuclide renography, because this study can provide differential renal function and an assessment of washout from the individual kidney. [p 2001]

4. **d. Spiral flap (Culp-DeWeerd) pyeloplasty.** The Culp and DeWeerd spiral flap is created from the renal pelvis and is used to repair the defect at the ureteropelvic junction. Such a flap is able to bridge the gap between the pelvis and healthy ureter over a distance of several centimeters. [p 2002]

5. **b. excising as much redundant renal pelvis as possible.** The portion of pelvis is excised, generally a diamond-shaped segment that is present within the traction sutures that were placed in the renal pelvis. It is better to leave too much renal pelvis than too little, especially when resecting along the medial aspect of the renal pelvis. Infundibula can be encountered if one is not careful. [p 2002]

6. **d. transureteroureterostomy.** Lack of drainage for a prolonged period would necessitate further intervention, including an endopyelotomy, redo pyeloplasty, or even ureterocalicostomy. [p 2004]

Chapter 58

Ectopic Ureter, Ureterocele, and Other Anomalies of the Ureter

Richard N. Schlussel • Alan B. Retik

Questions

1. All of the following are possible drainage sites for an ectopic ureter in a female except which site?

    a. Fallopian tube
    b. Uterus
    c. Rectum
    d. Vagina

2. Inadequate interaction between the ureteral bud and metanephric blastema will most likely lead to which of the following conditions?

    a. Dysplasia
    b. Hydronephrosis
    c. Reflux
    d. Ureteral ectopia

3. How is the relationship between the upper and lower pole orifices in a complete ureteral duplication best described?

    a. The upper pole orifice is cephalad and lateral to the lower orifice.
    b. The upper pole ureter joins the lower pole ureter just before entry into the bladder.
    c. The upper pole orifice is caudal and medial to the lower pole orifice.
    d. The upper pole orifice and lower pole orifice sit transversely side by side.

4. All of the following are considered contributors to vesicoureteral reflux except:

    a. lateral ureteral insertion.
    b. lax bladder neck.
    c. poorly developed trigone.
    d. gaping ureteral orifice.

5. What is the most common site of drainage of an ectopic ureter in a male?

    a. Vas deferens
    b. Anterior urethra
    c. Seminal vesicle
    d. Posterior urethra

6. Which voiding pattern is most often seen in a girl with an ectopic ureter?

    a. Urge incontinence
    b. Stress incontinence
    c. Continuous incontinence
    d. Interrupted urinary stream

7. Which of the following findings is most likely present on an excretory urogram in a patient with an ectopic ureter in a duplicated system?

    a. Nonvisualization of the lower pole of the kidney
    b. Medially displaced lower pole of the kidney
    c. Filling defect in the bladder
    d. Tortuous lower pole ureter

8. Which of the following anatomic derangements will not be seen in a patient with single-system ectopic ureters?

a. A poorly developed bladder neck
b. Decreased bladder capacity
c. A Hutch diverticulum
d. Trigone underdevelopment

9. Ureteroceles are most often associated with all of the following except:
   a. smoking during pregnancy.
   b. white race.
   c. female gender.
   d. duplicated kidneys.

10. All of the following can be caused by a ureterocele. Which is the least likely?
    a. Bladder outlet obstruction
    b. Upper pole obstruction
    c. Ipsilateral lower pole reflux
    d. Contralateral reflux

11. Which cystographic finding is most likely seen in a child with a ureterocele?
    a. Ureterocele eversion
    b. Reflux
    c. Midline filling defect
    d. Bilateral ureteroceles

12. A child undergoes open resection of a large ectopic ureterocele. After removal of her catheter, she has high postvoid residuals demonstrated on a sonogram. Which complication is most likely responsible?
    a. Persistent reflux
    b. A residual flap of the ureterocele in the urethra
    c. Neurapraxia secondary to bladder retraction
    d. Excessive buttressing of deficient detrusor at the bladder neck

13. What is the preferred method of endoscopic treatment of a ureterocele?
    a. Resection of the roof of the ureterocele
    b. Puncture of the ureterocele's urethral extension
    c. Puncture of the roof of the ureterocele
    d. Transverse incision at the base of the ureterocele

14. An adult is evaluated as a possible kidney donor. An excretory urogram demonstrates a round contrast agent–filled area at the bladder base with a thin radiolucent rim around it. What is the other most likely finding?
    a. A single-system kidney
    b. Marked opacification delay of the kidney
    c. Extension of a ureterocele to the bladder neck and urethra
    d. Reflux

15. A white infant is found to have a smooth interlabial mass on the posterior aspect of the urethra. What would be the most appropriate initial management?
    a. Chemotherapy
    b. Puncture of the mass
    c. Topical estrogen cream
    d. Observation

16. Which of the following areas of the ureter is least prone to ureteral stenosis?
    a. Immediately proximal to the ureterovesical junction
    b. At the level of the pelvic brim
    c. The ureteropelvic junction
    d. All are equal in incidence

17. Which of the following statements is true regarding ureteral duplications?
    a. The right side predominates.
    b. The left side predominates.
    c. Unilateral duplications outnumber bilateral duplications by a 6:1 ratio.
    d. Most commonly they have associated upper pole obstruction.

18. Which of the following statements regarding duplex kidneys is true?
    a. Duplex kidneys are the same size as single-system kidneys.
    b. The upper pole moiety is the more likely of the two to have a ureteropelvic junction obstruction.
    c. The duplex kidney arises as a consequence of two separate ureteric buds.
    d. The duplex kidney arises as a consequence of two separate metanephric blastemal entities arising near the mesonephric duct.

19. Anastomosis of an upper pole and lower pole ureter should not be done at the distal segments because of concerns of:
    a. injury to the ureteral nerve supply.
    b. to-and-fro peristalsis of urine into the bifid ureters.
    c. injury to the adjacent vas deferens.
    d. the possibility of causing vesicoureteral reflux.

20. Which of the following abnormalities are associated with inverted Y ureteral duplications?
    a. Urachal abnormalities
    b. Ectopic ureters
    c. Horseshoe kidneys
    d. Posterior urethral valves

21. What is the most common form of ureteral triplication?
    a. All three ureters joining to terminate in a single bladder orifice
    b. Three ureters joining to form two ureteral orifices
    c. Three ureters draining as three separate orifices
    d. One of the three ureters terminating ectopically, the other two draining orthotopically

22. Which of the following ureters is involved in preureteral vena cava and at which level?
    a. The right ureter at level L3–L4
    b. The right ureter at level L1
    c. The left ureter at level L3–L4
    d. The left ureter at level L1

23. Failure of atrophy of which vein leads to the formation of a preureteral vena cava?
    a. Posterior cardinal vein
    b. Subcardinal vein
    c. Supracardinal vein
    d. Umbilical artery

24. Which of the following types of ureterocele is associated with the lowest incidence of secondary procedures after endoscopic treatment?
    a. Ectopic ureterocele
    b. Ureterocele in a female patient
    c. Intravesical ureterocele
    d. Ureterocele associated with a duplicated system

25. What is the most common method of presentation of a ureterocele?

a. Incontinence
b. Urinary tract infection
c. Failure to thrive
d. Stranguria

26. In what percentage of cases is reflux associated with a ureterocele?

    a. 10% to 25%.
    b. 25% to 40%.
    c. 50% to 65%.
    d. 65% to 80%.

27. A patient with a suspected ectopic ureter has a renal moiety that is difficult to visualize on an ultrasonographic study. Which of the following tests is a sensitive method of detecting this moiety?

    a. Diethylenetriaminepentaacetic acid (DTPA) renal scanning
    b. MRI of the abdomen and pelvis
    c. Nuclear voiding cystourethrography
    d. Positron emission tomography

28. Voiding cystourethrography is performed on a patient with a known ureterocele. Which of the following images will most likely fail to depict the ureterocele?

    a. Beginning of the first cycle of filling
    b. Beginning of the second cycle of filling
    c. The lateral image
    d. Bladder filled to capacity

29. Which of the following factors is most likely associated with the need for a second operative procedure in ectopic ureteroceles?

    a. Single-system ureterocele
    b. Male sex
    c. Left-sided position
    d. Preoperative high-grade reflux

30. What is the incidence of reflux into a ureterocele after its endoscopic incision?

    a. 10%
    b. 30%
    c. 65%
    d. 90%

Answers

1. **c. Rectum.** An ectopic ureter draining into any of the female structures can rupture into the adjoining fallopian tube, uterus, upper vagina, or vestibule. [p 2009]

2. **a. Dysplasia.** These clinical and experimental observations combine to support the commonly held notion that dysplasia is the product of inadequate ureteric bud-to-blastema interaction. [p 2009]

3. **c. The upper pole orifice is caudal and medial to the lower pole orifice.** The lower pole orifice is more cranial and lateral to the caudad medial upper pole orifice. [p 2010]

4. **b. lax bladder neck.** It is owing to the combined effects of the lateral ureteral orifice position, the ureter's shortened submucosal course, the poorly developed trigone, and the abnormal morphology of the ureteral orifice that primary vesicoureteral reflux develops. [p 2013]

5. **d. Posterior urethra.** In the male, the posterior urethra is the most common site of the termination of the ectopic ureter. [p 2013]

6. **c. Continuous incontinence.** Continuous incontinence in a girl with an otherwise normal voiding pattern after toilet training is the classic symptom of an ectopic ureteral orifice. [p 2014]

7. **d. Tortuous lower pole ureter.** The upper pole displaces the lower pole downward and outward, the so-called drooping lily appearance. When the upper pole does not excrete contrast material and make the duplicated system readily apparent, there are several other clues to suggest that a duplicated system is present. First, the calyces of a lower pole are fewer in number than in the normal kidney. Second, the axis of the lowest to uppermost calyx does not point toward the midline. Third, the uppermost calyx of the lower pole unit is usually farther from the upper pole border than is the lowest calyx from the corresponding lower pole limit. In addition, the lower pole pelvis and the upper portion of its ureter may be farther from the spine than on the contralateral side, and the lower pole ureter may also be scalloped and tortuous secondary to its wrapping around a markedly dilated upper pole ureter (similar to the findings of upper pole hydroureteronephrosis seen in the child with a ureterocele in Fig. 58–33). [pp 2016, 2026]

8. **c. A Hutch diverticulum.** Because there is no formation of the trigone and base plate, a very wide, poorly defined, incompetent vesical neck results. In rare instances, bilateral single ectopic ureters are associated with agenesis of the bladder and urethra. This condition is usually, but not always, incompatible with life. Commonly, the involved kidneys are dysplastic or display varying degrees of hydronephrosis (see Fig. 58–26). The ureters are usually dilated, and reflux is often present. The bladder neck is incompetent; therefore, the child dribbles continuously. Because there is poor resistance, the bladder does not have the opportunity to distend with urine and therefore has a small capacity (see Fig. 58–27). [pp 2020–2023]

9. **a. smoking during pregnancy.** They occur most frequently in females (4:1 ratio) and almost exclusively in white people. Approximately 10% are bilateral. Eighty percent of all ureteroceles arise from the upper poles of duplicated systems. [p 2023]

10. **a. Bladder outlet obstruction.** Ultrasonographic study shows a dilated ureter emanating from a hydronephrotic upper pole (see Fig. 58–29). This finding should signal the examiner to image the bladder to determine whether a ureterocele is present. If the lower pole is associated with reflux, or if the ureterocele has caused delayed emptying from the ipsilateral lower pole, this lower pole may likewise be hydronephrotic. Similarly, the ureterocele may impinge on the contralateral ureteral orifice or obstruct the bladder neck and cause hydronephrosis in the opposite kidney. The upper pole parenchyma drained by the ureterocele will exhibit varying degrees of thickness and echogenicity. Increased echogenicity correlates with dysplastic changes. The bladder frequently displays a thin-walled cyst that is the ureterocele (see Fig. 58–30). Reflux may also be seen in the contralateral system if the ureterocele is large enough to distort the trigone and

the opposite ureteral submucosal tunnel. In one series, 35 of 127 patients (28%) had reflux in the contralateral unit. [pp 2024–2026]

11. **b. Reflux.** Voiding cystourethrography can demonstrate the size and location of the ureterocele as well as the presence or absence of vesicoureteral reflux. Assessing the severity of such reflux is crucial to future management. Reflux into the ipsilateral lower pole is commonly seen. [p 2025]

12. **b. A residual flap of the ureterocele in the urethra.** The authors of one study emphasized the need for passing a large catheter antegrade through the bladder neck to ascertain that all mucosal lips that might act as obstructing valves have been removed. [p 2029]

13. **d. Transverse incision at the base of the ureterocele.** Our preferred method of incising the ureterocele is similar to the one described by Rich and colleagues in 1990, that is, a transverse incision through the full thickness of the ureterocele wall using the cutting current. Making the incision as distally on the ureterocele and as close to the bladder floor as possible lessens the chance of postoperative reflux into the ureterocele. [p 2033]

14. **a. A single-system kidney.** Excretory urography often demonstrates the characteristic cobra-head (or spring-onion) deformity: an area of increased density similar to the head of a cobra with a halo or less dense shadow around it (see Fig. 58–42). The halo represents a filling defect, which is the ureterocele wall, and the oval density is contrast material excreted into the ureterocele from the functioning kidney. [p 2034]

15. **b. Puncture of the mass.** A ureterocele that extends through the bladder neck and the urethra and presents as a vaginal mass in girls is termed a prolapsing ureterocele. This mass can be distinguished from other interlabial masses (such as rhabdomyosarcoma, urethral prolapse, hydrometrocolpos, and periurethral cysts) by virtue of its appearance and location. The prolapsed ureterocele has a smooth round wall, as compared with the grapelike cluster that typifies rhabdomyosarcoma (see Fig. 58–28). The color may vary from pink to bright red to the necrotic shades of blue, purple, or brown. The ureterocele usually slides down the posterior wall of the urethra, and hence, the urethra can be demonstrated anterior to the mass and can be catheterized. The short-term goal is to decompress the ureterocele. The prolapsing ureterocele may be manually reduced back into the bladder; however, even if this is successful, the prolapse is likely to recur. Upper pole nephrectomy (as previously described) combined with aspiration of the ureterocele from above is usually effective in achieving decompression. [pp 2024, 2034]

16. **b. At the level of the pelvic brim.** Three areas of the ureter are particularly liable to ureteral stenosis. They are, in order of decreasing frequency, the distal ureter just above the extravesical junction, the ureteropelvic junction, and rarely, the midureter at the pelvic brim. [p 2035]

17. **c. Unilateral duplications outnumber bilateral duplications by a 6:1 ratio.** Unilateral duplication occurs about six times more often than bilateral duplication, with the right and left sides being involved about equally. [p 2040]

18. **c. The duplex kidney arises as a consequence of two separate ureteric buds.** If two separate ureteric buds originate from the mesonephric duct, two complete and separate interactions will develop between the ureter and the metanephric blastema. The result is two separate renal units and collecting systems, ureters, and ureteral orifices. [p 2041]

19. **b. to-and-fro peristalsis of urine into the bifid ureters.** Bifid ureter is often clinically unimportant, but stasis and pyelonephritis do occur. When the Y junction is extravesical, free to-and-fro peristalsis of urine from one collecting system to the other may appear, with preferential retrograde waves passing into slightly dilated limbs instead of down the common stem. [p 2042]

20. **b. Ectopic ureters.** One of the distal ureteral limbs not uncommonly ends in an ectopic ureter or ureterocele. [p 2043]

21. **a. All three ureters joining to terminate in a single bladder orifice.** In the classification used by most investigators, there are four varieties of triplicate ureter. In one variety, all three ureters unite and drain through a single orifice. This appears to be the most common form encountered. [p 2043]

22. **a. The right ureter at level L3–L4.** This disorder involves the right ureter, which typically deviates medially behind (dorsal to) the inferior vena cava, winding about and crossing in front of it from a medial to a lateral direction, to resume a normal course distally, to the bladder. Excretory urography often fails to visualize the portion of the ureter beyond the J hook (i.e., extending behind the vena cava), but retrograde ureteropyelography demonstrates an S curve to the point of obstruction (see Fig. 58–53), with the retrocaval segment lying at the level of L3 or L4. [pp 2044–2045]

23. **b. Subcardinal vein.** If the subcardinal vein in the lumbar portion fails to atrophy and becomes the primary right-sided vein, the ureter is trapped dorsal to it. [p 2045]

24. **c. Intravesical ureterocele.** One study concluded that intravesical ureteroceles fared better than ectopic ureteroceles with regard to decompression (93% versus 75%), preservation of upper pole function (96% versus 47%), newly created reflux (18% versus 47%), and need for secondary procedures (7% versus 50%). [p 2031]

25. **b. Urinary tract infection.** Many ureteroceles are still diagnosed clinically. The most common presentation is that of an infant who has a urinary tract infection or urosepsis. [p 2023]

26. **c. 50% to 65%.** In various series, the incidences of reflux reported were 49%, 59%, 67%, 54%, and 65%. [p 2025]

27. **b. MRI of the abdomen and pelvis.** Occasionally, the renal parenchyma is difficult to locate and may be identified only by alternative imaging studies. In such cases in which an ectopic ureter is strongly suspected because of incontinence yet no definite evidence of the upper pole renal segment is found, CT or MRI has demonstrated the small, poorly functioning upper pole segment (see Fig. 58–21). [pp 2017–2018]

28. **d. Bladder filled to capacity.** Images should be obtained from early in the filling phase because some ureteroceles may efface later in filling and may not be seen. [p 2026]

29. **d. Preoperative high-grade reflux.** One study noted that infants who will likely need a secondary procedure include those with high-grade reflux or a prolapsed ureterocele. Another study found that the reoperation rate varied on the basis of the degree of preoperative reflux. If there was no reflux, only 20% required reoperation. If there was low-grade reflux versus high-grade reflux, 30% versus 53% required reoperation, respectively. [p 2029]

30. **b. 30%.** In one study, incision of the ectopic ureterocele appeared to be mostly successful with regard to decompression, but it did not achieve the goal of correcting preexisting reflux and resulted in a significant incidence of reflux into the ureterocele itself (30%). [p 2032]

Chapter 59

Vesicoureteral Reflux and Megaureter

Anthony Atala • Michael A. Keating

Questions

1. The incidence of reflux is best estimated at more than:

    a. 0.1%.
    b. 1%.
    c. 3%.
    d. 5%.
    e. 10%.

2. Which of the following statements regarding reflux is NOT true?

    a. Antenatally detected reflux is associated with a male preponderance.
    b. Antenatally detected reflux is usually low grade in boys when compared with that in girls.
    c. Antenatally detected reflux is usually bilateral in boys when compared with that in girls.
    d. When reflux is detected antenatally, renal impairment is frequently present at birth and is likely due to congenital dysplasia.
    e. The vast majority of reflux detected later in life occurs in females.

3. When the natural history of reflux is considered in relation to race, which of the following statements is true?

    a. White girls are 10 times more likely to have reflux than their black American counterparts when evaluated for asymptomatic bacteriuria; however, once reflux is discovered, its grade and chance of spontaneous resolution are similar for both races.
    b. White girls are 10 times less likely to have reflux than their black American counterparts when evaluated for asymptomatic bacteriuria; however, once reflux is discovered, its grade and chance of spontaneous resolution are similar for both races.
    c. White girls are 10 times more likely to have reflux than their black American counterparts when evaluated for asymptomatic bacteriuria; however, once reflux is discovered, the chance of spontaneous resolution is greater for black girls.
    d. White girls are 10 times less likely to have reflux than their black American counterparts when evaluated for asymptomatic bacteriuria; however, once reflux is discovered, the chance of spontaneous resolution is greater for black girls.
    e. The incidence and grades of reflux are similar for both white and black American girls.

4. Primary reflux is a congenital anomaly of the ureterovesical junction with which of the following characteristics?

    a. A deficiency of the longitudinal muscle of the extravesical ureter results in an inadequate valvular mechanism.
    b. A deficiency of the longitudinal muscle of the intravesical ureter results in an inadequate valvular mechanism.
    c. A deficiency of the circumferential muscle of the extravesical ureter results in an inadequate valvular mechanism.
    d. A deficiency of the circumferential muscle of the intravesical ureter results in an inadequate valvular mechanism.
    e. A deficiency of the longitudinal and circumferential muscles of the intravesical ureter results in an inadequate valvular mechanism.

5. What is the ratio of tunnel length to ureteral diameter found in normal children without reflux?

    a. 5:1
    b. 4:1
    c. 3:1
    d. 2:1
    e. 1:1

6. Which of the following statements is true regarding children with non-neurogenic neurogenic bladders?

    a. Constriction of the urinary sphincter occurs during voiding in a voluntary form of detrusor-sphincter dyssynergia.
    b. Gradual bladder decompensation and myogenic failure result from incomplete emptying.
    c. Gradual bladder decompensation and myogenic failure result from increasing amounts of residual urine.
    d. All of the above.
    e. None of the above.

7. What is the most common urodynamic abnormality in patients with reflux?

    a. Uninhibited bladder contractions
    b. Hypertonic bladder
    c. Very low filling pressures
    d. All of the above
    e. None of the above

8. The complex anatomic relationships required of the ureterovesical junction may be gradually damaged by which of the following?

    a. Decreases in bladder wall compliance
    b. Detrusor decompensation
    c. Incomplete emptying
    d. All of the above
    e. None of the above

9. What does the initial management of functional causes of reflux involve?

    a. Surgical treatment
    b. Medical treatment

c. Observation only
  d. All of the above
  e. None of the above

10. Signs or symptoms of voiding dysfunction include:
   a. dribbling.
   b. urgency.
   c. incontinence.
   d. curtseying behavior in girls in an attempt to suppress bladder contractions.
   e. all of the above.

11. Treatment of bladder dysfunction and instability, regardless of its severity or cause, is directed at:
   a. dampening uninhibited bladder contractions.
   b. dilating the urethral sphincter.
   c. lowering intravesical pressures.
   d. all of the above.
   e. a and c only.

12. There is a strong association between the presence of reflux in patients with neuropathic bladders and intravesical pressures of greater than:
   a. 10 cm H_2O.
   b. 20 cm H_2O.
   c. 40 cm H_2O.
   d. 60 cm H_2O.
   e. 80 cm H_2O.

13. Bladder infections and their accompanying inflammation can also cause reflux by what mechanism?
   a. Lessening compliance
   b. Elevating intravesical pressures
   c. Distorting and weakening the ureterovesical junction
   d. All of the above
   e. None of the above

14. Which system provides the current standard for grading reflux based on the appearance of contrast in the ureter and upper collecting system during voiding cystourethrography?
   a. The Heikel and Parkkulainen system
   b. The International Classification system
   c. The Dwoskin and Perlmutter system
   d. The National Classification system
   e. The Dwoskin and Parkkulainen system

15. Which of the following statements is true regarding accurately grading reflux with coexistent ipsilateral obstruction?
   a. It is not possible.
   b. It is facilitated by obtaining a renal scan.
   c. It is facilitated by obtaining an ultrasonographic scan.
   d. It is facilitated by obtaining an excretory urogram.
   e. It is facilitated by obtaining a radionuclide cystogram.

16. Which of the following statements is true regarding the presence of fever?
   a. It may be an indicator of upper urinary tract involvement.
   b. It may not always be a reliable sign of upper urinary tract involvement.
   c. It increases the likelihood of discovering vesicoureteral reflux.
   d. All of the above.
   e. None of the above.

17. Complete evaluations that include voiding cystography and ultrasonography are required of which type of patient?
   a. Any child younger than 5 years of age with a documented urinary tract infection
   b. Febrile children with a urinary tract infection, regardless of age
   c. Any boy with a urinary tract infection unless he is sexually active or has a past urologic history
   d. All of the above
   e. None of the above

18. Which of the following statements is true regarding screening of older children who present with asymptomatic bacteriuria?
   a. They can be screened initially with ultrasonography.
   b. They can be screened initially with cystography.
   c. They can be screened initially with excretory urography.
   d. They can be screened initially with a renal scan.
   e. They do not require any screening studies.

19. Which of the following statements is true regarding cystography?
   a. Cystography performed with a Foley catheter or while the patient is under anesthesia produces static studies that inaccurately screen for reflux or sometimes exaggerate its degree because of bladder overfilling.
   b. Cystography performed in the presence of excessive hydration may mask low grades of reflux because diuresis can blunt the retrograde flow of urine.
   c. Cystograms may show reflux only during active infections when cystitis weakens the ureterovesical junction with edema or by increasing intravesical pressures.
   d. Cystograms obtained during active infections can overestimate the grade of reflux because the endotoxins produced by some gram-negative organisms can paralyze ureteral smooth muscle and exaggerate ureteral dilatation.
   e. All of the above.

20. Which of the following statements is true regarding radionuclide cystography?
   a. It provides similar anatomic detail to that obtained with fluoroscopic cystography.
   b. It is an accurate method for detecting and following reflux.
   c. It is associated with more radiation exposure than is fluoroscopic cystography.
   d. It is a less sensitive test than fluoroscopic cystography.
   e. It provides more anatomic detail than fluoroscopic cystography.

21. Which of the following statements is true regarding ultrasonography?
   a. It is the diagnostic study of choice to initially evaluate the upper urinary tracts of patients with suspected or proven vesicoureteral reflux.
   b. It can effectively rule out reflux.
   c. It should be performed every 2 to 3 years in patients with reflux who are medically managed.
   d. It is the study of choice for assessing renal function.
   e. An ultrasonogram showing intermittent dilatation of the renal pelvis or ureter confirms the presence of reflux.

22. What is the best study for the detection of pyelonephritis and cortical renal scarring?
   a. Diethylenetriaminepentaacetic acid (DTPA) renal scan
   b. Dimercaptosuccinic acid (DMSA) renal scan
   c. Mercaptoacetyltriglycine (MAG3) renal scan
   d. Pyelogram
   e. Renal ultrasonographic scan

23. Which of the following statements is true regarding urodynamic studies?
   a. They are indicated in any child suspected of having a

secondary cause for reflux (valves, neurogenic bladder, non-neurogenic neurogenic bladder, voiding dysfunction).
   b. They should be performed without the use of prophylactic antibiotics in children with secondary reflux.
   c. They help direct therapy in patients with secondary reflux.
   d. All of the above.
   e. a and c only.

24. The term *reflux nephropathy* encompasses a number of radiologic changes of the kidney associated with reflux, including which of the following?
    a. Focal thinning of renal parenchyma overlying a clubbed, distorted calyx.
    b. Generalized calyceal dilatation with parenchymal atrophy.
    c. Impaired renal growth, associated with either focal scarring or global atrophy.
    d. All of the above.
    e. None of the above.

25. Which of the following accurately describes what happens during ureteral development?
    a. A ureteral bud that is medially (caudally) positioned from a normal takeoff at the trigone offers an embryologic explanation for primary reflux.
    b. A ureteral bud that is laterally (cranially) positioned from a normal takeoff at the trigone offers an embryologic explanation for primary reflux.
    c. A ureteral bud that fails to meet with the renal blastema offers an embryologic explanation for primary reflux.
    d. A ureteral bud that is laterally (cranially) positioned is often obstructed.
    e. A ureteral bud that fails to meet with the renal blastema is often obstructed.

26. Renal scarring in the presence of reflux likely involves:
    a. high intravesical pressures with sterile urine.
    b. low intravesical pressures with sterile urine.
    c. infection.
    d. all of the above.
    e. none of the above.

27. Which of the following statements is true regarding hypertension?
    a. In children and young adults, it is most commonly caused by reflux nephropathy.
    b. It is not related to the grade of reflux or severity of scarring.
    c. It is not associated with abnormalities of Na^+,K^+-ATPase activity.
    d. All of the above.
    e. None of the above.

28. Which of the following factors might contribute to the effects of reflux on renal growth?
    a. The congenital dysmorphism often associated with, but not caused by, reflux
    b. The number and type of urinary infections and their resultant nephropathy
    c. The quality of the contralateral kidney and its implications for compensatory hypertrophy
    d. The grade of reflux in the affected kidney
    e. All of the above

29. With regard to renal growth and reflux, which of the following statements is true?
    a. With the exception of those kidneys that are developmentally arrested, most studies implicate infection as the cause for altered renal growth.
    b. Successful antireflux surgery can accelerate renal growth.
    c. Successful antireflux surgery may not allow the affected kidneys to return to normal size.
    d. All of the above.
    e. None of the above.

30. The anatomy of patients with ureteral duplication typically follows the Weigert-Meyer rule, in which:
    a. the upper pole ureter enters the bladder distally and medially and the lower pole ureter enters the bladder proximally and laterally.
    b. the upper pole ureter enters the bladder proximally and medially and the lower pole ureter enters the bladder distally and laterally.
    c. the upper pole ureter enters the bladder distally and laterally and the lower pole ureter enters the bladder proximally and medially.
    d. the upper pole ureter enters the bladder proximally and laterally and the lower pole ureter enters the bladder distally and medially.
    e. the upper pole ureter enters the bladder superior to the lower pole ureter.

31. Which of the following statements is true regarding vesicoureteral reflux?
    a. It is infrequently associated with complete ureteral duplications.
    b. It may occur into either ureter of a duplicated system.
    c. It more often involves the ureter from the upper pole in a duplicated system.
    d. It resolves less frequently in patients with double ureters.
    e. All of the above.

32. Which of the following statements regarding reflux is true?
    a. The reflux associated with small paraureteral diverticula resolves at rates similar to those of primary reflux and can be managed accordingly.
    b. The reflux associated with paraureteral large diverticula is less likely to resolve and usually requires surgical correction.
    c. The reflux associated with diverticula, in which the ureter enters the diverticulum, regardless of size, should be corrected surgically.
    d. All of the above.
    e. None of the above.

33. Which of the following accurately describes the state of the bladder during pregnancy?
    a. Urine volume decreases in the upper collecting system as the physiologic dilatation of pregnancy evolves.
    b. Bladder tone increases because of edema and hyperemia.
    c. Bladder changes predispose the patient to bacteriuria.
    d. All of the above.
    e. None of the above.

34. During pregnancy, the presence of vesicoureteral reflux in a system already prone to bacteriuria may lead to increased morbidity. What is an additional risk factor?
    a. Renal scarring
    b. Tendency to get urinary infections
    c. Hypertension
    d. Renal insufficiency
    e. All of the above

35. Which of the following is an indication for surgical management of vesicoureteral reflux?
    a. Breakthrough urinary tract infections despite prophylactic antibiotics
    b. Noncompliance with medical management

c. Reflux associated with congenital abnormalities at the ureterovesical junction
   d. Failure of renal growth, new renal scars, or deterioration of renal function on serial ultrasonograms and/or renal scans
   e. All of the above

36. A variety of techniques have been described for the correction of vesicoureteral reflux. How are these anatomically categorized?
    a. Extravesical
    b. Intravesical
    c. Combined extravesical and intravesical
    d. All of the above
    e. None of the above

37. Common to each type of surgical repair for reflux is:
    a. the creation of a valvular mechanism that enables ureteral compression with bladder filling and contraction.
    b. the creation of a mucosal tunnel for reimplantation having adequate muscular backing.
    c. the creation of a tunnel length of three times the ureteral diameter.
    d. all of the above.
    e. none of the above.

38. How can complete ureteral duplications with reflux be best managed surgically?
    a. By separating the ureters and reimplanting them separately
    b. By a common sheath repair in which both ureters are mobilized with one mucosal cuff
    c. By performing an upper to lower ureteroureterostomy and reimplanting the lower ureter
    d. By performing a lower to upper ureteroureterostomy and reimplanting the upper ureter
    e. None of the above

39. Early postoperative obstruction can occur after a ureteral reimplant due to:
    a. edema.
    b. subtrigonal bleeding.
    c. mucus plugs.
    d. blood clots.
    e. all of the above.

40. If early postoperative obstruction occurs after a ureteral reimplant, what would the best management involve?
    a. Immediate nephrostomy tube placement
    b. Immediate placement of a ureteral stent
    c. Initial observation and diversion for unabating symptoms
    d. Placement of both a nephrostomy tube and a ureteral stent
    e. Reoperation

41. Which of the following statements is true regarding persistent reflux after ureteral reimplantation?
    a. It may be due to unrecognized secondary causes of reflux, such as neuropathic bladder and severe voiding dysfunction.
    b. It seldom results from a failure to provide adequate muscular backing for the ureter within its tunnel.
    c. It may be repaired surgically using minor submucosal advancements.
    d. All of the above.
    e. None of the above.

42. What does a successful transureteroureterostomy require?
    a. That the recipient ureter be minimally mobilized
    b. That there be no angulation of the donor ureter under the sigmoid mesentery
    c. That a tension-free, widely spatulated anastomosis be created
    d. All of the above
    e. None of the above

43. Which of the following statements is true regarding the laparoscopic approach for ureteral reimplantation?
    a. The advantages of this approach over open surgery include smaller incisions, less discomfort, brief hospitalizations, and quicker convalescence.
    b. As with other laparoscopic procedures, experience is essential to the success of this approach.
    c. Costs may be increased because of lengthier surgery and the expense of disposable equipment.
    d. All of the above.
    e. None of the above.

44. Which of the following statements is true regarding primary obstructive megaureter?
    a. It is caused by an aperistaltic juxtavesical segment 3 to 4 cm long that is unable to propagate urine at acceptable rates of flow.
    b. It most commonly occurs with neurogenic and non-neurogenic voiding dysfunction or infravesical obstructions such as posterior urethral valves.
    c. It may be due to acute infections, nephropathies, and other medical conditions that cause significant increases in urinary output that overwhelm maximal peristalsis.
    d. It is diagnosed when reflux, obstruction, and secondary causes of dilatation are ruled out.
    e. None of the above.

45. Which of the following statements is true regarding secondary obstructive megaureter?
    a. It is caused by an aperistaltic juxtavesical segment 3 to 4 cm long that is unable to propagate urine at acceptable rates of flow.
    b. It most commonly occurs with neurogenic and non-neurogenic voiding dysfunction or infravesical obstructions such as posterior urethral valves.
    c. It may be due to acute infections, nephropathies, and other medical conditions that cause significant increases in urinary output that overwhelm maximal peristalsis.
    d. It is diagnosed once reflux, obstruction, and secondary causes of dilatation are ruled out.
    e. None of the above.

46. Which of the following statements is true regarding secondary nonobstructive, nonrefluxing megaureter?
    a. It is caused by an aperistaltic juxtavesical segment 3 to 4 cm long that is unable to propagate urine at acceptable rates of flow.
    b. It most commonly occurs with neurogenic and non-neurogenic voiding dysfunction or infravesical obstructions such as posterior urethral valves.
    c. It may be due to acute infections, nephropathies, and other medical conditions that cause significant increases in urinary output that overwhelm maximal peristalsis.
    d. It is diagnosed once reflux, obstruction, and secondary causes of dilatation are ruled out.
    e. None of the above.

47. Which of the following statements is true regarding primary nonobstructive, nonrefluxing megaureter?
    a. It is caused by an aperistaltic juxtavesical segment 3 to

222 PEDIATRIC UROLOGY

   4 cm long that is unable to propagate urine at acceptable rates of flow.
   b. It most commonly occurs with neurogenic and non-neurogenic voiding dysfunction or infravesical obstructions such as posterior urethral valves.
   c. It may be due to acute infections, nephropathies, and other medical conditions that cause significant increases in urinary output that overwhelm maximal peristalsis.
   d. It is diagnosed once reflux, obstruction, and secondary causes of dilatation are ruled out.
   e. None of the above.

48. Which of the following statements is true regarding primary refluxing megaureters?
   a. They often improve with the ablation of valves or medical management of neurogenic bladder.
   b. Surgical management is appropriate during infancy, regardless of the chances for resolution.
   c. Surgery remains the recommendation for persistent high-grade reflux in older children and adults.
   d. All of the above.
   e. None of the above.

49. Which of the following statements is true regarding primary obstructive, nonrefluxing megaureters?
   a. As long as renal function is not significantly affected and urinary infections do not become a problem, expectant management is preferred.
   b. Antibiotic suppression is appropriate in most cases.
   c. Close radiologic surveillance is appropriate in most cases.
   d. All of the above.
   e. None of the above.

50. Which of the following statements is true regarding the surgical management of megaureters?
   a. Ureteral tailoring is usually necessary to achieve the proper length-diameter ratio required of successful reimplants.
   b. Plication or infolding is useful for the more severely dilated ureter.
   c. Excisional tapering is preferred for the moderately dilated ureter.
   d. Narrowing the ureter may theoretically lead to less effective peristalsis.
   e. Patients usually have such massively dilated and tortuous ureters that straightening with removal of excess length and proximal revision become necessary.

Answers

1. **e. 10%.** The overall incidence of reflux is probably best estimated at more than 10%. [p 2054]

2. **b. Antenatally detected reflux is usually low grade in boys when compared with that in girls.** The reflux is usually high grade and bilateral in boys when compared with reflux in girls. [p 2055]

3. **a. White girls are 10 times more likely to have reflux than their black American counterparts when evaluated for asymptomatic bacteriuria; however, once reflux is discovered, its grade and chance of spontaneous resolution are similar for both races.** The majority of studies on reflux come from North America, northern Europe, and Scandinavia. White girls are 10 times more likely to have reflux than their black American counterparts when evaluated for asymptomatic bacteriuria. Black girls are also less likely to have reflux when evaluated for urinary infection (12% in blacks versus 41% in whites). However, once reflux is discovered, its grade and chance of spontaneous resolution are similar for both races. [p 2055]

4. **b. A deficiency of the longitudinal muscle of the intravesical ureter results in an inadequate valvular mechanism.** Primary reflux is a congenital anomaly of the ureterovesical junction in which a deficiency of the longitudinal muscle of the intravesical ureter results in an inadequate valvular mechanism. [p 2057]

5. **a. 5:1.** In Paquin's novel study, a 5:1 tunnel length-ureteral diameter ratio was found in normal children without reflux. [p 2057]

6. **d. All of the above.** On the far end of this spectrum are children with non-neurogenic neurogenic bladders. Here, constriction of the urinary sphincter occurs during voiding in a voluntary form of detrusor-sphincter dyssynergia. Gradual bladder decompensation and myogenic failure result from incomplete emptying and increasing amounts of residual urine. [p 2058]

7. **a. Uninhibited bladder contractions.** The most common urodynamic abnormality in patients with reflux is uninhibited bladder contractions. These were found in 75% of girls with reflux in one series. [p 2058]

8. **d. All of the above.** Decreases in bladder wall compliance, detrusor decompensation, and incomplete emptying gradually damage the complex anatomic relationships required of the ureterovesical junction. [p 2058]

9. **b. Medical treatment.** The initial management of functional causes of reflux is medical. It is imperative that clinicians inquire about and determine the voiding patterns of children with reflux. [p 2058]

10. **e. all of the above.** In addition to a careful physical examination, signs or symptoms of voiding dysfunction include dribbling, urgency, and incontinence. Girls often exhibit curtseying behavior and boys will squeeze the penis in an attempt to suppress bladder contractions. [p 2058]

11. **e. a and c only.** Treatment of bladder dysfunction and instability, regardless of its severity or cause, is directed at dampening uninhibited contractions and lowering intravesical pressures. [p 2059]

12. **c. 40 cm H_2O.** There is a strong association between intravesical pressures of greater than 40 cm H_2O and the presence of reflux in patients with myelodysplasia and neuropathic bladders. [p 2059]

13. **d. All of the above.** Bladder infections (urinary tract infections) and their accompanying inflammation can also cause reflux by lessening compliance, elevating intravesical pressures, and distorting and weakening the ureterovesical junction. [p 2060]

14. **b. The International Classification System.** The Heikel and Parkkulainen system gained popularity in Europe a few years before the Dwoskin and Perlmutter system became widely accepted in the United States. The International Classification System devised in 1981 by the International Reflux

Study represents a melding of the two. It provides the current standard for grading reflux based on the appearance of contrast in the ureter and upper collecting system during voiding cystourethrography. [p 2060]

15. **a. It is not possible.** Accurately grading reflux is impossible with coexistent ipsilateral obstruction. [p 2061]

16. **d. All of the above.** The presence of fever may be an indicator of upper urinary tract involvement but is not always a reliable sign. However, if fever (and presumably pyelonephritis) is present, the likelihood of discovering vesicoureteral reflux is significantly increased. [p 2061]

17. **d. All of the above.** Complete evaluations that include voiding cystourethrography and ultrasonography are required of three groups: any child younger than 5 years of age with a documented urinary tract infection; febrile children with a urinary tract infection, regardless of age; and any boy with a urinary tract infection unless he is sexually active or has a past urologic history. [p 2062]

18. **a. They can be screened initially with ultrasonography.** Older children who present with asymptomatic bacteriuria or urinary tract infections that manifest solely with lower tract symptoms can be screened initially with ultrasonography alone, reserving cystography for those with abnormal upper tracts or recalcitrant infections. [p 2062]

19. **e. All of the above.** Excessive hydration may mask low grades of reflux because diuresis can blunt the retrograde flow of urine. Some reflux is demonstrated only during active infections when cystitis weakens the ureterovesical junction with edema or by increasing intravesical pressures. In addition, cystograms obtained during active infections can overestimate the grade of reflux because the endotoxins produced by some gram-negative organisms can paralyze ureteral smooth muscle and exaggerate ureteral dilatation. [p 2063]

20. **b. It is an accurate method for detecting and following reflux.** Nuclear cystography is the scintigraphic equivalent of conventional cystography. Although the technique does not provide the anatomic detail of fluoroscopic studies, it is an accurate method for detecting and following reflux. [p 2063]

21. **a. It is the diagnostic study of choice to initially evaluate the upper urinary tracts of patients with suspected or proven vesicoureteral reflux.** Ultrasonography has replaced the excretory urogram (intravenous pyelogram) as the diagnostic study of choice to initially evaluate the upper urinary tracts of patients with suspected or proven vesicoureteral reflux. [p 2064]

22. **b. Dimercaptosuccinic acid (DMSA) renal scan.** Renal scintigraphy with technetium 99m–labeled DMSA is the best study for detection of pyelonephritis and the cortical renal scarring that sometimes results. [p 2065]

23. **e. a and c only.** Urodynamic studies are indicated in any child suspected of having a secondary cause for reflux (e.g., valves, neurogenic bladder, non-neurogenic neurogenic bladder, voiding dysfunction), and they help direct therapy. [pp 2066–2067]

24. **d. All of the above.** The term *reflux nephropathy* encompasses a number of radiologic changes of the kidney associated with reflux. These include (1) focal thinning of renal parenchyma overlying a clubbed, distorted calyx; (2) generalized calyceal dilatation with parenchymal atrophy; and (3) impaired renal growth, associated with either focal scarring or global atrophy. [p 2067]

25. **b. A ureteral bud that is laterally (cranially) positioned from a normal takeoff at the trigone offers an embryologic explanation for primary reflux.** As Mackie and Stevens have suggested, a ureteral bud that is laterally (cranially) positioned from a normal takeoff at the trigone offers an embryologic explanation for primary reflux, whereas those inferiorly (caudally) positioned are often obstructed. [p 2067]

26. **d. all of the above.** Hodson and colleagues' early work implicated sterile reflux and a high-pressure "water-hammer" effect as a significant cause of renal scarring. More recent evidence in animal studies, with the availability of newer imaging modalities, indicate that low-pressure sterile reflux into previously normal kidneys may lead to focal, chronic interstitial inflammation and fibrosis. The majority of clinical and experimental studies also underscore the importance of infection in the evolution of most renal scars. [p 2068]

27. **a. In children and young adults, it is most commonly caused by reflux nephropathy.** Reflux nephropathy is the most common cause of severe hypertension in children and young adults, although the actual incidence is unknown. [p 2071]

28. **e. All of the above.** Factors that might contribute to the effects of reflux on renal growth include the congenital dysmorphism often associated with (30% of cases), but not caused by, reflux; the number and type of urinary infections and their resultant nephropathy; the quality of the contralateral kidney and its implications for compensatory hypertrophy; and the grade of reflux in the affected kidney. [p 2071]

29. **d. All of the above.** With the exception of those kidneys that are developmentally arrested, most studies implicate infection as the cause for altered renal growth. Successful antireflux surgery can accelerate renal growth but may not allow affected kidneys to return to normal size. [p 2072]

30. **a. the upper pole ureter enters the bladder distally and medially and the lower pole ureter enters the bladder proximally and laterally.** The anatomy of patients with ureteral duplication typically follows the Weigert-Meyer rule wherein the upper pole ureter enters the bladder distally and medially and the lower pole ureter enters the bladder proximally and laterally. [p 2073]

31. **b. It may occur into either ureter of a duplicated system.** Although urine may reflux into either ureter, it more commonly involves the ureter from the lower pole because of its lateral position and shorter submucosal tunnel. [p 2073]

32. **d. All of the above.** Reflux associated with small diverticula resolves at rates similar to those of primary reflux and can be managed accordingly. In contrast, reflux found with paraureteral large diverticula is less likely to resolve and usually requires surgical correction. In any case, when the ureter enters the diverticulum, regardless of size, surgery is recommended. [p 2074]

33. **c. Bladder changes predispose the patient to bacteriuria.** Bladder tone decreases because of edema and hyperemia, changes that predispose the patient to bacteriuria. In addition, urine volume increases in the upper collecting system as the physiologic dilatation of pregnancy evolves. [p 2076]

34. **e. All of the above.** It seems logical to assume that during pregnancy the presence of vesicoureteral reflux in a system already prone to bacteriuria would lead to increased morbidity. Maternal history also becomes a factor if past reflux, renal scarring, and a tendency to get urinary infections are included. Women with hypertension and an element of renal failure are particularly at risk. [p 2076]

35. **e. All of the above.** Typical indications for antireflux sur-

gery include (1) breakthrough urinary tract infections despite prophylactic antibiotics; (2) noncompliance with medical management; (3) severe grades (4 or 5) of reflux, especially with pyelonephritic changes; (4) failure of renal growth, new renal scars, or deterioration of renal function on serial ultrasonograms and/or renal scans; (5) reflux that persists in girls as full linear growth is approached at puberty; and (6) reflux associated with congenital abnormalities at the ureterovesical junction (e.g., bladder diverticula). [p 2081]

36. **d. All of the above.** A variety of techniques have been described for the correction of vesicoureteral reflux. These are anatomically categorized as extravesical, intravesical, or combined, depending on the approach to the ureter and suprahiatal or infrahiatal, in description of the position of the new submucosal tunnel in relation to the original hiatus. [p 2081]

37. **a. the creation of a valvular mechanism that enables ureteral compression with bladder filling and contraction.** Common to each technique is the creation of a valvular mechanism that enables ureteral compression with bladder filling and contraction, thus re-enacting normal anatomy and function. A successful ureteroneocystostomy provides a submucosal tunnel for reimplantation having sufficient length and adequate muscular backing. A tunnel length of five times the ureteral diameter is cited as necessary for eliminating reflux. [p 2081]

38. **b. By a common sheath repair in which both ureters are mobilized with one mucosal cuff.** Approximately 10% of children undergoing antireflux surgery have an element of ureteral duplication. The most common configuration is a complete duplication that results in two separate orifices. This is best managed by preserving a cuff of bladder mucosa that encompasses both orifices. Because the pair typically share blood supply along their adjoining wall, mobilization as one unit with a "common sheath" preserves vascularity and minimizes trauma. [pp 2088–2089]

39. **e. all of the above.** Early after surgery, various degrees of obstruction can be expected of the reimplanted ureter. Edema, subtrigonal bleeding, and bladder spasms all possibly contribute. Mucus plugs and blood clots are other causes. Most postoperative obstructions are mild and asymptomatic and resolve spontaneously. More significant obstructions are usually symptomatic. Affected children typically present 1 to 2 weeks after surgery with acute abdominal pain, nausea, and vomiting. [p 2090]

40. **c. Initial observation and diversion for unabating symptoms.** The large majority of perioperative obstructions subside spontaneously, but placement of a nephrostomy tube or ureteral stent sometimes becomes necessary for unabating symptoms. [p 2090]

41. **a. It may be due to unrecognized secondary causes of reflux, such as neuropathic bladder and severe voiding dysfunction.** Other than technical errors, failure to identify and treat secondary causes of reflux is a common cause of the reappearance of reflux. Foremost among these secondary causes are unrecognized neuropathic bladder and severe voiding dysfunction. [p 2091]

42. **d. All of the above.** Historically, hesitation to use a transureteroureterostomy stemmed from the potential to affect the recipient ureter, which should be normal. This is not a problem if (1) the recipient ureter is minimally mobilized, (2) there is no angulation of the donor ureter under the sigmoid mesentery, and (3) a tension-free, widely spatulated anastomosis is created. [pp 2091–2092]

43. **d. All of the above.** The advantages of this approach over open surgery include smaller incisions, less discomfort, brief hospitalizations, and quicker convalescence. As with other laparoscopic procedures, a learning curve needs to be broached, and experience is essential to the success of this approach. Laparoscopic reimplantation requires a team with at least two surgeons; the repair is converted from an extraperitoneal to an intraperitoneal approach; many of the available instruments are less than ideal for use in children; operative time is greater than with open techniques; and cost is increased because of lengthier surgery and the expense of disposable equipment. [p 2094]

44. **a. It is caused by an aperistaltic juxtavesical segment 3 to 4 cm long that is unable to propagate urine at acceptable rates of flow.** It is generally agreed that the cause of primary obstructive megaureter is an aperistaltic juxtavesical segment 3 to 4 cm long that is unable to propagate urine at acceptable rates of flow. [p 2097]

45. **b. It most commonly occurs with neurogenic and non-neurogenic voiding dysfunction or infravesical obstructions such as posterior urethral valves.** This form of megaureter most commonly occurs with neurogenic and non-neurogenic voiding dysfunction or infravesical obstructions such as posterior urethral valves. [p 2098]

46. **c. It may be due to acute infections, nephropathies, and other medical conditions that cause significant increases in urinary output that overwhelm maximal peristalsis.** Significant ureteral dilatation can result from acute urinary tract infections accompanied by bacterial endotoxins that inhibit peristalsis. Resolution is expected with appropriate antibiotic therapy. Nephropathies and other medical conditions that cause significant increases in urinary output that overwhelm maximal peristalsis can also lead to progressive ureteral dilatation as collecting systems comply to handle the output from above. These include lithium toxicity, diabetes insipidus or mellitus, sickle cell nephropathy, and psychogenic polydipsia. [p 2098]

47. **d. It is diagnosed once reflux, obstruction, and secondary causes of dilatation are ruled out.** Once reflux, obstruction, and secondary causes of dilatation are ruled out, the designation of primary nonrefluxing, nonobstructed megaureter is appropriate. [p 2098]

48. **c. Surgery remains the recommendation for persistent high-grade reflux in older children and adults.** Routinely recommending surgery in newborns and infants with grades IV to V reflux no longer applies. Instead, medical management is appropriate during infancy and is continued if a trend to resolution is noted. Otherwise, surgery remains the recommendation for persistent high-grade reflux in older children and adults. [p 2101]

49. **d. All of the above.** Most clinicians now believe that as long as renal function is not significantly affected and urinary infections do not become a problem, expectant management is preferred. Antibiotic suppression and close radiologic surveillance are appropriate in most cases. [p 2103]

50. **a. Ureteral tailoring is usually necessary to achieve the proper length-diameter ratio required of successful reimplants.** Ureteral tailoring (excision or plication) is usually necessary to achieve the proper length-diameter ratio required of successful reimplants. Narrowing the ureter also theoretically enables its walls to coapt properly, leading to more effective peristalsis. Revising the distal segment intended for reimplantation is all that is usually required. [pp 2103–2104]

Chapter 60

Prune-Belly Syndrome

Edwin A. Smith • John R. Woodard

Questions

1. Common findings in the prune-belly syndrome include all but which of the following?

   a. Deficiency of abdominal wall musculature
   b. Urinary tract dilatation
   c. Palpable undescended testes
   d. Urachal pseudodiverticulum
   e. Vesicoureteral reflux

2. Which of the following statements regarding the prognosis of patients with prune-belly syndrome is NOT true?

   a. The patient will likely be infertile.
   b. A substantial risk of renal failure exists.
   c. Testicular descent will not occur spontaneously.
   d. The male "pseudo-prune" phenotype is not protected from renal failure.
   e. Chronic constipation and ineffective cough may result from abdominal wall laxity.

3. Complications involving which of the following organ systems are most likely to threaten the early survival of an infant with prune-belly syndrome?

   a. Cardiac
   b. Renal
   c. Pulmonary
   d. Gastrointestinal
   e. Endocrine

4. Ureteral dysfunction in prune-belly syndrome is related to all of the following except:

   a. ureteral dilatation with failure of luminal coaptation during peristalsis.
   b. reduced smooth muscle population.
   c. failure of propagation of an electrical conduction due to increased fibrous connective tissue.
   d. more severe proximal ureteral dysfunction with failure to conduct a urinary bolus from the renal pelvis.
   e. abnormal myofilament content in smooth muscle cells.

5. Urodynamic bladder evaluation in prune-belly syndrome is primarily characterized by bladder enlargement with:

   a. elevated voiding pressures and detrusor-sphincter dyssynergia.
   b. high-amplitude uninhibited contractions.
   c. poorly contractile detrusor or myogenic failure.
   d. poor compliance.
   e. absent sensation.

6. With regard to sexual function, prune-belly syndrome is most commonly associated with:

   a. normal erectile function and semen analysis but retrograde ejaculation.
   b. low levels of testosterone, follicle-stimulating hormone, and luteinizing hormone.
   c. normal levels of testosterone, normal to elevated levels of luteinizing hormone, and normal development of secondary sex characteristics.
   d. elevated levels of testosterone, luteinizing hormone, and follicle-stimulating hormone.
   e. normal secondary sex characteristics but impaired libido.

7. A management strategy of observation in the prune-belly syndrome is strongly supported by which finding?

   a. That spontaneous improvement in dilatation of the urinary tract generally occurs after puberty
   b. That vesicoureteral reflux occurs at low pressures and does not represent a threat to renal parenchyma
   c. That the risk of obstruction after ureteral reimplantation always outweighs the benefit
   d. That operative risks in this patient population are excessive
   e. None of the above

8. Which statement is most accurate when considering management of the lower urinary tract in the prune-belly patient?

   a. Reduction cystoplasty is indicated when bladder capacity becomes greater than expected for age.
   b. Internal urethrotomy improves postvoid residual urine volumes without risk of incontinence.
   c. Reduction cystoplasty permanently improves bladder dynamics.
   d. Internal urethrotomy should be specifically based on pressure-flow studies.
   e. Routine intermittent catheterization should be used to improve postvoid residual urine volumes in all patients.

9. Which statement regarding orchiopexy in the patient with prune-belly syndrome is true?

   a. It requires a microvascular testicular autotransplantation due to the high intra-abdominal position.
   b. It has been shown to maintain endocrine function but has no potential to preserve spermatogenesis.
   c. It can be best accomplished by transperitoneal mobilization before 1 year of age.
   d. It should never involve the use of the Fowler-Stephens technique because of the unreliability of collateral testicular blood supply.
   e. It is performed if spontaneous descent fails to occur by 2 years of age.

10. Arguments offered in favor of fetal urinary tract obstruction as the underlying cause of prune-belly syndrome have included all of the following except which one?

    a. Patients occasionally demonstrate urethral atresia or posterior urethral valves, producing gross dilatation of the bladder and hydroureteronephrosis.
    b. The testes fail to descend because of mechanical blockade from bladder distention.

c. The presence of renal parenchymal dysplasia relates to obstruction during renal development.
d. Megalourethra produces functional obstruction because of redundant urethral folds.
e. Maldevelopment of the abdominal wall is secondary to the pressure effects of the distended urinary tract and urinary ascites.

11. The most appropriate initial management of the newborn with prune-belly syndrome includes:

   a. percutaneous drainage of the upper urinary tract after stabilization.
   b. stabilization and then vesicostomy if anesthetic risk permits.
   c. stabilization and then bilateral cutaneous ureterostomy if anesthetic risk permits.
   d. evaluation of pulmonary status and voiding cystourethrogram to rule out posterior urethral valves and reflux.
   e. evaluation of pulmonary status, renal ultrasonographic study, and prophylactic antibiotics.

12. The prostatic urethra in prune-belly syndrome:

   a. is dilated and associated with bladder neck hypertrophy on a voiding cystogram.
   b. is sometimes associated with congenital urethral obstruction resulting in megalourethra.
   c. is associated with a hypoplastic prostate with decreased epithelium and increased smooth muscle.
   d. results in retrograde ejaculation.
   e. none of the above.

Answers

1. **c. Palpable undescended testes.** Bilateral cryptorchidism is a central feature of the syndrome, and in most patients both testes are intra-abdominal, overlying the ureters at the pelvic brim near the sacroiliac level. [p 2120]

2. **d. The male "pseudo-prune" phenotype is protected from renal failure.** Although it is exceptionally rare to encounter a normal urinary tract in association with the characteristic abdominal wall defect in a male, the converse is not unusual. Some patients (with pseudo–prune-belly syndrome) with a normal or relatively normal abdominal wall exhibit many or all of the internal urologic features. These features may include dysplastic or dysmorphic kidneys or may include dilated and tortuous ureters. One report noted eight boys with relatively mild external features of the syndrome, five of whom progressed to renal failure, evidence that these children remain vulnerable to renal deterioration. [p 2124]

3. **c. Pulmonary.** The most urgent matters are actually those concerned with cardiopulmonary function. Pulmonary complications including pulmonary hypoplasia, pneumomediastinum, pneumothorax, and cardiac abnormalities must be excluded. [p 2124]

4. **d. more severe proximal ureteral dysfunction with failure to conduct a urinary bolus from the renal pelvis.** The proximal ureter usually displays a more normal appearance, an important feature when considering corrective surgery. [p 2118]

5. **c. poorly contractile detrusor or myogenic failure.** Usually, the cystometrogram reveals excellent detrusor compliance; the end-filling pressure assumes a normal value; and the bladder functions well as a reservoir. However, bladder sensation during filling is shifted to the right with a delayed first sensation to void, and bladder capacity may be more than double the normal volume. Less consistent and less favorable results are seen with the voiding profile. The compressor capabilities of the detrusor are diminished by the frequent presence of vesicoureteral reflux and reduced detrusor contractility. [p 2119]

6. **c. normal levels of testosterone, normal to elevated levels of luteinizing hormone, and normal development of secondary sex characteristics.** Little information is available on sexual function in men with prune-belly syndrome. Preserved Leydig cell function usually allows for normal testosterone levels, although often in the presence of elevated luteinizing hormone levels. Erection and orgasm are apparently normal, but no cases of paternity have been reported. The potential for fertility in these patients is compromised not only by testicular abnormalities but also by multiple extratesticular factors. [p 2121]

7. **e. None of the above.** The obvious implication of different studies was that a more aggressive approach was necessary to improve the fate of the infant with prune-belly syndrome. With the recognition that infection and progressive renal insufficiency are the factors that most often pose the greatest threat to quality of life and survival, surgical reconstruction to normalize the anatomy and function of the genitourinary tract was advocated. Early retailoring of the urinary system to reduce stasis and eliminate reflux or obstruction has included ureteral shortening, tapering and vesicoureteral reimplantation, and reduction cystoplasty. Reconstruction is best delayed until the child is approximately 3 months old, to allow for pulmonary maturation. This approach has been successful in achieving anatomic and functional improvement. [p 2125]

8. **d. Internal urethrotomy should be specifically based on pressure-flow studies.** Some initial improvement in voiding dynamics can be achieved by aggressive bladder remodeling. However, with long-term follow-up, there has been no evidence that this improvement is maintained, and excessive bladder volumes tend to recur with time. Internal urethrotomy is indicated in the rare patient with true anatomic urethral obstruction or in patients with urodynamic evidence of urethral obstruction by pressure-flow studies. [pp 2128–2129]

9. **c. It can be best accomplished by transperitoneal mobilization before 1 year of age.** Orchiopexy in all patients is now generally performed during infancy in an effort to maintain the germ cell population and protect spermatogenesis. In the neonate and in patients up to at least 6 months of age, transabdominal complete mobilization of the spermatic cord almost always allows the testis to be positioned in the dependent portion of the scrotum without dividing the vascular portion of the spermatic cord. The Fowler-Stephens technique for performing orchiopexy in patients with intra-abdominal testes has become part of the standard urologic armamentarium. [p 2131]

10. **d. Megalourethra produces functional obstruction because of redundant urethral folds.** The cause of prune-belly syndrome remains unknown. Some investigators have suggested that both the abdominal wall defect and the intra-

abdominal cryptorchidism are secondary to distention of the urinary tract during early fetal development. Obstruction in the posterior urethra is a possible cause of this distention and would explain the predominance of male patients. Congenital megalourethra, characterized by dilatation of the anterior urethra without distal obstruction, occurs with increased frequency in this syndrome. [pp 2117, 2120]

11. **e. evaluation of pulmonary status, renal ultrasonographic study, and prophylactic antibiotics.** The most urgent matters are those concerned with cardiopulmonary function. After stabilization, urologic evaluation proceeds with physical examination and ultrasonography. Imaging requiring catheterization, and the potential for introduction of bacteria should be avoided unless the results are needed for immediate clinical decision-making. Attention to sterile technique is crucial if invasive studies are performed. Once introduced, infection in a static system may be difficult to eradicate. [p 2124]

12. **d. results in retrograde ejaculation.** The characteristically wide bladder neck merges with a grossly dilated prostatic urethra, so that the junction is nearly imperceptible both radiographically and by gross inspection. The prostatic urethra does, however, taper to a relatively narrow membranous urethra at the urogenital diaphragm. Retrograde ejaculation is common. [pp 2120–2121]

Chapter 61

Exstrophy, Epispadias, and Other Bladder Anomalies

John P. Gearhart

Questions

1. What is the incidence of classic bladder exstrophy?

    a. 1 in 100,000 live births
    b. 1 in 70,000 live births
    c. 1 in 50,000 live births
    d. 1 in 5000 live births
    e. 1 in 60,000 live births

2. What is the risk of bladder exstrophy in the offspring of individuals with bladder exstrophy and epispadias?

    a. 1 in 70 live births
    b. 1 in 100 live births
    c. 1 in 200 live births
    d. 1 in 50 live births
    e. 1 in 500 live births

3. The main theory of embryologic maldevelopment in exstrophy is that of:

    a. abnormal underdevelopment of the cloacal membrane, preventing medial migration of the mesoderm tissue and proper lower abdominal wall development.
    b. abnormal overdevelopment of the cloacal membrane, preventing medial migration of the mesodermal tissue and proper lower abdominal wall development.
    c. abnormal infiltration of ectoderm into the cloacal membrane.
    d. abnormal infiltration of mesoderm into the cloacal membrane.
    e. abnormal invasion of endoderm into the cloacal membrane.

4. In evaluation of the skeletal defects of bladder exstrophy, Sponseller and colleagues found that with classic bladder exstrophy there is a mean external rotation of the posterior aspect of the pelvis of 12 degrees on each side, retroversion of the acetabulum, and a mean 18 degree rotation of the anterior pelvis, along which of the following?

    a. 80% shortening of the pubic rami
    b. 20% shortening of the pubic rami
    c. 30% shortening of the pubic rami
    d. no abnormality of the pubic rami
    e. 40% shortening of the pubic rami in addition to a significant pubic symphyseal diastasis

5. What is the incidence of inguinal hernia in patients with bladder exstrophy?

    a. 100% of boys and 90% of girls
    b. 50% of boys and 50% of girls
    c. 81% of boys and 10% of girls
    d. 40% of boys and 20% of girls
    e. 100% of boys and 100% of girls

6. By using MRI to examine the erectile bodies in males with bladder exstrophy, it was found that the anterior corporeal length in males with bladder exstrophy is almost:

    a. 20% shorter than that of normal control subjects.
    b. 30% shorter than that of normal control subjects.
    c. 50% shorter than that of normal control subjects.
    d. 40% shorter than that of normal control subjects.
    e. 70% shorter than that of normal control subjects.

7. By using MRI to examine the prostate in adult males born with bladder exstrophy, it was found that the volume, weight, and maximum cross-section of the prostate:

    a. appeared normal compared with published results from control subjects.
    b. appeared smaller than normal compared with normal published results from control subjects.
    c. appeared larger than normal compared with published results from control subjects.
    d. appeared the same as those of normal control subjects.
    e. were infantile compared with normal published results from control subjects.

8. Which of the following accurately describes the vagina in the female patient with bladder exstrophy?

   a. Not only shorter than normal but of smaller caliber
   b. Shorter than normal but of normal caliber
   c. Longer than normal but of normal caliber
   d. Longer than normal but of smaller caliber
   e. Longer than normal and of wider caliber

9. Which of the following is correct regarding the true anatomic defect seen in classic bladder exstrophy?

   a. It is easy to evaluate in the nursery.
   b. It is easily appreciated while the child is taking a bottle.
   c. It cannot often be totally appreciated unless the child is relaxed under anesthesia.
   d. It is easily evaluated with ultrasonography prenatally.
   e. It is easy to evaluate in the nursery with the child under sedation.

10. Vesicoureteral reflux in the patient with closed bladder exstrophy occurs in what percentage of patients?

    a. 70%
    b. 30%
    c. 10%
    d. 100%
    e. 50%

11. In the pseudoexstrophy defect, the characteristic musculoskeletal defect of exstrophy is:

    a. present with multiple major defects of the lower urinary tract.
    b. present with no major defect of the urinary tract.
    c. present along with epispadias.
    d. present along with imperforate anus.
    e. present along with an omphalocele.

12. The characteristic prenatal appearance of bladder exstrophy includes which of the following: (1) absence of bladder filling; (2) low-set umbilicus; (3) widening of the pubic ramus; (4) diminutive genitalia; (5) lower abdominal mass that increases in size as the pregnancy progresses.

    a. 1 and 2
    b. 1 and 3
    c. 1 and 4
    d. 1 and 5
    e. All of the above.

13. What is the appropriate time for bladder neck reconstruction in a child with bladder exstrophy?

    a. At 2 years of age when the child has a 60-ml bladder capacity
    b. At 3 years of age when the child has a 60-ml bladder capacity
    c. At any age when the parents are ready
    d. When the child has an adequate bladder capacity and is motivated to participate in a postoperative voiding program
    e. When the child can tolerate 4 to 5 hours of anesthesia

14. What is(are) the best treatment option(s) at the time of birth in a child whose bladder template is judged to be too small to undergo closure?

    a. Excision of the bladder with a nonrefluxing colon conduit
    b. Excision of the bladder with ureterosigmoidostomy
    c. Giving the child 4 to 6 months to see whether the bladder template will grow
    d. Attempted closure regardless of the size of the bladder
    e. Bladder closure, augmentation, ureteral reimplantation, and a continence procedure in infancy

15. In the newborn patient with bladder exstrophy and a good-sized bladder template with significant pubic diastasis, osteotomy should be performed in what group of patients?

    a. All patients
    b. Patients with a greater than 5 cm pubic diastasis
    c. Patients who have a less than 5 cm pubic diastasis
    d. Only patients whose pubic bones can be brought together easily under anesthesia by pressure on the greater trochanters
    e. Those patients who not only have a diastasis but in whom adequate pubic apposition cannot easily be made under anesthesia

16. After closure of classic bladder exstrophy and after healing has occurred, the suprapubic tube should be removed under what conditions?

    a. After a normal intravenous pyelography (IVP) result is obtained
    b. After a normal voiding cystourethrographic (VCUG) result is obtained
    c. After an ultrasonographic scan is obtained
    d. After a dimercaptosuccinic acid (DMSA) renal scan is obtained
    e. After a diethylenetriamine penta-acetic acid (DTPA) renal scan is obtained

17. After bladder exstrophy closure in the newborn period and during the "incontinent interval" before bladder neck reconstruction, bladder capacity should be measured on a yearly basis. How are the best values for adequately predicting bladder growth obtained?

    a. With VCUG performed with the patient awake
    b. With a nuclear cystogram obtained with the patient awake
    c. With a gravity cystogram obtained with the patient under anesthesia
    d. By measurement of bladder capacity after IVP is performed
    e. With VCUG performed in the radiology department with the patient under light sedation

18. After initial primary bladder closure in the newborn, what should be done if recurrent urinary tract infections occur?

    a. VCUG should be performed.
    b. Immediate bladder exploration should be undertaken.
    c. A DMSA renal scan should be obtained.
    d. Cystoscopy should be performed.
    e. Bladder CT should be performed.

19. Regardless of the technique chosen for epispadias repair, the key concerns that must be addressed include:

    a. correction of dorsal chordee.
    b. urethral reconstruction.
    c. glandular reconstruction and penile skin closure.
    d. all of the above.
    e. b and c.

20. In a patient with bladder exstrophy who undergoes more than one closure of the bladder and urethral defect, what is the chance of having adequate bladder capacity for later bladder neck reconstruction?

    a. 60%
    b. 50%
    c. 80%
    d. 30%
    e. 70%

21. Information gleaned from most major series of bladder neck reconstruction indicates that the most important factor to

predict success and eventual continence after bladder neck reconstruction includes:

   a. age of the child.
   b. motivation of the parents.
   c. motivation of the child and the parents.
   d. bladder capacity at the time of bladder neck reconstruction.
   e. number of prior bladder infections.

22. After bladder neck reconstruction, within what time period do the majority of patients achieve daytime continence?

   a. 2 years
   b. 1 year
   c. 3 years
   d. 18 months
   e. 4 years

23. After a failed bladder closure in the newborn period, an appropriate time period should elapse before attempting a secondary repair. What should this time period be?

   a. 2 months
   b. 4 months
   c. 12 months
   d. 6 months
   e. 18 months

24. The risks of ureterosigmoidostomy in the exstrophy population include:

   a. pyelonephritis and hyperkalemic acidosis.
   b. pyelonephritis, hyperkalemic acidosis, and rectal incontinence.
   c. pyelonephritis, hyperkalemic acidosis, rectal incontinence, and ureteral obstruction.
   d. pyelonephritis, hyperkalemic acidosis, rectal incontinence, and delayed development of malignancy.
   e. pyelonephritis, hyponatremia, and rectal incontinence.

25. Sexual function and libido in male and female exstrophy patients are:

   a. normal in males, abnormal in females.
   b. normal in females and abnormal in males.
   c. normal in both males and females.
   d. normal only in females.
   e. normal only in males.

26. What is the most common complication following pregnancy in female exstrophy patients?

   a. Toxemia
   b. Cervical cancer
   c. Cervical and uterine prolapse
   d. Painful delivery
   e. Rectal prolapse

27. Psychological studies of male and female children with bladder exstrophy find that:

   a. all have clinical psychopathology.
   b. they do not have clinical psychopathology.
   c. only males have clinical psychopathology.
   d. only females have clinical psychopathology.
   e. half of males and half of females have clinical psychopathology.

28. What is the incidence of cloacal exstrophy?

   a. 1 in 400,000 live births
   b. 1 in 500,000 live births
   c. 1 in 100,000 live births
   d. 1 in 50,000 live births
   e. 1 in 750,000 live births

29. According to Muecke, what is the embryologic event that leads to cloacal exstrophy?

   a. Inadequate small cloacal membrane
   b. Abnormally large perigenital tubercles
   c. Abnormally extensive cloacal membrane
   d. Abnormal endodermal migration
   e. Abnormal ectodermal migration

30. In cloacal exstrophy, upper tract anomalies occur in what percentage of patients?

   a. 20% to 30%
   b. 41% to 60%
   c. 50% to 60%
   d. 70% to 80%
   e. 100%

31. What is the incidence of omphalocele associated with cloacal exstrophy?

   a. 40%
   b. 50%
   c. 95%
   d. 20%
   e. 70%

32. In the patient with cloacal exstrophy, hindgut remnants should be preserved to:

   a. enlarge the bladder.
   b. enlarge the vagina during infancy.
   c. enlarge the vagina during adolescence.
   d. provide additional length of bowel for fluid absorption.
   e. allow either bladder augmentation or vaginal reconstruction.

33. What is the incidence of male epispadias?

   a. 1 in 150,000 live births
   b. 1 in 200,000 live births
   c. 1 in 100,000 live births
   d. 1 in 117,000 live births
   e. 1 in 200,000 live births

34. What is the incidence of reflux in patients with complete epispadias?

   a. 10% to 20%
   b. 20% to 30%
   c. 50% to 60%
   d. 70% to 80%
   e. 30% to 40%

35. In the complete epispadias group, what is the predominant indicator of eventual continence?

   a. Length of the urethral groove
   b. Type of epispadias repair
   c. Bladder capacity at the time of bladder neck reconstruction
   d. Length of the epispadiac penis
   e. Presence of spinal abnormalities

36. Female epispadias is a rare congenital anomaly occurring in:

   a. 1 in 110,000 female births.
   b. 1 in 240,000 female births.
   c. 1 in 484,000 female births.
   d. 1 in 350,000 female births.
   e. 1 in 512,000 female births.

37. Acquired bladder diverticula are usually:

a. single and not associated with bladder outlet obstruction.
b. multiple and not associated with bladder outlet obstruction.
c. multiple and associated with bladder outlet obstruction.
d. on the dome of the bladder.
e. in females and usually single.

38. Which genitourinary anomaly is most commonly associated with the Ehlers-Danlos syndrome?

    a. Agenesis of the bladder
    b. Congenital bladder diverticula
    c. Posterior urethral valves
    d. Neurogenic bladder
    e. Urachal diverticulum

39. In the child born with a patent urachus, what is the most effective diagnostic test to elucidate this condition?

    a. MRI of the urachal tract
    b. CT of the urachal tract
    c. IVP
    d. Fistulography of the urachal tract
    e. VCUG

40. What is the most appropriate therapy for a patent urachus?

    a. Excision of a cuff of bladder
    b. Excision of the patent urachus and cuff of bladder
    c. Laparoscopic fulguration of the urachal tract
    d. Laparoscopic fulguration of the urachal tract and dome of the bladder
    e. Partial cystectomy

Answers

1. **c. 1 in 50,000 live births.** The incidence of bladder exstrophy has been estimated as being between 1 in 10,000 and 1 in 50,000. [p 2138]

2. **a. 1 in 70 live births.** Shapiro determined that the risk of bladder exstrophy in the offspring of individuals with bladder exstrophy and epispadias is 1 in 70 live births, a 500-fold greater incidence than in the general population. [p 2138]

3. **b. abnormal overdevelopment of the cloacal membrane, preventing medial migration of the mesodermal tissue and proper lower abdominal wall development.** The theory of embryonic maldevelopment in exstrophy held by Marshall and Muecke is that the basic defect is an abnormal overdevelopment of the cloacal membrane, preventing medial migration of the mesenchymal tissue and proper lower abdominal wall development. [p 2138]

4. **c. 30% shortening of the pubic rami.** Sponseller and colleagues found that patients with classic bladder exstrophy have a mean external rotation of the posterior aspect of the pelvis of 12 degrees on each side, retroversion of the acetabulum, and a mean 18-degree external rotation of the anterior pelvis, along with 30% shortening of the pubic rami. [p 2140]

5. **c. 81% of boys and 10% of girls.** Connelly and colleagues, in a review of 181 children with bladder exstrophy, reported inguinal hernias in 81.8% of boys and 10.5% of girls. [p 2141]

6. **c. 50% shorter than that of normal control subjects.** With the use of MRI to examine adult men with bladder exstrophy and comparison of this result with that from age- and race-matched control subjects, it was found that the anterior corporeal length in male patients with bladder exstrophy is almost 50% shorter than that of normal control subjects. [p 2142]

7. **a. appeared normal compared with published results from control subjects.** The volume, weight, and maximum cross-sectional area of the prostate appeared normal compared with published results from control subjects. [p 2142]

8. **b. Shorter than normal but of normal caliber.** The vagina is shorter than normal, hardly greater than 6 cm in depth, but of normal caliber. [p 2143]

9. **c. It cannot often be totally appreciated unless the child is relaxed under anesthesia.** The depth of the extension of bladder that may be sequestered below the fascial defect cannot often be appreciated unless the infant is totally relaxed under anesthesia. [p 2144]

10. **d. 100%.** Reflux in the closed exstrophy bladder occurs in 100% of cases, and subsequent surgery is usually required at the time of bladder neck reconstruction. [p 2145]

11. **b. present with no major defect of the urinary tract.** The presence of a characteristic musculoskeletal defect of the exstrophy anomaly with no major defect in the urinary tract has been named pseudoexstrophy. [p 2145]

12. **e. All of the above.** In a review of 25 prenatal ultrasonographic examinations with the resulting birth of a newborn with classic bladder exstrophy, several observations were made: (1) absence of bladder filling; (2) a low-set umbilicus; (3) widening pubis ramus; (4) diminutive genitalia; and (5) a lower abdominal mass that increases in size as the pregnancy progresses and as the intra-abdominal viscera increase in size. [p 2146]

13. **d. When the child has an adequate bladder capacity and is motivated to participate in a postoperative voiding program.** The surgical approach for bladder exstrophy includes bladder neck reconstruction along with an antireflux procedure at about the age of 4 to 5 years, when the child has achieved an adequate bladder capacity for bladder neck reconstruction and is motivated to participate in a postoperative voiding program. [p 2147]

14. **c. Giving the child 4 to 6 months to see whether the bladder template will grow.** Ideally, waiting for the bladder template to grow for 4 to 6 months in the child with a small bladder is not as risky as submitting a small bladder template to closure in an inappropriate setting, resulting in dehiscence and allowing the fate of the bladder to be sealed at that point. [p 2150]

15. **e. Those patients who not only have a diastasis but in whom adequate pubic apposition cannot easily be made under anesthesia.** If the pelvis is not malleable or if the pubic bones are greater than 4 cm apart at the time of the initial examination under anesthesia, osteotomy should be performed, even if it is closed before 72 hours of age. [p 2151]

16. **c. After an ultrasonographic scan is obtained.** Prior to removal of the suprapubic tube, 4 weeks postoperatively, the bladder outlet is calibrated by a urethral catheter or a urethral sound to ensure free drainage. A complete ultrasono-

graphic examination is obtained to ascertain the status of the renal pelves and ureters, and appropriate urinary antibiotics are administered to treat any bladder contamination that might be present after removal of the suprapubic tube. [p 2158]

17. **c. With a gravity cystogram obtained with the patient under anesthesia.** Cystoscopy and a cystogram obtained at yearly intervals will detect bilateral reflux in nearly 100% of patients and will provide an estimate of bladder capacity. [p 2158]

18. **d. Cystoscopy should be performed.** An important caveat is that if there are recurrent urinary tract infections, or if the bladder is distended on an ultrasonographic study, cystoscopy should be performed and the posterior urethra should be carefully examined anteriorly for erosion of the intrapubic stitch, which may be the cause of the recurrent infections. [p 2159]

19. **d. all of the above.** Regardless of the surgical technique chosen for reconstruction of the penis in bladder exstrophy, four key concerns must be addressed to ensure a functional and cosmetically pleasing penis: (1) correction of dorsal chordee; (2) urethral reconstruction; (3) glandular reconstruction; and (4) penile skin closure. [p 2159]

20. **a. 60%.** In one study, if a patient underwent two closures, the chance of having an adequate bladder capacity for bladder neck reconstruction was 60%. [p 2168]

21. **d. bladder capacity at the time of bladder neck reconstruction.** The most important long-term factor gleaned from a review of all these series is the fact that bladder capacity at the time of bladder neck reconstruction is a very important determinant of eventual success. [p 2170]

22. **b. 1 year.** The vast majority of patients achieve daytime continence in the first year after bladder neck reconstruction. [p 2171]

23. **d. 6 months.** Dehiscence, which may be precipitated by incomplete mobilization of the pelvic diaphragm, and inadequate pelvic immobilization postoperatively, wound infection, abdominal distention, or urinary tube malfunction, necessitates a 6-month recovery period prior to a second attempt at closure. [p 2172]

24. **d. pyelonephritis, hyperkalemic acidosis, rectal incontinence, and delayed development of malignancy.** However, this form of diversion should not be offered until one is certain that anal continence is normal and after the family has been made aware of the potential serious complications, including pyelonephritis, hyperkalemic acidosis, rectal incontinence, ureteral obstruction, and delayed development of malignancy. [p 2173]

25. **c. normal in both males and females.** Sexual function and libido in exstrophy patients are normal. [p 2174]

26. **c. Cervical and uterine prolapse.** The main complication following pregnancy was cervical and uterine prolapse, which occurred frequently. [p 2175]

27. **b. they do not have clinical psychopathology.** The conclusions of this long-term study were that children with exstrophy do not have clinical psychopathology. [p 2175]

28. **a. 1 in 400,000 live births.** Fortunately, cloacal exstrophy is exceedingly rare, occurring in 1 in 200,000 to 400,000 live births. [p 2176]

29. **c. Abnormally extensive cloacal membrane.** According to Muecke, an abnormally extensive cloacal membrane produces a wedge effect, serving as a mechanical barrier to mesodermal migration, which results in impaired development of the abdominal wall, failure of fusion of the paired genital tubercles, and diastasis pubis. [p 2176]

30. **b. 41% to 60% of patients.** Upper urinary tract anomalies occurred in 41% to 60% of patients in Diamond's review. [p 2177]

31. **c. 95%.** In Diamond's series, the incidence of omphalocele was 88%, with a majority of all series reporting 95% or greater. [p 2177]

32. **d. provide additional length of bowel for fluid absorption.** With the recognition of the metabolic changes in patients with ileostomy, an attempt is always made to use the hindgut remnant to provide additional length of bowel for fluid absorption. [p 2179]

33. **d. 1 in 117,000 live births.** Male epispadias is a rare anomaly, with a reported incidence of 1 in 117,000 males. [p 2181]

34. **e. 30% to 40%.** The ureterovesical junction is inherently deficient in complete epispadias, and reflux has been reported between 30% and 40% in a number of series. [p 2182]

35. **c. Bladder capacity at the time of bladder neck reconstruction.** In the epispadias group, much as in the exstrophy group, bladder capacity is the predominant indicator of eventual continence. [p 2183]

36. **c. 1 in 484,000 female births.** Female epispadias is a rare congenital anomaly occurring in 1 in 484,000 female patients. [p 2184]

37. **c. multiple and associated with bladder outlet obstruction.** Acquired bladder diverticula are usually multiple and associated with bladder outlet obstruction. [p 2189]

38. **b. Congenital bladder diverticula.** Congenital bladder diverticula have been described in children with Ehlers-Danlos syndrome and Menkes syndrome. [p 2189]

39. **d. Fistulography of the urachal tract.** Analysis of the periumbilical fluid for creatinine and urea is useful in differentiating a patent urachus from other conditions (e.g., omphalitis, granulation of a healing umbilical stump, patent omphalomesenteric duct, infected umbilical vessel, or external urachal sinus), and a fistulogram obtained with the use of radiopaque contrast material is often diagnostic. [pp 2190–2191]

40. **b. Excision of the patent urachus and cuff of bladder.** A more modern series by Cilento and colleagues (1998) recommended excision of both the anomaly and a cuff of bladder routinely. [p 2192]

Chapter 62

Surgical Technique for One-Stage Reconstruction of the Exstrophy-Epispadias Complex

Richard W. Grady • Michael E. Mitchell

Questions

1. Single-stage reconstruction using the complete primary exstrophy repair technique offers several advantages over staged reconstruction. Which of the following is NOT an advantage?

   a. The possibility of correcting the penile, bladder, and bladder neck abnormalities of bladder exstrophy with one operation.
   b. The potential to achieve urinary continence without bladder neck reconstruction.
   c. Correction of vesicoureteral reflux at the time of surgery.
   d. Lower complication rates than previous attempts at single-stage reconstruction.

2. What is the most important aspect of single-stage reconstruction using the complete primary exstrophy repair technique?

   a. Re-establishment of normal anatomic relationships
   b. Bladder neck reconstruction at the time of primary surgery
   c. Osteotomy at the time of single-stage reconstruction
   d. Simultaneous epispadias repair

3. All of the following postoperative factors have been shown to increase the success of reconstruction for bladder exstrophy except which one?

   a. Immobilization with, for example, external fixators, Buck's traction, or a spica cast
   b. Prolonged NPO (nothing by mouth) status to avoid abdominal distention
   c. Urinary diversion through ureteral stenting and suprapubic urinary drainage
   d. Adequate nutritional support

4. Single-stage reconstruction using the complete primary exstrophy repair technique can be safely performed for what reason?

   a. The neurovascular bundles of the corporeal bodies lie laterally rather than dorsally on the corporeal bodies.
   b. The cavernosal bodies and urethral wedge are not actually separated from each other with this technique.
   c. The blood supply to the corporeal bodies and urethral wedge are independent of each other.
   d. The blood supply is quickly re-established once the components are reassembled.

5. What are the proximal limits of dissection using the complete primary exstrophy repair technique?

   a. The intersymphyseal band
   b. The muscles of the pelvic floor complex
   c. The rectum
   d. The corpora spongiosa

6. What is the most important factor weighing against the use of a single-stage reconstruction technique for cloacal exstrophy?

   a. A large omphalocele
   b. A wide pubic diastasis
   c. A concomitant myelomeningocele
   d. Complete separation of the corpora cavernosa

7. Which of the following is a possible complication of the complete primary exstrophy repair technique?

   a. Myogenic bladder failure
   b. Testicular atrophy
   c. Urethrocutaneous fistula
   d. Hip dislocation

8. Penile disassembly during the complete primary repair for exstrophy in the boy is best initiated where?

   a. Along the dorsolateral aspect of the urethral plate
   b. At the anterior base of the penis
   c. Along the side of the penis over the neurovascular bundles
   d. With a circumcising incision on the ventral aspect of the penis

Answers

1. **c. Correction of vesicoureteral reflux at the time of surgery.** The single-stage anatomic approach offers many advantages. It offers the possibility of correction of the penile abnormalities, bladder abnormalities, and bladder neck abnormalities in one setting. These new techniques also have a lower complication rate than those reported in older series of single-stage reconstruction efforts. Finally, urinary continence can be achieved for many of these patients without the need for further bladder neck reconstruction. [p 2198]

2. **a. Re-establishment of normal anatomic relationships.** This technique effectively moves the bladder, bladder neck, and urethra posteriorly, thus positioning the proximal urethra within the pelvic diaphragm in an anatomically normal position. [p 2198]

3. **b. Prolonged NPO (nothing by mouth) status to avoid abdominal distention.** Postoperative factors that appear to have a direct impact on the success of initial closure include (1) postoperative immobilization; (2) use of postoperative antibiotics; (3) ureteral stenting catheters; (4) adequate postoperative pain management; (5) avoidance of abdominal distention; (6) adequate nutritional support; and (7) secure fixation of urinary drainage catheters. [p 2200]

4. **c. The blood supply to the corporeal bodies and urethral wedge are independent of each other.** The corporeal bodies may be completely separated from each other because they have a separate blood supply (see Fig. 62–8). It is important to keep the underlying corpora spongiosa with the urethral plate; the blood supply to the urethral plate is based on this corporeal tissue, which should appear wedge-shaped after its dissection from the adjacent corpora cavernosa. [p 2202]

5. **b. The muscles of the pelvic floor complex.** Deep incision of the intersymphyseal ligaments posterior and lateral to each side of the urethral wedge is absolutely necessary to allow the bladder to achieve a posterior position in the pelvis (see Fig. 62–9). This dissection should be carried until the pelvic floor musculature becomes visible. [p 2202]

6. **a. A large omphalocele.** A large omphalocele, in particular, will make single-stage closure hazardous. [p 2204]

7. **c. Urethrocutaneous fistula.** As is the case with any operation, operative complications can occur following complete primary exstrophy repair. These include urethrocutaneous fistula formation. In our experience, these fistulas often close spontaneously with proper urinary diversion. Dehiscence of the primary closure can also occur. After complete primary exstrophy repair, if the bladder and urethra have been adequately dissected, fascial dehiscence should not jeopardize the bladder and urethral closure. This is in marked contrast to the devastating consequences of wound dehiscence following a staged primary closure. Following complete primary exstrophy repair, some patients develop bladder and kidney infections. They should be appropriately evaluated to ensure that they have no evidence of outlet obstruction. We routinely maintain our patients on suppressive antibiotic therapy if they have vesicoureteral reflux. Other complications that have been reported following complete primary exstrophy repair include atrophy of the corpora cavernosa and urethra. These complications can occur if the blood supply to the corporeal bodies or urethral wedge are damaged during dissection. [p 2205]

8. **d. With a circumcising incision on the ventral aspect of the penis.** We begin the penile dissection along the ventral aspect of the penis as a circumcising incision (see Fig. 62–6). This should precede dissection of the urethral wedge from the corporeal bodies because it is easier to identify Buck's fascia ventrally. [p 2201]

Chapter 63

Posterior Urethral Valves and Other Urethral Anomalies

Edmond T. Gonzales, Jr.

Questions

1. What is a type I posterior urethral valve?
   a. A fold of tissue running between the bladder neck and verumontanum
   b. A web of tissue at the level of the bulbar urethra
   c. A membrane of tissue from the proximal verumontanum dorsally to the bladder neck
   d. A diaphragm of tissue with a central lumen at the level of the membranous urethra
   e. A membrane of tissue from the verumontanum to the membranous urethra

2. A lesion in the urethra is located at the bulbar urethra and is described as a diaphragm of tissue with a central lumen. This is best defined as a:
   a. type II valve.
   b. type I valve.
   c. type III valve.
   d. anterior urethra valve.
   e. plica colliculi.

3. What is the most common form of clinical presentation of a school-aged boy with posterior urethral valves?
   a. Sepsis
   b. Failure to thrive
   c. Hypertension
   d. Incontinence
   e. Weak urinary stream

4. When renal dysplasia is associated with posterior urethral valves, it is best characterized by:
   a. microcystic and most severe findings in the peripheral cortical zone.
   b. medullary loss and fibrosis of the cortex.
   c. diffuse heterotopic cartilage and macrocysts.
   d. glomerulosclerosis and cartilage formation.
   e. nephrogenic rests and macrocystic changes.

5. What is the most important determinant of ultimate renal outcome in a child with valves?

a. Presence of vesicoureteral reflux
b. Bladder function
c. Occurrence of infections
d. Presence of renal dysplasia
e. Degree of hydronephrosis at presentation

6. A newborn with posterior urethral valves is found to have bilateral grade 4 reflux and undergoes successful valve ablation. Because of the reflux, which procedure should this child undergo?

    a. Bilateral ureteral reimplantation
    b. Vesicostomy
    c. Bilateral ureterostomies
    d. End-cutaneous ureterostomies
    e. Observation and another voiding cystourethrogram

7. The urodynamic character of the bladder in a boy with posterior urethral valves prior to valve ablation is best described as:

    a. myogenic failure.
    b. hypertonic.
    c. dyssynergic.
    d. hyperreflexic.
    e. compliant.

8. What is a significant predictor of eventual end-stage renal failure in an adolescent with posterior urethral valves?

    a. Absence of vesicoureteral reflux
    b. Prior urinary diversion
    c. Need for intermittent catheterization
    d. Urinary incontinence
    e. Continued hydronephrosis

9. A newborn boy with posterior urethral valves and bilateral grade 5 reflux has had a bladder catheter in place for 4 days and his serum creatinine value is 0.7 mg/dl. Renal ultrasonography shows moderately severe hydroureteronephrosis, similar to his initial study. He is metabolically stable. What is the best management?

    a. Continued bladder catheterization
    b. Transurethral valve ablation
    c. Vesicostomy
    d. Bilateral ureteral reimplantation and valve ablation
    e. Bilateral proximal ureterostomies

10. The anatomy of an anterior urethral valve indicates that it is usually:

    a. a urethral diverticulum.
    b. a dilated duct of Cowper's gland.
    c. insufficiency of the corpus spongiosum.
    d. a diaphragmatic web across the urethra.
    e. a form of urethral duplication.

11. A newborn boy is found to have a urinary stream from a urethral meatus located in the glans and a stream from the perineum. What does this most likely represent?

    a. Congenital urethrocutaneous fistula to the perineum, which should be resected
    b. A form of imperforate anus with rectourethral fistula
    c. Urethral duplication with functional perineal urethra
    d. Severe hypospadias
    e. A cloacal anomaly with urethral duplication

Answers

1. **e. A membrane of tissue from the verumontanum to the membranous urethra.** A type I urethral valve is an obstructing membrane that arises from the posterior and inferior edge of the verumontanum and radiates distally toward the membranous urethra, inserting anteriorly near the proximal margin of the membranous urethra. [p 2209]

2. **c. type III valve.** Type III valves are believed to represent incomplete dissolution of the urogenital membrane. The obstructing membranes are situated distal to the verumontanum, at the level of the membranous urethra. These lesions have been classically described as discrete ring-like membranes with a central aperture. [p 2210]

3. **d. Incontinence.** Patients presenting during the toddler years are more likely to have somewhat better renal function and generally present because of urinary infection or voiding dysfunction. Boys of school age, the least common age for presentation, more often will have voiding dysfunction, which is generally recognized as urinary incontinence, as their primary complaint. [p 2212]

4. **a. microcystic and most severe findings in the peripheral cortical zone.** Renal parenchymal dysplasia is commonly associated with urethral valves. The renal dysplasia seen in association with urethral valves tends to be microcystic in nature and develops most severely in the peripheral cortical zone. It has long been suspected that this dysplasia is a result of the primitive metanephric blastema maturing in the presence of high intraluminal pressures. [p 2214]

5. **d. Presence of renal dysplasia.** Regardless of the mechanism that initiates abnormal parenchymal histology, it is clear that the development of dysplasia is an early embryologic event. The presence of renal dysplasia is the single most significant abnormality that will determine ultimate renal function, and it is perhaps the only aspect of this congenital disorder over which the clinician has no influence. [p 2214]

6. **e. Observation and another voiding cystourethrogram.** The presence of vesicoureteral reflux should not in itself influence the initial management of children with posterior urethral valves. In about one third of cases, the reflux will resolve spontaneously after obstruction is eliminated. [p 2217]

7. **b. hypertonic.** In one study of 16 infants, all patients had urodynamic testing before valve ablation and were followed postoperatively with serial urodynamic studies. In all boys preoperatively, the bladder was small in capacity and hypercontractile. After destruction of the valves, the bladder capacity increased, although the bladder continued to show some instability and some boys demonstrated incomplete emptying. A report of a second series of boys followed into late adolescence indicated that the pattern of bladder abnormality changed as the children got older and progressed from instability during infancy to myogenic failure in older boys. [p 2217]

8. **d. Urinary incontinence.** One study that followed a series of children with urethral valves into adolescence observed that those children who were incontinent during childhood ultimately developed more severe degrees of renal insufficiency during adolescence than did children who had dem-

onstrated normal urinary control. The researchers proposed that children who were incontinent had more severe bladder dysfunction than did those children who had normal urinary control. [p 2217]

9. **b. Transurethral valve ablation.** In the presence of normal or satisfactory renal function (most often described as a serum creatinine value of less than 1.0 mg/dl in the newborn after several days of catheter drainage, although a healthy neonate at 4 weeks of age may have a serum creatinine value of 0.2 to 0.4 mg/dl), endoscopic destruction of the valves would be considered. [p 2218]

10. **a. a urethral diverticulum.** An anterior urethral valve, in nearly all cases, is actually a congenital urethral diverticulum. During voiding, the diverticulum expands, ballooning ventrally and distally beneath the thinned corpus spongiosum. The flap-like dorsal margin of the diverticulum then extends into the urethral lumen, occluding urinary flow (an obstructing valve). [p 2225]

11. **c. Urethral duplication with functional perineal urethra.** Urinary flow is preferentially through the perianal urethral opening, and the ventral urethra is generally considered the more normal urethra, because it traverses the sphincter mechanism. [p 2228]

Chapter 64

Voiding Dysfunction in Children: Neurogenic and Non-Neurogenic

Stuart B. Bauer • Stephen A. Koff • Venkata R. Jayanthi

Questions

1. What is the risk in the United States of having a child with spina bifida?
   a. 1:500
   b. 1:750
   c. 1:1000
   d. 1:1250
   e. 1:1500

2. Which of the following statements about the neurologic lesion in myelodysplasia is true?
   a. The neurologic lesion is predictable from the height of the bony defect.
   b. Children with similar bony levels have similar neurologic lesions.
   c. Children with thoracic-level lesions often have intact sacral cord function.
   d. Children with sacral cord lesions usually have normal bladder function.
   e. The neurologic lesion at birth is stable and does not change throughout childhood.

3. The urodynamic findings of newborns with myelodysplasia are best characterized by:
   a. bladder reflexia.
   b. bladder areflexia.
   c. normal sphincter innervation.
   d. detrusor sphincter synergy.
   e. detrusor sphincter dyssynergy.

4. How is grade IV/V vesicoureteral reflux in children with myelodysplasia best managed?
   a. Credé voiding
   b. Anticholinergic medication alone
   c. Clean intermittent catheterization (CIC) plus anticholinergic medication
   d. Antireflux surgery
   e. Antibiotics alone

5. Urinary incontinence in children with myelodysplasia is treated initially with:
   a. intermittent catheterization plus alpha-sympathomimetics.
   b. intermittent catheterization plus alpha-sympatholytics.
   c. intermittent catheterization plus anticholinergics.
   d. bladder neck reconstruction.
   e. augmentation cystoplasty.

6. Which of the following statements is true about occult spinal dysraphism (OSD)?
   a. Ninety percent of children with OSD have a cutaneous back lesion overlying the lower spine.
   b. Most infants have a neurologic deficit.
   c. Most older children have normal urodynamic function.
   d. The incidence of neurourologic lesions is stable throughout childhood.
   e. Urinary incontinence is rarely noted in untreated older children.

7. Which of the following statements regarding the diagnosis of sacral agenesis is NOT true?
   a. Insulin-dependent mothers have a 1% chance of having a child with sacral agenesis.
   b. The diagnosis is often made only after the child fails to toilet train at a reasonable age.
   c. The appearance of the lower back and gluteal cleft are rarely suggestive of the diagnosis.
   d. A lateral film of the lower spine most easily confirms the diagnosis of sacral agenesis.
   e. MRI reveals a characteristic cutoff to the spinal cord at the level of T12.

8. Which of the following statements is true regarding imperforate anus?

a. It is usually an isolated lesion.
b. Renal abnormalities are seen in more than one third of the children, especially those with high lesions.
c. Girls are affected more often than boys.
d. Spinal cord anomalies occur in less than 10% of affected children.
e. Neurogenic bladder dysfunction is rare, even in cases of a spinal cord abnormality.

9. Which of the following statements is true regarding cerebral palsy?

   a. It is rarely seen in premature infants with low birth weight.
   b. It is unusual in those children who had an infection or seizure in early childhood.
   c. It is often the consequence of a period of anoxia in early infancy.
   d. It is never the result of maternal infection during later pregnancy.
   e. It is a progressive neurologic disorder.

10. The mechanism of spinal cord injuries in children differs from that in adults in which of the following ways?

    a. The upper cervical vertebrae acting as a fulcrum for the head
    b. The delayed support of paraspinous muscles and ligaments
    c. The horizontal versus the vertical orientation of the facet joints of the upper vertebral bodies
    d. All of the above
    e. None of the above

11. What is the best way to manage the child after the initial insult from a spinal cord injury?

    a. Check urine residuals and, if they are low, continue observation.
    b. Begin intermittent catheterization as soon as feasible after the injury has occurred.
    c. Start antibiotics to prevent urinary infection once the child has stabilized.
    d. Initiate anticholinergic agents along with intermittent catheterization early in the course of treatment.
    e. All of the above.

Non-Neurogenic Dysfunction
Stephen A. Koff • Venkata R. Jayanthi

12. Which of the following statements best characterizes bladder emptying in the newborn child?

    a. Bladder function is similar to that in the older child and adult.
    b. Coordination between bladder and sphincter is usually present.
    c. Most voiding occurs while the infant is awake.
    d. Bladder emptying is neither complete nor coordinated.
    e. Residual urine volume after voiding is usually normal (<10% capacity).

13. Which of the following statements best characterizes bladder and sphincter function in the normal male infant?

    a. Voiding generally occurs at pressures that are lower than those in adults.
    b. Bladder instability occurs commonly (>35%).
    c. Voluntary control over the sphincter muscles develops in utero.
    d. Continence depends on developing control over bladder smooth muscle.
    e. More complete bladder emptying occurs in the supine position.

14. Because functional obstruction occurs during voiding rather than filling, which pattern of dysfunctional elimination is potentially most harmful to the urinary tract?

    a. The unstable bladder
    b. Infrequent voiding syndrome
    c. Small-capacity hypertonic bladder
    d. The urgency incontinence syndrome
    e. The non-neurogenic neurogenic bladder

15. A 6-year-old boy who presents with urgency and day and night incontinence is suspected of having bladder instability. Ultrasonographic study shows no hydronephrosis. Voiding cystourethrography (VCUG) reveals grade I left-sided reflux. In addition to antibiotic prophylaxis, an empirical trial of an anticholinergic agent is planned. Which of the following diagnostic features would suggest that anticholinergic medication is not appropriate?

    a. History of urinary tract infection (UTI) 18 months ago
    b. Bladder wall thickening
    c. Left-sided bladder diverticulum
    d. Squatting to keep from wetting
    e. Presence of residual urine

16. Children with bladder instability who develop the most severe functional urinary obstruction often do NOT display which of the following factors?

    a. Normal voiding pressure
    b. Bladder wall thickening
    c. Urinary incontinence
    d. Reflux
    e. UTI

17. Which of the following therapies is inappropriate for treating a 7-year-old girl with bladder instability, grade 2 bilateral reflux, and recurrent UTI?

    a. Prophylactic antibiotics to prevent UTI
    b. Laxatives to treat constipation
    c. Anticholinergic medication for bladder instability
    d. Frequent voiding program for bladder instability
    e. Forcing fluids to prevent UTI

18. Fecal retention and constipation are often associated with which of the following urinary tract abnormalities?

    a. UTI
    b. Bladder instability
    c. Increased residual urine volume
    d. Vesicoureteral reflux
    e. All of the above

19. When severe urinary frequency (voiding every 30 minutes) suddenly develops in a toilet-trained boy and occurs only in the daytime, without incontinence or a UTI:

a. the most likely diagnosis is meatal stenosis.
b. VCUG is required for evaluation.
c. neurologic investigation for cord tethering is needed.
d. symptoms should resolve in a few weeks or months.
e. anticholinergic medication is usually effective therapy.

20. Which of the following statements best characterizes children with nocturnal enuresis?

    a. There is a 15% spontaneous resolution rate.
    b. It is more common in girls than in boys.
    c. Most enuretics wet during the daytime and nighttime.
    d. Encopresis is common in enuretics until 9 years of age.
    e. Enuretics who become dry by 12 years of age do not relapse.

21. What is the most constant urodynamic finding in children with monosymptomatic nocturnal enuresis (MNE)?

    a. Nocturnal bladder instability
    b. Normal urodynamic examination
    c. A small functional bladder capacity
    d. Detrusor-sphincter dyssynergia
    e. A weak striated muscle sphincter

22. What is the most common cause for MNE?

    a. Sleeping too deeply
    b. An abnormality in vasopressin secretion
    c. Bladder instability during sleep
    d. Genetic predisposition
    e. A delay in development

23. Evaluation of the child with nocturnal enuresis requires a history, physical examination, and urinalysis. In addition, it is important to perform a genitourinary ultrasonographic study to screen the urinary tract of the child who also has:

    a. daytime incontinence.
    b. bedwetting every night of the week.
    c. no family history of bedwetting.
    d. postvoiding incontinence.
    e. an attention deficit disorder (e.g., attention-deficit hyperactivity disorder).

24. What does the most effective form of cure for MNE involve?

    a. Desmopressin (DDAVP)
    b. Urinary alarm
    c. Imipramine
    d. Bladder training
    e. Bladder-stretching exercises

Answers

1. **c. 1:1000.** The incidence had been reported as 1 per 1000 births in the United States. [p 2234]

2. **c. Children with thoracic-level lesions often have intact sacral cord function.** Children with thoracic and upper lumbar meningoceles often have complete reconstitution of the spine in the sacral area, and these individuals frequently have intact sacral reflex arc function. [p 2236]

3. **a. bladder reflexia.** Urodynamic studies in the newborn period have shown that 57% of infants have bladder contractions. [p 2237]

4. **c. Clean intermittent catheterization (CIC) plus anticholinergic medication.** In children with high-grade reflux, CIC is begun to ensure complete emptying. Children with detrusor hypertonicity with or without hydroureteronephrosis are also started with oxybutynin to lower intravesical pressure. When reflux has been managed in this manner, there has been a dramatic response, with reflux resolving in 30% to 55% of individuals. [p 2240]

5. **c. intermittent catheterization plus anticholinergics.** Initial attempts at achieving continence include CIC and drug therapy designed to maintain low intravesical pressures. [pp 2241–2242]

6. **a. Ninety percent of children with OSD have a cutaneous back lesion overlying the lower spine.** In more than 90% of children, there is a cutaneous abnormality overlying the lower spine. [p 2245]

7. **c. The appearance of the lower back and gluteal cleft are rarely suggestive of the diagnosis.** The only clue, besides a high index of suspicion, is flattened buttocks and a low short gluteal cleft. [p 2248]

8. **b. Renal abnormalities are seen in more than one third of the children, especially those with high lesions.** Urinary tract abnormalities have been noted in 26% to 52% of affected children, with renal agenesis (primarily left-sided) and vesicoureteral reflux the most common associated findings. [p 2251]

9. **c. It is often the consequence of a period of anoxia in early infancy.** The condition is usually due to a perinatal infection, or a period of anoxia that affects the central nervous system. [p 2253]

10. **d. All of the above.** The horizontal versus the vertical orientation of the facet joints in vertebral bodies that predisposes to anteroposterior subluxation in children, the delayed supportive effect of the paraspinous musculature and ligaments, and the relative heaviness of the head, which causes a fulcrum of maximal flexion of the upper cervical region in infants and young children, all contribute to a high degree of hypermobility that predisposes the child's spinal cord to ischemic necrosis. [p 2254]

11. **b. Begin intermittent catheterization as soon as feasible after the injury has occurred.** An indwelling Foley catheter is passed into the bladder and left in place for as short a time as possible, until the patient is stable and aseptic intermittent catheterization can be started safely on a regular basis. [p 2255]

12. **d. Bladder emptying is neither complete nor coordinated.** Bladder emptying is neither complete nor coordinated; it often takes two or three small voidings to completely empty the bladder, and residual urine volumes of up to 30% of capacity are typical. [p 2262]

13. **d. Continence depends on developing control over bladder smooth muscle.** Direct volitional control over the spinal reflex that controls the detrusor smooth muscle must develop for the child to be able to voluntarily initiate or inhibit detrusor contraction. [p 2262]

14. **e. The non-neurogenic neurogenic bladder.** Patients with non-neurogenic neurogenic bladder demonstrate a functional

obstruction that occurs during voiding to produce severe clinical manifestations that are as prominent as those observed in patients with true neurogenic bladder disease. [p 2263]

15. **e. Presence of residual urine.** Children with bladder instability void normally to completion without residue, so the occurrence of a large residual urine volume should make the diagnosis suspect. [p 2268]

16. **c. Urinary incontinence.** Paradoxically, up to one third of children with bladder instability have no incontinence. [p 2268]

17. **e. Forcing fluids to prevent UTI.** The practice of forcing fluids to children with bladder instability is inappropriate therapy; it will cause the bladder to rapidly overfill to exceed threshold volumes. [p 2269]

18. **e. All of the above.** It has been noted that fecal retention was associated with reflux, hydronephrosis, enuresis, and UTI. Radiographic alteration of the shape of the bladder neck and urethra by the fecal mass and abnormal voiding patterns with a hesitant and interrupted stream were observed. [p 2270]

19. **d. symptoms should resolve in a few weeks or months.** The daytime urinary frequency syndrome occurs relatively commonly. It is characterized by the development of sudden, severe and often dramatic daytime urinary frequency without incontinence in healthy young children (mean age 4.5 years) without any identifiable antecedent illness or injury and with no history of UTI. The natural history is one of spontaneous resolution after several months. [p 2273]

20. **a. There is a 15% spontaneous resolution rate.** More girls than boys are dry both day and night by the age of 2 years, and nocturnal enuresis is 50% more common in boys than in girls. Nocturnal enuresis has a spontaneous resolution rate of 15% per year, so that by age 15 years it persists in only 1% of the population (see Table 64–11). [p 2273]

21. **c. A small functional bladder capacity.** The single most important urodynamic observation in MNE is a reduced bladder capacity. This reduction has been shown to be functional, not anatomic, by measurements of bladder capacity obtained with the patient under anesthesia. [p 2273]

22. **e. A delay in development.** In most children, MNE represents a delay in development, and each of the physiologic alterations tends to improve with time and to resolve spontaneously. [p 2275]

23. **a. daytime incontinence.** A carefully obtained history, a physical examination, and a urinalysis are sufficient for most children with primary MNE. The goal of evaluation is to identify children who require further study. Clues such as a history of urinary infection, diurnal incontinence, or obstructive symptoms or subtle signs of neuropathy must be pursued. In their absence, there is generally no indication for radiographic studies or cystoscopy, because the incidence of associated uropathology is so low. [p 2277]

24. **b. Urinary alarm.** In controlled studies, the urinary alarm is superior to drug therapy, imipramine, or DDAVP, with a cure rate of 60% to 100% (80% in the authors' experience) after discontinuation. When compared directly with DDAVP, the alarm cure rate is significantly better, and after therapy, the relapse rate with DDAVP is 10 times greater. [p 2279]

Chapter 65

Hypospadias

Alan B. Retik • Joseph G. Borer

Questions

1. When is the level of the hypospadiac defect most appropriately defined?
   a. At diagnosis in the absence of penile curvature
   b. After correction of penile curvature (orthoplasty), when necessary
   c. At any time before repair
   d. Both a and b are correct.

2. Embryologically, the endodermal differentiation theory purports that the distal glanular portion of the urethra is formed by:
   a. differentiation of ectodermal tissue into stratified squamous epithelium.
   b. an invagination of surface epithelium of ectodermal origin.
   c. differentiation of endodermal tissue into stratified squamous epithelium.
   d. closure of the urethral folds in the dorsal midline.

3. Disruption of the normal endocrine milieu as a possible cause of hypospadias has been supported by which of the following?
   a. Maternal progestin intake during pregnancy
   b. An increased rate of hypospadias in male offspring conceived by in vitro fertilization
   c. An 8.5-fold higher rate of hypospadias in one of monozygotic male twins compared with singleton live male births
   d. All of the above

4. Recent developments regarding the etiology of penile curvature noted on histologic evaluation of boys with hypospadias include which of the following?
   a. Subepithelial biopsy of the urethral plate revealing well-vascularized smooth muscle and collagen
   b. Findings that differ from those of a fetus with hypospadias
   c. A band of dense fibrous tissue composed of abortive corpus spongiosum
   d. "Scar" tissue of epithelial origin

5. All of the following are causes of penile curvature without hypospadias. Which is thought to be the least common?
   a. Skin tethering
   b. Fibrotic dartos tissue
   c. A congenitally short urethra
   d. Corporeal disproportion

6. Two independent and well-established congenital anomaly registries in the United States have shown trends in hypospadias prevalence that are best summarized in which of the following statement(s)?
   a. A near-doubling of hypospadias rates has occurred in the most recent decade compared with immediately preceding decades.
   b. The prevalence for hypospadias is approximately 1 in every 250 live male births.
   c. There has been a three- to fivefold increase in the occurrence of severe hypospadias.
   d. All of the above.

7. Which of the following findings on physical examination should raise the suspicion of an intersex state in a presumed male with hypospadias?
   a. Midpenile shaft hypospadias with otherwise normal examination findings
   b. Bilateral cryptorchidism in a patient without hypospadias
   c. Either unilateral or bilateral cryptorchidism with any degree of hypospadias
   d. Distal hypospadias with descended, palpably normal gonads, and a normal-appearing scrotum

8. Which of the following statements regarding imaging in patients with hypospadias is true?
   a. Voiding cystourethrography (VCUG) may aid in the management of severe hypospadias.
   b. A "genitogram" is indicated for the patient with severe hypospadias and nonpalpable gonads.
   c. Because of the high incidence of concomitant pathology, all patients with hypospadias should undergo some form of radiologic evaluation of the upper urinary tract.
   d. Both a and b are true.

9. Preoperative androgen stimulation or administration in patients with severe hypospadias has had all of the following results except which one?
   a. Decreased penile size (from normal) in adulthood
   b. An approximately 50% increase in penile size compared with preadministration measurement as noted by several investigators
   c. Hormonal levels that return to normal shortly after cessation of treatment
   d. No appreciable lasting undesirable side effects of treatment

10. Preferably, local tissue flaps used for urethral reconstruction have all of the following characteristics except which one?
    a. Axial blood supply preserved within dartos fascia
    b. Thin, nonhirsute, and reliably tailored tissue
    c. Blood supply and drainage via the internal iliac vessels
    d. If an island flap type, maintenance of vascular and division of cutaneous continuity

11. Which of the following statements regarding tissue grafts is true?
    a. They rely on inosculation, defined as the diffusion of nutrient material from the adjacent graft host bed into the graft during the first 48 hours after placement.
    b. They rely on imbibition, defined as the formation of new and permanent vascularization of the graft.
    c. They survive in a graft host bed after successful completion of a process called "take."
    d. By definition, they imply use of transferred tissue with an intact blood supply and drainage.

12. In various forms, perhaps the single most important adjunctive measure to urethroplasty for the purpose of decreasing the risk of postoperative urethrocutaneous fistula formation is the use of:
    a. a compressive penile dressing.
    b. autologous dermal graft for orthoplasty.
    c. postoperative urinary diversion with an indwelling urethral catheter.
    d. subcutaneous (dartos) tissue second-layer neourethral coverage.

13. Appropriate statements regarding intraoperative hemostasis include all of the following except which one?
    a. Liberal use of monopolar electrocautery is encouraged in the well-vascularized glans and other penile tissues.
    b. Intermittent use of a tourniquet at the base of the penis may optimize visualization of tissues during urethroplasty.
    c. Bipolar electrocautery may have advantages over monopolar technology.
    d. In general, methods of achieving hemostasis without causing permanent tissue devitalization are preferred.

14. Ketoconazole may be used to eliminate postoperative penile erections in adolescent and adult males after hypospadias repair. Which of the following best describes the method of action for ketoconazole?
    a. It decreases production of cholesterol.
    b. It inhibits conversion of androstenedione to testosterone.
    c. It reduces both adrenal and testicular androgen production through the inhibition of the enzyme 17,20-desmolase.
    d. It directly inhibits 5α-reductase activity.

15. Ideal conditions for the MAGPI (meatoplasty and glanuloplasty) hypospadias repair technique include which of the following?
    a. Glanular hypospadias with adequate urethral mobility and no penile curvature
    b. Distal hypospadias with or without mild penile curvature, regardless of urethral characteristics
    c. Middle and distal hypospadias with no penile curvature
    d. All distal hypospadias not amenable to repair by tubularization techniques

16. Characteristics of the tubularized, incised plate (TIP) urethroplasty technique for hypospadias repair include which of the following?
    a. The TIP urethroplasty technique is a modification of the Thiersch-Duplay technique of hypospadias repair.
    b. The TIP urethroplasty technique incorporates a longitudinal urethral plate "relaxing incision" to allow tension-free tubularization of the neourethra.
    c. The TIP urethroplasty technique is applicable to only distal hypospadias defects.
    d. Both a and b are correct.

17. The onlay island flap technique for hypospadias repair is best summarized by which of the following statements?
    a. Use of the onlay island flap technique is limited to middle and anterior hypospadias.
    b. Since introduction of the onlay island flap technique in 1987, its applicability has expanded to include proximal hypospadias defects.

c. A high complication rate has prohibited generalized use of the onlay island flap technique.
d. Popularity of this technique and its excellent results are due to a highly efficient take process.

18. Although a "two-stage" hypospadias repair is controversial, indications for such a repair may include which of the following?

    a. Parental request
    b. Penoscrotal hypospadias with mild to moderate curvature
    c. Middle hypospadias in the patient with a previously failed hypospadias repair
    d. The patient with a scrotal or perineal hypospadias, severe curvature, and a small penis

19. An accurate statement(s) regarding general principles of reoperative hypospadias repair includes which of the following?

    a. Attempts at reoperative hypospadias surgery should not be undertaken less than approximately 6 months after previous failure of repair.
    b. The first choice of method for a repeated hypospadias repair involves use of extragenital tissue as a free graft.
    c. No attempt at repair should be entertained until all edema, infection, and/or inflammation have resolved and healing is complete.
    d. Both a and c are correct.

20. What is the role of the postoperative use of uroflowmetry?

    a. It will ensure long-term patency of the repair if normal parameters are documented in the immediate postoperative period.
    b. It may identify an asymptomatic urethral stricture in some patients.
    c. It has been helpful in determining viability of tissue used in complex, posterior hypospadias repair.
    d. It should be compared with routine preoperative uroflowmetry for all patients who undergo hypospadias repair.

Answers

1. **d. both a and b are correct.** Culp, in 1959, was perhaps the first to classify the level of hypospadias after any necessary treatment of penile curvature (orthoplasty) and realize the importance of this method. In 1973, Barcat more formally proposed designating the location of the hypospadiac meatus, and thus the true extent of the urethral defect requiring repair, after orthoplasty. [pp 2285–2286]

2. **c. differentiation of endodermal tissue into stratified squamous epithelium.** One study provided further support for the endodermal differentiation theory using tissue recombinant grafting techniques, which suggest that under the correct cellular signaling conditions, endodermally derived epithelium (urethral plate) differentiates into the stratified squamous epithelial phenotype present in the fully developed distal glanular urethra. [p 2287]

3. **d. all of the above.** A study investigating pathogenetic mechanisms that might have interfered with fetal testicular differentiation and/or function found a history of maternal progestin intake early in pregnancy, either for treatment of threatened abortion or in combination with estrogen for pregnancy testing. When the position of the urethral meatus was compared with the week of gestation at which progestin therapy was begun, a positive correlation was noted for more proximal hypospadias in mothers treated in the first month of pregnancy. Further support of an endocrine disruptor origin for hypospadias may be provided by markedly increased rates of hypospadias in male offspring conceived by in vitro fertilization (progesterone given early for pregnancy support). Also, another group noted an 8.5-fold higher rate of hypospadias in one of monozygotic male twins compared with singleton live male births. These authors suggested that this strong association of monozygotic twinning and hypospadias may be due to an inability of a single placenta and reduced human chorionic gonadotropin levels to meet the requirements of two developing male fetuses. [pp 2289–2291]

4. **a. subepithelial biopsy of the urethral plate revealing well-vascularized smooth muscle and collagen.** A report has challenged most of the historical tenets that typically vilified the urethral plate as the sole source or a contributing factor in chordee or penile curvature. Using light microscopy and routine staining techniques, these investigators showed that subepithelial biopsy of the urethral plate in 17 boys with hypospadias, including 5 with curvature and 4 with penoscrotal defects, revealed well-vascularized smooth muscle and collagen without fibrous bands or dysplastic tissue. These results were consistent with histologic findings at autopsy in a boy with proximal hypospadias and a fetus with distal hypospadias. [p 2290]

5. **c. a congenitally short urethra.** One report evenly divided the cause of congenital penile curvature without hypospadias in a series of 87 patients into three categories: (1) skin tethering, (2) fibrotic dartos and Buck's fasciae, and (3) corporeal disproportion. According to these authors, a congenitally short urethra was a rare cause of isolated curvature. [p 2291]

6. **d. all of the above.** In 1997, two independent and well-established surveillance systems in the United States, the Metropolitan Atlanta Congenital Defects Program (MACDP) and the nationwide Birth Defects Monitoring Program (BDMP), reported near-doubling of hypospadias rates in the most recent decade compared with immediately preceding decades. As measured by the BDMP, hypospadias rates increased from 2.02 per 1000 male births in 1970 to 3.97 per 1000 male births in 1993. In other words, approximately 1 in every 250 live male births involved hypospadias. The rate of severe hypospadias increased three- to fivefold from 0.11 per 1000 male births in 1968 to between 0.27 and 0.55 per 1000 male births per year from 1990 to 1993 as recorded by the MACDP. [p 2291]

7. **c. either unilateral or bilateral cryptorchidism with any degree of hypospadias.** A high index of suspicion for an intersex state is important for a finding of a presumed male with any degree of hypospadias and cryptorchidism. [p 2292]

8. **d. both a and b are true.** In general, the literature does not support routine imaging of the urinary tract with either ultrasonography or intravenous urography for evaluation of children with isolated hypospadias, particularly when the hypospadiac meatus is middle or anterior in location. Retrograde injection of radiographic contrast material into the presumed urethral meatus (genitogram) is an essential component of the intersex evaluation when such an evaluation is deemed appropriate. Preoperative evaluation is more extensive in patients with posterior hypospadias and at our institution includes VCUG in those with a scrotal or perineal defect to

evaluate the frequent presence and extent of a prostatic utricle. [pp 2292–2295]

9. **a. decreased penile size (from normal) in adulthood.** In one report, testosterone enanthate was administered intramuscularly (2 mg/kg body weight), 5 and 2 weeks before reconstructive penile surgery. The authors noted a 50% increase in penile size and an increase in available skin and local vascularity in all patients. A near-doubling (from 3 to 5 cm) of the mean transverse length of the inner prepuce was also noted in some patients. In addition, the authors reported minimal side effects and a return of plasma testosterone levels to within the normal range for age within 6 months after therapy. Others have employed variations in the total dose and schedule of testosterone enanthate administration, using 25 mg intramuscularly once weekly for a total of either two or three injections. Other investigators have employed a 4-week period of local penile stimulation with daily application of dihydrotestosterone cream before hypospadias or epispadias repair. These authors reported a mean increase in penile circumference and length by 50% of pretreatment measurements, without any lasting side effects or gonadotropin level perturbation, or effects in the pubertal or postpubertal period. Hormonal manipulation, at any age, is not without risk. Caution must be exercised with regard to neonatal administration of human chorionic gonadotropin, in that evidence obtained from an experimental rat micropenis model supports delaying hormonal therapy until the pubertal period. However, one study of boys with congenital hypogonadotropic hypogonadism and micropenis concluded that one or two short courses of testosterone therapy in infancy and childhood (puberty) augmented adult penile size into the normal range. These results refute the theoretical concern, and experimental evidence, that testosterone treatment in infancy or childhood impairs penile growth in adolescence and compromises adult penile length. The conclusion that prepubertal exogenous testosterone administration does not adversely affect ultimate penile growth has been supported by the study of men with true precocious puberty or congenital adrenal hyperplasia, and by the study of growth and androgen receptor status of testosterone-stimulated human fetal penile tissue in vitro. [pp 2295–2296]

10. **c. blood supply and drainage via the internal iliac vessels.** Local tissue flaps used for urethral reconstruction must be thin, nonhirsute, and reliably tailored. These flaps are properly termed fasciocutaneous flaps, and the extended fascial system is called the dartos fascia. The vessels of the fasciocutaneous flap are preserved within the fascia, which provides a conduit for smaller arteries and veins. Axial blood supply and drainage are typically provided by branches of the deep and superficial external pudendal vessels, which are medial branches of the femoral vessels. The term *island flap* implies maintenance of vascular and division of cutaneous continuity. [pp 2299–2300]

11. **c. survive in a graft host bed after successful completion of a process called *take*.** The term *graft* implies that tissue has been excised from one location and transferred to a graft host bed, where a new blood supply develops by a process called *take*. As with all free grafts, a well-vascularized recipient site is crucial for optimal graft survival. The initial phase of take, called *imbibition*, relies on diffusion of nutrient material from the adjacent graft host bed into the graft and requires approximately 48 hours. This is followed by the second phase of take, inosculation, which is the formation of new and permanent vascularization of the graft, also requiring approximately 48 hours. [p 2300]

12. **d. subcutaneous (dartos) tissue second-layer neourethral coverage.** Second-layer coverage of the neourethra with the use of various vascularized flaps has significantly decreased urethrocutaneous fistula as a complication of hypospadias repair. [p 2300]

13. **a. liberal use of monopolar electrocautery is encouraged in the well-vascularized glans and other penile tissues.** On the basis of the hypothesis that some complications such as urethrocutaneous fistula and repair breakdown are, in part, a result of ischemic tissue necrosis, use of electrocautery should be limited, if used at all, during hypospadias repair. The current of monopolar cautery is dispersed to the remote grounding site, generally along the vessels, and in this way may irreparably damage tissue microvasculature. Other practitioners employing electrocautery may prefer the bipolar variant and the use of fine-point neurologic forceps. We favor injection of a vasoconstrictive agent (epinephrine diluted 1:200,000 with lidocaine [Xylocaine]) deep to proposed glanular incision(s), as well as intermittent use of a tourniquet at the base of the penis during urethroplasty. Other options for effective temporary hemostasis without permanent tissue devitalization include intermittent compression with gauze soaked in iced saline and/or epinephrine solution. [pp 2302–2303]

14. **c. reduces both adrenal and testicular androgen production through the inhibition of the enzyme 17,20-desmolase.** Ketoconazole reduces adrenal and testicular androgen production through the inhibition of 17,20-desmolase, thereby preventing the conversion of cholesterol to testosterone. [p 2304]

15. **a. glanular hypospadias with adequate urethral mobility and no penile curvature.** Glanular and some coronal hypospadias defects are amenable to the meatoplasty and glanuloplasty (MAGPI) technique (see Fig. 65–12), with excellent functional and cosmetic results, provided that there is adequate urethral mobility and no penile curvature. [pp 2305 and 2307]

16. **d. both a and b are correct.** A modification of the Thiersch-Duplay technique has been described by Snodgrass. The tubularized incised plate (TIP) urethroplasty combines modifications of the previously described techniques of urethral plate incision and tubularization. The concept of a urethral plate "relaxing incision" as an adjunct to hypospadias repair to allow tension-free neourethral tubularization was also described simultaneously by Pervovic. [p 2307]

17. **b. since introduction of the onlay island flap technique in 1987, its applicability has expanded to include proximal hypospadias defects.** Among the most commonly used techniques for repair of middle hypospadias is the onlay island flap (onlay, OIF) technique. Since its introduction for the repair of subcoronal and midshaft hypospadias, use of this technique has expanded in frequency and for indications to include more proximal defects as well. One 1994 study reported use of the technique in 374, or 33%, of the total hypospadias repairs during a 5-year period. Complications requiring reoperation occurred in 32 (8.6%) of 374 patients. Twenty-three (6%) of the patients developed a urethrocutaneous fistula. [p 2312]

18. **d. the patient with a scrotal or perineal hypospadias, severe curvature, and a small penis.** Because the majority of hypospadias can be repaired with a one-stage procedure, the use of two-stage techniques for repair of posterior hypospadias is controversial. In the setting of scrotal or perineal hypospadias, severe curvature and a small penis, we prefer to perform a two-stage repair. [p 2319]

19. **d. both a and c are correct.** In general, attempts at reoperative hypospadias surgery should not be undertaken less than 6 months after the previous failure of repair. Certainly, no

attempt at repair should be considered until all edema, infection, and/or inflammation have resolved and healing is complete. When possible, the use of immediately adjacent or local pedicled, well-vascularized tissue is preferred for reoperative hypospadias surgery. [p 2324]

20. **b. may identify an asymptomatic urethral stricture in some patients.** At some centers, this noninvasive study is a postoperative evaluation routine and has been of value in identifying asymptomatic urethral stricture in some patients. [p 2325]

Chapter 66

Abnormalities of the Genitalia in Boys and Their Surgical Management

Jack S. Elder

Questions

1. In the male, development of the external genitalia is stimulated by which substance(s)?

    a. Testosterone
    b. Dihydrotestosterone (DHT)
    c. Human chorionic gonadotropin
    d. Luteinizing hormone and follicle-stimulating hormone
    e. Maternal progesterone

2. In the male, what do the genital swellings become?

    a. The glans penis
    b. The urethra
    c. The penile shaft
    d. The scrotum
    e. The penis and scrotum

3. In a term male neonate, approximately how long is the mean stretched penile length?

    a. 2.5 cm
    b. 3.0 cm
    c. 3.5 cm
    d. 4.0 cm
    e. 4.5 cm

4. What is the approximate incidence of hypospadias?

    a. 1:50
    b. 1:125
    c. 1:250
    d. 1:500
    e. 1:1000

5. An 8-year-old boy has never been able to retract his foreskin. He has not had balanitis or balanoposthitis but experiences mild penile discomfort during erections. What is the most appropriate management?

    a. Application of topical corticosteroid cream
    b. Forceful retraction of the foreskin
    c. "Preputioplasty" (dorsal slit)
    d. Circumcision
    e. Observation

6. In a newborn undergoing circumcision, what risk is associated with EMLA cream for local anesthesia?

    a. Hepatic toxicity
    b. Cardiac arrhythmia
    c. Allergic reaction
    d. Prolonged bleeding time
    e. Methemoglobinemia

7. A newborn male undergoes circumcision and nearly all of the penile skin and foreskin is removed. What is the most appropriate therapy?

    a. Suture the skin edges together
    b. Split-thickness skin graft
    c. Full-thickness skin graft
    d. Application of adherent gauze and antibiotic ointment
    e. Application of small intestine submucosa graft

8. During a newborn circumcision, half of the glans is amputated and the urethra is transected. What is the most appropriate treatment?

    a. Split-thickness skin graft
    b. Application of adherent gauze and antibiotic ointment and insertion of a Foley catheter
    c. Suturing of excised tissue to penis, a nonmicroscopic repair
    d. Suturing of excised tissue to penis, a microscopic repair
    e. Coverage of raw glans with penile shaft skin

9. What is the normal size of the urethral meatus of a 2-year-old boy usually?

    a. 6 Fr
    b. 8 Fr
    c. 10 Fr
    d. 12 Fr
    e. 14 Fr

10. Which of the following statements is true regarding a micropenis in a term male newborn?

    a. It increases the likelihood of urinary tract infection.
    b. It is best managed by gender reassignment.
    c. It has a normal circumference but short length.
    d. It is less than 1.9 cm stretched length.
    e. It is unlikely to respond to testosterone stimulation until puberty.

11. What is the most common cause of micropenis?
    a. Hypogonadotropic hypogonadism
    b. Growth hormone deficiency
    c. Primary testicular failure
    d. Androgen insensitivity syndrome
    e. Inadequate human chorionic gonadotropin in utero

12. Micropenis is associated with:
    a. ear anomalies.
    b. cardiac anomalies.
    c. midline brain defects.
    d. myelodysplasia.
    e. VATER syndrome.

13. If a newborn male with micropenis is given three monthly intramuscular injections of testosterone enanthate, 25 mg, what is the result?
    a. The penis is unlikely to increase in size.
    b. Bone age will be higher than normal.
    c. Puberty will occur at an earlier age.
    d. The penis should still increase in size at puberty.
    e. The adult body habitus will probably be eunuchoid.

14. A male newborn with complete penoscrotal transposition and a normal scrotum commonly has which condition?
    a. Urinary tract abnormality
    b. Cardiac abnormality
    c. Sex chromosome abnormality
    d. Non–sex chromosome abnormality
    e. Tethered spinal cord

15. A newborn male has a strawberry hemangioma of the scrotum. At 6 months, the lesion is noted to have doubled in size. What is the appropriate management?
    a. Observation
    b. Surgical excision
    c. Neodymium:yttrium-aluminum-garnet laser therapy
    d. Argon laser therapy
    e. KTP laser therapy

Answers

1. **b. Dihydrotestosterone (DHT).** In the male embryo, differentiation of the external genitalia occurs between weeks 9 and 13 of gestation and requires production of testosterone by the testes as well as conversion of testosterone into DHT under the enzymatic influence of 5α-reductase in the genital anlagen. [p 2334]

2. **d. The scrotum.** Under the influence of DHT, the genital tubercle differentiates into the glans penis, the genital folds become the shaft of the penis, and the genital swellings migrate inferomedially, fusing in the midline to become the scrotum. [p 2334]

3. **c. 3.5 cm.** In a normal term male neonate, the penis is 3.5 ± 0.7 cm in stretched length and 1.1 ± 0.2 cm in diameter. [p 2334]

4. **c. 1:250.** A urethral deformity such as hypospadias or epispadias occurs in approximately 1 in 250 males. [p 2334]

5. **a. Application of topical corticosteroid cream.** In boys older than 4 or 5 years of age and those who develop balanitis or balanoposthitis, application of a topical corticosteroid cream (e.g., 0.1% dexamethasone) to the foreskin three or four times daily for 6 weeks loosens the phimotic ring in two thirds of the boys and usually allows the foreskin to be retracted manually. [p 2335]

6. **e. Methemoglobinemia.** The prilocaine in EMLA cream poses a risk for methemoglobinemia, although the risk is quite low. [p 2336]

7. **d. Application of adherent gauze and antibiotic ointment.** If too much penile shaft skin is removed, application of antibiotic ointment and adherent gauze to the open wound usually yields a satisfactory result. Typically, most of the skin will grow back and bridge the defect. [p 2337]

8. **c. Suturing of excised tissue to penis, a nonmicroscopic repair.** The most serious circumcision complications include urethral injury and removal of part of the glans or part or all of the penile shaft. Partial glans removal has been reported to occur with a Mogen clamp; in these cases, the excised tissue should be preserved and immediately sutured back to the penis. A microscopic repair is unnecessary. [p 2337]

9. **c. 10 Fr.** [p 2338]

10. **d. It is less than 1.9 cm stretched length.** Micropenis is defined as a normally formed penis that is at least 2.5 standard deviations below the mean in size (see Fig. 66–5A). Typically, the ratio of the length of the penile shaft to its circumference is normal. In general, the penis of a term newborn should be at least 1.9 cm long. Stretched penile length is used because it correlates more closely with erectile length than the relaxed length of the penis. [p 2340]

11. **a. Hypogonadotropic hypogonadism.** The most common cause of micropenis is failure of the hypothalamus to produce an adequate amount of gonadotropin-releasing hormone. This condition, termed *hypogonadotropic hypogonadism*, may result from hypothalamic dysfunction, such as Kallmann's syndrome (genito-olfactory dysplasia), Prader-Willi syndrome, Lawrence-Moon-Biedl syndrome, and the CHARGE association. [p 2341]

12. **c. midline brain defects.** Other major causes include congenital pituitary aplasia and midline brain defects such as agenesis of the corpus callosum and occipital encephalocele. [p 2341]

13. **d. The penis should still increase in size at puberty.** A report on eight boys with micropenis who were treated with androgens both at birth and at puberty showed that the final penile stretched length averaged 10.3 cm, and all were in the normal range. [p 2342]

14. **a. Urinary tract abnormality.** When there is complete penoscrotal transposition and a normal scrotum, as many as 75% of infants have a significant urinary tract abnormality, and a renal sonogram and voiding cystourethrogram should be obtained. [p 2346]

15. **a. Observation.** Strawberry hemangiomas, the most common type of genital hemangioma, result from proliferation of immature capillary vessels. Although the lesions may undergo a period of rapid growth lasting 3 to 6 months, gradual involution is common, and most lesions require no treatment. [p 2349]

Chapter 67

Abnormalities of the Testes and Scrotum and Their Surgical Management

Francis X. Schneck • Mark F. Bellinger

Questions

1. Most adolescent varicoceles evaluated by urologists are:

   a. painful.
   b. a cosmetic concern.
   c. asymptomatic.
   d. associated with an ipsilateral hydrocele.
   e. bilateral.

2. What is the most likely cause of testicular injury from varicocele?

   a. Elevated scrotal temperature
   b. Testicular hypoxia
   c. Effect of adrenal metabolites
   d. Altered levels of spermatic vein testosterone
   e. Testicular hypertension

3. What is the upper limit of difference in testis volume between right and left?

   a. 1 ml
   b. 2 ml
   c. 3 ml
   d. 4 ml
   e. 5 ml

4. Hydrocele formation after varicocele ligation is least likely to occur after which of the following procedures?

   a. Retroperitoneal ligation
   b. Subinguinal ligation
   c. Laparoscopic ligation
   d. Microscopic inguinal ligation
   e. Transvenous embolization

5. Irreversible ischemic injury of the testicular parenchyma begins how soon after torsion of the spermatic cord?

   a. 1 hour
   b. 2 hours
   c. 4 hours
   d. 6 hours
   e. 8 hours

6. One of the best physical findings indicative of torsion of the spermatic cord is:

   a. high-riding testis.
   b. absence of the cremasteric reflex.
   c. transverse lie of the testis.
   d. absent Doppler sounds.
   e. inflammatory hydrocele.

7. After manual detorsion of the spermatic cord, which of the following is appropriate management?

   a. Color Doppler ultrasonographic examination
   b. Radionuclide scan
   c. Doppler examination of the testis and spermatic cord
   d. Discharge of the patient and arrangement of an office re-evaluation in 1 week
   e. Immediate scrotal exploration

8. An adolescent is evaluated for a prior history of self-limited intermittent episodes of severe unilateral scrotal pain and swelling. Physical examination findings are normal. What is the most appropriate course of action?

   a. Color Doppler ultrasonographic examination
   b. Reassessment in 6 months
   c. Elective scrotal exploration
   d. Radionuclide scrotal imaging
   e. Immediate scrotal exploration

9. When diagnosis of a torsion of the appendix epididymis is made, which of the following is optimal management?

   a. Observation
   b. Color Doppler examination
   c. Radionuclide scrotal imaging
   d. Immediate exploration
   e. Cord block and manual detorsion

10. Most boys with sterile urine and a clinical diagnosis of epididymitis will be found to have which of the following conditions?

    a. Unilateral renal agenesis
    b. A large prostatic utricle
    c. Urethral stricture disease
    d. Persistent vasoureteral fusion
    e. Radiographically normal urinary tracts

11. If the cause of neonatal scrotal swelling appears to be an acute postnatal event, what is the most appropriate course of action to follow in a healthy neonate?

    a. Prompt surgical exploration of the affected testis
    b. Prompt surgical exploration of the affected testis with contralateral scrotal exploration
    c. Color Doppler imaging of the scrotum
    d. Radionuclide testicular scan
    e. Observation

12. What is the major gene responsible for male sexual differentiation?

    a. *TDF*
    b. *SOX*
    c. *WT-1*

d. *SRY*
e. *ZFY*

13. During male sexual development, androgens mediate the differentiation of all of these structures except which one?

    a. Seminal vesicles
    b. Ureter
    c. Epididymis
    d. Vas deferens
    e. Ejaculatory ducts

14. Testosterone and müllerian-inhibiting substance are produced by the fetal testis at what gestational week?

    a. 5th
    b. 8th
    c. 10th
    d. 12th
    e. 23rd

15. What is the incidence of cryptorchidism at 1 year of age?

    a. 10%
    b. 3%
    c. 1%
    d. 0.3%
    e. 0.1%

16. What is the most important determining factor of cryptorchidism at 1 year of age?

    a. Gestational age at delivery
    b. Birth weight
    c. Maternal smoking history
    d. Family history of cryptorchidism
    e. Asian descent

17. In utero testosterone deficiency can be due to all of the following except:

    a. loss of function mutations involved with testosterone biosynthesis.
    b. impaired gonadotropin-releasing hormone receptor function.
    c. decreased luteinizing hormone (LH).
    d. increased inhibin B.
    e. impaired LH receptor function.

18. Patients with cryptorchidism demonstrate impaired biosynthesis of which of the following hormones in the first year of life?

    a. Follicle-stimulating hormone
    b. Testosterone
    c. Müllerian-inhibiting substance
    d. Gonadotropin-releasing hormone
    e. Inhibin A

19. All of the following structures have been theorized to aid in testicular descent except which one?

    a. Gubernaculum
    b. Genitofemoral nerve
    c. Epididymis
    d. Processus vaginalis
    e. Scrotum

20. Histologic findings in cryptorchid testes include all of the following except:

    a. decreased number of Leydig cells.
    b. delayed appearance of adult dark spermatogonia.
    c. early disappearance of gonocytes.
    d. degeneration of Sertoli cells.
    e. reduced total germ cell counts.

Answers

1. **c. asymptomatic.** Most adolescent varicoceles are asymptomatic. [p 2386]

2. **a. Elevated scrotal temperature.** The presence of varicosities impedes this countercurrent exchange mechanism, perhaps a crucial alteration in normal homeostasis because it is considered that elevated scrotal temperature associated with varicocele formation can inhibit spermatogenesis. [p 2385]

3. **b. 2 ml.** In adults and adolescents, testis size (volume) should be approximately equal bilaterally, with the normal differential not being more than 2 ml or 20% volume. [p 2386]

4. **e. Transvenous embolization.** Hydrocele formation is related to failure to preserve spermatic vessels associated with the spermatic cord and its vessels. Hydrocele formation seems most common after retroperitoneal ligation, especially when a mass ligation technique is used, and is least likely to occur after transvenous embolization. [p 2388]

5. **c. 4 hours.** Irreversible ischemic injury to the testicular parenchyma may begin as soon as 4 hours after occlusion of the cord. [p 2379]

6. **b. absence of the cremasteric reflex.** The absence of a cremasteric reflex is a good indicator of torsion of the cord. [p 2380]

7. **e. Immediate scrotal exploration.** It should always be kept in mind that manual detorsion may not totally correct the rotation that has occurred, and prompt exploration is usually still indicated. [p 2380]

8. **c. Elective scrotal exploration.** If the suspicion is strong that episodes of intermittent torsion and spontaneous detorsion have occurred, our experience has been that the finding of a bellclapper deformity at exploration can be expected. Elective scrotal exploration should be performed, with scrotal fixation of both testes. [p 2381]

9. **a. Observation.** When the diagnosis of a torsed appendage is confirmed clinically or by imaging, nonoperative management will allow most cases to resolve spontaneously. [p 2382]

10. **e. Radiographically normal urinary tracts.** The majority of boys with epididymitis have sterile urine and apparently radiographically normal urinary tracts. [p 2382]

11. **b. Prompt surgical exploration of the affected testis with contralateral scrotal exploration.** Clearly, if the cause of scrotal swelling appears to be related to an acute postnatal event, all efforts should be made to pursue prompt surgical intervention. Exploration, when elected, should be carried out through an inguinal incision to allow for the most efficacious treatment of other potential or unexpected causes of scrotal swelling. If torsion is confirmed, contralateral scrotal exploration with testicular fixation should be carried out. [p 2384]

12. **d. SRY.** Although the *SRY* gene appears to be primarily responsible for male sexual differentiation through complex interactions involving both activation and repression of other male-specific genes, little is known about its mode of action or downstream target genes, which convert the bipotential gonad into the testis. [p 2354]

13. **b. Ureter.** Androgens (testosterone, dihydroxytestosterone) mediate the differentiation of the paired wolffian ducts into the seminal vesicles, epididymis, vas deferens, and ejaculatory ducts. [p 2354]

14. **b. 8th.** During the 8th week, the fetal testis begins to secrete testosterone and müllerian-inhibiting substance independent of pituitary hormonal regulation. [p 2355]

15. **c. 1%.** By 1 year of age, the incidence of cryptorchidism declines to about 1% and remains constant throughout adulthood. [p 2357]

16. **b. Birth weight.** Accurate analysis of data concludes that birth weight alone is the principal determinant of cryptorchidism at birth and at 1 year of life, independent of the length of gestation. [p 2357]

17. **d. increased inhibin B.** In utero testosterone deficiency can be due to decreased LH, impaired function of the gonadotropin-releasing hormone or LH receptors, and loss of function mutations in the proteins involved in testosterone biosynthesis. [p 2359]

18. **c. Müllerian-inhibiting substance.** One report found that patients with cryptorchidism do not demonstrate a surge in the first year of life and that mean müllerian-inhibiting substance serum concentrations in cryptorchid boys are significantly lower than those in control subjects. [p 2360]

19. **e. Scrotum.** The testes lie dormant within the abdomen until about the 23rd week of gestation, during which time the processus vaginalis continues its elongation into the scrotum. The testis, epididymis, and gubernaculum have been observed to descend en masse through the inguinal canal posterior to the patent processus vaginalis. The theoretical association uniting normal testicular descent to epididymal function is based on the observations that epididymal abnormalities often accompany cryptorchidism. Data have also been presented that the genitofemoral nerve induced testicular descent and gubernacular differentiation. [pp 2356 and 2361–2363]

20. **c. early disappearance of gonocytes.** The histopathologic hallmarks associated with cryptorchidism are evident between 1 and 2 years of age and include decreased numbers of Leydig cells, degeneration of Sertoli cells, delayed disappearance of gonocytes, delayed appearance of adult dark (Ad) spermatogonia, failure of primary spermatocytes to develop, and reduced total germ cell counts. The earliest postnatal histologic abnormality in cryptorchid testes was hypoplasia of the Leydig cells, which was observed from the first month of life. [pp 2362–2363]

Chapter 68

Sexual Differentiation: Normal and Abnormal

David A. Diamond

Questions

1. What is the testis-determining factor (TDF)?
    a. It is synonymous with the H-Y antigen.
    b. It is located on the short arm of the Y chromosome adjacent to the pseudoautosomal boundary.
    c. It is a zinc finger gene on the Y chromosome, known as ZFY.
    d. It was genetically mapped by the study of patients with Klinefelter's and Turner's syndromes.
    e. It is synonymous with *SRY* in humans.

2. Which of the following statements is true regarding müllerian-inhibiting substance (MIS)?
    a. It acts systemically to produce müllerian regression.
    b. It is secreted by the fetal Leydig cells.
    c. It functions normally in patients with hernia uteri inguinale.
    d. It is secreted at 7 to 8 weeks of gestation, representing the initial endocrine function of the fetal testis.
    e. It is secreted by the fetal testis at 10 weeks of gestation, after testosterone production has begun.

3. Which of the following statements is true regarding fetal testosterone?
    a. It results in regression of the müllerian ducts.
    b. It is produced primarily by the adrenal gland.
    c. It acts locally to virilize the urogenital sinus and genital tubercle.
    d. It acts locally to virilize the internal wolffian duct structures.
    e. It enters target tissue by active diffusion.

4. Which of the following statements is true regarding dihydrotestosterone (DHT)?
    a. It produces virilization of wolffian duct structures.
    b. It is converted by 5α-reductase to testosterone in target tissues.
    c. It produces virilization of the urogenital sinus.
    d. It acts locally to produce regression of müllerian structures.
    e. It is secreted in large quantities by the fetal testis.

5. Which of the following statements is true regarding patients with Klinefelter's syndrome?

   a. They have at least one X and two Y chromosomes.
   b. They are at increased risk for development of adenocarcinoma of the breast.
   c. They undergo replacement of Leydig cells with hyaline.
   d. They are characteristically fertile.
   e. They bear little resemblance to XX males.

6. The streak gonad of Turner's syndrome:

   a. can descend to the scrotum.
   b. has a reduced number of oocytes.
   c. in the presence of a Y chromosome results in increased risk for development of seminoma.
   d. is located in the round ligament.
   e. in the presence of a Y chromosome results in risk for development of gonadoblastoma.

7. Which of the following statements is true regarding patients with "pure" gonadal dysgenesis?

   a. They frequently have chromosomal anomalies.
   b. They are at lesser risk for gonadal tumors than are patients with Turner's syndrome.
   c. They lack the somatic defects associated with Turner's syndrome.
   d. They have gonadal histology different from that of patients with Turner's syndrome.
   e. They derive similar benefit from synthetic growth hormone as do patients with Turner's syndrome.

8. What is the common denominator in all cases of Denys-Drash syndrome?

   a. Gonadoblastoma
   b. Nephropathy with early-onset proteinuria
   c. Wilms' tumor
   d. Caliceal blunting
   e. Progressive renal failure

9. Which of the following statements is true regarding patients with embryonic testicular regression or bilateral vanishing testes syndromes?

   a. They have normal testosterone and elevated estradiol levels.
   b. They have normal testosterone but decreased DHT levels.
   c. They have castrate testosterone and elevated gonadotropin levels.
   d. They have castrate testosterone and normal gonadotropin levels.
   e. They have normal follicle-stimulating hormone but decreased luteinizing hormone levels.

10. Which of the following statements is true regarding the ovotestis in true hermaphroditism?

    a. It cannot descend from the retroperitoneum.
    b. It is found in the minority of patients.
    c. It can be unilateral or bilateral.
    d. It has testicular and ovarian elements randomly distributed.
    e. It is impossible to cleave surgically.

11. An important consideration for gender assignment in the true hermaphrodite is:

    a. that these patients have the potential for fertility.
    b. the impossibility of precisely dividing an ovotestis surgically.
    c. that malignant degeneration of gonads does not occur.
    d. the familial pattern of inheritance of the disorder.
    e. unresponsiveness of the external genitalia to testosterone.

12. Which of the following statements is true regarding the 21-hydroxylase deficiency in congenital adrenal hyperplasia (CAH)?

    a. It accounts for 99% of CAH cases.
    b. It occurs as a result of gene inactivation in the majority of cases.
    c. It presents with simple virilization in 75% of cases and salt wasting in 25% of cases.
    d. It presents with a predictable phenotype.
    e. It is transmitted in an autosomal dominant pattern.

13. Prenatal treatment of patients with CAH with dexamethasone:

    a. will result in appropriate therapy in seven of eight at-risk fetuses.
    b. may be initiated after a diagnosis of CAH is confirmed.
    c. entails no risk to the fetus.
    d. has clearly been demonstrated to be effective.
    e. acts by suppressing maternal corticotropin.

14. Which of the following statements is true regarding enzymatic disorders of testosterone biosynthesis?

    a. They are transmitted in an autosomal dominant pattern.
    b. They are associated with persistent müllerian structures.
    c. They present clinically with a predictable phenotype.
    d. They may involve impaired glucocorticoid and mineralocorticoid synthesis.
    e. They may be associated with fertility.

15. Which of the following statements is true regarding patients with complete androgen insensitivity?

    a. They are appropriately raised as female.
    b. They have normal wolffian duct structures.
    c. They have persistent müllerian duct structures.
    d. They should undergo orchiectomy as early as possible.
    e. They have a 2% incidence of inguinal hernia.

16. What is Reifenstein's syndrome?

    a. The group of defects in testosterone biosynthesis that result in male pseudohermaphroditism
    b. A form of 5α-reductase deficiency
    c. A name assigned to patients with evidence of defective MIS elaboration in utero
    d. A disorder of androgen receptor quantity or function
    e. An autosomal recessively transmitted disorder

17. Which of the following statements is true regarding patients with 5α-reductase deficiency?

    a. Fertility is an important issue in gender assignment.
    b. Isoenzymes I and II are abnormal.
    c. Serum testosterone levels are normal, but there is a decreased testosterone/DHT ratio.
    d. Masculinization occurs at puberty.
    e. Prostatic enlargement occurs at puberty.

18. Which of the following statements is true regarding patients with persistent müllerian duct syndrome?

    a. They have absent wolffian duct structures.
    b. They represent a homogeneous disorder of the MIS receptor.
    c. They should undergo routine removal of müllerian structures.
    d. They experience a high incidence of transverse testicular ectopia.
    e. They are uniformly infertile.

19. Which of the following statements is true regarding Mayer-Rokitansky-Küster-Hauser syndrome?

a. It presents most commonly with infertility.
b. It is a homogeneous disorder entailing congenital absence of the uterus and vagina.
c. It is associated with a spectrum of ovarian abnormalities.
d. It has associated upper urinary tract anomalies, primarily with the atypical disorder.
e. It is associated with persistent wolffian duct structures.

20. In an unambiguous newborn with hypospadias and a unilateral cryptorchid testis:

a. midshaft location of the urethral meatus is an important risk factor for an intersex disorder.
b. impalpability of the cryptorchid testis carries a 50% risk of intersex disorder.
c. palpability of the cryptorchid testis effectively rules out an intersex disorder.
d. perineal hypospadias is not a risk factor for an intersex disorder.
e. a difference in tissue texture of the poles of the cryptorchid gonad is suggestive of tumor.

Answers

1. **b. It is located on the short arm of the Y chromosome adjacent to the pseudoautosomal boundary.** Deletion maps based on the genomes of these individuals were constructed by a number of laboratories, and TDF was mapped to the most distal aspect of the Y-unique region of the short arm of the Y chromosome, adjacent to the pseudoautosomal boundary (see Fig. 68–1). [p 2396]

2. **d. It is secreted at 7 to 8 weeks of gestation, representing the initial endocrine function of the fetal testis.** The initial endocrine function of the fetal testes is the secretion of MIS by the Sertoli cells at 7 to 8 weeks of gestation. [p 2400]

3. **d. It acts locally to virilize the internal wolffian duct structures.** It was clearly demonstrated that androgen is essential for virilization of wolffian duct structures, the urogenital sinus, and genital tubercle. Testosterone, the major androgen secreted by the testes, enters target tissues by passive diffusion. The local source of androgen is important for wolffian duct development, which does not occur if testosterone is supplied only via the peripheral circulation. [p 2400]

4. **c. It produces virilization of the urogenital sinus.** In some cells, such as those in the urogenital sinus, testosterone is converted to DHT by intracellular 5α-reductase. Testosterone or DHT then binds to a high-affinity intracellular receptor protein, and this complex enters the nucleus where it binds to acceptor sites on DNA, resulting in new messenger RNA and protein synthesis. Therefore, in tissues equipped with 5α-reductase at the time of sexual differentiation, such as prostate, urogenital sinus, and external genitalia, DHT is the active androgen. [p 2400]

5. **b. They are at increased risk for development of adenocarcinoma of the breast.** Gynecomastia, which can be quite marked, is a common pubertal development in patients with Klinefelter's syndrome. As a result, these patients are at eight times the risk for developing breast carcinoma relative to normal males. [p 2404]

6. **e. in the presence of a Y chromosome results in risk for development of gonadoblastoma.** In patients with occult Y chromosomal material, the risk of gonadoblastoma, an in situ germ cell cancer, is approximately 30%. [p 2405]

7. **c. They lack the somatic defects associated with Turner's syndrome.** Patients with 46,XX "pure" gonadal dysgenesis are closely related to those with Turner's syndrome. Because these subjects exhibit none of the somatic stigmata associated with Turner's syndrome and their condition entails gonadal dysgenesis only, it has been regarded by some authors as pure. [p 2406]

8. **b. Nephropathy with early-onset proteinuria.** The full triad of the syndrome includes nephropathy, characterized by the early onset of proteinuria and hypertension, and progressive renal failure in the majority. Because incomplete forms of the syndrome may occur, the nephropathy has become regarded as the common denominator of the syndrome. [p 2407]

9. **c. They have castrate testosterone and elevated gonadotropin levels.** The diagnosis can be made on the basis of a 46,XY karyotype and castrate levels of testosterone despite persistently elevated serum luteinizing hormone and follicle-stimulating hormone levels. [p 2409]

10. **c. It can be unilateral or bilateral.** True hermaphrodites are individuals having both testicular tissue with well-developed seminiferous tubules and ovarian tissue with primordial follicles, which may take the form of one ovary and one testis or, more commonly, one or two ovotestes. [pp 2409–2410]

11. **a. that these patients have the potential for fertility.** The most important aspect of management in true hermaphroditism is gender assignment. [p 2411]

12. **b. It occurs as a result of gene inactivation in the majority of cases.** Mutations leading to gene conversion of the active CYP21 gene into the inactive gene occur in 65% to 90% of cases of the classic disorder (salt wasting and simple virilizing) and all cases of nonclassic 21-hydroxylase deficiency. [p 2412]

13. **d. has clearly been demonstrated to be effective.** A number of series have established the effectiveness of prenatal treatment of CAH with dexamethasone. [p 2414]

14. **d. They may involve impaired glucocorticoid and mineralocorticoid synthesis.** A defect in any of the five enzymes required for the conversion of cholesterol to testosterone can cause incomplete (or absent) virilization of the male fetus during embryogenesis. The first three enzymes (cholesterol side chain cleavage enzyme, 3β-hydroxysteroid dehydrogenase, and 17α-hydroxylase) are present in both the adrenals and the testes. Therefore, their deficiency results in impaired synthesis of glucocorticoids and mineralocorticoids in addition to testosterone. [p 2415]

15. **a. They are appropriately raised as female.** It is of great interest that currently, all studies of patients with complete androgen insensitivity support an unequivocal female gender identity, consistent with androgen resistance of brain tissue as well. To date, there has been no report of a patient raised as a female who needed gender reassignment to male. [p 2418]

16. **d. A disorder of androgen receptor quantity or function.** Androgen receptor studies in cultured fibroblasts have demonstrated two forms of receptor defect in the partial androgen insensitivity syndrome. These include a reduced number of normally functioning androgen receptors, and normal receptor number but decreased binding affinity. [p 2418]

17. **d. Masculinization occurs at puberty.** At puberty, partial masculinization occurs with an increase in muscle mass, development of male body habitus, increase in phallic size, and onset of erections. [p 2420]

18. **d. They experience a high incidence of transverse testicular ectopia.** Persistent müllerian duct syndrome is thought to be etiologically important in transverse testicular ectopia, occurring in 30% to 50% of cases. [p 2420]

19. **d. It has associated upper urinary tract anomalies, primarily with the atypical disorder.** Urinary tract anomalies occur more commonly in patients with the atypical form of the disorder than in patients with the typical syndrome. [p 2421]

20. **b. impalpability of the cryptorchid testis carries a 50% risk of intersex.** With a unilateral cryptorchid testis, the incidence of intersex was 30% overall—15% if the undescended testis was palpable and 50% if impalpable. [p 2421]

Chapter 69

Surgical Management of Intersexuality, Cloacal Malformations, and Other Abnormalities of the Genitalia in Girls

Richard C. Rink • Martin Kaefer

Questions

1. What is the crucial period in embryogenesis for the formation of the terminal bowel, kidney, paramesonephric ductal system, and lumbosacral spine?

   a. 4 to 6 weeks
   b. 8 to 10 weeks
   c. 10 to 14 weeks
   d. 14 to 18 weeks
   e. >18 weeks

2. Which of the following is NOT true regarding vaginal agenesis (müllerian aplasia)?

   a. It occurs with an incidence of approximately 1 in 5000 live female births.
   b. Serum follicle-stimulating hormone and luteinizing hormone levels can be expected to be abnormally high.
   c. Embryologically it results from a failure of the sinovaginal bulbs to develop and form the vaginal plate.
   d. It is a condition associated with renal abnormalities.
   e. It is a condition associated with skeletal abnormalities.

3. Skeletal anomalies are found in what percentage of patients with Meyer-Rokitansky-Küster-Hauser syndrome?

   a. 10% to 20%
   b. 25% to 35%
   c. 40% to 60%
   d. 70% to 90%
   e. 0% (they are not seen in association with the syndrome)

4. What is the most common cause of primary amenorrhea?

   a. Testicular feminization
   b. Vaginal agenesis
   c. Mixed gonadal dysgenesis
   d. Imperforate hymen
   e. Transverse vaginal septum

5. Which of the following statements is NOT true regarding the genitalia of women with Meyer-Rokitansky-Küster-Hauser syndrome?

   a. In approximately 10% of patients, a normal but obstructed uterus or rudimentary uterus with functional endometrium is present.
   b. Normal fallopian tubes are seen in approximately 35% of patients.
   c. The ovaries are not functional in the majority of patients.
   d. The hymenal fringe is usually present along with a small vaginal pouch.
   e. The labia majora are typically normal in appearance.

6. Which of the following is NOT true regarding the construction of a bowel vagina?

   a. Failure to develop an adequate space between the rectum and bladder can result in compromised blood flow to the segment used for vaginal construction.
   b. In general, colon is preferred over ileum because of its lower incidence of associated postoperative stenosis.
   c. When compared with the McIndoe procedure, the bowel vagina suffers from a higher incidence of postoperative stenosis.
   d. An advantage of a bowel vagina over the McIndoe procedure includes the lubricating properties of mucus (which may help to facilitate intercourse).
   e. One specific indication for the use of ileum is a previous history of pelvic radiation.

7. Uterus didelphys with unilateral imperforate vagina most commonly presents with which condition?

a. Primary amenorrhea
b. Cyclical abdominal pain associated with normal cyclical menstruation
c. Renal anomalies contralateral to the side of the obstruction
d. Anomalies of the axial skeleton
e. Constipation

8. Urethral prolapse is most commonly seen in young females of which ethnic background?

   a. African American
   b. White
   c. Asian
   d. Hispanic
   e. American Indian

9. In most cases of labial adhesions, which of the following is true?

   a. They are believed to occur because of a relative state of hyperestrogenism.
   b. They should be treated with surgical lysis.
   c. They require no treatment.
   d. They occur secondary to sexual abuse.
   e. They have associated renal anomalies.

10. What is the mean age of a child with vaginal rhabdomyosarcoma?

    a. <2 years
    b. 2 to 4 years
    c. 4 to 8 years
    d. 8 to 12 years
    e. >12 years

11. Urogenital sinus anomalies are most often seen in intersex states, most commonly in association with which condition?

    a. Congenital adrenal hyperplasia
    b. Mixed gonadal dysgenesis
    c. True hermaphroditism
    d. Cloacal anomalies

12. Cloacal anomalies have been diagnosed by antenatal ultrasonography. What is the common finding in all reports?

    a. Ascites
    b. Distended rectum
    c. Distended bladder
    d. Distended vagina

13. What is the most common vaginal anatomy in cloacal malformation?

    a. Single vagina, single uterus
    b. Single vagina, double uterus
    c. Two vaginas, two uteri
    d. Two vaginas, one uterus

14. Which of the following is not part of the normal evaluation of a child born with a cloacal anomaly?

    a. Genitography
    b. MRI of the head
    c. Echocardiography
    d. MRI of the spine

15. Neonatal vaginoplasty combined with clitoroplasty and labioplasty has all of the following advantages except which one?

    a. It allows phallic skin for vaginal reconstruction.
    b. Maternal estrogens increase vaginal thickness and vascularity.
    c. Tissues are less scarred.
    d. Vaginal stenosis is clearly less.

16. The cut-back vaginoplasty is appropriate for only which condition?

    a. Labial fusion
    b. Low vaginal confluence
    c. High vaginal confluence
    d. Vaginal atresia

17. Surgical management of cloacal malformations involves all of the following steps except which one?

    a. Decompression of the gastrointestinal tract
    b. Decompression of the genitourinary tract
    c. Vaginostomy
    d. Definitive repair of the cloaca

18. Fecal continence after cloacal reconstruction is most closely related to:

    a. the level of rectal confluence.
    b. associated urinary anomalies.
    c. neurologic status.
    d. the type of repair.

Answers

1. **a. 4 to 6 weeks.** Laboratory data with teratogens support the concept of a key event occurring between the 4th and 5th weeks of gestation that results in an error in the simultaneous development of the terminal bowel, kidney, bladder, paramesonephric ductal system, and lumbosacral spine. [p 2430]

2. **b. Serum follicle-stimulating hormone and luteinizing hormone levels can be expected to be abnormally high.** Vaginal agenesis, which occurs with an incidence of approximately 1 in 5000 live female births, is the congenital absence of the proximal portion of the vagina in an otherwise phenotypically (i.e., normal secondary sexual characteristics), chromosomally (i.e., 46,XX), and hormonally (i.e., normal luteinizing hormone and follicle-stimulating hormone levels) intact female. It results from a failure of the sinovaginal bulbs to develop and form the vaginal plate. Hauser brought further attention to the frequent association of renal and skeletal anomalies in these patients and stressed the differences between patients with these findings and those with testicular feminization. [pp 2431–2432]

3. **a. 10% to 20%.** Associated congenital abnormalities of the skeletal system have been described in 10% to 20% of cases. [p 2432]

4. **c. Mixed gonadal dysgenesis.** Meyer-Rokitansky-Küster-Hauser syndrome is in fact secondary only to gonadal dysgenesis as a cause of primary amenorrhea. [p 2432]

5. **c. The ovaries are not functional in the majority of patients.** Although occasionally cystic, the ovaries were almost always present and functional. [p 2432]

6. **c. When compared with the McIndoe procedure, the bowel vagina suffers from a higher incidence of postoperative stenosis.** A high incidence of postoperative vaginal

stenosis necessitates postoperative vaginal dilatation. [p 2433]

7. **b. Cyclical abdominal pain associated with normal cyclical menstruation.** As with other obstructive disorders, the patient may present with cyclical or chronic abdominal pain. However, unlike other obstructive processes, duplication anomalies with unilateral obstruction are not associated with primary amenorrhea. [p 2437]

8. **a. African American.** This entity, which was first described by Solinger in 1732, occurs most often in prepubertal black girls and postmenopausal white women. [p 2441]

9. **c. They require no treatment.** Most children do not require treatment unless one of the aforementioned symptoms (urine pooling within the vagina, which may lead to postvoid dribbling; perineal irritation; physical findings of sexual abuse) occurs. [p 2439]

10. **a. <2 years.** The mean age of patients with primary vaginal tumors is younger than 2 years. [p 2442]

11. **a. Congenital adrenal hyperplasia.** Urogenital sinus abnormalities are most often seen in intersex states, most commonly in association with congenital adrenal hyperplasia, which has been noted to have an incidence as frequent as 1 in 500 in the nonclassic mild forms. [p 2443]

12. **d. Distended vagina.** The common finding in all reports has been a cystic pelvic mass between the bladder and rectum, representing a distended vagina. [p 2448]

13. **c. Two vaginas, two uteri.** In Hendren's report on 154 patients with cloacal anomalies, 66 patients had one vagina, 68 had two vaginas, and the vagina was absent in 20. The incidence of vaginal duplication is even higher in our own patient population. The uterus anomaly generally is similar to the vaginal, that is, two vaginas with two uteri. [p 2448]

14. **b. MRI of the head.** The frequency of associated organ system abnormalities requires further radiographic evaluation. Echocardiography should always be done. MRI to evaluate the lumbosacral spine and to evaluate pelvic anatomy and musculature is necessary. [p 2449]

15. **d. Vaginal stenosis is clearly less.** Other investigators, including our group, have thought that vaginoplasty, regardless of the vaginal location, is best combined with clitoroplasty in a single stage. This allows the redundant phallic skin to be used in the reconstruction, adding flexibility for the surgeon, which is compromised when the skin has been previously mobilized. Furthermore, we and others have noted that maternal estrogen stimulation of the child's genitalia results in thicker vaginal tissue, which is better vascularized, making vaginal mobilization more easily performed. [p 2450]

16. **a. Labial fusion.** The cut-back vaginoplasty is rarely used and is appropriate only for simple labial fusion (see Fig. 69–35). [p 2450]

17. **c. Vaginostomy.** Surgical management now involves four basic steps: (1) decompression of the gastrointestinal tract, (2) decompression of the genitourinary tract, (3) correction of nephron destructive or potentially lethal urinary anomalies, and (4) definitive repair of the cloaca. [p 2460]

18. **c. neurologic status.** Fecal continence is directly related to neurologic status. [p 2463]

Chapter 70

Pediatric Urologic Oncology

Michael Ritchey

Questions

1. Which chromosomal abnormality is associated with an adverse prognosis in neuroblastoma?

   a. Mutation of chromosome 11p15
   b. Absence of the *MDR* gene
   c. Mutation of the *p53* gene
   d. Deletion of the short arm of chromosome 1
   e. Loss of heterozygosity (LOH) for chromosome 11p13

2. Which of the following statements is true regarding in situ neuroblastoma?

   a. It invariably progresses to clinical neuroblastoma.
   b. It usually regresses spontaneously.
   c. It is associated with deletion of chromosome 11.
   d. It can usually be detected on newborn screening.
   e. It is frequently associated with amplification of the N-*myc* oncogene.

3. Which of the following statements is true regarding ganglioneuroma?

   a. It is a stroma-rich tumor by the Shimada classification.
   b. It is most commonly located in the adrenal gland.
   c. It is often found secondary to symptoms from metastatic disease.
   d. It is associated with acute myoclonic encephalopathy.
   e. It is associated with an unfavorable prognosis.

4. Which of the following statements is true regarding screening for neuroblastoma?

   a. It has improved survival in patients with neuroblastoma.
   b. It has decreased the number of children older than 1 year of age with advanced stage disease.
   c. It has identified more tumors with amplified N-*myc* oncogene expression.
   d. It discovers tumors with an improved prognosis.
   e. It is widely performed in the United States.

5. Which clinical feature is associated with a favorable prognosis in neuroblastoma?

   a. Age greater than 2 years
   b. Thoracic location of the primary tumor
   c. N-*myc* amplification

d. Chromosome 1p deletion
e. Stroma-poor histology

6. A 1-month-old girl is found to have a right suprarenal mass on abdominal ultrasonographic examination. The mass measures 4 cm in diameter. Imaging evaluation detects liver metastases. Results of a skeletal survey are normal. The physical examination reveals multiple subcutaneous skin nodules. The mass is removed and confirmed to be neuroblastoma. Analysis of the tumor reveals no N-*myc* amplification. What is the next best step?

   a. Observation
   b. Irradiation to the tumor bed
   c. Vincristine, cyclophosphamide, and doxorubicin
   d. Vincristine, cyclophosphamide, and irradiation to the tumor bed
   e. Autologous bone marrow transplantation after chemotherapy and total body irradiation

7. A 3-year-old girl has vaginal rhabdomyosarcoma. Her mother has a history of breast cancer. Which condition does this patient most likely have?

   a. Beckwith-Wiedemann syndrome (BWS)
   b. Li-Fraumeni syndrome
   c. Perlman syndrome
   d. Fragile X syndrome
   e. Sotos' syndrome

8. A 3-year-old boy has prostatic rhabdomyosarcoma. Which of the following is an unfavorable prognostic feature of this tumor?

   a. Alveolar histologic type
   b. Embryonal histologic type
   c. LOH for chromosome 11p15
   d. A botryoid pattern
   e. Spindle cell variant

9. A 1-year-old girl previously had partial cystectomy for rhabdomyosarcoma of the bladder. After completion of vincristine, dactinomycin, and cyclophosphamide chemotherapy, biopsy of the bladder reveals rhabdomyoblasts. Abdominal and chest CT results are negative. What is the next step?

   a. Radiation therapy
   b. Continue chemotherapy
   c. Cystectomy with diversion
   d. Observation
   e. Change in chemotherapy regimen

10. A 4-year-old boy has paratesticular rhabdomyosarcoma found by biopsy of his spermatic cord lesion. The best next step is radical orchiectomy and:

    a. Vincristine, dactinomycin, and cyclophosphamide chemotherapy
    b. Retroperitoneal lymph node dissection
    c. Retroperitoneal lymph node sampling
    d. Radiation therapy to the retroperitoneum
    e. Cisplatin, etoposide, and vincristine chemotherapy

11. A 3-year-old boy had undergone treatment for hypospadias and undescended testis as an infant. He develops renal insufficiency. Renal biopsy is consistent with a membranoproliferative glomerulonephritis. What is appropriate management before renal transplantation?

    a. Voiding cystourethrography
    b. Gonadal biopsy
    c. Observation
    d. Bilateral nephrectomy
    e. Serial renal ultrasonographic studies

12. The WAGR (Wilms' tumor, aniridia, genital anomalies, mental retardation) syndrome is most frequently associated with:

    a. deletion of chromosome 11.
    b. advanced-stage Wilms' tumor.
    c. neonatal presentation of Wilms' tumor.
    d. renal insufficiency.
    e. familial predisposition to Wilms' tumor.

13. A 2-year-old boy has a palpable right-sided abdominal mass. CT shows this to be a solid lesion. On physical examination, the patient's right arm and leg are noted to be slightly longer. What is the most probable diagnosis?

    a. Wilms' tumor
    b. Neuroblastoma
    c. Angiomyolipoma
    d. Nephroblastomatosis
    e. Renal call carcinoma

14. A newborn is identified with BWS. A renal ultrasonographic scan is obtained. Which clinical finding most predicts the risk of subsequent Wilms' tumor development?

    a. Hepatomegaly
    b. Hemihypertrophy
    c. Nephromegaly
    d. Mutation at chromosome 11p13
    e. Family history of Wilms' tumor

15. A 6-month-old girl is diagnosed with aniridia. Ultrasonographic scans are obtained every 3 months. This will result in:

    a. increased survival.
    b. detection of lower stage renal tumor.
    c. decreased incidence of bilateral tumors.
    d. decreased surgical morbidity.
    e. detection of tumors smaller than 3 cm in diameter.

16. A deletion of chromosome 11 has been found most frequently in patients with Wilms' tumor who have which condition?

    a. Aniridia
    b. Bilateral tumors
    c. Hemihypertrophy
    d. Denys-Drash syndrome
    e. BWS

17. A 5-year-old boy undergoes nephrectomy for a solid renal mass. Pathology reveals stage 1 favorable histologic type Wilms' tumor. An increased risk for tumor relapse is associated with:

    a. tumor aneuploidy on flow cytometry.
    b. deletion of chromosome 11p13.
    c. duplication of chromosome 1.
    d. LOH for chromosome 16q.
    e. elevated serum ferritin level.

18. A 2-year-old girl undergoes a left nephrectomy for Wilms' tumor. A solitary left pulmonary lesion is noted on a chest CT scan. The pathologic studies show favorable histologic type but with capsular penetration. What is the most important prognostic feature?

    a. Capsular presentation
    b. Histologic subtype
    c. Absence of lymph node involvement
    d. Age at presentation
    e. Presence of pulmonary metastasis

19. Which feature is associated with worse survival in children with Wilms' tumor?

a. Diffuse anaplasia
b. Diffuse tumor spill
c. Incomplete tumor resection
d. Tumor spread to periaortic lymph nodes
e. Lung metastasis

20. An increased risk for metachronous Wilms' tumor is associated with:

    a. anaplastic histologic type.
    b. clear cell sarcoma.
    c. blastemal predominant pattern.
    d. renal sinus invasion.
    e. nephrogenic rests.

21. A 6-year-old boy has a solid abdominal mass noted on an ultrasonographic scan. A right-sided varicocele is present on the physical examination. What is the next best step?

    a. Abdominal CT
    b. MRI of the abdomen
    c. Chest CT
    d. Intravenous pyelogram
    e. Arteriogram

22. A 1-year-old boy undergoes nephrectomy for Wilms' tumor. Which finding has the most adverse impact on survival?

    a. Hilar lymph node involvement
    b. Renal sinus invasion
    c. Capsular penetration
    d. Local tumor spill
    e. Renal vein thrombus

23. Which factor is NOT predictive of local tumor relapse in children with Wilms' tumor?

    a. Local tumor spill
    b. Unfavorable histologic type
    c. Incomplete tumor removal
    d. Absence of lymph node sampling
    e. Capsular penetration

24. A 4-year-old girl undergoes removal of a Wilms' tumor with favorable histologic type. Imaging evaluation reveals multiple pulmonary metastases. Treatment should include vincristine, dactinomycin, and:

    a. chest irradiation.
    b. doxorubicin (Adriamycin).
    c. Adriamycin and chest irradiation.
    d. Adriamycin, cyclophosphamide, and irradiation therapy.
    e. Adriamycin, etoposide, and VP-16.

25. A 3-month-old boy undergoes removal of a 300 g Wilms' tumor of the right kidney. The pathologic analysis shows diffuse anaplasia and tumor confined to the kidney. Lymph nodes were negative. What is the next step?

    a. Observation
    b. Vincristine and dactinomycin
    c. Vincristine, dactinomycin, and irradiation of tumor beds
    d. Doxorubicin, vincristine, dactinomycin, and irradiation to the tumor bed
    e. Ifosfamide, VP-16, and doxorubicin

26. A 5-year-old girl presents with hematuria. CT reveals a right abdominal mass with extension of tumor thrombus into the suprahepatic vena cava. What is the best next step?

    a. Chemotherapy
    b. Irradiation therapy
    c. Open biopsy followed by chemotherapy
    d. Preoperative chemotherapy and radiation therapy
    e. Primary surgical removal of the kidney and tumor thrombus

27. A 2-year-old boy is found to have bilateral Wilms' tumor. There is a tumor occupying more than 50% of the left kidney and a smaller tumor in the upper pole of the right kidney. What is the best next step?

    a. Left nephrectomy and right renal biopsy
    b. Bilateral partial nephrectomy
    c. Right partial nephrectomy and left renal biopsy
    d. Bilateral renal biopsies
    e. Chemotherapy

28. A 1-year-old girl has a stage III Wilms' tumor. During the course of chemotherapy, she develops an enlarged heart and evidence of congestive heart failure. Which drug is most likely responsible for these findings?

    a. Dactinomycin
    b. Etoposide
    c. Vincristine
    d. Cyclophosphamide
    e. Doxorubicin

29. A 1-year-old boy undergoes left radical nephrectomy for a large renal mass. Which pathologic feature is associated with the worst prognosis?

    a. Diffuse anaplasia stage I
    b. Focal anaplasia stage III
    c. Rhabdoid tumor of the kidney stage III
    d. Clear cell sarcoma of the kidney stage III
    e. Favorable histologic type stage IV

30. A newborn boy was noted to have a left renal mass on a prenatal ultrasonographic scan. Postnatal evaluation confirms a 5-cm solid mass in the lower pole of the left kidney. The right kidney is normal. Chest radiographic and CT results of the chest are negative for metastatic disease. The mass was completely removed by a radical nephrectomy. What is the next step in treatment?

    a. 1200 cGy abdominal irradiation to the left flank
    b. Observation only
    c. Dactinomycin and vincristine for 10 weeks
    d. Dactinomycin and vincristine for 18 weeks
    e. 2000 cGy abdominal irradiation plus dactinomycin and vincristine for 18 weeks

31. The tuberous sclerosis complex is associated with the development of angiomyolipoma and cystic renal disease. These patients have been found to have an abnormality on which chromosome?

    a. 1
    b. 13
    c. 9
    d. 11
    e. 7

32. A 3-month-old boy undergoes removal of a solid yolk-sac tumor. The margins of resection are negative for tumor. Chest and abdominal CT results show no signs of metastatic disease. Two weeks postoperatively, the serum alpha-fetoprotein value is 35. What is the next step?

    a. Chemotherapy
    b. Retroperitoneal lymph node dissection
    c. Observation
    d. Retroperitoneal lymph node sampling
    e. Abdominal radiation

33. A 2-year-old boy has a left upper pole testicular mass that is cystic on an ultrasonographic scan. Excision of the lesion is done via an inguinal approach, leaving the lower half of the testis. Frozen section demonstrates clear margins. Final pathologic analysis reveals teratoma, and the margins are

negative for tumor. Assays for serum alpha-fetoprotein and β-human chorionic gonadotropin are negative. Chest and abdominal CT results are negative. What is the next step?

   a. Radical orchiectomy and modified retroperitoneal lymph node dissection
   b. Observation
   c. Radical orchiectomy and combination chemotherapy
   d. Radical orchiectomy
   e. Radical orchiectomy and abdominal irradiation

34. A 2-year-old boy undergoes left orchiectomy. Pathologic examination reveals a yolk-sac tumor confined to the testis. CT results of the chest and abdomen are negative. No preoperative tumor markers were done. At 4 weeks after surgery, tumor markers are negative. What is the next step?

   a. Lymph node dissection
   b. Observation
   c. Chemotherapy
   d. Staining of the tumor for alpha-fetoprotein
   e. Retroperitoneal lymph node sampling

35. A 6-year-old, phenotypic boy with hypospadias and bilateral cryptorchidism has a 3-cm lower abdominal mass. The karyotype is XO/XY. At abdominal exploration, a tumor is found in the right gonad. Right orchiectomy is performed. Frozen section reveals gonadoblastoma. What is the best next step?

   a. Left orchiopexy
   b. Retroperitoneal lymph node sampling
   c. Left orchiectomy
   d. Chemotherapy
   e. Observation

Answers

1. **d. Deletion of the short arm of chromosome 1.** Deletion of the short arm of chromosome 1 is found in 70% to 80% of neuroblastomas and is an adverse prognostic marker. The deletions are of different size, but in a series of eight cases, a consensus deletion included the segment 1p36.1–2, suggesting that genetic information related to neuroblastoma tumorigenesis is located in this segment. [p 2470]

2. **b. It usually regresses spontaneously.** In 1963, Beckwith and Perrin coined the term *in situ neuroblastoma* for small nodules of neuroblastoma cells found incidentally within the adrenal gland, which are histologically indistinguishable from neuroblastoma. In infants younger than 3 months of age undergoing postmortem examination, neuroblastoma in situ was found in 1 of 224 infants. This represents an incidence of in situ neuroblastoma approximately 40 to 45 times greater than the incidence of clinical tumors, suggesting that these small tumors regress spontaneously in most cases. However, more recent studies have shown that these neuroblastic nodules are found in all fetuses studied and generally regress. [p 2470]

3. **a. It is a stroma-rich tumor by the Shimada classification.** The Shimada classification is an age-linked histopathologic classification. One of the important aspects of the Shimada classification is determining whether the tumor is stroma-poor or stroma-rich. Patients with stroma-poor tumors with unfavorable histopathologic features have a very poor prognosis (less than 10% survival). Stroma-rich tumors can be separated into three subgroups: nodular, intermixed, and well differentiated. Tumors in the last two categories more closely resemble ganglioneuroblastoma or immature ganglioneuroma and have a higher rate of survival. [p 2470]

4. **d. It discovers tumors with an improved prognosis.** The goal of screening programs is to detect disease at an earlier stage and decrease the number of older children with advanced stage disease and thus improve survival. An increased number of infants younger than 1 year of age have been diagnosed with the mass screening program, and most of these patients have lower stage tumors. Regrettably, the number of children older than 1 year of age with advanced stage disease has not decreased. [p 2471]

5. **b. Thoracic location of the primary tumor.** The site of origin is of significance, with a better survival rate noted for nonadrenal primary tumors. Most children with thoracic neuroblastoma present at a younger age with localized disease and have improved survival even when corrected for age and stage. [p 2472]

6. **a. Observation.** The generally favorable behavior of stage IV-S disease has been explained with the development of biologic markers. The vast majority of these infants have tumors with entirely favorable markers explaining their nonmalignant behavior. A small percentage, however, have adverse markers, and it is these children who have progressive disease to which they often succumb. Resection of the primary tumor is not mandatory. Although excellent survival has been reported after surgery, information regarding histologic prognostic factors was not available for all of these patients. A more recent review was performed of a large cohort of 110 infants with stage IV-S disease. The entire cohort of infants had an estimated 3-year survival rate of 85% ± 4%. This survival rate was significantly decreased, however, to 68% ± 12% for infants who were diploid, 44% ± 33% for those who were N-*myc* amplified, and 33% ± 19% for those with unfavorable histology tumors. Of note, there was no statistical difference in survival rate for infants who underwent complete resection of their primary tumor compared with those with partial resection or only biopsy. Patients with extensive metastatic disease who are N-*myc*-positive represent a high-risk group. These patients should be considered for a more aggressive treatment with multimodal therapy as per the Risk Group classification. [p 2474]

7. **b. Li-Fraumeni syndrome.** Subgroups of children with a genetic predisposition to the development of rhabdomyosarcoma have been identified. The Li-Fraumeni syndrome associates childhood sarcomas with mothers who have an excess of premenopausal breast cancer and with siblings who have an increased risk of cancer. A mutation of the p53 tumor suppressor gene was found in the tumors in all patients with this syndrome. [p 2475]

8. **a. Alveolar histologic type.** The second most common form is alveolar, which occurs more commonly in the trunk and extremity than in genitourinary sites and has a worse prognosis. Alveolar rhabdomyosarcoma also has a higher rate of local recurrence and spread to regional lymph nodes, bone marrow, and distant sites. [p 2476]

9. **d. Observation.** If tumor is shrinking during chemotherapy, and another biopsy after completing radiotherapy shows maturing rhabdomyoblasts without frank tumor cells, total cystectomy can be postponed or avoided all together. [p 2479]

10. **a. Vincristine, dactinomycin, and cyclophosphamide.** Before effective chemotherapy, surgery alone produced a 50% 2-year relapse-free survival rate. With current multimodal treatment, survival rates of 90% are expected. Currently, the Intergroup Rhabdomyosarcoma Study Group recommends that children 10 years of age and older undergo ipsilateral retroperitoneal lymph node dissection before chemotherapy. [pp 2479–2480]

11. **d. Bilateral nephrectomy.** One specific association of male pseudohermaphroditism, renal mesangial sclerosis, and nephroblastoma is the Denys-Drash syndrome. The majority of these patients progress to end-stage renal disease. A specific mutation of the 11p13 Wilms' tumor gene has been identified in these children. Although XY individuals have been reported most often, the syndrome has been reported in genotypic/phenotypic females. One should have a high index of suspicion for the development of renal failure and Wilms' tumor in patients with male pseudohermaphroditism. [p 2481]

12. **a. deletion of chromosome 11.** Aniridia and Wilms' tumor are most commonly associated in patients with the WAGR syndrome. These patients also have an abnormality of chromosome 11 with a germline deletion at band p13. [p 2481]

13. **a. Wilms' tumor.** BWS is characterized by excess growth at the cellular, organ (macroglossia, nephromegaly, hepatomegaly), or body segment (hemihypertrophy) levels. Most cases of BWS are sporadic, but up to 15% exhibit heritable characteristics with apparent autosomal dominant inheritance. The risk of nephroblastoma in children with BWS and hemihypertrophy is estimated to be 4% to 10%. [p 2482]

14. **c. Nephromegaly.** Children with BWS found to have nephromegaly (kidneys greater than or equal to the 95th percentile of age-adjusted renal length) are at the greatest risk for the development of Wilms' tumor. [p 2482]

15. **b. detection of lower stage renal tumor.** Screening with serial renal ultrasonographic scans has been recommended in children with aniridia, hemihypertrophy, and BWS. Review of most studies suggests that 3 to 4 months is the appropriate screening interval. Tumors detected by screening will generally be at a lower stage. [p 2482]

16. **a. Aniridia.** Approximately 50% of patients with WAGR syndrome and a constitutional deletion on chromosome 11 will develop Wilms' tumor. [p 2481]

17. **d. LOH for chromosome 16q.** LOH for a portion of chromosome 16q has been noted in 20% of Wilms' tumors. A study of 232 patients registered on the National Wilms Tumor Study Group (NWTSG) found LOH for 16q in 17% of the tumors. Patients with tumor-specific LOH for chromosome 16q had a statistically significantly poorer 2-year relapse-free and overall survival rate than did those patients without LOH for chromosome 16q. [pp 2487–2488]

18. **b. Histologic subtype.** Markers associated with unfavorable outcome include nuclear atypia (anaplasia), focal or diffuse, and sarcomatous tumors (rhabdoid and clear cell type). The latter two tumor types, however, are tumor categories distinct from Wilms' tumor. These unfavorable features occurred in approximately 10% of patients but accounted for almost half of the tumor deaths in early NWTSG studies. [pp 2483–2484]

19. **a. Diffuse anaplasia.** Anaplasia is associated with resistance to chemotherapy. This is evidenced by the similar incidence of anaplasia (5%) in the NWTSG and International Society of Paediatric Oncology studies. Although the presence of anaplasia has clearly been demonstrated to carry a poor prognosis, patients with stage I anaplastic Wilms' tumor as well as those with higher stages and focal rather than diffuse anaplasia seem to have a more favorable outcome. This confirms the observation that anaplasia is more a marker of chemoresistance than inherent aggressiveness of the tumor. [p 2484]

20. **e. nephrogenic rests.** NWTSG investigators demonstrated the clinical importance of nephrogenic rests. Multiple rests in one kidney usually imply that nephrogenic rests are present in the other kidney. Children younger than 12 months of age diagnosed with Wilms' tumor who also have nephrogenic rests, in particular perilobar nephrogenic rests, have a markedly increased risk of developing contralateral disease and require frequent and regular surveillance for several years. [pp 2485–2486]

21. **b. MRI of the abdomen.** Compression or invasion of adjacent structures may result in an atypical presentation. Extension of Wilms' tumor into the renal vein and inferior vena cava (IVC) can cause varicocele, hepatomegaly due to hepatic vein obstruction, ascites, and congestive heart failure. Such symptoms are found in less than 10% of patients with intracaval or atrial tumor extension. [p 2486]

22. **a. Hilar lymph node involvement.** The most important determinants of outcome in children with Wilms' tumor are histopathology and tumor stage. Accurate staging of Wilms' tumor allows treatment results to be evaluated and enables universal comparisons of outcomes. The staging system used by the NWTSG (see Table 70–9) is based primarily on the surgical and histopathologic findings. Examination for extension through the capsule, residual disease, vascular involvement, and lymph node involvement is essential to properly assess the extent of the tumor. [p 2487]

23. **e. Capsular penetration.** One study identified risk factors for local tumor recurrence as tumor spillage, unfavorable histology, incomplete tumor removal, and absence of any lymph node sampling. The 2-year survival rate after abdominal recurrence was 43%, emphasizing the importance of the surgeon in performing careful and complete tumor resection. [p 2488]

24. **c. Adriamycin and chest irradiation.** Patients with stage III favorable histologic type tumors and stage II–III focal anaplasia are treated with dactinomycin, vincristine, and doxorubicin and 10.8 Gy abdominal irradiation. Patients with stage IV favorable histologic type tumors receive abdominal irradiation based on the local tumor stage and 12 Gy to both lungs. [p 2489]

25. **b. Vincristine and dactinomycin.** Accrual of patients for the NWTS-5 study should have been completed in late 2001. A portion of the study examining the role of surgery alone for children younger than 2 years of age with stage I favorable histologic type tumors weighing less than 550 g has already been suspended. This study was based on preliminary observations of favorable outcomes on small numbers of such patients when postoperative adjuvant therapy had been omitted. It was suspended when the number of tumor relapses exceeded the limit allowed by the design of the study and the recommendation was made that all children with stage I tumors receive dactinomycin and vincristine. [p 2489]

26. **c. Open biopsy followed by chemotherapy.** The current recommendations from the NWTSG are that preoperative chemotherapy is of benefit in patients with bilateral involvement, inoperable at surgical exploration, and IVC extension above the hepatic veins. All other patients should undergo primary nephrectomy. [p 2490]

27. **c. Right partial nephrectomy and left renal biopsy.** Partial nephrectomy or wedge excision can be performed at the initial operation, only if all tumors can be removed with pres-

ervation of two thirds or more of the renal parenchyma on both sides. Bilateral biopsies are obtained to confirm the presence of Wilms' tumor in both kidneys and to define the histologic type. [pp 2491–2492]

28. **e. Doxorubicin.** In recent years, there has been increasing concern regarding the risk of congestive heart failure in children who receive treatment with anthracyclines such as doxorubicin. In addition to the acute cardiotoxicity, cardiac failure can develop many years after treatment. [pp 2492–2493]

29. **c. Rhabdoid tumor of the kidney stage III.** Typical clinical features include early age at diagnosis (median age of <16 months), resistance to chemotherapy, and high mortality rate. Unlike Wilms' tumor, which typically metastasizes to the lungs, abdomen/flank, and liver, rhabdoid tumor of the kidney, which also metastasizes to these sites, is distinguished by its propensity to metastasize to the brain. [p 2493]

30. **b. Observation only.** The most important aspect of the recognition of these tumors as a separate entity is the usually excellent outcome with radical surgery only. [p 2493]

31. **c. 9.** Two genes have been identified in the tuberous sclerosis complex on chromosome 9 (*TSC1*) and chromosome 16 (*TSC2*). It has been postulated that these genes act as tumor suppressor genes and that the LOH of *TSC1* or *TSC2* may explain the progressive growth pattern of renal lesions seen in these patients. [p 2494]

32. **c. Observation.** It is important to note that an elevated alpha-fetoprotein level after orchiectomy for yolk-sac tumor in an infant does not always represent persistent disease. Normal adult reference laboratory values for alpha-fetoprotein cannot be used in young children, as alpha-fetoprotein synthesis continues after birth. Normal adult levels (<10 mg/ml) are not reached until 8 months of age. [p 2497]

33. **b. Observation.** Prepubertal mature teratomas have a benign clinical course, which contrasts with the clinical behavior of teratomas in adults, which have the propensity to metastasize. This benign behavior has led to the consideration of testicular-sparing procedures rather than radical orchiectomy. [p 2497]

34. **b. Observation.** The initial treatment for yolk-sac tumor is radical inguinal orchiectomy. This treatment is curative in most children. Routine retroperitoneal lymph node dissection and adjuvant chemotherapy are not indicated. [pp 2497–2498]

35. **c. Left orchiectomy.** Early gonadectomy is advocated, as tumors have been reported in children younger than 5 years of age. In patients with mixed gonadal dysgenesis who are reared as males, all streak gonads and undescended testes should be removed. Scrotal testes can be preserved because they are less prone to tumor development. [p 2499]

Chapter 71

Urinary Tract Reconstruction in Children

Mark C. Adams • David B. Joseph

Questions

1. What is the most common diagnosis in children that results in significant bladder or sphincter dysfunction and that requires reconstructive surgery?

    a. Bladder exstrophy or epispadias
    b. Posterior urethral valves
    c. Cloacal anomalies
    d. Prune-belly syndrome
    e. Spinal dysraphism

2. What was the most important contribution to the field of pediatric reconstructive surgery?

    a. Mitrofanoff's description of a continent abdominal wall stoma using appendix
    b. The introduction of clean intermittent catheterization (CIC) by Lapides
    c. Goodwin's description of ileal reconfiguration
    d. Development of several effective means to increase bladder outlet resistance
    e. Recognition that a dilated ureter could be used for bladder augmentation

3. Normal bladder compliance is based on which of the following factors?

    a. Ample collagen type II
    b. The inverse relationship of bladder volume and bladder pressure
    c. Bladder unfolding, elasticity, and viscoelasticity
    d. Subepithelial matrix bridges associated with collagen
    e. Hypertrophic bladder bundles interspersed with collagen

4. Chronically elevated bladder filling pressures may cause hydronephrosis, vesicoureteral reflux, and impaired renal function. The lowest threshold to typically cause problems is chronic bladder pressure of more than:

    a. 20 cm H_2O.
    b. 30 cm H_2O.
    c. 40 cm H_2O.
    d. 50 cm H_2O.
    e. 60 cm H_2O.

5. How are upper urinary tract changes associated with a poorly compliant, hyperreflexic bladder initially treated?

    a. Autoaugmentation
    b. Pharmacologic management and intermittent catheterization
    c. Ileal augmentation

d. Sigmoid augmentation
e. Gastric augmentation

6. Before reconstructive surgery, bladder capacity and compliance can best be determined by urodynamics using:

   a. carbon dioxide as an irrigant at a slow fill rate (<10% of capacity per minute).
   b. body temperature saline at a slow fill rate (<10% of capacity per minute).
   c. body temperature saline at a fast fill rate (>10% of capacity per minute).
   d. cooled saline at a slow fill rate (<10% of capacity per minute).
   e. cooled saline at a fast fill rate (>10% of capacity per minute).

7. Before urinary tract reconstruction to achieve urinary continence, it is most important to:

   a. confirm a normal upper urinary tract.
   b. identify a highly compliant bladder.
   c. document the presence or absence of vesicoureteral reflux.
   d. ensure acceptance and compliance with intermittent catheterization.
   e. document a serum creatinine value less than 1.4 mg/dl.

8. Mechanical bowel preparation should be performed in patients planned for which procedure?

   a. Ileocystoplasty
   b. Sigmoid cystoplasty
   c. Gastrocystoplasty
   d. Ureterocystoplasty
   e. All of the above

9. All of the following steps aid in achieving a good result with transureteroureterostomy (TUU) except which one?

   a. Careful mobilization of the crossing ureter with periureteral tissue.
   b. Careful mobilization of the crossing ureter without angulation beneath the inferior mesenteric artery.
   c. Careful mobilization of the recipient ureter to meet the crossing one.
   d. Wide anastomosis of the crossing ureter to the posteromedial aspect of the recipient one.
   e. Water-tight anastomosis of the two ureters.

10. Creation of an antireflux mechanism is most difficult with which of the following intestinal segments?

    a. Stomach
    b. Ileum
    c. Cecum
    d. Transverse colon
    e. Sigmoid colon

11. Which of the following statements is true regarding the Young-Dees-Leadbetter bladder neck repair in children with neurogenic sphincter deficiency?

    a. It results in limited success because of a lack of muscle tone and activity of the native bladder neck.
    b. It can achieve successful continence results similar to those noted in children with bladder exstrophy.
    c. It does not often require bladder augmentation or intermittent catheterization.
    d. It is best performed in association with a Silastic sling.
    e. It limits the necessity for intermittent catheterization in children who could empty by a Valsalva maneuver preoperatively.

12. An ambulatory 15-year-old patient with lumbosacral myelomeningocele voids to completion with a low-pressure detrusor contraction, which is augmented by abdominal straining. However, urinary incontinence persists due to bladder neck and intrinsic sphincter dysfunction, which is refractory to pharmacologic management. What is the most appropriate form of operative intervention potentially avoiding the need for catheterization?

    a. Young-Dees-Leadbetter bladder neck repair
    b. Artificial urinary sphincter placement
    c. Fascial bladder neck sling placement
    d. Kropp bladder neck repair
    e. Pippi-Salle bladder neck repair

13. Which of the following is one of the most serious side effects associated with bladder neck repair?

    a. Recurrent urolithiasis
    b. Recurrent cystitis
    c. Inability to spontaneously void
    d. The associated need for augmentation cystoplasty
    e. The unmasking of detrusor hostility, resulting in upper urinary tract changes

14. Fascial slings to increase outflow resistance in the pediatric population can be expected to:

    a. produce better results in girls than in boys with neurogenic sphincteric incompetence.
    b. produce results dependent on the type of fascial or cadaveric tissue used.
    c. produce results dependent on the configuration of the sling and wrap used.
    d. produce results that rarely include the need for bladder augmentation and intermittent catheterization.
    e. produce results complicated by a significant rate of urethral erosion.

15. Which of the following is a relative contraindication to the use of the artificial urinary sphincter to achieve adequate outflow resistance and continence?

    a. Neurogenic bladder dysfunction
    b. Bladder exstrophy or epispadias
    c. Inability to empty the bladder by spontaneous voiding
    d. An associated need for bladder augmentation
    e. Prepubertal age

16. What has been the most common complication of the Kropp technique of urethral lengthening and implantation?

    a. A fistula from the urethra to the bladder, resulting in incontinence
    b. Inability to spontaneously void, resulting in urinary retention
    c. Difficulty with intermittent catheterization, particularly in boys
    d. New vesicoureteral reflux
    e. Distal ureteral obstruction

17. Urinary continence without urethral leakage is most definitively achieved after which of the following bladder neck procedures?

    a. Young-Dees-Leadbetter bladder repair
    b. Artificial urinary sphincter placement
    c. Placement of a fascial sling with circumferential wrap
    d. Urethral lengthening and reimplantation
    e. Bladder neck division

18. What is the most important step in enterocystoplasty to avoid uninhibited pressure contractions postoperatively?

    a. Use of a large bowel segment for augmentation
    b. Reconfiguration of the intestinal segment

c. Excision of the majority of the diseased bladder
d. A stellate incision into the bladder to increase the circumference of the anastomosis to the bowel
e. Use of small mesenteric windows in the bowel to avoid vascular injury to the isolated segment

19. An antireflux mechanism may be constructed using ileum by each of the following except which one?

    a. An intussuscepted nipple valve
    b. A split nipple cuff of ureter
    c. Placement of the spatulated ureter into an incised mucosal trough as described by LeDuc
    d. A flap valve created beneath a tenia
    e. Placement of the ureter within a serosa-lined tunnel created between two limbs of ileum

20. The use of which of the following gastrointestinal segments for simple bladder augmentation in the neurogenic population is most commonly associated with permanent gastrointestinal side effects?

    a. Stomach
    b. Jejunum
    c. Ileum
    d. Ileocecal segment
    e. Sigmoid colon

21. Possible effects on gastrointestinal function after bladder augmentation include all of the following except which one?

    a. Early satiety
    b. Hyperchloremic metabolic acidosis
    c. Small bowel obstruction
    d. Chronic diarrhea
    e. Vitamin B_{12} deficiency with megaloblastic anemia

22. The vast majority of published reports regarding pediatric bladder augmentation suggest that which of the following bowel segments is the least likely to be associated with postoperative problems related to capacity and compliance?

    a. Gastric body
    b. Gastric antrum
    c. Ileum
    d. Cecum
    e. Sigmoid colon

23. In preoperative counseling before bladder augmentation, the risk of failure related to problems with capacity and compliance should be mentioned at which rate?

    a. <2%
    b. 5% to 10%
    c. 11% to 15%
    d. 16% to 20%
    e. >20%

24. Which serum metabolic pattern is most likely to be found after ileo- or colocystoplasty?

    a. Hypochloremic metabolic acidosis
    b. Hyperchloremic metabolic acidosis
    c. Hypochloremic metabolic alkalosis
    d. Hyperchloremic metabolic alkalosis
    e. Hyponatremic metabolic acidosis

25. Which serum metabolic problem is most likely to be found after gastrocystoplasty?

    a. Hypochloremic metabolic acidosis
    b. Hyperchloremic metabolic acidosis
    c. Hypochloremic metabolic alkalosis
    d. Hyperchloremic metabolic alkalosis
    e. Hyponatremic metabolic acidosis

26. Intermittent hematuria and dysuria after gastrocystoplasty are more likely to occur in patients with all of the following except:

    a. gastric body used in the bladder.
    b. persistent urinary incontinence.
    c. decreased renal function.
    d. a diagnosis of bladder exstrophy.
    e. neurogenic bladder dysfunction.

27. Bacteriuria should be treated after bladder augmentation if:

    a. the patient performs CIC.
    b. urinalysis demonstrates microscopic hematuria.
    c. the patient has noticed increased mucus production.
    d. the underlying diagnosis is posterior urethral valves.
    e. urine culture reveals growth of a urea-splitting organism.

28. Bladder calculi after augmentation cystoplasty have been recognized with more frequency and are likely due to mucus production and bacteriuria. Which segment is associated with the lowest incident of stone formation?

    a. Stomach
    b. Jejunum
    c. Ileum
    d. Cecum
    e. Sigmoid colon

29. What is the shortest time reported to develop an adenocarcinoma in the bladder after augmentation?

    a. 2 years
    b. 4 years
    c. 8 years
    d. 16 years
    e. 26 years

30. Factors associated with an increased risk of perforation after bladder augmentation include all of the following except which one?

    a. High outflow resistance
    b. Persistent hyperreflexia or uninhibited bladder contractions
    c. Use of sigmoid colon for augmentation
    d. An underlying diagnosis of bladder exstrophy
    e. An underlying diagnosis of neurogenic bladder dysfunction

31. Initial management of a patient found to have spontaneous perforation of an augmented bladder should include which of the following?

    a. Placement of a large-bore urethral catheter for drainage
    b. Placement of a large-bore suprapubic cystotomy tube for drainage
    c. Immediate surgical exploration and repair
    d. Serial abdominal examinations
    e. Urine culture

32. Pregnancy in women having undergone urinary reconstruction is best characterized by which of the following statements?

    a. Pregnancy is reasonable for women who have undergone urinary diversion but is contraindicated with augmentation cystoplasty.
    b. The mesenteric pedicle of the augmentation is typically found directly anterior to the uterus.
    c. The mesenteric pedicle of the augmentation has usually been found to be deflected laterally and has not compromised the vascular supply to the augmented segment.
    d. Pregnancy should be cautioned against in women with augmentation cystoplasty because of the reported loss of

the augmented segment secondary to ischemia from mechanical compression of the pedicle.
    e. Pregnancy is contraindicated in women after augmentation cystoplasty because of increased risk of systemic sepsis complicating the hydronephrosis of pregnancy and chronic bacteriuria associated with the augmented segment.

33. What is the major disadvantage of ureterocystoplasty at this time?
    a. It requires an intraperitoneal approach.
    b. Complete mobilization of the ureter may result in vascular compromise.
    c. The dilated ureter is not as compliant as a similar sized bowel segment.
    d. A dilated ureter is not available in many patients.
    e. Ureterocystoplasty precludes spontaneous voiding.

34. Which of the following should be considered a contraindication to autoaugmentation?
    a. A serum creatinine value greater than 1.4 ng/dl
    b. An associated need to perform CIC
    c. Vesicoureteral reflux
    d. Uninhibited bladder contractions
    e. Small bladder capacity

35. Which of the following is(are) an absolute contraindication(s) to ureterosigmoidostomy and its variants?
    a. Dilated ureters
    b. Anteriorly placed rectum associated with a diagnosis of bladder exstrophy
    c. History of recurrent pyelonephritis
    d. Fecal incontinence
    e. History of constipation

36. Which of the following statements best characterizes the use of nipple valves in efferent limb construction for pediatric continent diversion?
    a. Results with nipple valves in children have not approached those achieved for adults.
    b. Despite various modifications to secure the nipple, complication and reoperation rates have been higher than those associated with flap valves.
    c. Results are equivalent to those with any other continence mechanism.
    d. The most common complication is difficulty with catheterization.
    e. Stomal stenosis is the most common complication.

37. Which of the following statements regarding appendicovesicostomy is incorrect?
    a. A wide cecal cuff will help decrease the potential for stomal stenosis.
    b. A greater than 5:1 ratio of diameter to tunnel length is required for continence.
    c. The small, uniform lumen allows for easy catheterization.
    d. The right colon may need to be mobilized to adequately mobilize the appendix.
    e. Additional proximal length can be obtained by tubularizing a small portion of the cecum in continuity with the appendix.

38. Which of the following has been the most common complication of continent urinary diversion using the flap valve mechanism?
    a. Urinary incontinence caused by the inadequate length of the flap valve mechanism
    b. Urinary incontinence caused by persistently elevated reservoir pressure
    c. Appendiceal perforation with catheterization
    d. Appendiceal stricture or necrosis
    e. Stomal stenosis

39. A 12-year-old obese girl with spina bifida is undergoing reconstruction with creation of a stoma for antegrade continence enemas using the appendix, bladder neck sling, bladder augmentation, and construction of a continent catheterizable stoma for independent self-catheterization. Her upper urinary tract is normal. What is the best source of tissue for the continent urinary stoma?
    a. The distal right ureter after right-to-left TUU
    b. A tapered segment of small bowel of adequate length
    c. The right fallopian tube
    d. A gastric tube
    e. A tubularized bladder flap

40. In complex urinary undiversion for pediatric patients, which aspect is most likely to be associated with complications and require reoperation?
    a. Providing adequate outflow resistance
    b. Providing a compliant urinary reservoir
    c. Achieving an effective antireflux mechanism without upper tract obstruction
    d. Providing a reliable means of intermittent catheterization when necessary
    e. Achieving urinary and fecal continence

Answers

1. **e. Spinal dysraphism.** Most reconstructive procedures are now undertaken primarily to correct a problem in the native urinary tract (hydronephrosis, infection, incontinence) unresponsive to medical management or after temporary diversion. Children with bladder and sphincteric dysfunction represent some of the most complex cases seen in pediatric urology; among others, patients with diagnoses such as exstrophy, persistent cloaca and urogenital sinus, posterior urethral valves, bilateral single ectopic ureters, and prune-belly syndrome may be involved. For most pediatric urologists, patients with myelomeningocele make up the vast majority of patients requiring this type of surgical intervention. [p 2509]

2. **b. The introduction of clean intermittent catheterization (CIC) by Lapides.** One of the most important contributions in the care of children with bladder dysfunction came with the acceptance of clean intermittent catheterization described by Lapides and colleagues in 1972 and 1976, based on the work of Guttmann and Frankel. The effective use of CIC has allowed the application of augmentation and lower tract reconstruction to groups of patients who had not previously been candidates. The principle of intermittent catheterization allows the reconstructive surgeon to aggressively correct storage problems by providing an adequate reservoir and good outflow resistance. Good spontaneous voiding, while a goal, is not imperative because catheterization can be used for emptying. [p 2511]

3. **c. Bladder unfolding, elasticity, and viscoelasticity.** Multi-

ple factors contribute to the property of compliance. Initially the bladder is in a collapsed state, which allows for the storage of urine at low pressure by simply unfolding. As it expands, detrusor properties of elasticity and viscoelasticity take effect. Elasticity allows the detrusor muscle to stretch without an increase in tension until it reaches a critical volume. When filling is slow, as in a natural state, or stops, there is a rapid decay in this pressure known as stress relaxation. Normally, stress relaxation is in balance with the filling rate and prevents an increase in detrusor pressure. [p 2509]

4. **c. 40 cm H$_2$O.** Elevated passive filling pressure becomes clinically pathogenic when a pressure greater than 40 cm H$_2$O is chronically reached. Pressures at this level sustained over a period of time impair ureteral drainage, which may result in pyelocaliceal changes, hydroureteronephrosis, and decreased glomerular filtration rate. In addition, persistent elevation in filling pressure can result in acquired vesicoureteral reflux. [p 2510]

5. **b. Pharmacologic management and intermittent catheterization.** Pharmacologic management can play a role in decreasing filling pressure, particularly when hyperreflexic detrusor contractions are present. A combination of medications and intermittent catheterization has a positive impact, particularly in children with neurogenic dysfunction. [p 2510]

6. **b. body temperature saline at a slow fill rate (<10% of capacity per minute).** The testing medium and infusion rate can influence the results. Carbon dioxide is not as reliable as fluid infusion, particularly when evaluating bladder compliance and capacity. The most common fluids used for testing are saline and iodinated contrast material, both of which provide reproducible results. Use of testing media at body temperature is also appropriate. End filling pressure, and therefore bladder compliance, can be dramatically affected by simply changing the filling rate. One study suggested that the cystometrogram be performed at a fill rate of no greater than 10% per minute of the predicted bladder capacity for age. [p 2512]

7. **d. ensure acceptance and compliance with intermittent catheterization.** No test ensures that a patient will be able to void spontaneously and empty well after bladder augmentation or other reconstruction. Therefore, all patients must be prepared to perform CIC postoperatively. The native urethra should be examined for the ease of catheterization. Ideally, the patient should learn CIC and practice it preoperatively until the patient, family, and surgeon are comfortable that catheterization can and will be done reliably. Failure to catheterize and empty reliably after bladder reconstruction may result in upper tract deterioration, urinary tract infection, or bladder perforation despite a technically perfect operation. [p 2513]

8. **e. All of the above.** Each patient undergoes preoperative bowel preparation to minimize the potential risk of surgery if the use of any bowel is contemplated. Even when ureterocystoplasty or other alternatives are planned, intraoperative findings may dictate the need for use of a bowel segment. [p 2513]

9. **c. Careful mobilization of the recipient ureter to meet the crossing one.** If the native urinary bladder is small and adequate for only a single ureteral tunnel, TUU and a single reimplant may be helpful (see Fig. 71-1). Typically, the better ureter should be implanted into the bladder, draining the other across into it. The crossing ureter should be mobilized to swing gently across the abdomen to the donor side in a smooth course without tension. It should be carefully mobilized with all of its adventitia and as much periureteral tissue as possible to preserve blood supply. Care must be taken not to angulate the crossing ureter immediately beneath the inferior mesenteric artery. The crossing ureter is widely anastomosed to the posteromedial aspect of the recipient ureter. The recipient is not mobilized or brought medially to meet the end of the other ureter. [p 2514]

10. **b. Ileum.** The necessity of ureteral reimplantation into an intestinal segment may occasionally determine the segment to be used for bladder augmentation or replacement. Long experience with ureterosigmoidostomy and colon conduit diversion has established an effective means of creating antireflux into a colonic segment. If a gastric segment is used for bladder augmentation or replacement, ureters may be reimplanted into the stomach in a manner remarkably similar to that used in the native bladder. Creating an effective antireflux mechanism into an ileal segment is more difficult. The split nipple technique described by Griffith may prevent reflux at least at low reservoir pressure. [pp 2514, 2516]

11. **a. It results in limited success because of a lack of muscle tone and activity of the native bladder neck.** Reports of success with the Young-Dees-Leadbetter bladder neck reconstruction in children with neurogenic sphincter dysfunction are limited, not only in the number of series but in overall improvement of incontinence. Independent reviews of long-term results of this repair showed minimal success in individuals with neurogenic dysfunction. These authors speculated that the lack of success was due to a lack of muscle tone and activity in the wrapped muscle related to the neurogenic problem. [p 2517]

12. **b. Artificial urinary sphincter placement.** The artificial urinary sphincter has been recognized as a device that can result in prompt continence in selected children while preserving their ability to void spontaneously. [p 2519]

13. **e. The unmasking of detrusor hostility, resulting in upper urinary tract changes.** It is now recognized that occlusion of the bladder neck in children with neurogenic sphincter incompetence can result in the unmasking or development of detrusor hostility manifest by a decrease in bladder compliance or increase in detrusor hyperreflexia. Careful preoperative urodynamic assessment helps to identify only some of the children who are at risk. [pp 2520-2521]

14. **a. produce better results in girls than in boys with neurogenic sphincteric incompetence.** Fascial slings have been used more extensively and with better results in girls with neurogenic sphincter incompetence, although recently some success has been reported in boys. Overall long-term success with fascial slings in the neurogenic population has varied greatly from 40% to 100%. [p 2518]

15. **c. Inability to empty the bladder by spontaneous voiding.** The ultimate benefits of the artificial urinary sphincter include its ability to achieve a high rate of continence while maintaining the potential for spontaneous voiding. For practical purposes, when intermittent catheterization is required along with augmentation cystoplasty, using native tissue for continence eliminates the long-term concern for infection/erosion and the risk of mechanical failure. [p 2521]

16. **c. Difficulty with intermittent catheterization, particularly in boys.** One study examined the results in 23 children, 22 of whom had neurogenic sphincter incompetence, and noted continence in more than 90% of the children. The most common complication was difficult catheterization, particularly in boys. Less than half of the boys in this series catheterized through the native urethra; the majority did so via an abdominal wall stoma. [p 2523]

17. **e. Bladder neck division.** The ultimate procedure to increase bladder outlet resistance is to divide the bladder neck so that it is no longer in continuity with the urethra. This must be accompanied by creation of a continent abdominal wall stoma and should be performed only in patients who will reliably catheterize. [p 2523]

18. **b. Reconfiguration of the intestinal segment.** Two studies well demonstrated the advantages of opening a bowel segment on its antimesenteric border, which allows detubularization and reconfiguration of that intestinal segment. Reconfiguration into a spherical shape provides multiple advantages, including maximization of the volume achieved for any given surface area, blunting of bowel contractions, and improvement of overall capacity and compliance. [p 2525]

19. **d. A flap valve created beneath a tenia.** The split nipple technique described by Griffith may prevent reflux at least at low reservoir pressure. LeDuc and colleagues in 1987 described a technique in which the ureter is brought through a hiatus in the ileal wall. From that hiatus, the ileal mucosa is incised and the edges are mobilized so as to create a trough for the ureter. It may also be possible to create antireflux using a serosal-lined tunnel created between two limbs of ileum as described by Abol-Enein and Ghoneim in 1999. Reinforced nipple valves of ileum have been used extensively for antireflux with the Kock pouch. After several modifications by Skinner, good long-term results have been achieved. [p 2516]

20. **d. Ileocecal segment.** Reports of chronic diarrhea after bladder augmentation alone have been rare. Diarrhea can occur after removal of large segments of ileum from the gastrointestinal tract, although the length of the segments typically used for augmentation is rarely problematic unless other problems coexist. Removal of a segment from the gastrointestinal tract including the ileocecal valve is the most likely to cause diarrhea. One study noted that 10% of patients with neurogenic dysfunction have significant diarrhea after such displacement. [p 2532]

21. **b. Hyperchloremic metabolic acidosis.** Postoperative bowel obstruction is uncommon after augmentation cystoplasty, occurring in approximately 3% of patients after augmentation. The rate of obstruction is equivalent to that noted after conduit diversion or continent urinary diversion. Removal of the distal ileum from the gastrointestinal tract may therefore result in vitamin B_{12} deficiency and megaloblastic anemia. Certainly the terminal 15 to 20 cm of ileum should not be used for augmentation, although problems may arise even if that segment is preserved. Early satiety may occur after gastrocystoplasty but usually resolves with time. Disorders of gastric emptying should be extremely rare, particularly when using the body of the stomach. [p 2532]

22. **c. Ileum.** In continent urinary diversion, ileal reservoirs have been noted to have lower basal pressures and less motor activity. Any problems with pressure following augmentation cystoplasty usually occur from uninhibited contractions, apparently in the bowel segment. It is extremely rare not to achieve an adequate capacity or flat tonus limb unless a technical error has occurred with use of the bowel segment. Rhythmic contractions have been noted postoperatively with all bowel segments, although ileum seems the least likely to demonstrate remarkable urodynamic abnormalities, and stomach the most. [p 2533]

23. **b. 5% to 10%.** In perhaps the largest experience with pediatric bladder augmentation, Hollensbe and associates at Indiana University found that approximately 5% of several hundred patients after augmentation cystoplasty had significant uninhibited contractions causing clinical problems. Another study found that 6% of more than 300 patients required secondary augmentation of a previously augmented bladder for similar problems in long-term follow-up. [p 2533]

24. **b. Hyperchloremic metabolic acidosis.** The first recognized metabolic complication related to storage of urine within intestinal segments was the occasional development of hyperchloremic metabolic acidosis after ureterosigmoidostomy. Another study demonstrated the mechanisms by which acid is absorbed from urine in contact with intestinal mucosa. A later report noted that essentially every patient after augmentation with an intestinal segment had an increase in serum chloride and a decrease in serum bicarbonate level, although full acidosis was rare if renal function was normal. [p 2534]

25. **c. Hypochloremic metabolic alkalosis.** Gastric mucosa is a barrier to chloride and acid resorption and, in fact, secretes hydrochloric acid. The secretory nature of gastric mucosa may at times be detrimental to the patient and can result in two unique complications of gastrocystoplasty. Severe episodes of hypokalemic hypochloremic metabolic alkalosis after acute gastrointestinal illnesses have been noted in 5 of 37 patients after gastrocystoplasty. [p 2534]

26. **e. neurogenic bladder dysfunction.** Virtually all patients after gastrocystoplasty with normal sensation have occasional hematuria or dysuria with voiding or catheterization beyond that which is expected with other intestinal segments. All patients should be warned of this potential problem, although in most patients these symptoms are intermittent and mild and do not require treatment. The dysuria is certainly not as problematic in patients with neurogenic dysfunction. Certain authors believe that patients who are incontinent or have decreased renal function are at increased risk. Such problems can occur but are less frequent after antral cystoplasty in which there is a smaller load of parietal cells. [p 2535]

27. **e. urine culture reveals growth of a urea-splitting organism.** It appears that the use of CIC is a prominent factor in the development of bacteriuria in patients after augmentation cystoplasty. Every episode of asymptomatic bacteriuria does not require treatment in patients performing CIC. Bacteriuria should be treated for significant symptoms such as incontinence or suprapubic pain and may be treated for hematuria, foul-smelling urine, or remarkably increased mucus production. Bacteriuria should be treated if the urine culture demonstrates growth of a urea-splitting organism that may lead to stone formation. [p 2536]

28. **a. Stomach.** The majority of bladder stones in this patient population are struvite in composition, and bacteriuria has been thought to be an important risk factor. Stones have been noted after the use of all intestinal segments with no significant difference noted between small and large intestine. Struvite stones are less likely after gastrocystoplasty. [p 2536]

29. **b. 4 years.** Patients undergoing augmentation cystoplasty should be made aware of a potential increased risk of tumor development. Yearly surveillance of the augmented bladder with endoscopy should eventually be performed; the latency period until such procedures are necessary is not well defined. The earliest reported tumor after augmentation was found only 4 years after cystoplasty. [p 2537]

30. **d. An underlying diagnosis of bladder exstrophy.** The cause of delayed perforations within a bowel segment is unknown. One report indicated that perforations occur in bladders with significant uninhibited contractions following augmentation, as have others. High outflow resistance may

maintain bladder pressure rather than allowing urinary leakage and venting of the pressure, potentially increasing ischemia. The majority of patients suffering perforations following augmentation cystoplasty have had myelodysplasia. At Indiana University, perforations were noted in 32 of 330 patients undergoing cystoplasty an average of 4.3 years after augmentation. Analysis of this experience suggested that the use of sigmoid colon was the only significant increased risk. [pp 2537–2538]

31. **c. Immediate surgical exploration and repair.** The standard treatment of spontaneous perforation of the augmented bladder is surgical repair, as it is for intraperitoneal rupture of the bladder following trauma. The majority of patients with perforations have myelodysplasia and present late in the course of the disease because of impaired sensation. Increasing sepsis and death of the patient may result from a delay in diagnosis or treatment. [pp 2538–2539]

32. **c. The mesenteric pedicle of the augmentation has usually been found to be deflected laterally and has not compromised the vascular supply to the augmented segment.** Experience during pregnancy related to the pedicle of a prior bladder augmentation is very limited. Certain authors have noted that the mesenteric pedicle to bladder augmentations did not appear to be stretched at the time of cesarean section. In those cases, the pedicle was not located near the exposed anterior uterus but deflected laterally. Urinary tract infections may be problematic in women who have undergone urinary reconstruction, including bladder augmentation. Ureteral dilatation, increased residual urine, and diminished tone to the upper tract may all be important risk factors. [p 2539]

33. **d. A dilated ureter is not available in many patients.** Numerous series have reported good results following augmentation using ureters, some with follow-up as long as 8 years. The upper tracts have remained stable or improved in virtually all patients. Complications have been uncommon. The main disadvantage to ureterocystoplasty is the limited patient population with a nonfunctioning kidney draining into a megaureter. [p 2541]

34. **e. Small bladder capacity.** There has been concern that although these procedures usually improve compliance, increase in volume is "modest at best." In a report of 12 detrusorectomies, five patients were considered to have excellent results, two had acceptable results, and one was lost to follow-up. The main disadvantage of autoaugmentation is a limited increase in bladder capacity such that adequate preoperative volume may be the most important predictor of success. [pp 2542–2543]

35. **d. Fecal incontinence.** Before any variant of ureterosigmoidostomy is considered, competence of the anal sphincter must be ensured. Tests used to assess sphincter integrity include manometry, electromyography, and practical evaluation of the ability to retain an oatmeal enema in the upright position for a time period without soilage. Incontinence of a mixture of stool and urine results in foul soilage and must be avoided. [p 2546]

36. **b. Despite various modifications to secure the nipple, complication and reoperation rates have been higher than those associated with flap valves.** The greatest experience with nipple valves used to achieve urinary continence has been with the Kock pouch. Skinner and associates made a series of modifications to aid in maintenance of the efferent nipple. Even with experience and these modifications, a failure rate of 15% or higher can be expected. Equivalent results with the nipple valve and a Kock pouch have been achieved in children. [p 2546]

37. **b. A greater than 5:1 ratio of diameter to tunnel length is required for continence.** The appendix is an ideal natural tubular structure that can be safely removed from the gastrointestinal tract without significant morbidity. The small caliber of the appendix facilitates creation of a short functional tunnel with the bladder wall. Experience has shown that continence can be achieved with only a 2-cm appendiceal tunnel. [p 2547]

38. **e. Stomal stenosis.** Incontinence is a rare event with the Mitrofanoff principle and may result from inadequate length of the flap valve mechanism or persistently elevated reservoir pressure. The most common complication has been stomal stenosis, which has generally occurred in 10% to 20% of patients. Such stenosis resulting in difficult catheterization may occur early in the postoperative course and require formal revision. [p 2548]

39. **b. A tapered segment of small bowel of adequate length.** When the appendix is unavailable for use, other tubular structures can provide a similar mechanism for catheterization and continence. Mitrofanoff in 1980 described a similar technique using ureter. Woodhouse and MacNeily in 1994 as well as others have used the fallopian tube, which can accommodate catheterization. Monti has been credited with a novel modification of the tapered intestinal segment, which can be reimplanted according to the Mitrofanoff principle. Recognition should also be directed to another report of this procedure by Yang. [p 2548]

40. **c. Achieving an effective antireflux mechanism without upper tract obstruction.** The key to urinary undiversion is understanding the original pathologic condition that led to diversion. One report described a 26-year experience with urinary undiversion in 216 patients. In that series, management of the bladder was relatively straightforward and effective with bladder augmentation as necessary. Inadequate outflow resistance was usually treated with Young-Dees-Ledbetter bladder neck repair. Most complications were related to the ureters; 23 patients required reoperation for persistent reflux, whereas 10 did so for partial obstruction of the ureter. Those reoperation rates are indicative of the difficulty one faces in dealing with short, dilated, and scarred ureters, which may be present after urinary diversion. [pp 2554–2555]

Chapter 72

Pediatric Endourology and Laparoscopy

Steven G. Docimo • Craig A. Peters

Questions

1. Routine follow-up after a retrograde ureteroscopic stone removal in a 5-year-old girl should include which examination?

   a. Intravenous pyelography (IVP)
   b. Voiding cystourethrography
   c. Renal ultrasonography
   d. Dimercaptosuccinic acid (DMSA) scan
   e. Mercaptoacetyltriglycine (MAG3) diuretic renography

2. In a 12-month-old child, what is the most appropriate irrigating fluid to use during percutaneous nephrolithotripsy with electrohydraulic lithotripsy?

   a. Glycine
   b. Warmed glycine
   c. Warmed water
   d. Warmed saline
   e. Either warmed glycine or warmed water

3. A 4-year-old boy with a family history of calcium oxalate stone disease is found to have a 12-mm calculus in the left renal pelvis with no hydronephrosis. He has had no urinary tract surgery. What would be the first-line surgical approach to this stone?

   a. Shock wave lithotripsy
   b. Shock wave lithotripsy with a ureteral stent
   c. Minipercutaneous nephrolithotomy
   d. Ureteroscopy after "prestenting" to dilate the ureter
   e. Posterior lumbotomy approach to pyelolithotomy

4. A 2-year-old boy has had pyeloplasty, and now, 3 months later, has a nephrostomy tube in place for poor drainage. Which of the following is considered an absolute contraindication to percutaneous endopyelotomy?

   a. Differential renal function less than 20%
   b. Inability to cannulate the lumen of the ureteropelvic junction
   c. Renal pelvis greater than 50 ml
   d. Suspected crossing vessel
   e. None of the above

5. An 8-year-old boy with persistent right flank pain is found to have a 4-cm cystic structure containing a calcification in the lateral upper pole of his right kidney. It fills with contrast material on IVP. What is the best management?

   a. Open marsupialization
   b. Retrograde incision of diverticular neck and stone removal
   c. Observation
   d. Percutaneous stone removal and diverticular ablation
   e. Upper pole nephrectomy

6. What is the principal goal of diagnostic laparoscopy for a nonpalpable testis?

   a. Confirmation of the absence of the testis
   b. Documentation of the location and presence of the testis
   c. Preparation for a first-stage laparoscopic orchiopexy
   d. Preparation for a one-stage laparoscopic orchiopexy
   e. Documentation of passage of the testis through the internal inguinal ring

7. Before diagnostic laparoscopy for a nonpalpable testis, it is essential to:

   a. assess contralateral testicular size.
   b. obtain a pelvic ultrasonographic scan.
   c. obtain an abdominal MRI scan.
   d. perform a human chorionic gonadotropin (hCG) stimulation test.
   e. perform an examination with the patient under anesthesia.

8. What is the definition of a vanishing intra-abdominal testis?

   a. Atretic vas deferens, absence of spermatic vessels
   b. Atretic spermatic vessels with no vas deferens
   c. Presence of both spermatic vessels and vas ending blindly
   d. Absence of both vas deferens and spermatic vessels
   e. A fibrous nub of tissue at the internal inguinal ring

9. During a diagnostic laparoscopy for a nonpalpable testis, the vas deferens and thin spermatic vessels are seen to pass through the internal inguinal ring. What is the best next step?

   a. Conclude the procedure
   b. Perform a formal inguinal exploration for the testis
   c. Perform a perineal exploration for an ectopic testis
   d. Perform a low inguinal incision to remove the testicular nub
   e. Continue the laparoscopic exploration for an occult pelvic testis

10. The role of laparoscopy in children with intersex conditions is principally when:

    a. gonadal development may be abnormal or discordant with sex of rearing.
    b. müllerian structures are present.
    c. the external genitalia suggest the presence of 5α-reductase deficiency.
    d. congenital adrenal hyperplasia is suspected.
    e. gonadal function is deficient.

11. Which of the following is a significant functional consequence of pneumoperitoneum in children compared with adults?

a. Increased cardiac output
b. Reduced oxygen reserve
c. Increased urine output
d. Reduced CO_2 absorption
e. Increased cardiac irritability

12. During transperitoneal laparoscopic nephrectomy, a 2-year-old child's urine output falls to less than 0.2 ml/kg/hour. What is the most appropriate management?

    a. Immediate bolus of isotonic saline, 10 ml/kg
    b. Emergency treatment for CO_2 embolus
    c. Cessation of the procedure and conversion to open nephrectomy
    d. Continuation of the procedure and monitoring of postoperative urine output
    e. Increasing the intravenous fluid rate to 100 ml/hour

13. Which anatomic structure should be preserved during dissection for a laparoscopic orchidopexy?

    a. Umbilical ligament (medial umbilical ligament)
    b. Peritoneal triangle between the vas deferens and the spermatic vessels
    c. Appendix testis and its blood supply
    d. Anterior processus vaginalis
    e. Distal gubernaculum

14. Initial performance of a transperitoneal laparoscopic right nephrectomy includes:

    a. upper pole mobilization and control of the hilum.
    b. direct control of the hilar vessels.
    c. duodenal mobilization and hilar control.
    d. placement of a ureteral stent.
    e. lateral mobilization of the colon and medial reflection.

15. Which of the following is considered an absolute contraindication to laparoscopic surgery in a 10-year-old child?

    a. Ventriculoperitoneal shunt
    b. Previous abdominal surgery
    c. Peritoneal dialysis
    d. Renal insufficiency
    e. None of the above

Answers

1. **c. Renal ultrasonography.** After stent removal, ultrasonography is used to monitor upper tract dilatation, which may occur with ureteral obstruction. The timing of follow-up should be based on the complexity of the case but should not be delayed for more than 4 weeks after the stent is removed. If there is no hydronephrosis, IVP, MAG3, and DMSA scans are not needed. If significant dilatation is present, or if the child develops symptoms of obstruction, IVP is used to define the functional anatomy of the ureter. Vesicoureteral reflux is a theoretical complication of ureteral dilatation and manipulation but has not been reported to be a significant clinical issue. Routine cystography is not recommended. [p 2566]

2. **d. Warmed saline.** Irrigation solutions must be warmed to prevent hypothermia, which can occur quickly in young children. Saline should be used as an irrigant in all cases to avoid dilutional hyponatremia, which can also develop quickly in the small child if extravasation should occur. [p 2566]

3. **a. Shock wave lithotripsy.** Percutaneous access in children is used most commonly for stone removal. Because the ureter in the child is very distensible, allowing passage of relatively large stone fragments, extracorporeal shock wave lithotripsy (ESWL) is the first-line treatment for most renal calculi in children. There is no strict upper limit of stone burden that can be managed with ESWL in children, as there is in adults, although the larger the burden is, the less likely it is that success will be achieved with one procedure. [p 2568]

4. **b. Inability to cannulate the lumen of the ureteropelvic junction.** Endopyelotomy is generally acknowledged to be the procedure of choice after failed pyeloplasty in the adult and has a reasonable success rate. The same may be true in the pediatric population, although fewer cases have been reported. Endopyelotomy should be attempted only when a lumen is recognizable and can be cannulated. Considering the difficulty and morbidity of reoperative pyeloplasty, an attempt at endopyelotomy in most cases is reasonable. [p 2569]

5. **d. Percutaneous stone removal and diverticular ablation.** Because there are symptoms, treatment is needed. Open marsupialization and retrograde drainage are possible options but are more invasive and not always as effective as percutaneous ablation. Percutaneous intervention in children is based on obliteration and scarification of the epithelial lining of the diverticulum, rather than inducing drainage through opening of the neck of the diverticulum, as is often performed in adults. Any procedure intending to establish free drainage requires temporary indwelling stents and runs the risk of reclosure of the neck. The impact of each of these elements in the child is greater than in the adult. Laparoscopic marsupialization may be another option, although there is little experience with it. Upper pole nephrectomy would not be reasonable. [p 2570]

6. **b. Documentation of the location and presence of the testis.** The primary aims of diagnostic laparoscopy are to identify the presence or absence, location, and anatomy of the nonpalpable testis. [p 2571]

7. **e. perform an examination with the patient under anesthesia.** It is important to perform a careful examination with the patient under anesthesia to detect a small number of testes that were not detected in the office setting. One report indicated an 18% incidence of testes palpable under anesthesia but not palpated in the clinical setting. This obviously reduces the number of diagnostic laparoscopies that would reveal a testis that had descended into the inguinal canal. Imaging studies have not been able to definitively prove the absence of a testis and therefore are of little practical value. An hCG stimulation test is not useful for a unilateral nonpalpable testis. Contralaterally increased testicular size may suggest contralateral testicular absence but cannot be considered sufficient proof to avoid some form of exploration. [p 2571]

8. **c. Presence of both spermatic vessels and vas ending blindly.** On the affected side, three basic patterns may be seen. When the vas and the vessels dwindle away before the internal inguinal ring, a vanishing intra-abdominal testis is diagnosed. If either one is not seen, it is uncertain whether a

testis may be present in the abdomen and further exploration is required. Absence of both also suggests the need for further exploration. In the setting of a vanishing testis, there is never a testicular remnant seen intra-abdominally. [pp 2571–2572]

9. **d. Perform a low inguinal incision to remove the testicular nub.** The second common appearance is that of vas and vessels that pass through the inguinal ring. This pattern may look very similar to normal, but the important feature to examine is the appearance of the vessels. If the vas and vessels pass through the internal inguinal ring and they are atretic, it is presumed that a vanishing testis is present and a small, low inguinal exploration is performed at the level of the pubic tubercle. This permits confirmation of the diagnosis with excision of a nub of testis. [pp 2572, 2574]

10. **a. gonadal development may be abnormal or discordant with sex of rearing.** The principal use of diagnostic laparoscopy for intersex is for conditions in which gonadal development may be abnormal or discordant with the sex of rearing, including gonadal dysgenesis and hermaphroditism. It is of little benefit in cases of congenital adrenal hyperplasia. When persistent müllerian ductal structures should be removed, laparoscopy may be useful as well, although it is not universally so. [p 2574]

11. **b. Reduced oxygen reserve.** Intra-abdominal pressure is increased significantly, and with the common use of CO_2 as the insufflating agent, there is absorption of CO_2 across the peritoneum. There are also risks of CO_2 embolus. In children, the key differences from an anesthetic standpoint, relative to adults, is their decreased pulmonary reserve because of a relatively low functional residual capacity and lower oxygen reserve. [p 2577]

12. **d. Continuation of the procedure and monitoring of postoperative urine output.** As with adults, increased intra-abdominal pressure in children reduces urine output, although this is transient and has not been observed to cause any permanent renal injury. There is no need to increase normal fluid management, nor is there any reason to stop the procedure. A CO_2 embolus would present with acutely altered cardiorespiratory function. [p 2577]

13. **b. Peritoneal triangle between the vas deferens and the spermatic vessels.** The peritoneal dissection as described will leave a triangle of undisturbed tissue between the vas and the spermatic vessels. This has the theoretical advantage of preserving collateral vascularity between the vas and the spermatic vessels in case of spasm or inadvertent injury to the spermatic vessels. [p 2579]

14. **e. lateral mobilization of the colon and medial reflection.** In transperitoneal nephrectomy, the colon is first reflected from the kidney by incision of the lateral line of Toldt. In most cases, the ureter can be identified and used as a handle to lift the lower pole of the kidney. This facilitates access to the hilar vessels, which are then dissected free and independently ligated. [p 2583]

15. **e. None of the above.** Laparoscopically assisted surgery is widely applicable in patients who require bladder reconstruction and/or antegrade continence enema stoma. The majority of patients reported have had prior abdominal surgery, including ventriculoperitoneal shunt placement and bladder exstrophy closure. The benefit of laparoscopic mobilization is not just cosmetic; in theory, one would expect more rapid recovery and decreased intra-abdominal adhesions. Therefore, even patients with a prior midline incision might benefit. The presence of a ventriculoperitoneal shunt is not a contraindication to laparoscopic surgery and requires no special precautions or monitoring. [p 2587]

Chapter 73

Tissue Engineering Perspectives for Reconstructive Surgery

Anthony Atala

Questions

1. Currently, possible tissue replacements for reconstruction include which of the following?
   a. Native nonurologic tissues
   b. Homologous tissues
   c. Heterologous tissues
   d. Artificial biomaterials
   e. All of the above

2. What are the most common types of synthetic prostheses for urologic use made of?
   a. Latex
   b. Silicone
   c. Urethane
   d. Biodegradable polymers
   e. Polyvinyl

3. What does tissue engineering involve?
   a. The principles of cell transplantation
   b. The principles of materials science
   c. The use of matrices alone
   d. The use of matrices with cells
   e. All of the above

4. In tissue engineering, when autologous cells are used:
   a. donor tissue is dissociated into individual cells.
   b. cells are either implanted directly into the host or expanded in culture.
   c. cells are attached to a support matrix.
   d. the cells and matrix are implanted in vivo.
   e. all of the above.

5. Which of the following statements is true regarding biomaterials?

   a. They facilitate the localization and delivery of cells.
   b. They facilitate the localization and delivery of bioactive factors.
   c. They define a three-dimensional space for the formation of new tissues.
   d. They guide the development of new tissues with appropriate function.
   e. All of the above.

6. Types of biomaterials that have been utilized for engineering genitourinary tissues include which of the following?

   a. Naturally derived materials
   b. Acellular tissue matrices
   c. Synthetic polymers
   d. All of the above
   e. None of the above

7. Procedures and techniques that allow for the exclusion of nonurologic tissues during augmentation cystoplasty include which of the following?

   a. Autoaugmentation
   b. Ureterocystoplasty
   c. Tissue expansion
   d. Tissue engineering
   e. All of the above

8. In demucosalized intestinal segments for urinary reconstruction, removal of the mucosa and submucosa may lead to:

   a. contraction of the intestinal patch.
   b. mucosal regrowth.
   c. tissue necrosis.
   d. decreased vascularity.
   e. angiogenesis.

9. Permanent synthetic materials, when used in continuity with the urinary tract, have been associated with:

   a. mechanical failure.
   b. emboli.
   c. calculus formation.
   d. a and c.
   e. none of the above.

10. Urothelium is associated with:

    a. a high reparative capacity.
    b. an inherent capacity for artificial extracellular matrix attachment.
    c. frequent malignant differentiation.
    d. poor growth parameters.
    e. none of the above.

11. Major limitations in phallic reconstructive surgery include which of the following?

    a. The availability of adequate growth factors
    b. The availability of sufficient autologous tissue
    c. The availability of adequate surgical techniques
    d. All of the above
    e. None of the above

12. What is the most prevalent form of renal replacement therapy?

    a. Organ transplantation
    b. Dialysis
    c. Bioartificial hemofilters
    d. Bioartificial renal tubules
    e. Engineered functional renal structures

13. The ideal bulking substance for the endoscopic treatment of reflux and incontinence should have what characteristic?

    a. Easily injectable
    b. Nonantigenic
    c. Nonmigratory
    d. Volume stable
    e. All of the above

14. Which of the following statements regarding microencapsulated cells is true?

    a. They have a semipermeable barrier.
    b. They are protected from the host's immune system.
    c. They allow for physiologic release of substances.
    d. They provide a long-term delivery system of by-products.
    e. All of the above.

15. What are the most common cell sources for tissue engineering today?

    a. Embryonic stem cells
    b. Adult unipotent stem cells
    c. Autologous primary cells
    d. Stem cells derived from nuclear transfer techniques
    e. None of the above

Answers

1. **e. All of the above.** Whenever there is a lack of native urologic tissue, reconstruction may be performed with native nonurologic tissues (skin, gastrointestinal segments, or mucosa from multiple body sites), homologous tissues (cadaver fascia, cadaver or donor kidney), heterologous tissues (bovine collagen), or artificial materials (silicone, polyurethane, Teflon). [p 2594]

2. **b. Silicone.** The most common type of synthetic prostheses for urologic use is made of silicone. [p 2594]

3. **e. All of the above.** Tissue engineering follows the principles of cell transplantation, materials science, and engineering toward the development of biologic substitutes that would restore and maintain normal function. Tissue engineering may involve matrices alone, wherein the body's natural ability to regenerate is used to orient or direct new tissue growth, or the use of matrices with cells. [p 2594]

4. **e. All of the above.** When cells are used for tissue engineering, donor tissue is dissociated into individual cells, which either are implanted directly into the host or are expanded in culture, attached to a support matrix, and reimplanted after expansion. The implanted tissue can be heterologous, allogeneic, or autologous. [p 2594]

5. **e. All of the above.** Biomaterials facilitate the localization and delivery of cells and/or bioactive factors (e.g., cell adhesion peptides and growth factors) to desired sites in the body, define a three-dimensional space for the formation of new tissues with appropriate structure, and guide the development of new tissues with appropriate function. [p 2595]

6. **d. All of the above.** Generally, three classes of biomaterials have been used for engineering genitourinary tissues: naturally derived materials (e.g., collagen and alginate), acellular tissue matrices (e.g., bladder submucosa and small intestinal submucosa), and synthetic polymers (e.g., polyglycolic acid [PGA], polylactic acid [PLA], and poly(lactic-co-glycolic acid) [PLGA]). [p 2596]

7. **e. All of the above.** Because of the problems encountered with the use of gastrointestinal segments, numerous investigators have attempted alternative methods, materials, and tissues for bladder replacement or repair. These include autoaugmentation, ureterocystoplasty, methods for tissue expansion, seromuscular grafts, matrices for tissue regeneration, and tissue engineering using cell transplantation. [p 2598]

8. **a. contraction of the intestinal patch.** It has been noted that removal of only the mucosa may lead to mucosal regrowth, whereas removal of the mucosa and submucosa may lead to retraction of the intestinal patch. [p 2601]

9. **d. a and c.** Usually, permanent synthetic materials used for bladder reconstruction succumb to mechanical failure and urinary stone formation and degradable materials lead to fibroblast deposition, scarring, graft contracture, and a reduced reservoir volume over time. [p 2602]

10. **a. a high reparative capacity.** It has been well established for decades that the bladder is able to regenerate generously over free grafts. Urothelium is associated with a high reparative capacity. Bladder muscle tissue is less likely to regenerate in a normal manner. [p 2603]

11. **b. The availability of sufficient autologous tissue.** One of the major limitations of phallic reconstructive surgery is the availability of sufficient autologous tissue. [p 2605]

12. **b. Dialysis.** Although dialysis therapy is currently the most prevalent form of renal replacement therapy, the relatively high morbidity and mortality rates have prompted investigators to seek alternative solutions involving ex vivo systems. [p 2611]

13. **e. All of the above.** The ideal substance for the endoscopic treatment of reflux and incontinence should be injectable, nonantigenic, nonmigratory, volume stable, and safe for human use. [p 2614]

14. **e. All of the above.** Microencapsulated Leydig cells offer several advantages, such as serving as a semipermeable barrier between the transplanted cells and the host's immune system, as well as allowing for the long-term physiologic release of testosterone. [p 2615]

15. **c. Autologous primary cells.** Most current strategies for engineering urologic tissues involve harvesting of autologous cells from the host diseased organ. However, in situations in which extensive end-stage organ failure is present, a tissue biopsy may not yield enough normal cells for expansion. Under these circumstances, the availability of pluripotent stem cells may be beneficial. [p 2617]

SECTION X

ONCOLOGY

Chapter 74

Molecular Genetics and Cancer Biology

Adam S. Kibel • Joel B. Nelson

Questions

1. DNA is composed of all of the following elements except:
   a. a base, either a purine or a pyrimidine.
   b. a sugar, called ribose.
   c. a phosphate.
   d. two complementary strands.
   e. hydrogen bonds.

2. The physical chemistry of DNA bases requires:
   a. uracil to form a hydrogen bond with guanine.
   b. a purine to form a hydrogen bond with another purine.
   c. a pyrimidine to form a hydrogen bond with a purine.
   d. adenine to form a hydrogen bond with cytosine.
   e. thymine to form a hydrogen bond with guanine.

3. Which of the following does DNA expression require?
   a. Linear DNA to be converted into linear RNA, a process called translation
   b. Conversion of linear RNA into a linear set of amino acids, a process called transcription
   c. Protein synthesis exclusively within the nucleus
   d. Mitosis
   e. A mechanism to bridge the gap between the genetic code and protein synthesis

4. Which of the following statements about transcriptional regulation is NOT true?
   a. The two general components involved in transcriptional regulation are specific sequences in the RNA and proteins that interact with those sequences.
   b. In addition to the genetic information carried within the nucleotide sequence of DNA, it provides specific docking sites for proteins that enhance the activity of the transcriptional machinery.
   c. Specific sequences within the promoter or enhancer region of a gene are called response elements.
   d. DNA sequences, often referred to as consensus sequences, are found in many genes and respond in a coordinated manner to a specific signal.
   e. It is an important mechanism to ensure coordinated gene expression.

5. What is alternative splicing?
   a. A form of protein modification occurring after a mature polypeptide is produced
   b. A modification to DNA during meiosis
   c. A process of including or excluding certain exons in an mRNA transcript
   d. A process in which multiple genes can encode for a single polypeptide sequence
   e. A method of RNA degradation

6. Which of the following statements is true regarding the nuclear matrix?
   a. It has the same protein composition in every tissue type.
   b. It is the site of mRNA transcription.
   c. It has the same protein composition whether a cell is proliferating or undergoing differentiation.
   d. It provides a mechanism to trace the cell type of origin for a cancer, because the nuclear matrix is identical within tissue types.
   e. It is a form of DNA.

7. What happens in the process of translation?
   a. A message of four parts (the nucleotides A, U, C, G) is converted into 20 amino acids by using a functional group of three adjacent nucleotides called a codon.
   b. One amino acid is encoded by only one codon.
   c. Shifts in the reading frame are of no consequence in the production of the polypeptide chain because of the fidelity of template DNA.
   d. Single-base substitutions always encode for the identical amino acid, known as a polymorphism.
   e. The transfer of genetic information from the DNA to the RNA occurs.

8. Which of the following statements about ubiquitization is NOT true?
   a. Ubiquitization is an important regulatory mechanism of a cell, used in the efficient disposal of proteins.
   b. A small protein called ubiquitin is linked to a protein, tagging it for destruction.
   c. The proteosome is the site of protein-ubiquitin complex degradation.
   d. The proteosome has a cylindrical shape.
   e. Targeted inhibition of proteosome function appears to enhance cancer progression.

9. Which of the following statements about oncogenes is true?
   a. They are mutated forms of abnormal genes, known as proto-oncogenes.

b. They can be produced by an inactivating mutation of a proto-oncogene, resulting in the silencing of the gene.
c. They can be produced by gene amplification, resulting in many copies of the gene, or by chromosomal rearrangement.
d. They are always due to retroviruses, capable of inducing malignant transformation of normal cells.
e. They are endogenous cancer-fighting genes.

10. Which of the following statements about hypermethylation is true?
    a. It is a direct change to the DNA sequence, similar to a mutation.
    b. It occurs exclusively on cytosine nucleotides in the dinucleotide sequence CG.
    c. Somatic methylation of CpG dinucleotides in the regulatory regions of genes is very often associated with increased transcriptional activity, leading to increased expression of that gene.
    d. In cancer, hypermethylation is associated with enhanced activity of oncogenes, and demethylation may be an effective strategy for the treatment of cancer.
    e. Hypermethylation occurs outside of the CpG islands within the DNA sequence.

11. Von Hippel–Lindau (VHL) disease predisposes patients to which condition?
    a. Epididymal carcinoma
    b. Clear cell renal carcinoma
    c. Papillary renal cell carcinoma
    d. Adrenocortical carcinoma
    e. All of the above

12. Hereditary prostate carcinoma is estimated to account for what percentage of patients diagnosed with prostate cancer before 55 years of age?
    a. 0% to 20%
    b. 21% to 40%
    c. 41% to 60%
    d. 61% to 80%
    e. 81% to 100%

13. Wilms' tumor has been linked to which of the following hereditary tumor syndromes?
    a. WAGR syndrome
    b. Denys-Drash syndrome
    c. Beckwith-Wiedemann syndrome
    d. None of the above
    e. All of the above

14. Polymorphism with which of the following genes has been linked to prostate cancer?
    a. Vitamin D receptor
    b. 5α-reductase type II
    c. Androgen receptor
    d. None of the above
    e. All of the above

15. What are the two main points of control in the cell cycle?
    a. S and G_0
    b. S and G_2M
    c. M and G_1S
    d. G_1S and G_2M
    e. G_2 and M

16. The p53 tumor suppressor gene plays a crucial role in which of the following processes?
    a. apoptosis
    b. angiogenesis
    c. DNA replication
    d. mismatch repair
    e. signal transduction

17. Which of the following is an alternative splice variant of $p16^{INK4a}$?
    a. $p27^{kip1}$
    b. $p57^{kip2}$
    c. $p15^{INK4b}$
    d. $p14^{ARF}$
    e. $p21^{cip1}$

18. INK4 family members inhibit the activity of:
    a. cyclin D/cdk4.
    b. cyclin E/cdk2.
    c. cyclin A/cdk2.
    d. cyclin B/cdc2.
    e. all of the above.

19. Cyclin-cdk complexes primarily function at the G_1S boundary by which mechanism?
    a. Dephosphorylation of Rb
    b. Phosphorylation of mdm2
    c. Dephosphorylation of E2F
    d. Phosphorylation of E2F
    e. Phosphorylation of Rb

20. The regulatory proteins at the G_2M checkpoint respond to which of the following factors?
    a. Hypoxia
    b. Nutrient-poor environment
    c. DNA damage
    d. Cytokines
    e. All of the above

21. Nucleotide excision repair primarily protects the cell from DNA damage from which source?
    a. Reactive oxygen species
    b. DNA polymerase errors
    c. Double-stranded breaks
    d. Ultraviolet light
    e. All of the above

22. Which mismatch repair pathway heterodimer is responsible for single nucleotide mismatches?
    a. MSH2/MSH6
    b. MSH2/MSH3
    c. MSH3/MSH6
    d. MLH1/PMS2
    e. PMS2/MSH6

23. Which of the following genes have been linked to double-stranded break repair?
    a. *p53*
    b. *VHL*
    c. *BRCA1*
    d. *Rb*
    e. *PTEN*

24. Which of the following is a procaspase?
    a. TRAIL
    b. FLICE
    c. FAS
    d. TRID
    e. bcl-2

25. Ligand-dependent apoptosis is an attractive therapeutic target because:
    a. activation is independent of p53.
    b. activation is dependent on p53.

c. activation is independent of caspases.
  d. activation is dependent on caspases.
  e. activation is dependent on Rb.

26. p53-induced apoptosis is mediated through:
  a. APAF-1/caspase 9.
  b. CD95 receptor.
  c. TRAIL.
  d. bcl-2.
  e. p21^{cip1}.

27. How do proapoptotic bcl-2 family members function?
  a. By digesting the mitochondria
  b. By increasing the cellular membrane permeability
  c. By increasing the mitochondrial membrane permeability
  d. By directly activating executioner caspases
  e. By increasing nuclear membrane permeability

28. Telomerase immortalizes cells by:
  a. protecting the cells from DNA damage.
  b. stabilizing p53.
  c. allowing the cell to grow in a nutrient-poor environment.
  d. inhibiting apoptosis.
  e. maintaining chromosomal length.

29. Which of the following statements is true regarding epidermal growth factor (EGF)?
  a. It induces cell proliferation exclusively in epithelial cells.
  b. It is opposed in its actions by transforming growth factor-α.
  c. When inhibited by using an antibody directed against its receptor, it induces carcinogenesis.
  d. It acts as an inductive signal in embryogenesis.
  e. It acts only on the epidermis of the skin.

30. Which of the following statements is true regarding transforming growth factor-β?
  a. It is a positive regulator of stromal cell growth and simultaneously induces cell cycle arrest in epithelial and hematopoietic cell populations.
  b. It is a potent stimulator of the immune system.
  c. It is produced and secreted in an activated form.
  d. It acts to inhibit cancer, by inhibiting angiogenesis and growth of epithelial-derived carcinoma cells and stimulating production of extracellular matrix, limiting tumor growth.
  e. It appears to be of little importance in carcinogenesis.

31. The small bioactive peptides bombesin, endothelin-1, and neurotensin:
  a. act through specific, high-affinity receptor tyrosine kinases.
  b. may enhance prostate cancer progression through a decrease in the enzyme responsible for their degradation.
  c. act as classic tumor suppressors.
  d. have no functional counterparts in nonmammalian species.
  e. are endogenous toxins, resulting from ischemia.

32. Which of the following statements about receptors is NOT true?
  a. The response of a cell to all physiologic signals, whether a large protein, a peptide, a steroid, a fatty acid, or even a gas, is first through a specific receptor.
  b. All receptors are bound to the cell surface, with an extracellular ligand binding in the extracellular space, and the receptor-activating pathways within the cell.
  c. An autocrine signaling pathway implies that a cell produces a signal that acts back on the same cell.
  d. The three general classes of membrane-bound receptors are the ion-channel linked receptors, enzyme-linked receptors, and G-protein–linked receptors.
  e. A paracrine signaling pathway implies that a cell produces a signal that acts on another cell locally.

33. Which of the following statements is true regarding integrins?
  a. They are secreted endogenous hormones.
  b. They bridge the gap between the extracellular matrix and the cytoskeleton and act exclusively as a structural element.
  c. They are, at a basic level, heterotrimers, made of alpha, beta, and gamma chains.
  d. They are a large number of proteins, resulting from the alternative splicing of integrin mRNA.
  e. They produce a proliferative process called anoikis by maintaining the adherence of normal epithelial cells to the extracellular matrix.

34. Which of the following statements about E-cadherin is NOT true?
  a. Cadherins are responsible for cell-cell adhesion and tissue integrity.
  b. E-cadherin is dependent on its interaction with the catenins in linking to the actin cytoskeleton.
  c. There is considerable evidence for perturbations of the E-cadherin pathway in tumor progression and metastases.
  d. E-cadherin was originally called uvomorulin.
  e. In general, increased expression of E-cadherin results in cells that are more invasive, and this increased expression is characteristic of more aggressive cancers.

35. Hepatitis B virus and papillomaviruses are responsible for approximately what percentage of virus-induced malignancies?
  a. 20%
  b. 40%
  c. 60%
  d. 80%
  e. 100%

36. The viral protein E6 functions by inactivating:
  a. VHL.
  b. Rb.
  c. p16^{INK4a}.
  d. *p53*.
  e. E2F.

37. Human papillomavirus has been most convincingly linked to which of the following genitourinary malignancies?
  a. Testicular carcinoma
  b. Prostate carcinoma
  c. Renal carcinoma
  d. Bladder carcinoma
  e. Penile carcinoma

38. High-risk human papillomavirus subtypes include:
  a. HPV-11.
  b. HPV-16.
  c. HPV-18.
  d. HPV-33.
  e. all of the above.

39. Which of the following statements is true regarding angiogenesis?
  a. In normal tissues it is characterized by a predominance of angiogenesis inducers, constantly producing the new blood vessels required for tissue homeostasis.

b. It is required for a tumor larger than 2 cm, given the physical limitations of oxygen diffusion in solid tissue.
c. It results from angiogenesis activators, such as fibroblast growth factor-2 (FGF-2), which are sequestered in the extracellular matrix.
d. Inhibitors are activated immediately in wound healing and likely limit uncontrolled bleeding.
e. As a normal physiologic process, it appears to have almost no role in carcinogenesis.

40. Which of the following statements is true regarding angiogenesis activators?

    a. They are secreted by tumors themselves or are produced by infiltrating immune cells.
    b. Like vascular endothelial growth factor, they can be inhibited by hypoxia.
    c. They uniquely induce angiogenesis, lacking any other functions.
    d. They include endostatin and angiostatin.
    e. They include thrombospondin.

41. Which of the following statements about the general mechanisms through which angiogenesis inhibitors act is NOT true?

    a. Angiogenesis inhibitors may prevent tumor cell production of angiogenesis factors, such as interferon blockade of FGF-2 production.
    b. Angiogenesis inhibitors may neutralize angiogenesis factors, such as the action of suramin.
    c. Angiogenesis inhibitors may block the response of endothelial cells to angiogenic factors, such as the activity of thrombospondin on endothelial cells.
    d. Angiogenesis inhibitors may interfere with matrix formation required for vessels to sprout and grow through solid tissues, such as those factors isolated from cartilage.
    e. Angiogenesis inhibitors are key in maintaining the balance between normal and abnormal vessel formation.

42. Which of the following statements is true regarding the antibiotic angiogenesis inhibitors?

    a. They include roquinimex (linomide), which selectively inhibits both new blood vessel formation and established blood vessels.
    b. They include fumagillin, which induces late G_1 cell cycle arrest in endothelial cells.
    c. They include suramin, an antiparasitic compound that potently blocks the transcription and translation of FGF-2 alone.
    d. They include minocycline, a semisynthetic tetracycline with procollagenase activities.
    e. They act through inhibition of bacterial activity.

43. The angiogenesis inhibitors, which are proteolytic products of inactive molecules:

    a. include angiostatin, a protein cleaved from plasminogen, which renders the endothelium refractory to angiogenic stimuli.
    b. include angiostatin, which inhibits tumor growth, but with increasing toxicity and tumor resistance over time.
    c. include endostatin, a protein fragment of collagen XVIII, which inhibits endothelial cell proliferation but has no effect on established tumors.
    d. include endostatin, for which a likely mechanism of action is unknown.
    e. result in disseminated intravascular coagulopathy.

44. Which of the following statements is true regarding the other angiogenesis inhibitors?

    a. They include vascular endothelial growth factor and basic fibroblast growth factor.
    b. They include the interferons, which function only as antiangiogenic factors.
    c. They include thrombospondin, the ubiquitous adhesive glycoprotein that inhibits endothelial cell migration and induces endothelial cell apoptosis.
    d. They include matrix metalloproteinases, which are found in high concentrations in cartilage.
    e. They include the sedative thalidomide, the teratogen producing dysmelia (stunted limb growth), which appears to anesthetize endothelial cells.

45. Conditional knockout mice are useful genetic tools because:

    a. they recapitulate tumor syndromes exactly in humans.
    b. they allow induction of tumor formation in the adult.
    c. organ systems can be selectively targeted.
    d. none of the above.
    e. all of the above.

46. What is immunohistochemistry useful for?

    a. Identifying tumors of uncertain origin
    b. Identifying prognostic markers in tumors
    c. Identifying molecular targets for therapy
    d. All of the above
    e. None of the above

47. An isochromosome of 12p has been identified in which genitourinary malignancy?

    a. Testis carcinoma
    b. Prostate carcinoma
    c. Renal carcinoma
    d. Bladder carcinoma
    e. Penile carcinoma

48. What happens in rational drug discovery?

    a. A large number of compounds are screened for activity against a general target, such as cell division.
    b. Lead compounds are chosen based on activity in other systems or based on a history as a folk remedy.
    c. Screening for activity uses, as a first end point, measurements such as reduction in tumor size.
    d. Samples are often derived from brain tissue, hence the name "rational" drug.
    e. Compounds are designed to target a specific end point, receptor, or signaling pathway.

49. Which of the following statements about the rationale behind gene therapy is NOT true?

    a. In hereditary diseases characterized by a mutation of a single gene, such as cystic fibrosis, a correct copy of that gene can be replaced.
    b. In cancers known for a mutation of a tumor suppressor gene, such as p53, replacing a wild-type copy of that gene leads to programmed cell death.
    c. Expression of a foreign gene, followed by exposure to an otherwise harmless drug, can produce a toxin that kills the cell; an example of this approach is expression of the herpes simplex thymidine kinase gene followed by exposure to the antiviral drug ganciclovir.
    d. In the "suicide gene" approach, proapoptic genes are overexpressed, leading the cell to commit cellular suicide.
    e. Gene therapy is not expected to replace almost all other forms of medical and surgical therapy within the next 5 years.

50. Which of the following statements is true regarding gene therapy?

    a. It has been as easy to insert genes into target cells inside the body (in vivo) as it has been to insert genes into target cells outside the body (ex vivo).

b. Tissue-specific promoters and enhancers have been used to obtain gene expression only in those cells in which expression is desired.
c. Effective gene transfer has not been a major obstacle to systemic gene therapy.
d. Retroviruses, which transduce both dividing and nondividing cells, and adenoviruses, which transduce only dividing cells, are commonly used vectors, or vehicles to get genes into cells.
e. A myriad of examples of effective gene targeting and transfer in vivo already exists.

Answers

1. **b. a sugar, called ribose.** In a rudimentary form, DNA is the fusion of three different elements: a base (either a pyrimidine or a purine), a sugar (in the case of DNA called 2-deoxyribose; for RNA called ribose), and a phosphate (which links individual nucleotides together). The repeating connections between the phosphates and the sugars provide the backbone from which the information-carrying bases protrude. In its "resting" or nonreplicating form, this chain of elements forms a helix of two complementary strands; this double helix is held together by the hydrogen bonds. [pp 2626–2627]

2. **c. a pyrimidine to form a hydrogen bond with a purine.** The physical chemistry of the bases requires a purine to form a specific hydrogen bond with a pyrimidine. [p 2627]

3. **e. A mechanism to bridge the gap between the genetic code and protein synthesis.** The physical locations of DNA and its genetic code and protein synthesis and the manifestation of that code are separate: DNA is in the nucleus and protein synthesis is cytoplasmic. To bridge this gap, copies or transcripts of the DNA are made in the nucleus and the language of these transcripts is translated into the language of proteins. [p 2627]

4. **a. The two general components involved in transcriptional regulation are specific sequences in the RNA and proteins that interact with those sequences.** There are two general components involved in transcriptional regulation: specific sequences within the DNA and proteins that interact with those sequences. [p 2628]

5. **c. A process of including or excluding certain exons in an mRNA transcript.** In many genes, the RNA can undergo alternative splicing: certain exons can be included or excluded in the mRNA transcript. [p 2629]

6. **b. It is the site of mRNA transcription.** The nuclear matrix is the site of mRNA transcription. [p 2629]

7. **a. A message of four parts (the nucleotides A, U, C, G) is converted into 20 amino acids by using a functional group of three adjacent nucleotides called a codon.** The translation of a message made of four parts (the nucleotides A, U, C, G) into 20 amino acids uses a functional group of three adjacent nucleotides, called a codon. [p 2629]

8. **e. Targeted inhibition of proteosome function appears to enhance cancer progression.** Targeted inhibition of proteosome function has emerged as a novel antitumor strategy. [p 2630]

9. **c. They can be produced by gene amplification, resulting in many copies of the gene, or by chromosomal rearrangement.** There are at least three ways a proto-oncogene can be converted into an oncogene. First, a mutation can occur within the coding sequence, producing a permanently activated form of the gene. A second mechanism converting a proto-oncogene into an oncogene is through gene amplification. A third mechanism of oncogene formation is through chromosomal rearrangement. [p 2631]

10. **b. It occurs exclusively on cytosine nucleotides in the dinucleotide sequence CG.** DNA methylation occurs exclusively on cytosine nucleotides in the dinucleotide sequence CG. [p 2631]

11. **b. Clear cell renal carcinoma.** VHL is a hereditary tumor syndrome that predisposes patients to clear cell renal carcinoma, retinal angiomas, pheochromocytomas, hemangiomas of the central nervous system, epididymal cystadenomas, and pancreatic islet cell tumors. [p 2633]

12. **c. 41% to 60%.** Although the inherited form of prostate cancer is estimated to be responsible for only 9% of all prostate cancer, it is implicated in 43% of cases of disease diagnosed before 55 years of age. [p 2634]

13. **e. All of the above.** Hereditary Wilms' tumor accounts for approximately 1% of Wilms' tumor cases. The classic disease was first described by Fitzgerald and Hardin in 1955 and is characterized by bilateral and multicentric tumors. Wilms' tumor can also occur as part of the more complex tumor syndromes WAGR and Denys-Drash syndrome. WAGR syndrome is characterized by Wilms' tumor, aniridia, genitourinary abnormalities, gonadoblastoma, and mental retardation and was first described by Miller and colleagues in 1964. Denys-Drash syndrome is characterized by Wilms' tumor, genitourinary abnormalities, pseudohermaphroditism, and nephropathy and was first described in 1967. All three syndromes are caused, at least in part, by genetic abnormalities in the same gene, *WT1*. Wilms' tumor is also associated with Beckwith-Wiedemann syndrome. [p 2635]

14. **e. All of the above.** The link between prostate cancer and polymorphisms within genes important in steroid metabolism or function provides one of the best examples in genitourinary malignancies. The relationship between androgens and prostate cancer is well known. Although the androgen receptor has been targeted for the treatment of advanced prostate cancer for many years, it is only recently that the association between androgen receptor polymorphisms and prostate cancer has been identified. Shorter CAG repeat variants within the open reading frame have been linked to not only localized prostate cancer but also advanced and even lethal disease. Polymorphisms within the 5α-reductase type II gene have also been linked to aggressive prostate carcinoma. The known association between prostate cancer and vitamin D, coupled with the discovery that certain vitamin D receptor genotypes have altered activity, has stimulated interest in the effect of vitamin D receptor genotype on prostate cancer risk, and an association between the less active receptor variant and prostate cancer has been demonstrated. [p 2636]

15. **d. G_1S and G_2M.** The two main points of control are the G_1S and G_2M checkpoints. [p 2636]

16. **a. apoptosis.** Active p53 binds to the promoter region of p53 responsive genes and stimulates the transcription of

genes responsible for cell cycle arrest, repair of DNA damage, and apoptosis. p53 responds to DNA damage by inducing cell cycle arrest through p21^{cip1} and then transcriptionally activating DNA repair enzymes. If the cell cannot arrest growth and/or repair the DNA, p53 induces apoptosis. [p 2637]

17. **d. p14^{ARF}.** p14^{ARF} was originally identified as an alternative splice variant of the cdk inhibitor p16^{INK4a}. It has been demonstrated that p14^{ARF} functions not by acting as a cdk inhibitor but by degrading mdm2. [p 2637]

18. **a. cyclin D/cdk4.** The INK4 family of cdk inhibitors directly inhibits the assembly of cyclin D with cdk4 and cdk6 by blocking the phosphorylation of the cyclin D-cdk4/6 complex. This phosphorylation is necessary for activation of the complex. [p 2638]

19. **e. Phosphorylation of Rb.** Cyclin-cdk complexes phosphorylate Rb or its family members, p107 and p130. Phosphorylated Rb can no longer bind to members of the E2F family of transcription factors. Free E2F heterodimerizes with DP-1 or DP-2 and transcriptionally activates genes important in DNA replication, such as DNA polymerase-α and the cell cycle, such as E2F-1. [pp 2638–2639]

20. **c. DNA damage.** Unlike the G$_1$S checkpoint, which responds to a variety of extracellular signals in addition to DNA damage, G$_2$M appears to respond only to DNA damage and serves as an important point of control for replication errors. [p 2640]

21. **d. Ultraviolet light.** Nucleotide excision repair is a major defense against DNA damage caused by ultraviolet radiation and chemical exposure. [p 2641]

22. **a. MSH2/MSH6.** The MSH2/MSH3 heterodimer (MutSβ) mediates repair of insertions and deletions, whereas the MSH2/MSH6 heterodimer (MutSα) recognizes the single nucleotide mismatches in addition to insertions and deletions. [p 2642]

23. **c. BRCA1.** It is believed that the breast cancer susceptibility genes *BRCA1* and *BRCA2* play an important role in homologous recombination as well as sensing DNA damage. Both *BRCA1* and *BRCA2* are part of an enzymatic complex with *RAD51*- and *BRCA1*-associated RING domain 1 (BARD1). This complex is recruited by proliferating nuclear antigen (PCNA) to regions that have undergone DNA damage to repair DNA breaks. [p 2643]

24. **b. FLICE.** In turn, procaspase 8, or FLICE, binds to FADD via the death effector domain. Procaspase 8 oligomerization promotes autoactivation to caspase 8. [pp 2643–2644]

25. **a. activation is independent of p53.** The identification of ligand-dependent apoptosis receptors may have a profound impact on therapy. Most cancer therapies (e.g., chemotherapy and external beam radiotherapy) depend on p53 to induce apoptosis in the cancer cell. Because p53 is mutated in more than half of malignancies, p53-independent pathways for apoptosis are of great clinical interest. Because ligand-dependent apoptosis is independent of p53, this makes these receptors and ligands attractive novel treatment targets. [p 2644]

26. **a. APAF-1/caspase 9.** p53-induced apoptosis is dependent on the APAF-1/caspase 9 activation pathway (see Fig. 74–14). [p 2644]

27. **c. By increasing the mitochondrial membrane permeability.** Although each proapoptotic *bcl*-2 family member responds to different stimuli, the principal mechanism by which these family members induce cell death is by increasing mitochondrial membrane permeability. [p 2645]

28. **e. maintaining chromosomal length.** Telomerase immortalizes cells by maintaining the ends of the chromosomes, or telomeres, which normally shorten with each cell division. [p 2646]

29. **d. It acts as an inductive signal in embryogenesis.** EGF induces cell proliferation across a broad set of cell types, including those derived from all three embryonic tissues, ectoderm, mesoderm, and endoderm. It is not surprising, therefore, to find EGF acting as an inductive signal in embryogenesis. [p 2647]

30. **a. It is a positive regulator of stromal cell growth and simultaneously induces cell cycle arrest in epithelial and hematopoietic cell populations.** Transforming growth factor-β is a positive regulator of stromal cell growth, stimulates extracellular matrix production, and simultaneously induces cell cycle arrest in epithelial and hematopoietic cell populations. [p 2647]

31. **b. may enhance prostate cancer progression through a decrease in the enzyme responsible for their degradation.** In prostate cancer, the enzyme responsible for the degradation of these peptides, endopeptidase 24.11, is decreased in androgen-independent disease; loss of local peptide degradation may enhance the local concentrations of these bioactive peptides and enhance cancer progression. [p 2648]

32. **b. All receptors are bound to the cell surface, with an extracellular ligand binding in the extracellular space, and the receptor-activating pathways within the cell.** Most receptors are bound to the cell surface, with extracellular ligand binding in the extracellular space and the receptor-activating pathways within the cell. [p 2649]

33. **d. They are a large number of proteins, resulting from the alternative splicing of integrin mRNA.** Because of alternative splicing of integrin mRNA, there are large numbers of integrin combinations with different affinities to extracellular matrix and cellular proteins. [p 2650]

34. **e. In general, increased expression of E-cadherin results in cells that are more invasive, and this increased expression is characteristic of more aggressive cancers.** In human tumors, loss of E-cadherin or α-catenin expression is associated with more aggressive and metastatic disease in prostate cancer. [p 2651]

35. **d. 80%.** DNA viruses are believed to play much more of a role in human tumorigenesis than RNA viruses, with hepatitis B virus and papillomaviruses responsible for 80% of virus-induced malignancies. [p 2652]

36. **d. *p53*.** E6 appears to primarily function by targeting *p53* for ubiquitin-mediated degradation. Inactivation of *p53* blocks both cell cycle arrest and apoptosis and in doing so promotes the malignant phenotype. [p 2652]

37. **e. Penile carcinoma.** Human papillomavirus infection with high-risk subtypes has been linked to penile carcinoma. This virus has been detected in 15% to 80% of penile lesions. [p 2652]

38. **e. all of the above.** HPV-16 appears to be the dominant subtype and has been identified in up to 90% of human papillomavirus-positive lesions. HPV-11, HPV-18, and HPV-33 have also been identified in penile tumors. [pp 2652–2653]

39. **c. It results from angiogenesis activators, such as fibroblast growth factor-2 (FGF-2), which are sequestered in the extracellular matrix.** Many angiogenesis activators, such as FGF-2 (also known as basic fibroblast growth factor,

or bFGF), are also sequestered in the extracellular matrix, bound to heparin sulfate; degradation of the matrix by tumor-derived proteases releases these factors and stimulates endothelial cell proliferation. [p 2653]

40. **a. They are secreted by tumors themselves or are produced by infiltrating immune cells.** A host of factors identified as stimulating angiogenesis are secreted by the tumors themselves or by infiltrating immune cells, leading to new blood vessel formation. [p 2653]

41. **d. Angiogenesis inhibitors may interfere with matrix formation required for vessels to sprout and grow through solid tissues, such as those factors isolated from cartilage.** Angiogenesis inhibitors interfere with the matrix degradation required for vessels to sprout and grow through solid tissues, such as the matrix metalloproteinase inhibitor BB-94. [p 2654]

42. **b. They include fumagillin, which induces late G_1 cell cycle arrest in endothelial cells.** The small molecule derivatives of fumagillin, AMG-1470 and TMP-470, inhibit neovascularization via endothelial cell cycle arrest in late G_1 phase. [p 2654]

43. **a. include angiostatin, a protein cleaved from plasminogen, which renders the endothelium refractory to angiogenic stimuli.** Angiostatin, a 38-kD protein, is a cleaved internal fragment of the first four kringle domains of plasminogen. By rendering the endothelium refractory to angiogenic stimuli, systemically administered angiostatin inhibited primary tumor growth with no obvious toxicity or tumor resistance. [p 2655]

44. **c. They include thrombospondin, the ubiquitous adhesive glycoprotein that inhibits endothelial cell migration and induces endothelial cell apoptosis.** This protein was identified as thrombospondin, the ubiquitous adhesive glycoprotein, of which several protein fragments retained antiangiogenic qualities. Thrombospondin inhibits neovascularization in vivo and endothelial cell migration in vitro and induces apoptosis in endothelial cells. [p 2655]

45. **c. organ systems can be selectively targeted.** Selective deletion of genes once the mouse reached maturity became possible in 1988 when Sauer and Henderson demonstrated that the Cre protein isolated from bacteriophage could be used to induce recombination events in mammalian cells at genetically engineered sites. This allowed the mouse to develop normally until exposed to the protein, at which point the cells exposed would delete the gene of interest. Conditional knockouts of the *apc* gene are allowed to develop normally until adulthood. Exposure of the colonic mucosa to Cre leads to loss of the *apc* gene in some cells and the development of colon carcinoma. This more closely recapitulates the chain of events that leads to colon carcinoma. In the near future, additional conditional knockouts will be developed. [p 2657]

46. **d. All of the above.** Immunohistochemistry has several important uses in oncology. Immunohistochemistry is crucial to the accurate identification of tumors of uncertain origin, if conventional light microscopy cannot identify the tumor. This can be crucial for instituting proper therapy. For example, prostate-specific antigen staining has proved to be a useful adjunct in identifying adenocarcinomas of uncertain origin as prostatic. Cancer markers have also proved useful for identifying bladder tumors from metastatic lesions. A second use of immunohistochemistry is to stain for prognostic biomarkers. The subclassification of tumors into aggressive and indolent on the basis of the molecular profile has the potential to radically change practice. For example, prostate cancers of identical stage and grade can have variable clinical courses. The ability to identify patients with a poor prognosis and/or those who will respond to a particular treatment independent of grade and stage would be of significant clinical utility. Although still experimental, *p53* in bladder cancer is emerging as a potential independent indicator of aggressive disease and may prove useful for stratifying patients for neoadjuvant chemotherapy. Last, molecular identification of tumor targets for therapy will become increasingly prevalent in the near future. The best example of this is the use of immunohistochemistry to identify the presence of *her-2/neu* receptors in breast cancer. Not only does *her-2/neu* receptor provide prognostic information in breast cancer, but if the receptor is present it provides a molecular target for antibody therapy. Preliminary data have demonstrated that the antibody herceptin is effective in treating patients whose tumors express the receptor. [p 2658]

47. **a. Testis carcinoma.** The urologic malignancy most closely linked to a karyotypic abnormality is testis tumors. A 12p isochromosome was first identified in testis tumors in the 1980s, and experimentally this cytogenetic hallmark of testicular tumors has diagnostic and prognostic value. [p 2658]

48. **e. Compounds are designed to target a specific end point, receptor, or signaling pathway.** Rational drug discovery seeks to identify and exploit specific targets in a biochemical pathway. This may be through blocking a particular receptor-ligand interaction, through inhibiting the enzyme activity of a particular kinase or phosphatase, or through altering the final protein product of a gene. [p 2659]

49. **d. In the "suicide gene" approach, proapoptic genes are overexpressed, leading the cell to commit cellular suicide.** The suicide gene approach is also used when the bacterial enzyme cytosine deaminase is artificially expressed in mammalian cells, which will metabolize innocuous 5-fluorocytosine to the toxin 5-fluorouracil. [p 2660]

50. **b. Tissue-specific promoters and enhancers have been used to obtain gene expression only in those cells where expression is desired.** One approach to overcoming the problem of insertion of genes into the specific target cells in the body is the use of tissue-specific promoters and enhancers. [p 2660]

Chapter 75

Renal Tumors

Andrew C. Novick • Steven C. Campbell

Questions

1. What is the most accurate imaging study for characterizing a renal mass?
   a. Intravenous pyelography
   b. Ultrasonography
   c. CT with and without contrast enhancement
   d. MRI
   e. Renal arteriography

2. A hyperdense renal cyst may also be termed a:
   a. probable malignancy.
   b. Bosniak II cyst.
   c. Bosniak III cyst.
   d. Bosniak IV cyst.
   e. probable angiomyolipoma.

3. The primary indication for fine needle aspiration of a renal mass is which suspected clinical diagnosis?
   a. Renal cell carcinoma
   b. Renal oncocytoma
   c. Renal adenoma
   d. Renal metastasis
   e. Renal angiomyolipoma

4. Postoperative radiographic surveillance after radical nephrectomy for T1N0M0 renal cell carcinoma should comprise which studies?
   a. No imaging studies
   b. Chest radiograph yearly
   c. Chest radiograph and abdominal CT scan yearly
   d. Chest radiograph yearly and abdominal CT scan every 2 years
   e. Chest radiograph and abdominal CT scan every 2 years

5. The major disadvantage of partial nephrectomy compared with radical nephrectomy for localized low-stage renal cell carcinoma is the increased risk of:
   a. perioperative renal failure.
   b. perioperative hemorrhage.
   c. postoperative distant metastasis.
   d. postoperative tumor recurrence in remnant kidney.
   e. postoperative tumor recurrence in perirenal lymph nodes.

6. Following partial nephrectomy for pT2N0M0 renal cell carcinoma, it is necessary to perform surveillance abdominal CT scanning with what frequency?
   a. Never
   b. Every 6 months
   c. Every year
   d. Every 2 years
   e. Every 4 years

7. Following partial nephrectomy of a solitary kidney, what is the most effective method of screening for hyperfiltration nephropathy?
   a. Urinary dipstick test for protein
   b. 24-hour urinary protein measurement
   c. Iothalamate glomerular filtration measurement
   d. Serum creatinine measurement
   e. Renal biopsy

8. What is an important prerequisite for successful laparoscopic cryoablation of a renal tumor?
   a. Slow freezing
   b. Rapid thawing
   c. A single freeze-thaw cycle
   d. A double freeze-thaw cycle
   e. Freezing of tumor to a temperature of −10°C

9. What is the most accurate and preferred imaging modality for demonstrating the presence and extent of an inferior vena caval tumor thrombus?
   a. Abdominal ultrasonography
   b. Transesophageal ultrasonography
   c. CT
   d. MRI
   e. Contrast venacavography

10. In patients undergoing complete surgical excision of a renal cell carcinoma, the lowest 5-year survival rate is associated with which factor?
    a. Perinephric fat involvement
    b. Microvascular renal invasion
    c. Subdiaphragmatic inferior vena caval involvement
    d. Intra-atrial tumor thrombus
    e. Lymph node involvement

11. A 45-year-old man has a 5 cm renal cell carcinoma in the upper pole of a solitary left kidney and a single 2 cm left lower lung metastasis. What is the best treatment?
    a. Initial immunotherapy, then partial nephrectomy
    b. Partial nephrectomy, then immunotherapy
    c. Staged partial nephrectomy and pulmonary lobectomy
    d. Simultaneous partial nephrectomy and pulmonary lobectomy
    e. Simultaneous radical nephrectomy and pulmonary lobectomy

12. What is the approximate overall objective response rate to interleukin-2 monotherapy in patients with metastatic renal cell carcinoma?
    a. 5%
    b. 10%
    c. 15%
    d. 20%
    e. 25%

13. Which treatment will yield the highest response rate in patients with metastatic renal cell carcinoma?

a. Interleukin-2
b. Interferon-α
c. Interleukin-2 and 5-fluorouracil
d. Interferon-α and dendritic cell
e. Interleukin-2 and interferon-α

14. Which of the following statements is true of a diagnosis of renal adenoma?

    a. It can be made primarily on the basis of histologic criteria.
    b. It can be rendered only if tumor size is less than 1.0 cm.
    c. It is commonly made at autopsy.
    d. It requires specific immunohistochemical staining.
    e. It can be confirmed by electron microscopy.

15. A healthy 62-year-old man is referred after renal biopsy of a 3.0 cm centrally located renal mass. The biopsy is interpreted as renal oncocytoma. The other kidney is normal, the serum creatinine level is 1.0 mg/dl, and there is no evidence of metastatic disease. What is the best next step?

    a. Observation with follow-up abdominal CT in 3 months
    b. Radical nephrectomy
    c. Laparoscopic exposure and renal cryoablative therapy
    d. Partial nephrectomy
    e. Observation with follow-up renal ultrasonography in 6 to 12 months

16. Tuberous sclerosis is similar to von Hippel–Lindau disorder in which of the following respects?

    a. Propensity toward development of seizure disorders
    b. Similarity of cutaneous lesions
    c. Common development of adrenal tumors
    d. Frequent involvement of cerebral cortex with vascular lesions
    e. Mode of genetic transmission

17. A 48-year-old woman with a history of seizure disorder presents with recurrent gross hematuria and left flank pain. Abdominal CT shows a large left perinephric hematoma associated with a 3.0 cm left renal angiomyolipoma. There are also multiple right renal angiomyolipomas ranging in size from 1.5 to 6.5 cm. What is the best management of the left renal lesion?

    a. Selective embolization
    b. Radical nephrectomy
    c. Observation
    d. Partial nephrectomy
    e. Laparoscopic exposure and renal cryoablative therapy

18. Which of the following statements is true regarding multiloculated cystic nephromas?

    a. They are complex cystic lesions that are typically classified as Bosniak II.
    b. They are malignant 2% to 5% of the time.
    c. They are more common in men than in women.
    d. They are characterized by bimodal age distribution.
    e. They are readily differentiated from renal cell carcinoma on the basis of appropriate imaging studies.

19. Which environmental factor is most generally accepted as a risk factor for renal cell carcinoma?

    a. Radiation therapy
    b. Antihypertensive medications
    c. Tobacco use
    d. Diuretics
    e. High-fat diet

20. Which of the following manifestations is restricted to certain families with the von Hippel–Lindau disorder?

    a. Renal cell carcinoma
    b. Pancreatic cysts or tumors
    c. Epididymal tumors
    d. Pheochromocytoma
    e. Inner ear tumors

21. Renal cell carcinoma develops in what percentage of patients with the von Hippel–Lindau disorder?

    a. 0% to 20%
    b. 21% to 40%
    c. 41% to 60%
    d. 61% to 80%
    e. 81% to 100%

22. What is the most common cause of death in patients with the von Hippel–Lindau syndrome?

    a. Renal failure
    b. Cerebellar hemangioblastoma
    c. Unrelated medical disease
    d. Pheochromocytoma
    e. Renal cell carcinoma

23. The von Hippel–Lindau syndrome tumor suppressor protein regulates the expression of which of the following mediators of biologic aggressiveness for renal cell carcinoma?

    a. Basic fibroblast growth factor
    b. Vascular endothelial cell growth factor
    c. Epidermal growth factor receptor
    d. Hepatocyte growth factor (scatter factor)
    e. P-glycoprotein (multiple drug resistance efflux protein)

24. What do the hereditary papillary renal cell carcinoma syndrome and von Hippel–Lindau syndrome have in common?

    a. The mode of genetic transmission
    b. Chromosome 3 abnormalities
    c. A propensity toward tumor formation in multiple organ systems
    d. Inactivation of a tumor suppressor gene
    e. Nearly complete penetrance

25. Mutation of the *met* proto-oncogene in hereditary papillary renal cell carcinoma leads to:

    a. increased expression of hepatocyte growth factor.
    b. increased sensitivity to vascular endothelial growth factor.
    c. inactivation of a tumor suppressor gene that regulates cellular proliferation.
    d. constitutive activation of the receptor for hepatocyte growth factor.
    e. increased expression of vascular endothelial growth factor.

26. P-glycoprotein is a transmembrane protein that is involved in:

    a. immunotolerance.
    b. resistance to high-dose interleukin-2 therapy.
    c. resistance to cisplatin therapy.
    d. resistance to radiation therapy.
    e. efflux of large hydrophobic compounds, including many cytotoxic drugs.

27. What is the primary proangiogenic molecule in conventional renal cell carcinoma?

    a. Basic fibroblast growth factor
    b. Hepatocyte growth factor
    c. Vascular endothelial cell growth factor
    d. Epidermal growth factor
    e. Transforming growth factor-β

28. Which of the following is most likely to demonstrate an infiltrative growth pattern?

    a. Sarcomatoid variants of conventional renal cell carcinoma
    b. High-grade granular variants of conventional renal cell carcinoma
    c. High-grade papillary renal cell carcinoma
    d. Moderate-grade transitional cell carcinoma of the renal pelvis
    e. Classic variant of chromophobe cell carcinoma

29. What is the most common mutation identified in sporadic conventional renal cell carcinoma?

    a. Activation of the *met* proto-oncogene
    b. Activation of the von Hippel–Lindau tumor suppressor gene
    c. Inactivation of the von Hippel–Lindau tumor suppressor gene
    d. Inactivation of *p53*
    e. Inactivation of genes on chromosome 9

30. Which of the following cytogenetic abnormalities is among those commonly associated with papillary renal cell carcinoma?

    a. Trisomy of chromosome 7
    b. Trisomy of the Y chromosome
    c. Loss of chromosome 17
    d. Loss of all or parts of chromosome 3
    e. Loss of chromosome 7

31. What percentage of renal cell carcinomas are chromophobe cell carcinomas?

    a. 0% to 2%
    b. 4% to 5%
    c. 8% to 10%
    d. 12% to 15%
    e. 18% to 25%

32. Most renal medullary cell carcinomas are:

    a. found in patients with sickle cell disease.
    b. diagnosed in the fifth decade of life.
    c. responsive to high-dose chemotherapy.
    d. genetically and histologically similar to papillary renal cell carcinoma.
    e. metastatic at the time of diagnosis.

33. Which paraneoplastic syndrome associated with renal cell carcinoma can often be managed or palliated medically?

    a. Polycythemia
    b. Stauffer's syndrome
    c. Neuropathy
    d. Hypercalcemia
    e. Cachexia

34. A healthy 64-year-old man is found to have a 6.0 cm solid, heterogeneous mass in the hilum of the right kidney. CT of the abdomen and pelvis shows interaortocaval lymph nodes enlarged to 2.5 cm. A chest radiograph and a bone scan have negative results, and the contralateral kidney is normal. The serum creatinine level is 1.0 mg/dl. What is the next best step?

    a. Right radical nephrectomy and regional or extended lymph node dissection
    b. Abdominal exploration, sampling of the enlarged lymph nodes, and possible radical nephrectomy pending frozen section analysis
    c. CT-guided percutaneous biopsy of the lymph nodes
    d. CT-guided percutaneous biopsy of the tumor mass
    e. Systemic immunotherapy followed by radical nephrectomy

35. What is the most versatile and informative study for the assessment of venous tumor thrombus associated with renal cell carcinoma?

    a. CT
    b. Doppler ultrasonography
    c. MRI
    d. Vena cavography
    e. Transesophageal echography

36. Which of the following patients would be a good candidate for percutaneous biopsy of a renal mass?

    a. A 42-year-old man with a 2.5-cm Bosniak III complex renal cyst
    b. An 88-year-old man with angina and a 1.7-cm solid, enhancing renal mass
    c. A 32-year-old woman with bilateral solid, enhancing renal masses ranging in size from 1.5 to 4.0 cm
    d. A 48-year-old woman with a 3.5-cm solid, enhancing renal mass with fat density present
    e. A 38-year-old woman with a fever, a urinary tract infection, and a 3.5–cm solid, enhancing renal mass

37. A 67-year-old man undergoes radical nephrectomy and inferior vena caval thrombectomy (level 2 thrombus). The primary tumor is otherwise confined to the kidney, and the lymph nodes are not involved. What is the approximate 5-year cancer-free survival rate?

    a. 15% to 25%
    b. 26% to 35%
    c. 36% to 45%
    d. 46% to 60%
    e. 61% to 75%

38. Important prognostic factors for patients with metastatic renal cell carcinoma include which of the following?

    a. Age
    b. Performance status
    c. Degree of renal function
    d. Primary tumor size
    e. Tumor grade

39. What is the most common form of renal sarcoma?

    a. Liposarcoma
    b. Rhabdosarcoma
    c. Fibrosarcoma
    d. Leiomyosarcoma
    e. Angiosarcoma

40. Which of the following statements about renal lymphoma is true?

    a. Five to 10% of all lymphomas involving the kidney are primary tumors.
    b. The radiographic patterns manifested by renal lymphoma are diverse and can be difficult to differentiate from renal cell carcinoma.
    c. Percutaneous biopsy is rarely indicated if renal lymphoma is suspected.
    d. Renal failure associated with renal lymphoma is most often due to extensive parenchymal replacement by the malignancy.
    e. The most common pattern of renal involvement is from direct extension from adjacent retroperitoneal lymph nodes.

Answers

1. **c. CT with and without contrast enhancement.** A dedicated (thin-slice) renal CT scan remains the single most important radiographic image for delineating the nature of a renal mass. In general, any renal mass that enhances with administration of intravenous contrast material on CT scanning should be considered a renal cell carcinoma until proved otherwise. [p 2675]

2. **b. Bosniak II cyst.** Category II lesions are minimally complicated cysts that are benign but have some radiologic findings that cause concern. Classic hyperdense renal cysts are small (<3 cm), round, and sharply marginated and do not enhance after administration of contrast material. [p 2677]

3. **d. Renal metastasis.** Fine needle aspiration or biopsy is of limited value in the evaluation of renal masses. The major problem with this technique is the high incidence of falsely negative biopsies in patients with renal malignancy. The primary indication for needle aspiration or biopsy of a renal mass occurs when a renal abscess or infected cyst is suspected, or when differentiating renal cell carcinoma from metastatic malignancy or renal lymphoma. [p 2676]

4. **a. No imaging studies.** Surveillance for recurrent malignancy after radical nephrectomy for renal cell carcinoma can be tailored according to the initial pathologic tumor stage. All patients should be evaluated with a medical history, physical examination, and selected blood studies on a yearly or twice-yearly basis. For patients with T1N0M0 tumors, routine postoperative radiographic imaging is not necessary because of the low risk of recurrent malignancy. [p 2705]

5. **d. postoperative tumor recurrence in remnant kidney.** The major disadvantage of nephron-sparing surgery is the risk of postoperative local tumor recurrence in the operated kidney, which has occurred in up to 10% of patients. [p 2706]

6. **d. Every 2 years.** Surveillance for recurrent malignancy after nephron-sparing surgery for renal cell carcinoma can be tailored according to the initial pathologic tumor stage. A yearly chest radiograph is recommended after nephron-sparing surgery for T2N0M0 tumors because the lung is the most common site of postoperative metastasis. Abdominal or retroperitoneal tumor recurrence is uncommon in the latter group, particularly early after nephron-sparing surgery, and these patients require only occasional follow-up abdominal CT; the authors recommend that this be done every 2 years. [pp 2706–2707]

7. **b. 24-hour urinary protein measurement.** Patients who undergo nephron-sparing surgery for renal cell carcinoma may be left with a relatively small amount of renal tissue. The patients are at risk for developing long-term renal functional impairment from hyperfiltration renal injury. Because proteinuria is the initial manifestation of the phenomenon, a 24-hour urinary protein measurement should be obtained yearly in patients with a solitary remnant kidney to screen for hyperfiltration nephropathy. [pp 2707–2708]

8. **d. A double freeze-thaw cycle.** Renal cryosurgery is an emerging nephron-sparing treatment option for renal cell carcinoma. The aim of cryosurgery is to ablate the same predetermined volume of tissue that would have been removed had a conventional surgical excision been performed. Established critical prerequisites for successful cryosurgery include rapid freezing, gradual thawing, and a repetition of the freeze-thaw cycle. [p 2710]

9. **d. MRI.** MRI is a noninvasive and accurate modality for demonstrating both the presence and the distal extent of vena caval involvement, and this has become the preferred diagnostic study at most centers. [p 2712]

10. **e. Lymph node involvement.** In most studies, the presence of lymph node or distant metastases has carried a dismal prognosis that is not appreciably altered by radical surgical extirpation. [p 2713]

11. **d. Simultaneous partial nephrectomy and pulmonary lobectomy.** The subset of patients with metastatic renal cell carcinoma and a solitary metastasis, estimated at between 1.6% and 3.2% of patients, may derive benefit from nephrectomy with resection of the metastatic lesion. [p 2715]

12. **c. 15%.** A recent review of clinical results in 1714 patients treated with interleukin-2 monotherapy indicated an overall objective response rate of 15.4%. [p 2716]

13. **e. Interleukin-2 and interferon-α.** The single-agent activity of interferon-α and interleukin-2 in patients with metastatic renal cell carcinoma, and preclinical observations indicating that these cytokines may have synergistic antitumor activity led to studies examining their combined use in the treatment of this disease. A recent review of 1411 patients receiving interferon-α and interleukin-2 in phase I or II trials indicated an overall objective response rate of 20.6%, with a 4.4% complete response rate. [p 2717]

14. **c. It is commonly made at autopsy.** Small, evidently benign, solid renal cortical lesions have been found at autopsy with an incidence of 7% to 23% and have been designated renal adenomas. [p 2680]

15. **b. Radical nephrectomy.** Most renal oncocytomas cannot be differentiated from malignant renal cell carcinomas on the basis of clinical or radiographic means. Given these uncertainties about a preoperative diagnosis, most authors have emphasized the need to treat these tumors aggressively with exploration and nephron-sparing surgery or radical nephrectomy dependent on the clinical circumstances. [p 2681]

16. **e. Mode of genetic transmission.** Approximately 20% of angiomyolipomas are found in patients with the tuberous sclerosis (TS) syndrome, an autosomal dominant disorder characterized by mental retardation, epilepsy, and adenoma sebaceum, a distinctive skin lesion. [p 2681]

17. **a. Selective embolization.** Most patients with acute or potentially life-threatening hemorrhage will require total nephrectomy if exploration is done, and if the patient has TS, bilateral disease, pre-existing renal insufficiency, or other medical or urologic disease that could affect renal function in the future, selective embolization should be considered. In such circumstances, selective embolization can temporize and in many cases will prove to be definitive treatment. [p 2683]

18. **d. They are characterized by bimodal age distribution.** Multiloculated cystic nephroma is a characteristic renal lesion with a bimodal age distribution and a benign clinical course. [p 2683]

19. **c. Tobacco use.** The only generally accepted environmental risk factor for renal cell carcinoma is tobacco use, although the relative associated risks have been modest, ranging from 1.4 to 2.3 when compared with controls. All forms of tobacco use have been implicated, with risk increasing with cumulative dose or pack-years. [p 2686]

20. **d. Pheochromocytoma.** The familial form of the common

clear cell variant of renal cell carcinoma is the von Hippel–Lindau syndrome. Major manifestations include the development of renal cell carcinoma, pheochromocytoma, retinal angiomas, and hemangioblastomas of the brain stem, cerebellum, or spinal cord. Penetrance for all of these traits is far from complete, and some, such as pheochromocytomas, tend to be clustered in certain families but not in others. [p 2687]

21. **c. 41% to 60%.** Renal cell carcinoma develops in about 50% of patients with von Hippel–Lindau syndrome and is distinctive for early age at onset, often developing in the third, fourth, or fifth decades of life, and for bilateral and multifocal involvement. [p 2687]

22. **e. Renal cell carcinoma.** With improved management of the central nervous system manifestations of the disease, renal cell carcinoma has now become the most common cause of mortality in patients with von Hippel–Lindau syndrome. [p 2687]

23. **b. Vascular endothelial cell growth factor.** Data suggest that inactivation or mutation of the von Hippel–Lindau gene leads to dysregulated expression of hypoxia inducible factor-1, an intracellular protein that plays an important role in regulating cellular responses to hypoxia, starvation, and other stresses. This in turn leads to a several-fold upregulation of the expression of vascular endothelial growth factor (VEGF), the primary proangiogenic growth factor in renal cell carcinoma, contributing to the pronounced neovascularity associated with this carcinoma. [p 2688]

24. **a. The mode of genetic transmission.** Studies of families with hereditary papillary renal cell carcinoma have demonstrated an autosomal dominant mode of transmission. [p 2688]

25. **d. constitutive activation of the receptor for hepatocyte growth factor.** Missense mutations of the *met* proto-oncogene at 7q31 were found to segregate with the disease, implicating it as the relevant genetic locus. The protein product of this gene is the receptor tyrosine kinase for the hepatocyte growth factor (also known as scatter factor), which plays an important role in the regulation of the proliferation and differentiation of epithelial and endothelial cells in a wide variety of organs, including the kidney. Most of the mutations in hereditary papillary renal cell carcinoma have been found in the tyrosine kinase domain of *met* and apparently lead to constitutive activation. [p 2688]

26. **e. efflux of large hydrophobic compounds including many cytotoxic drugs.** P-glycoprotein is a 170-kDa transmembrane protein expressed by 80% to 90% of renal cell carcinomas that acts as an energy-dependent efflux pump for a wide variety of large hydrophobic compounds including several cytotoxic drugs. [p 2690]

27. **c. Vascular endothelial cell growth factor.** The primary angiogenesis inducer in clear cell renal cell carcinoma appears to be VEGF, which is suppressed by the wild-type von Hippel–Lindau protein under normal conditions and is dramatically upregulated during tumor development. [p 2690]

28. **a. Sarcomatoid variants of conventional renal cell carcinoma.** Most renal cell carcinomas are round to ovoid and circumscribed by a pseudocapsule of compressed parenchyma and fibrous tissue rather than a true histologic capsule. Unlike upper tract transitional cell carcinomas, most renal cell carcinomas are not grossly infiltrative, with the notable exception of some sarcomatoid variants. [p 2691]

29. **c. Inactivation of the von Hippel–Lindau tumor suppressor gene.** Chromosome 3 alterations and von Hippel–Lindau mutations are common in conventional renal cell carcinoma, and mutation or inactivation of this gene has been found in 75% of sporadic cases. [p 2693]

30. **a. Trisomy of chromosome 7.** The cytogenetic abnormalities associated with papillary renal cell carcinoma are characteristic and include trisomy of chromosomes 7 and 17 and loss of the Y chromosome. [pp 2693–2694]

31. **b. 4% to 5%.** Chromophobe cell carcinoma is a distinctive histologic subtype of renal cell carcinoma that appears to be derived from the cortical portion of the collecting duct. It represents 4% to 5% of all renal cell carcinomas. [p 2694]

32. **e. metastatic at the time of diagnosis.** Renal medullary carcinoma is a relatively new histologic subtype of renal cell carcinoma that occurs almost exclusively in association with sickle cell trait. It is typically diagnosed in young African Americans, often in the third decade of life. Many cases are both locally advanced and metastatic at the time of diagnosis. Most patients have not responded to therapy and have succumbed to their disease in a few to several months. [p 2695]

33. **d. Hypercalcemia.** Hypercalcemia has been reported in up to 13% of patients with renal cell carcinoma and can be due to either paraneoplastic phenomena or osteolytic metastatic involvement of the bone. The production of parathyroid hormone–like peptides is the most common paraneoplastic cause, although tumor-derived 1,25-dihydroxyvitamin D_3 and prostaglandins may contribute in a minority of cases. Medical management includes vigorous hydration followed by diuresis with furosemide and the selective use of corticosteroids and/or calcitonin. [p 2696]

34. **a. Right radical nephrectomy and regional or extended lymph node dissection.** Identification of tumors with early nodal involvement, which is facilitated by an extensive lymph node dissection, allows them to be classified as N+ rather than N0, which would improve outcome results for both groups. The N0 group is improved by the removal of a small proportion of patients who actually have positive nodes, and the N+ group is improved by the addition of a subgroup with very early nodal involvement. [p 2703]

35. **c. MRI.** MRI is now established as the premier study for the evaluation and staging of inferior vena caval tumor thrombus. It provides reliable information about both the cephalad and the caudad extents of the thrombus and can often distinguish bland from tumor thrombus. In addition, MRI is noninvasive and does not place the patient at risk for contrast nephropathy. [p 2701]

36. **e. A 38-year-old woman with a febrile urinary tract infection and a 3.5-cm solid, enhancing renal mass.** Patients with flank pain, a febrile urinary tract infection, and a renal mass may be considered for percutaneous biopsy or aspiration to establish a diagnosis of renal abscess rather than malignancy. [p 2701]

37. **d. 46% to 60%.** Venous involvement was once thought to be a poor prognostic finding for renal cell carcinoma, but more recent studies suggest that most patients with tumor thrombi can be salvaged with an aggressive surgical approach. These studies document 45% to 69% 5-year survival rates for patients with venous tumor thrombi as long as the tumor is otherwise confined to the kidney. [p 2702]

38. **b. Performance status.** Systemic metastases portend a particularly poor prognosis for renal cell carcinoma, with 1-year survival of less than 50%, 5-year survival of 5% to 30%, and 10-year survival of 0% to 5%. For patients with asynchronous metastases, the metastasis-free interval has proved to be a useful prognosticator, as it reflects the tempo of disease progression. Other important prognostic factors for pa-

tients with systemic metastases include performance status, the number and sites of metastases, anemia, and hypercalcemia. [p 2703]

39. **d. Leiomyosarcoma.** Leiomyosarcoma is the most common histologic subtype of renal sarcoma, accounting for 50% to 60% of such tumors. [p 2720]

40. **b. The radiographic patterns manifested by renal lymphoma are diverse and can be difficult to differentiate from renal cell carcinoma.** CT is the radiographic modality of choice for the diagnosis of renal lymphoma and for monitoring the response to therapy. Renal lymphoma can present as multiple distinct renal masses; a solitary renal mass, which can be difficult to differentiate from renal cell carcinoma; diffuse renal infiltration; or direct invasion of the kidney from enlarged retroperitoneal nodes. [pp 2720–2721]

Chapter 76

Urothelial Tumors of the Urinary Tract

Edward M. Messing

Questions

1. Members of which of the following American demographic groups are most likely to die from bladder cancer if they contract it?
   a. White women
   b. White men
   c. African-American women
   d. African-American men
   e. Hispanic women

2. Under-reporting of bladder cancer is not likely to explain the differences in this disease's incidence in various demographic groups in the United States for which of the following reasons?
   a. The national Surveillance, Epidemiology, and End Result database keeps very accurate statistics.
   b. There are relatively similar incidences in all geographic regions.
   c. Bladder cancer is rarely found incidentally.
   d. The disease is rare in the elderly, in whom other illnesses prove fatal before bladder cancer is diagnosed.
   e. There are many noninvasive ways to achieve an accurate diagnosis.

3. *p53* abnormalities in bladder cancer are frequently associated with:
   a. hypermethylation of the *p53* gene's promoter.
   b. nuclear overexpression of the p53 protein.
   c. loss of heterozygosity of chromosome 9q.
   d. low-grade papillary superficial tumors.
   e. primarily those cancers not related to cigarette smoking.

4. Progress in identifying the early genetic abnormalities of low-grade papillary superficial bladder cancer has been hindered by which of the following?
   a. The predominance of *p53* abnormalities in these tumors
   b. Genomic instability associated with these tumors
   c. The molecular fingerprint of smoking-related mutations
   d. The frequent loss of all of chromosome 9
   e. The slow rate of growth of these tumors in situ

5. The product of the retinoblastoma gene (*pRb*) effect on the cell cycle:
   a. is associated with trisomy of chromosome 7.
   b. is mediated through *bcl*-2.
   c. is controlled by p16.
   d. is unaltered by its phosphorylation status.
   e. acts primarily on the $G_2 \rightarrow M$ transition.

6. In former cigarette smokers, a significant decline in the risk of developing bladder cancer does not occur until smoking has been discontinued for how long?
   a. 1 year
   b. 2 to 4 years
   c. 5 to 9 years
   d. 10 to 20 years
   e. 21 to 30 years

7. Which of the following statements is true of urothelial (transitional cell) cancers associated with cigarette smoking and/or industrial carcinogen exposures?
   a. They tend to be far more aggressive than those arising in patients without these exposures.
   b. They are more indolent than are those arising in patients without these exposures.
   c. They are about as likely to be as aggressive and indolent as those arising in patients without these exposures.
   d. They are less often associated with abnormalities in the *p53* gene than are cancers arising in patients without these exposures.
   e. They are likely to be caused by the same chemical carcinogen, acrolein.

8. Which of the following is a recently documented urothelial mutagen associated with ingestion of herbal preparations used for weight reduction?
   a. 4-Aminobiphenyl
   b. Arsenic
   c. Phenacetin
   d. Aristolochic acid
   e. Acrolein

9. Which of the following is the strongest argument against there being a directly inherited form of most cases of bladder cancer?

a. Polymorphisms in enzymes involved in mutagen activation and detoxification seem not to be important in bladder cancer development.
b. More distant relatives have a higher likelihood of contracting bladder cancer than closer relatives.
c. Familial clusters of bladder cancer have not been reported.
d. Blackfoot disease–related bladder cancer has a very large male predominance.
e. Chinese weight-reducing herb–associated urothelial cancer occurs almost exclusively in females.

10. Which of the following is a normal anatomic structure that confounds the accurate staging of bladder cancer on transurethral resection specimens?

    a. Glycosaminoglycan layer
    b. Basal lamina
    c. Lamina propria
    d. Muscularis mucosae
    e. Muscularis propria

11. What is the nonmalignant lesion associated with prior, concurrent, or subsequent bladder cancer?

    a. Overactive atypia
    b. Inverted papilloma
    c. Malacoplakia
    d. Nephrogenic adenoma
    e. Cystitis cystica

12. Abnormalities of which of the following genes or gene products often occur in carcinoma in situ?

    a. *erb*B-2
    b. *pRb*
    c. DBCCR1
    d. *p53*
    e. *ras*-p21

13. Low-grade urothelial cancer in the 1998 World Health Organization (WHO) and the International Society of Urological Pathology (ISUP) classification is the same lesion as which of the following?

    a. Papillary urothelial tumor of low malignant potential
    b. Urothelial papilloma
    c. Grade 1 transitional cell carcinoma
    d. Grade 2 transitional cell carcinoma
    e. Grade 3 transitional cell carcinoma

14. Which of the following statements is true regarding bilharzial squamous cell carcinoma of the bladder?

    a. It generally occurs in individuals who are older than those in whom nonbilharzial squamous cell carcinoma of the bladder occurs.
    b. It occurs more commonly in females than does nonbilharzial squamous cell carcinoma of the bladder.
    c. It less frequently has distant metastases than does nonbilharzial squamous cell carcinoma of the bladder.
    d. It is more responsive to systemic chemotherapy than is nonbilharzial squamous cell carcinoma of the bladder.
    e. It is a common sequela of infections with all species of schistosomes that are pathogenic in humans.

15. Genetic aberrations frequently occur in which of the following pairs of genes in both squamous cell and transitional cell carcinomas of the bladder?

    a. *Rb* and *bcl-2*
    b. *p53* and *p16*
    c. *H-ras* and *p27*
    d. *Rb* and *erb*B-2
    e. *DBCCR1* and *p53*

16. Which of the following statements is true regarding urachal carcinoma?

    a. It is usually transitional cell carcinoma.
    b. If nonmetastatic, it is best treated by partial cystectomy.
    c. It responds well to radiation therapy.
    d. It is usually adenocarcinoma.
    e. It is usually squamous cell carcinoma.

17. The existence of both clonal and multiclonal origins of urothelial cancer's occurrences and recurrences is supported by:

    a. molecular fingerprinting of tumors and remote urothelium.
    b. the development of late recurrences after tumor-free intervals of more than 5 years.
    c. the success of immediate postresection intravesical therapy.
    d. relative consistency between phenotypes of recurrent and initial tumors.
    e. the success of intravesical bacille Calmette-Guérin started several weeks after transurethral resection.

18. Which biologic process does not enable cancer cells to invade and metastasize?

    a. Proliferation
    b. Motility
    c. Expression of proteolytic enzymes
    d. Apoptosis
    e. Neoangiogenesis

19. The normal expression of which intracellular adhesion molecule provides a barrier to invasion?

    a. Urokinase plasminogen activator
    b. Autocrine motility factor receptor
    c. Vascular endothelial growth factor
    d. E-cadherin
    e. Matrix metalloproteinase-2 (MMP-2)

20. Which of the following statements is true regarding bladder cancer metastases?

    a. They rarely develop before muscularis propria invasion occurs.
    b. They involve primarily perivesical nodes.
    c. They involve the liver more commonly than pelvic nodes.
    d. They almost never appear in bone.
    e. They frequently result from transurethral resection.

21. What proportion of newly diagnosed urothelial cancers are high-grade tumors?

    a. Less than 20%
    b. 21% to 29%
    c. 30% to 39%
    d. 40% to 49%
    e. 50% to 59%

22. Nuclear expression of *p53* detected immunohistochemically:

    a. is a poor surrogate for abnormalities of the *p53* gene.
    b. cannot be seen unless both alleles of *p53* are deleted or mutated.
    c. predicts a poor response to systemic therapy with cisplatin-containing regimens.
    d. is commonly found in low-grade urothelial tumors in young adults.
    e. is not detected in formalin-fixed, paraffin-embedded specimens.

23. Increased expression of which of the following markers is not associated with a worse prognosis?

    a. Endothelial growth factor receptor
    b. *p53*

c. pRb
d. E-cadherin
e. MMP-2

24. Aberrations of which chromosome or chromosome segment is associated most closely with papillary low-grade, superficial urothelial tumors?

    a. 17p
    b. 13q
    c. 9q
    d. 9p
    e. 7

25. Which of the following statements is true of hematuria caused by bladder cancer?

    a. It is usually accompanied by discomfort and painful voiding.
    b. It is intermittent.
    c. It occurs in a minority of patients with bladder cancer.
    d. It commonly causes anemia.
    e. When grossly visible, it occurs primarily only in the initial phase of the urinary stream.

26. A patient with hematuria undergoes cystoscopy, and a lesion with the typical appearance of a low-grade, superficial papillary urothelial tumor is identified. What is the chief benefit of sending a urinary or bladder wash specimen for cytologic examination?

    a. To confirm the cystoscopic impression
    b. To determine whether upper urinary tract imaging is needed
    c. To identify as yet invisible high-grade cancer
    d. To decide whether cystoscopic resection or biopsy is needed
    e. To serve as a baseline for follow-up

27. The rarity of finding urothelial cancer incidentally at autopsy indicates what?

    a. That bladder cancer screening is likely to detect tumors that normally would have gone unrecognized throughout the lifetime of patients
    b. That underdiagnosis is contributing to differences in the reported incidences of bladder cancer among people of different sexes, races, and ages
    c. That there is a very brief presymptomatic period in which tumors are diagnosable before they cause symptoms
    d. That bladder cancer screening could safely be performed once every 3 to 5 years
    e. That high-grade cancers grow much more rapidly than low-grade ones

28. It is important for a bladder cancer screening instrument to be able to detect low-grade urothelial cancers with as great a sensitivity as for high-grade cancers, because:

    a. both of these tumors have similar likelihoods of causing morbidity.
    b. low-grade cancers often become high-grade ones if their diagnosis is delayed.
    c. the effectiveness of a screening program depends on diagnosing more cancers in a screened than in an unscreened population.
    d. confidence in the screening program will be seriously undermined if any bladder cancers are undiagnosed.
    e. low-grade cancers are more readily controlled by endoscopic means than are high-grade ones.

29. Of the following, which is the diagnostic test most likely not to detect low-grade cancers?

    a. Multiple Hemastix strips
    b. Telomerase activity in urine
    c. Lewis immunocytology
    d. Bladder Tumor Antigen (BTA) stat
    e. Immunocytology

30. Determining the specificity of all bladder cancer diagnostic tests is complicated by which of the following factors?

    a. Inability to detect very small tumors
    b. Detection of cancer not yet cystoscopically visible
    c. Inability to detect low-grade tumors
    d. Controversy about criteria for papillary urothelial tumors of low malignant potential
    e. Positive results caused by inflammation

31. In individuals exposed to known bladder carcinogens, a positive "marker" test:

    a. is usually less sensitive than in patients with sporadic bladder cancer.
    b. may detect molecular alterations induced by the carcinogen that are not necessarily associated with malignant transformation.
    c. must be evaluated more thoroughly than in nonexposed individuals.
    d. has been shown to effectively reduce bladder cancer mortality in exposed individuals.
    e. is not related to cumulative carcinogen exposure.

32. What is a major benefit of fluorescent cystoscopy following intravesical instillation of 5-aminolevulinic acid (ALA)?

    a. It is used to treat tumors with photodynamic therapy.
    b. It permits resection of endoscopically invisible tumors.
    c. It enables treatment of tumors with the use of local anesthesia.
    d. It shortens the time of transurethral resection.
    e. It does not require special instrumentation.

33. Which of the following statements is true regarding transurethral biopsy of normal-appearing bladder urothelium?

    a. It is of value when there are multifocal low-grade superficial bladder tumors and negative urinary cytologic results.
    b. It is of value when there is multifocal high-grade superficial urothelial cancer.
    c. It helps management of multifocal invasive bladder cancer.
    d. It is very important preceding planned partial cystectomy.
    e. It is not helpful when there are positive cytologic results and low-grade papillary cancer.

34. For prognosis and planned therapy, what is the most important distinction between levels of invasiveness of a urothelial tumor?

    a. Between epithelium and lamina propria
    b. Between superficial and deep lamina propria
    c. Between lamina propria and muscularis propria
    d. Between superficial and deep muscularis propria
    e. Between muscularis propria and perivesical fat

35. Tests needed to appropriately stage and evaluate muscle-invading urothelial cancer include all of the following except which one?

    a. CT of the abdomen and pelvis
    b. Intravenous urography
    c. Nuclear bone scan
    d. Chest CT
    e. Serum creatinine assay

36. Invasion of bladder cancer into deep detrusor muscle is

which of the following T stages in the 1997 American Joint Committee on Cancer Staging-International Union Against Cancer (AJC-UICC) system?

a. T1
b. T2a
c. T2b
d. T3a
e. T3b

37. Strategies and nonprescription agents for which there are substantial data indicating efficacy in preventing urothelial cancer include which of the following?

a. Vitamin D supplements
b. Selenium dietary supplements
c. Switching from unfiltered to filtered cigarettes
d. High consumption of fluids
e. High-fiber diet

38. Of the following uncommon bladder malignancies, which one has the most aggressive behavior and most ominous prognosis?

a. Nonurachal adenocarcinoma
b. Carcinosarcoma
c. Primary bladder lymphoma
d. Leiomyosarcoma
e. Embryonal rhabdomyosarcoma

39. Upper tract urothelial cancer associated with Balkan endemic nephropathy tends to be:

a. unilateral.
b. solitary.
c. of low histologic grade.
d. of high histologic grade.
e. predictable in its pattern of inheritance.

40. Upper tract cancers associated with ingestion of Chinese herbs, analgesic abuse, and Balkan nephropathy all have what in common?

a. They occur only after 10 to 20 years of exposure to suspected agents.
b. They are transitional cell carcinomas exclusively.
c. They are usually unilateral.
d. They occur only in individuals affected with interstitial nephropathy.
e. They are more common in cigarette smokers.

41. Which carcinogenic agent is believed to be responsible for urothelial cancer associated with Chinese herb ingestion?

a. Phenacetin
b. Aminobyphenyl
c. Acrolein
d. Arsenic
e. Aristolochic acid

42. What is the most common location for upper tract urothelial cancer?

a. Renal pelvis and calyces
b. Ureteropelvic junction
c. Upper ureter
d. Midureter
e. Lower ureter

43. Microscopic stage T3 urothelial cancer of the upper urinary tract has the best prognosis if it arises where?

a. In the renal pelvis and calyces
b. In the ureteropelvic junction
c. In the upper ureter
d. In the midureter
e. In the lower ureter

44. Upper tract squamous cell carcinomas are associated with all of the following except which one?

a. Diffuse papillary calcifications
b. Chronic bacteriuria
c. Upper tract calculi
d. Analgesic abuse
e. Cyclophosphamide exposure

45. Available evidence concerning uniclonal versus multiclonal etiologies of multiple recurrent upper tract urothelial cancers indicates:

a. a multiclonal origin of most high-grade cancers.
b. a uniclonal origin of most low-grade cancers.
c. the frequent presence of a cancer field defect on a molecular genetic level.
d. the presence of a cancer field defect on a molecular epigenetic level only.
e. that field cancerization on a histologic level is unusual cephalad to high-grade cancers.

46. A 60-year-old man during a microhematuria evaluation was found by intravenous urography to have an intraluminal midureteral filling defect and moderate unilateral hydroureteronephrosis above the filling defect. At cystoscopy, no abnormalities were seen in the bladder; retrograde urography revealed no other lesions in either upper tract; and on ureteroscopy the lesion looked like a papillary urothelial tumor. Voided urinary cytology showed a few "atypical cells," but an attempted biopsy of the lesion had insufficient tissue. A metastatic work-up had negative results. What is the next step?

a. Obtain upper tract irrigation for cytology
b. Repeat ureteroscopy and redo biopsy of the lesion until confirmation is obtained
c. Perform a biopsy through a percutaneous nephrostomy and an anterograde approach
d. Plan and carry out definitive therapy
e. Obtain washings via anterograde access

47. An HIV-positive cigarette smoker who has taken large quantities of phenacetin-containing analgesics for more than 10 years and recently started treatment with the protease inhibitor indinavir has hematuria and a renal pelvic filling defect detected by intravenous urography. This lesion has soft tissue density on CT scans, and bladder urine has highly suspicious cells on cytologic inspection. What is the most appropriate next step?

a. Nephroureterectomy and bladder cuff
b. Ureteropyeloscopy
c. Abdominal MRI
d. Percutaneous nephrostomy and pyeloscopy
e. Discontinuation of indinavir, hydration, and reimaging in 3 months

Answers

1. **c. African-American women.** There is some evidence that this increased risk in whites is primarily limited to noninvasive cancers, which implies a later diagnosis of tumors in African Americans. However, recent genetic and epidemiologic evidence indicates that African Americans may have a more aggressive form of other malignancies. Men have higher 5-year survival rates than women, with this difference in mortality being particularly impressive in African-American women (5-year survival rates of white men, 84%; black men, 71%; white women, 76%; black women, 51%). [p 2733]

2. **c. Bladder cancer is rarely found incidentally.** Because it "always" causes symptoms or signs, bladder cancer is almost always diagnosed before patients die. Thus, it almost never goes undiagnosed, as other malignancies often do. [p 2733]

3. **b. nuclear overexpression of the p53 protein.** The p53 protein exists in a multimeric form, and abnormal chains (from a mutated allele) lead to a nonfunctional protein but one that is not degraded as rapidly as is wild-type p53. Thus, the altered form collects in the nucleus and is readily detectable by immunohistochemistry. In addition, because the wild-type p53 protein functions as a tetramer, the altered product of a mutant allele stabilizes (permitting nuclear accumulation) but inactivates the tetrameric protein (resulting in tumorigenesis), even when the nonmutated allele is expressed normally. This dominant negative effect offers a theoretical hurdle to genetic therapeutic strategies that attempt to insert a wild-type p53 gene into tumors with mutated p53 alleles. [p 2736]

4. **d. The frequent loss of all of chromosome 9.** An entire copy of chromosome 9 is frequently lost, making molecular analysis of specific deleted genes on this chromosome very difficult. [p 2736]

5. **c. is controlled by p16.** Unphosphorylated pRb binds to and inactivates the transcription factor E2F. When pRb is phosphorylated, E2F is released to induce expression of genes needed for mitogenesis. p16 inhibits the cyclin-dependent kinases, which phosphorylate pRb. [p 2736]

6. **d. 10 to 20 years.** That the reduction of risk takes far longer for bladder cancer than for lung or esophageal cancer indicates that bladder cancer carcinogens in cigarette smokers are usually activated and detoxified via different mechanisms than those in patients with other cancers, in whom the carcinogen reaches the target directly, without metabolism. [p 2738]

7. **c. They are about as likely to be as aggressive and indolent as those arising in patients without these exposures.** However, when p53 mutations in bladder tumors of smokers were compared with those in bladder cancers of patients who never smoked, differences in the types or sites of mutations were not seen, although a higher number of mutations occurred in smokers. This suggests that smoking might increase the number of mutations in urothelial cells without necessarily directing the site or type of mutation that occurs. This type of analysis correlates closely with the elegant case control study of Hayes and co-workers, who found that although exposure to industrial carcinogens and smoking clearly correlated with an increased risk for developing bladder cancer, with the exception of young patients, these exposures did not correlate with any particular bladder cancer phenotype. Thus, assuming that low-grade superficial and high-grade rapidly invasive transitional cell carcinomas have different fundamental "genetic pathways," the two best described environmental carcinogenic exposures for bladder cancer predispose for developing each of these genetic alterations in similar proportions to those seen in the nonexposed population. [p 2739]

8. **d. Aristolochic acid.** A Chinese herb (containing *Stephania tetrandra* and *Magnolia officinalis*) that was imported into Belgium as a popular weight reduction aid used primarily by women became responsible for an epidemic of interstitial nephropathy, presumably because of contamination with *Aristolochia fangchi*, which had been substituted for *S. tetrandra*. Subsequently, patients with Chinese herb nephropathy have been reported to be at much higher risk for developing transitional cell carcinoma, primarily of the upper urinary tract but also in the bladder. A major mechanism in transitional cell cancer appears to be the development of aristolochic acid–related DNA adducts in the urothelium of both the upper-urinary tract and bladder. [p 2741]

9. **b. More distant relatives have a higher likelihood of contracting bladder cancer than closer relatives.** Perhaps the most compelling evidence in this regard comes from the work of Kiemeney and co-workers, who studied the records of more than 12,000 relatives of 190 patients diagnosed with transitional cell cancer in Iceland between 1983 and 1992 and found that although the risk of developing transitional cell carcinoma was slightly elevated in relatives (observed-to-expected odds ratio 1.24, 95% confidence interval 0.90 to 1.67), this ratio was greater among second- and third-degree than among first-degree relatives. This result argues strongly against a straightforward genetic mechanism being responsible. [p 2741]

10. **d. Muscularis mucosae.** Part of the reason for discrepancies in the interpretation of histologic sections among different pathologists assessing tumor grade and depth of infiltration is related to the smooth muscle fibers of the tunica muscularis mucosae in the lamina propria of the bladder wall, which may be confused with detrusor muscle. [pp 2744, 2760]

11. **b. Inverted papilloma.** Rare cases of malignant transformation of inverted papillomas have been reported. However, there is a more common association of inverted papilloma occurring in patients with coexistent transitional cell carcinoma elsewhere in the bladder or with histories of such tumors. [p 2742]

12. **d. p53.** p53 abnormalities occur in more than half of high-grade urothelial cancers. Its aberration in carcinoma in situ indicates that this is a precursor lesion for high-grade, but not low-grade, urothelial cancer. [p 2743]

13. **d. Grade 2 transitional cell carcinoma.** Moderately differentiated (grade 2) tumors (see Fig. 76–5) have a wider fibrovascular core, a greater disturbance of the base-to-surface cellular maturation, and a loss of cell polarity, compared with well-differentiated tumors. The nuclear/cytoplasmic ratio is higher, with more nuclear pleomorphism and prominent nucleoli. Mitotic figures are more frequent. These have been termed low-grade urothelial carcinoma in the new WHO/ISUP classification. [pp 2744, 2745–2746]

14. **c. It less frequently has distant metastases than does nonbilharzial squamous cell carcinoma of the bladder.**

These cancers occur in patients who are, on the average, 10 to 20 years younger than patients with transitional cell carcinoma. Bilharzial cancers are exophytic, nodular, fungating lesions that are usually well differentiated and have a relatively low incidence of lymph node and distant metastases. Whether the low incidence of distant metastases is due to capillary and lymphatic fibrosis resulting from chronic schistosomal infection or the relatively low histologic grade of these tumors is not clear. Nonbilharzial squamous cell cancers are usually caused by chronic irritation from urinary calculi, long-term indwelling catheters, chronic urinary infections, or bladder diverticula. [p 2746]

15. **b. p53 and p16.** As with aggressive urothelial (transitional cell) cancer, squamous cell cancers often have p16 and p53 abnormalities, although the mechanisms of gene silencing often differ between the two tumor types. [p 2747]

16. **d. It is usually adenocarcinoma.** Urachal carcinomas are extremely rare tumors that arise outside the bladder and are usually adenocarcinomas, although they may be primary transitional cell or squamous carcinomas and, rarely, even sarcomas. They are rarely responsive to radiotherapy, and, because of their infiltrative nature under the epithelium, they often have extensions that are overlooked so that partial cystectomy is unsuccessful. [p 2747]

17. **a. molecular fingerprinting of tumors and remote urothelium.** The other answers primarily support either clonal (c and d) or multiclonal (b) theories or are unrelated to clonality (e). [pp 2747–2748]

18. **d. Apoptosis.** Apoptosis, programmed cell death in a cancer cell, impedes metastases. [pp 2735, 2736, 2748]

19. **d. E-cadherin.** Major intracellular adhesion molecules, such as E-cadherin and the transmembrane protein family of integrins, also appear to be important barriers against invasion that can become disrupted in invasive tumors. [pp 2748, 2749]

20. **a. They rarely develop before muscularis propria invasion occurs.** It is very unusual for patients to have metastases without concomitant or prior muscularis propria–invading cancer. [pp 2749, 2755]

21. **d. 40% to 49%.** Forty percent to 45% of newly diagnosed bladder cancers are high-grade lesions, more than half of which are muscle invading or more extensive at the time of diagnosis. [p 2750]

22. **d. is commonly found in low-grade urothelial tumors in young adults.** Peculiarly, the majority of patients younger than 30 years of age with bladder cancer, despite almost all having low-grade superficial papillary cancers, have nuclear overexpression of p53 (which in older individuals is almost always overexpressed in only high-grade cancers). [p 2750]

23. **d. E-cadherin.** E-cadherin, an extracellular matrix protein connecting the environment to the cytoskeleton, is deleted or deficient in cancers likely to invade and metastasize. The other markers are all overexpressed in high-grade cancers. [p 2748]

24. **c. 9q.** Several loci on 9q, particularly in 9q32-34, which includes DBCCR1, have been best described with low-grade, superficial tumors. The other aberrations are all associated with high-grade disease. [p 2750]

25. **b. It is intermittent.** Often only one in three to five voidings in patients with active bladder cancer have any hematuria. [pp 2753–2754]

26. **c. To identify as yet invisible high-grade cancer.** High-grade cancer cells in a cytology specimen are very unlikely to come from a low-grade cancer. Thus, a high-grade cancer or carcinoma in situ producing these cells is probably somewhere in the urinary tract. [p 2755]

27. **c. That there is a very brief presymptomatic period in which tumors are diagnosable before they cause symptoms.** The failure to find bladder cancer incidentally implies that from the time a tumor is large enough to be diagnosed until it causes symptoms is sufficiently brief that death from unrelated causes rarely occurs in that interval. Thus, the disease is not likely to be incidentally found (symptoms or signs occur rapidly). [pp 2734, 2755]

28. **d. confidence in the screening program will be seriously undermined if any bladder cancers are undiagnosed.** If a screening participant has a negative test result and shortly thereafter has hematuria recognized and a bladder tumor (even a low-grade superficial one) diagnosed, participants and primary care physicians who do not recognize that only high-grade cancers are likely to be lethal will lose confidence in the screening test and program and will drop their support for it. Thus, screening must detect low- and high-grade cancers equally well. [p 2756]

29. **d. BTA stat.** The others all detect low-grade cancers also, almost as well as high-grade cancers. [pp 2756–2757]

30. **b. Detection of cancer not yet cystoscopically visible.** Specificity is the number of true-negative results divided by the sum of the number of true-negative plus false-positive results. If tests can detect tumors too small to be endoscopically visible (and hence before they can be diagnosed), false-positive rates will appear to increase, enlarging the denominator and reducing specificity. Although inflammatory lesions can cause some bladder cancer detection tests (e.g., hematuria) to be positive (answer e), several tests are *not* affected by inflammation, so that this is not a generic problem in determining specificity for *all* bladder cancer tests. [pp 2757–2758]

31. **b. may detect molecular alterations induced by the carcinogen that are not necessarily associated with malignant transformation.** Studies have been limited because of a combination of factors, including incomplete information about previous exposures, changing production standards, and difficulties with compliance and follow-up. Additionally, the possibility of the chemical exposures themselves causing abnormal test results without leading to diagnosable malignancy is uncertain. Even when a positive biomarker test precedes the appearance of overt malignancy, whether the positive test indicates the presence of (1) a premalignant field change that may be reversed by cessation of carcinogen exposure, (2) irreversible changes in the urothelium, or (3) true malignant transformation that was not yet clinically detectable is not clear. [pp 2758–2759]

32. **b. It permits resection of endoscopically invisible tumors.** ALA, when administered intravesically in conjunction with fluorescent cystoscopy using blue light at 375 to 440 nm, can enable detection of lesions invisible with white light cystoscopy. In the largest series to date, the authors claimed that this procedure increased sensitivity in detecting small tumors and carcinoma in situ from 77% with white light to nearly 98% with fluorescent cystoscopy. [p 2759]

33. **d. It is very important preceding planned partial cystectomy.** Regardless of the questionable wisdom of performing selected site urothelial biopsies for most bladder tumors, these biopsies are required if partial cystectomy is contem-

plated, or if urinary cytology indicates the presence of high-grade cancer and cystoscopically no tumors are seen or all lesions look like low-grade superficial papillary tumors. [p 2759]

34. **c. Between lamina propria and muscularis propria.** The first treatment decision based on tumor stage is whether the patient has a superficial or muscle invasive tumor. [p 2760]

35. **d. Chest CT.** Chest CT may be too sensitive in detecting small pulmonary lesions that are not metastases. Because standard films do not have the sufficient resolution to demonstrate small granulomas, but rather detect only lesions larger than 1 cm in diameter, routine chest radiographs rather than CT scans are usually relied on to rule out pulmonary metastases in bladder cancer patients. [p 2761]

36. **c. T2b.** In the AJC-UICC system, muscle-invading tumors, depending on whether there is superficial or deep muscle invasion, are classified as stage T2a or T2b, respectively. [p 2762]

37. **d. High consumption of fluid.** Not surprisingly, dilution of carcinogenic agents in the urine by increasing fluid ingestion protects against bladder cancer, with a relative risk of 0.51 for the highest quartile of chronic fluid ingestion compared with the lowest. [p 2763]

38. **b. Carcinosarcoma.** Carcinosarcomas are highly malignant tumors containing both malignant mesenchymal and epithelial elements. The common presenting symptom is gross, painless hematuria. The prognosis is uniformly poor despite aggressive treatment with cystectomy, radiation, and/or chemotherapy. [p 2764]

39. **c. of low histologic grade.** The urothelial tumors associated with Balkan nephropathy are generally of low grade and are more often multiple and bilateral than are upper tract transitional cell cancers of other causes. This nephropathy, although familial, is not obviously inherited, and environmental agents have not been identified. [p 2766]

40. **d. They occur only in individuals affected with interstitial nephropathy.** It has been recognized that phenacetin alone is not the only culprit in analgesic nephropathy and that almost all cases occurred in patients taking combination preparations that often included caffeine, codeine, acetaminophen, and aspirin or other salicylates. This may explain in part the variability of risks for cancer. Nearly half of patients with end-stage renal failure resulting from *A. fangchi*–induced nephropathy, which produces interstitial fibrosis not unlike Balkan nephropathy, who agreed to undergo "prophylactic" bilateral nephroureterectomies had urothelial cancers, more than 90% of which were in the ureters and/or renal pelves. Despite this aggressive management approach, 18% of the upper tract cancers were already invasive. Moreover, in the patients who did not actually have urothelial cancer, more than 90% had at least moderate dysplasia in the renal pelves and/or ureters. [pp 2766–2767]

41. **e. Aristolochic acid.** A third chronic nephropathy, associated with ingestion of Chinese herbs for weight reduction inadvertently contaminated with *A. fangchi*, causes urothelial carcinoma resulting from DNA adducts formed by aristolochic acid. [p 2767]

42. **a. Renal pelvis and calyces.** Urothelial cancers of the renal pelvis and calyces are roughly four times as common as ureteral cancers. The most common site of ureteral cancer is in the lower third of the ureter. Upper ureteral cancers are the least common. [pp 2765, 2768]

43. **a. In the renal pelvis and calyces.** Patients with renal pelvic and calyceal cancers extending microscopically beyond the collecting system have a far better prognosis than do patients with ureteral cancers invading beyond the ureter. Guinan and colleagues suggested that in reviewing the Illinois tumor registry data, patients with stage T3 renal pelvic carcinomas had a far better prognosis than those with stage T3 ureteral carcinomas, in part because the renal parenchyma may serve as a barrier against further dissemination. Further complicating the issue was the rather detailed analysis by Fujimoto and colleagues, who found that patients with renal pelvic cancers who had microscopic involvement of the collecting duct with or without minimal renal parenchymal invasion or with minimal microscopic invasion of the renal parenchyma (less than 5-mm extension) with no collecting duct involvement had a far better prognosis than those with extensive parenchymal extension. [p 2769]

44. **e. Cyclophosphamide exposure.** Upper tract squamous cell carcinomas are frequently associated with infected staghorn calculi that have been present for a long time. In addition, diffuse papillary calcification, especially related to analgesic abuse, is associated with squamous cell carcinomas. Patients characteristically present with advanced disease. [p 2768]

45. **c. the frequent presence of a cancer field defect on a molecular genetic level.** Analyses from histologically normal-appearing urothelium throughout the ipsilateral upper tract and bladder that is remote from even low-grade papillary tumors usually reveal the identical signature alterations in microsatellite loci that appear in tumors. The remaining answers are incorrect. [p 2768]

46. **d. Plan and carry out definitive therapy.** Radiologic and ureteroscopic evidence of malignancy is sufficient to proceed with definitive treatment, assuming that there is a normal contralateral ureter and kidney. [p 2772]

47. **b. Ureteropyeloscopy.** Indinavir stones are lucent on radiographs and CT scans and can cause cytologic results that should raise suspicions or are positive. Distinction between urothelial cancer and this stone is crucial, but a waiting period of 3 months to re-evaluate is too long in case there is urothelial cancer. MRI may not always distinguish this stone from tumors. Ultrasonography (not a choice in this question) can distinguish stone from tumor in most circumstances, but direct inspection is most accurate. [p 2771]

Chapter 77

Management of Superficial Bladder Cancer

Stanley Bruce Malkowicz

Questions

1. When a transurethral resection (TUR) of a bladder lesion demonstrates high-grade T1 disease:

    a. the finding is often an overstaging error because of cautery artifact.
    b. detrusor perforation occurs more frequently.
    c. another TUR is appropriate in the absence of detectable muscularis propria.
    d. urine cytology will generally demonstrate atypia.
    e. p53 staining is rarely positive.

2. Which of the following statements is true of random bladder biopsy samples obtained during TUR of bladder tumor?

    a. They are difficult to interpret because of crush artifact.
    b. They are associated with a high degree of bladder perforation.
    c. They generally demonstrate muscularis mucosae.
    d. They rarely provide additional clinical information.
    e. They confound flow cytometry data because of inflammation.

3. Which of the following statements is true of laser therapy for superficial bladder cancer?

    a. It is optimally performed with a CO_2 laser.
    b. It is associated with a high degree of bladder perforation.
    c. It is associated with fewer recurrences at the treatment site compared with TUR.
    d. It requires more anesthesia than does conventional TUR of bladder tumor.
    e. It results in a higher tumor progression rate compared with TUR.

4. During bacille Calmette-Guérin (BCG) therapy, the initial catheterization is traumatic. What is the best response?

    a. To administer quinolone antibiotics and proceed with therapy
    b. To abort the procedure and re-evaluate the patient's status in 1 week
    c. To administer BCG and monitor the patient for positive urine culture results and fever
    d. To abort the procedure and administer interferon-α_{2a} for the remainder of the treatment course
    e. To administer keyhole-limpet hemocyanin for one dose and then resume BCG administration for the remainder of the treatment course

5. The effect of BCG on superficial tumor progression is best represented by which of the following statements?

    a. BCG administration has no effect on tumor progression.
    b. A decrease in tumor progression is noted only when BCG is administered with intravesical chemotherapy.
    c. BCG decreases the progression of high-grade disease but has little impact on the progression of low-grade lesions.
    d. BCG has an initial impact on tumor progression that is less evident on long-term follow-up.
    e. Intravesical chemotherapy has a greater effect on tumor progression than does BCG therapy.

6. Antimycobacterial therapy is necessary during BCG treatment if a patient demonstrates which of the following signs and symptoms?

    a. Any temperature higher than 38.5°C
    b. Diastolic blood pressure less than 80 mm Hg
    c. Dysuria with microscopic hematuria
    d. Arthralgias and headache
    e. Any temperature higher than 39.5°C, or a temperature higher than 38.5°C for more than 24 hours

7. Immediate intravesical chemotherapy after TUR is associated with:

    a. decreases in tumor recurrence during an intermediate follow-up period.
    b. significant bladder contracture and dysuria.
    c. a decrease in the progression rate of high-grade lesions.
    d. thrombocytopenia and leukocytopenia of short duration.
    e. a decrease in occurrence of carcinoma in situ but no change in papillary tumor recurrence.

8. The current recommended schedules for bladder tumor surveillance are based on:

    a. the lack of tumor progression in Ta lesions after 5 years.
    b. the introduction of modern tumor markers for following bladder tumors.
    c. authority opinion.
    d. the association of early recurrence with tumor progression.
    e. patterns of recurrence in clinical trials.

9. The contemporary role for bladder tumor markers in the monitoring of patients with diagnosed superficial bladder tumors is best described by:

    a. routine monitoring of patients who have carcinoma in situ with BTA, NMP22, or HA-HAase tests.
    b. microsatellite deletion assays in patients who experience an early recurrence at the first 3-month follow-up assessment.
    c. lack of a routine role for bladder tumor markers in follow-up of patients with superficial disease.
    d. proven value of quantitative but not qualitative markers in the follow-up of patients.
    e. standard use of a panel of markers, including cytology once yearly.

10. Monitoring of the upper urinary tracts is best managed in patients with superficial transitional cell carcinoma by:
    a. serial follow-up with voided urine cytology.
    b. yearly or bi-yearly intravenous urograms in patients with high-grade lesions treated with BCG.
    c. renal ultrasonography yearly for 5 years.
    d. follow-up studies triggered by microscopic or gross hematuria.
    e. no routine follow-up after 3 years.

Answers

1. **c. another TUR is appropriate in the absence of detectable muscularis propria.** In the evaluation of T1 tumors specifically, another TUR can demonstrate findings of worse prognosis (concomitant tumor in situ, extensive T1 grade 3 disease, or disease of higher grade than T1) in up to 25% of specimens. Given the borderline status of high-grade T1 lesions, another TUR is appropriate, especially if no muscle is identified on the initial pathologic study. [p 2786]

2. **d. They rarely provide additional clinical information.** Older studies suggest a useful prognostic role for random biopsies. More recent work indicates that the additional value provided by biopsies from random sites of normal-appearing tissue at the time of resection appears to be minimal and, theoretically, the process may aid tumor implantation. Select biopsies of suspicious areas, however, are an important part of a complete evaluation. [p 2787]

3. **c. It is associated with fewer recurrences at the treatment site compared with TUR.** Although early reports suggested lower tumor recurrence rates, a prospective randomized series demonstrated no difference with regard to recurrence. This series demonstrated fewer recurrences at the site of treatment (3 of 44), a finding noted in earlier investigations. [p 2787]

4. **b. To abort the procedure and re-evaluate the patient's status in 1 week.** The presence of gross hematuria or a likely bacterial infection is a contraindication for administration of BCG because toxicity is associated with intravascular inoculation. Similarly, catheterization should be atraumatic and administration should be performed under gravity drainage. In the event of a traumatic catheterization, the treatment should be delayed for several days. Optimally, the patient should retain the solution for 2 hours. [p 2790]

5. **d. BCG has an initial impact on tumor progression that is less evident on long-term follow-up.** The available data suggest that BCG can effect an early delay in progression of high-risk bladder cancer, yet the long-term advantage of this therapy cannot be adequately assessed because of the small numbers of study patients at risk over 10 to 15 years. [p 2790]

6. **e. Any temperature higher than 39.5°C, or a temperature higher than 38.5°C for more than 24 hours.** A low-grade fever and/or slight malaise may occur in a large proportion of patients. If a temperature greater than 38.5°C persists for more than 24 hours and does not resolve with antipyretic therapy or if a temperature greater than 39.5°C is encountered, treatment with isoniazid (300 mg daily for 3 months) is necessary. [p 2792]

7. **a. decreases in tumor recurrence during an intermediate follow-up period.** In all of these studies, the side effects were minimal and the therapeutic advantage was demonstrated when the agent was delivered within 6 hours of the TUR. Although it is difficult to draw the conclusion that the natural history of these lesions has been permanently altered, the positive effect of decreasing recurrence rate and prolonging the recurrence-free interval for an intermediate time interval seems apparent. [p 2794]

8. **c. authority opinion.** The classic recommendation for cystoscopic surveillance in superficial disease has been every 3 months for the first year, every 6 months for the second year, and yearly thereafter. Regimens of greater intensity have also been suggested for potentially more aggressive lesions. These are authority-based opinions with little empirical backing that have persisted for many years. [p 2796]

9. **c. lack of a routine role for bladder tumor markers in follow-up of patients with superficial disease.** At the present time, there is no well-defined, established role for the use of these markers in the routine follow-up of bladder cancer patients. Well-designed prospective studies will be required to demonstrate the safety and economy of marker-directed follow-up care for individual patients. [p 2797]

10. **b. yearly or bi-yearly intravenous urograms in patients with high-grade lesions treated with BCG.** The cumulative evidence suggests that those patients with high-risk superficial disease successfully treated with BCG require close, lifelong observation of the upper tracts with routine intravenous urograms on a yearly basis or at the detection of a positive urine cytology result. Few data support such intense follow-up in low-risk patients, yet evaluation of the upper tracts on a 3- to 4-year schedule is reasonable. [p 2797]

Chapter 78

Management of Invasive and Metastatic Bladder Cancer

Mark Schoenberg

Questions

1. Which of the following statements is NOT true with regard to staging of invasive bladder cancer?

   a. Bimanual examination is highly predictive of the presence of extravesical disease if a mass is palpable after transurethral resection.
   b. CT and MRI are equivalent methods of noninvasive axial imaging for prediction of nodal involvement.
   c. Bone scanning is a useful routine staging tool for asymptomatic patients with clinically organ-confined invasive bladder cancer.
   d. The utility of positron emission tomography in staging bladder tumors is limited by concentration of the fluorodeoxyglucose agent in the lumen of the bladder.

2. Which of the following statements is true regarding nerve-sparing cystoprostatectomy?

   a. It is more likely to result in local recurrence than is standard cystectomy.
   b. It is accomplished by high lateral ligation of the pedicles of the prostate gland adjacent to the seminal vesicles.
   c. It is associated with potency rates higher than 50% in men aged 75 years and older when both nerves are preserved.
   d. It is associated with inferior stage-for-stage disease-specific survival compared with standard cystectomy.

3. In a 34-year-old female patient with T2N0Mx bladder cancer who undergoes radical cystectomy, which of the following is true?

   a. Excision of the anterior vaginal wall is required.
   b. The urethra is usually involved in the tumor diathesis.
   c. Orthotopic reconstruction is not recommended if the trigone is diffusely involved by carcinoma in situ.
   d. Classic anterior exenteration would not require removal of the uterus.

4. Which of the following statements is true regarding radical cystectomy?

   a. It results in disease-free survival rates that decline with increasing stage of disease.
   b. It is best for patients with moderate local nodal disease appreciated via preoperative imaging.
   c. It produces overall survival rates that have been shown in prospective trials to exceed those obtained with bladder-sparing protocols.
   d. It results in bowel obstruction requiring operative correction in 20% of patients.

5. Which of the following statements is true regarding pelvic lymphadenectomy in the context of radical cystectomy?

   a. It can result in long-term disease-free survival in patients with N1 bladder cancer.
   b. It is routinely recommended for patients with palpable adenopathy above the aortic bifurcation.
   c. It will usually identify metastatic disease contralateral to the patient's known tumor.
   d. It provides limited staging information that cannot be obtained from axial imaging studies performed preoperatively.

6. Which of the following statements is true regarding neoadjuvant chemotherapy for bladder cancer?

   a. It generally relies on normal renal function.
   b. It provides a relative advantage to patients with disease of T3 stage or greater.
   c. It has been associated with improved disease-specific survival rates in randomized U.S. trials.
   d. All of the above.

7. Which of the following statements is true regarding adjuvant chemotherapy?

   a. It improves disease-specific outcome in patients undergoing cystectomy.
   b. It is most appropriate for patients with disease of less than stage pT2.
   c. It is better tolerated than neoadjuvant chemotherapy.
   d. None of the above.

8. Which of the following statements is true regarding transurethral resection?

   a. It can achieve a long-term disease-free survival rate in patients with invasive bladder cancer equivalent to that achieved with standard surgical therapy.
   b. It is unlikely to achieve disease-free survival in patients with T2N0Mx bladder cancer.
   c. As a form of monotherapy for invasive bladder cancer, it is most likely to be successful if residual disease is only microscopic.
   d. None of the above.

9. Which of the following statements is true regarding bladder preservation protocols?

   a. They are indicated for all stages of clinically organ-confined bladder cancer.
   b. They are equally effective whether hydronephrosis is present or absent.
   c. They are flawed by reliance on clinical staging.
   d. They achieve 5-year disease-specific survival rates similar to those obtained with radical cystectomy.

10. Each of the following statements is true of systemic chemotherapy for bladder cancer except which one?

a. It is reserved for the treatment of patients with measurable metastatic bladder cancer.
b. It is usually more successful if a multiagent regimen as opposed to a single-agent protocol is used.
c. It often includes methotrexate, cisplatin, doxorubicin, and bleomycin.
d. All of the above.

11. Salvage cystectomy is appropriate:

    a. when residual disease is limited to the true pelvis.
    b. and is most likely to achieve the greatest chance of disease-free survival when the patient's response to chemotherapy is incomplete.
    c. for patients who have received radiation to the pelvis and chemotherapy, but it is never safe to perform orthotopic reconstruction in this setting.
    d. none of the above.

12. A 41-year-old otherwise healthy male patient with T2N0Mx transitional cell carcinoma of the bladder:

    a. should have a preoperative bone scan because his alkaline phosphatase level is normal.
    b. is not a candidate for bladder preservation on the basis of age.
    c. has an approximately 5% risk of positive lymph nodes at the time of radical cystectomy.
    d. should have ureteral frozen section analysis at the time of cystectomy.

Answers

1. **c. Bone scanning is a useful routine staging tool for asymptomatic patients with clinically organ-confined invasive bladder cancer.** Several studies from the last two decades substantiate the impression that, in general, preoperative bone scanning is not necessary for patients with clinically organ-confined muscle invasive bladder carcinoma. [p 2804]

2. **b. It is accomplished by high lateral ligation of the pedicles of the prostate adjacent to the seminal vesicles.** A key technical point to observe intraoperatively when performing nerve-sparing cystoprostatectomy is high lateral ligation of the pedicles of the bladder and prostate, as these tissues coalesce near the seminal vesicles. [p 2805]

3. **c. Orthotopic reconstruction is not recommended if the trigone is diffusely involved by carcinoma in situ.** Female patients with overt cancer at the bladder neck and urethra, diffuse carcinoma in situ, or a positive margin at surgery are poor candidates for orthotopic reconstruction and should be treated by immediate en bloc urethrectomy as part of the radical cystectomy. [p 2806]

4. **a. It results in disease-free survival rates that decline with increasing stage of disease.** Pathologic stage of disease correlates significantly with patient outcome after intervention. Nowhere is this more clearly delineated than in the contemporary literature on radical cystectomy with pelvic lymphadenectomy for clinically organ-confined bladder cancer. Long-term survival is uniformly better for patients with pathologically organ-confined disease (see Table 78–2). Although the results of radical cystectomy for patients with clinically organ-confined disease appear unimpeachable, radical cystectomy performed in the context of locoregional disease or malignant pelvic adenopathy is more controversial. [pp 2805, 2807]

5. **a. It can result in long-term disease-free survival in patients with N1 bladder cancer.** Pelvic lymphadenectomy provides insight into the local extent of disease. In addition, patients with very limited nodal burden experience unexpectedly high rates of long-term survival in the absence of additional interventions. [p 2807]

6. **d. All of the above.** Utilizing cis-platin-based therapy, trials have shown a trend toward improved long-term disease-specific survival rates in some younger patients and in those with lesions greater than stage T3. [p 2808]

7. **d. None of the above**. There is no evidence to suggest that the administration of adjuvant chemotherapy to patients with organ-confined bladder cancer (T1-T2) will provide either a survival advantage or an improvement in local control after cystectomy. [p 2809]

8. **a. It can achieve long-term disease-free survival in patients with invasive bladder cancer equivalent to that achieved with standard surgical therapy.** In one study, a large group of patients was treated by transurethral resection with a negative tumor bed and peripheral biopsies after complete "radical" transurethral resection. The 5-year disease-specific survival statistics were impressively similar to those reported for radical cystectomy. [p 2810]

9. **d. They achieve 5-year disease-specific survival rates similar to those obtained with radical cystectomy.** One study treated 106 patients with T2-4NxM0 bladder cancer by transurethral resection, neoadjuvant chemotherapy (methotrexate, cisplatin, and vinblastine), and subsequent radiation therapy. Patients not responding were treated by radical cystectomy. These authors reported a 52% overall survival rate. Of the patients completing the full course of therapy, 75% retained bladders free of disease with a median follow-up of 64 months. Subsequent studies by other investigators have lent support to these conclusions. [p 2810]

10. **c. It often includes methotrexate, cisplatin, doxorubicin, and bleomycin.** The most commonly employed agents are methotrexate, vinblastine, doxorubicin (Adriamycin), and cisplatin. [p 2813]

11. **d. none of the above.** Patients electing conservative or primarily nonsurgical forms of therapy for invasive or locoregionally advanced bladder cancer may require subsequent definitive surgical intervention when conservative treatment has produced a partial response and residual disease remains clinically confined to the bladder. Another study found that orthotopic reconstruction is safe and effective in selected patients undergoing salvage surgery. Resection appears to help patients who have had a complete response to systemic therapy, but surgery for residual extravesical disease confers no long-term survival advantage and is generally to be discouraged. [p 2813]

12. **d. should have ureteral frozen section analysis at the time of cystectomy.** Analysis of the ureteral margin at the time of cystectomy before urinary tract reconstruction is standard contemporary practice. The rationale for this procedure is that carcinoma and particularly carcinoma in situ can involve the distal ureteral margin. Urologists have historically resected positive margins to effect clearance of all documented cancer, assuming that this would provide better long-term local disease control. [p 2806]

Chapter 79

Surgery of Bladder Cancer

V. Keith Jiminez • Fray F. Marshall

Questions

1. Which of the following statements regarding the arterial supply to the bladder is true?

    a. The inferior vesical artery arises from the posterior trunk of the internal iliac artery.
    b. The superior vesical artery arises from the anterior trunk of the internal iliac artery.
    c. The majority of the blood supply to the bladder is derived from the obturator artery.
    d. The inferior gluteal artery sends no branches to the bladder.
    e. The bladder cannot be mobilized substantially because of its tenuous blood supply.

2. Which of the following statements regarding cold-cup biopsy of bladder lesions is true?

    a. It is useful for biopsy of large bladder tumors.
    b. Lesions on the inside of the bladder neck are most amenable to cold-cup biopsy.
    c. It is difficult to do through a standard cystoscope.
    d. It requires suprapubic pressure if the lesion is located on the trigone.
    e. It allows for better tissue procurement without coagulation defects when compared with standard loop resection.

3. Tumor characteristics that would allow for transurethral resection as the sole treatment for muscle-invasive disease include which of the following?

    a. High grade
    b. Multifocal
    c. Papillary
    d. Tumor base larger than 2 cm
    e. Sessile

4. A suitable bowel preparation for a radical cystectomy should include all of the following except which one?

    a. A cathartic such as GoLYTELY
    b. Erythromycin
    c. Gentamicin
    d. Neomycin
    e. A clear liquid diet

5. What is the cephalad limit to a pelvic lymphadenectomy?

    a. Peritoneal reflection
    b. Bifurcation of the common iliac artery
    c. Vas deferens
    d. Median umbilical ligament
    e. Node of Cloquet

6. What is the mortality rate associated with radical cystectomy in most modern series?

    a. 0.1% to 0.2%
    b. 1% to 3%
    c. 5% to 7%
    d. 9% to 11%
    e. 15% to 17%

7. What is the incidence of urethral recurrence after radical cystoprostatectomy?

    a. 0.5% to 4%
    b. 4% to 18%
    c. 19% to 28%
    d. 29% to 37%
    e. 39% to 48%

8. Which of the following statements regarding urethrectomy is true?

    a. The dissection is much easier if carried out several weeks after radical cystectomy.
    b. Drainage is not recommended after urethrectomy.
    c. The bulbar urethral arteries should be carefully preserved throughout the dissection.
    d. When a urethrectomy is performed, the best position for the patient is the exaggerated lithotomy.
    e. It is necessary to split the glans to remove all of the transitional cell epithelium.

9. Which of the following statements regarding urethral involvement in bladder cancer in the female patient is true?

    a. Female patients have a much higher incidence of urethral involvement than do male patients.
    b. Orthotopic bladder substitution can rarely be used in the female patient because of the risk of urethral recurrence.
    c. Intraoperative frozen section is the best way to determine whether the urethra is suitable for orthotopic substitution.
    d. Involvement of tumor at the bladder neck always signifies urethral involvement.
    e. The incidence of urethral involvement in female patients has been shown to be consistently above 15%.

10. A complete anterior exenteration in the female includes all of the following procedures except which one?

    a. Cystectomy
    b. Hysterectomy
    c. Bilateral pelvic lymphadenectomy
    d. Pubovaginal sling
    e. Partial vaginectomy

11. All of the following can be considered indications for simple cystectomy except which one?

    a. Pyocystis in a neurogenic bladder
    b. Colovesical fistula after urinary diversion
    c. Urachal adenocarcinoma
    d. Hemorrhagic cystitis resulting from cyclophosphamide use
    e. Feelings of pain and incomplete emptying in patients with prior supravesical diversions

12. What is the advantage of partial cystectomy over total cystectomy in the management of bladder cancer?

a. More accurate staging
b. Improved survival
c. The preservation of bladder and sexual function
d. The possibility of using surveillance cystoscopy
e. Lower recurrence rates of tumor

13. Which of the following is a contraindication to partial cystectomy?

a. Tumor location at the dome of the bladder
b. Grade I transitional cell carcinoma
c. Tumor within a bladder diverticulum
d. Multifocal tumor associated with multifocal carcinoma in situ
e. Urachal adenocarcinoma

Answers

1. **b. The superior vesical artery arises from the anterior trunk of the internal iliac artery.** The urinary bladder has a rich blood supply derived from the superior and inferior vesical branches that arise from the anterior trunk of the internal iliac artery and by smaller branches from the obturator and internal gluteal arteries. [p 2820]

2. **e. It allows for better tissue procurement without coagulation defects when compared with standard loop resection.** If the bladder lesion is small, it may be amenable to cold-cup biopsy and fulguration. This technique has the advantage of tissue procurement without coagulation defects from the resectoscope. [p 2821]

3. **c. Papillary.** No randomized studies have compared transurethral resection alone with cystectomy. However, there is probably a small subset of patients with stage T2 transitional cell carcinoma who may be candidates for resection therapy alone. These patients are likely to have tumors that are small, solitary, papillary, moderately differentiated, less than 2 cm in diameter at the tumor base, and stage T2 or minimal stage T3a. [p 2822]

4. **c. Gentamicin.** Clear liquids are recommended for the 2 days before surgery. Polyethylene glycol-electrolyte solution (GoLYTELY) is given on the day before surgery, and oral antibiotics containing both neomycin and erythromycin base, 1 g each, are administered in three doses on the day before surgery. [p 2824]

5. **b. Bifurcation of the common iliac artery.** The bifurcation of the common iliac artery is the cephalad limit of the dissection. [p 2825]

6. **b. 1% to 3%.** The operative mortality rate for radical cystectomy has been shown to be between 1% and 3% in most modern series. [p 2828]

7. **b. 4% to 18%.** The incidence of urethral recurrence has been documented in prior studies to be between 4% and 18%. [p 2829]

8. **d. When a urethrectomy is performed, the best position for the patient is the exaggerated lithotomy.** The urethrectomy from the perineal approach is most easily performed with the patient in the exaggerated lithotomy position. [p 2830]

9. **c. Intraoperative frozen section is the best way to determine whether the urethra is suitable for orthotopic substitution.** An intraoperative frozen section of the proximal urethra should now be considered the best way to determine whether a female patient is a suitable candidate for orthotopic reconstruction. [p 2833]

10. **d. Pubovaginal sling.** The anterior approach has advantages in that it allows for simultaneous pelvic lymphadenectomy, cystectomy, urethrectomy, hysterectomy, salpingo-oophorectomy, and partial vaginectomy if clinically indicated for extensive carcinomatous involvement. [pp 2833–2835]

11. **c. Urachal adenocarcinoma.** Various benign conditions that may warrant simple cystectomy include pyocystis, neurogenic bladder, severe urinary incontinence, severe urethral trauma, large vesical fistula, cyclophosphamide cystitis, and radiation cystitis after treatment of other pelvic malignancies. [p 2839]

12. **c. The preservation of bladder and sexual function.** The benefits of partial cystectomy include complete pathologic staging of the tumor and pelvic lymph nodes, as well as preservation of both bladder and sexual function. [p 2841]

13. **d. Multifocal tumor associated with multifocal carcinoma in situ.** Absolute contraindications to partial cystectomy would include multifocal carcinoma in situ. [p 2841]

Chapter 80

Management of Urothelial Tumors of the Renal Pelvis and Ureter

Arthur I. Sagalowsky • Thomas W. Jarrett

Questions

1. Which factor is the major determinant of the type of treatment for upper tract urothelial tumors?

   a. Size
   b. Number
   c. Stage and grade
   d. Contralateral renal function
   e. Level of lesion

2. What is(are) the most common symptom(s) of localized upper tract tumors?

   a. None, inasmuch as such tumors are incidental findings
   b. Flank pain
   c. Different from bladder cancer
   d. Dysuria and hematuria
   e. Weight loss and fatigue

3. Which of the following statements is true regarding flank pain in patients with upper tract tumors?

   a. It is rare.
   b. It signifies invasive disease.
   c. It indicates invasion into adjacent structures.
   d. It correlates with stage.
   e. None of the above.

4. In patients with upper tract tumors, what is the most common finding on imaging studies of the urinary tract?

   a. A mass
   b. A filling defect
   c. Hydronephrosis
   d. Nonfunction
   e. Delayed function

5. The majority of renal pelvis tumors are of which type?

   a. Papillary and invasive
   b. Papillary and noninvasive
   c. Sessile and invasive
   d. Sessile and noninvasive
   e. Mixed papillary and sessile

6. Most ureteral tumors are:

   a. sessile.
   b. high grade and noninvasive.
   c. low grade and noninvasive.
   d. medium grade and low stage.
   e. low grade and invasive.

7. What is the most common location of ureteral tumors?

   a. The ureteropelvic junction
   b. Proximal
   c. Middle
   d. Distal
   e. Intramural

8. After complete conservative treatment of a ureteral tumor (i.e., segmental excision or endoscopic ablation), which of the following is true?

   a. Ipsilateral recurrence is common.
   b. Recurrence is rare.
   c. Recurrence would most likely be contralateral.
   d. Recurrence signifies incomplete initial therapy.
   e. Recurrence in the renal pelvis is common.

9. What is the major factor predisposing to recurrence of upper tract tumors?

   a. Incomplete therapy
   b. Multifocal field change
   c. Implantation during instrumentation
   d. Normal ureteral peristalsis
   e. Periureteral spread

10. What is the outcome in patients with multifocal upper tract tumors?

    a. Determined mainly by stage
    b. Poor without early radical surgery
    c. Poor independent of stage
    d. Determined by the rate of recurrence
    e. Poor regardless of the extent of surgery

11. What is the single most important determinant of outcome in the treatment of upper tract tumors?

    a. Grade
    b. Stage
    c. Early diagnosis
    d. Extent of surgery
    e. Size and focality of lesion

12. What is the earliest site of spread of proximal ureteral tumors?

    a. Lung and bone
    b. Liver and bone
    c. Lung and liver
    d. Pelvic nodes
    e. Para-aortic nodes

13. Reasons to consider nephron-sparing surgery for patients with upper tract tumors include all of the following except which one?

    a. Bilateral tumors
    b. Unreliable follow-up
    c. Balkan nephropathy

d. Diabetic nephropathy
e. Solitary kidney

14. A 60-year-old diabetic man is diagnosed with a 4-cm, grade 2 to 3/3 transitional cell tumor of the renal pelvis. His serum creatinine value is 2.2 mg/dl. What is the recommended treatment?

    a. Ureteroscopic ablation
    b. Antegrade percutaneous resection
    c. Pyelotomy and tumor excision
    d. Radical nephroureterectomy
    e. Ileal ureteral substitution

15. A 57-year-old man with a grade 3, stage T2 tumor of the proximal ureter is undergoing radical nephroureterectomy. Correct management of the ureter requires which of the following?

    a. Ligation and division as far as exposure allows
    b. Ureterectomy in continuity with the kidney
    c. Ligation and division at the juxtavesical portion
    d. Complete distal ureterectomy with a bladder cuff
    e. Ligation and division 4 cm distal to the tumor, and a negative margin on frozen section.

16. Which statement is most correct regarding the role of lymphadenectomy in conjunction with radical nephroureterectomy?

    a. It should not be performed.
    b. It is helpful for determining prognosis.
    c. It is associated with high morbidity rate.
    d. It decreases the occurrence of distant relapse.
    e. It is therapeutic.

17. A 46-year-old woman has a 2.5 cm stage Ta, grade 2 transitional cell tumor of the midureter. Initial treatment consists of "complete" ureteroscopic laser ablation of the tumor. Six months later, there is a recurrent 2-cm tumor of the same stage and grade at the same location in the ureter. What should the next step in management be?

    a. Segmental ureterectomy
    b. Nephroureterectomy
    c. Ureteroscopic ablation
    d. Antegrade resection
    e. Antegrade resection followed by instillation of mitomycin

18. A 38-year-old man has a brief episode of gross hematuria. His initial evaluation included the following evaluations, all of whose results were normal: bladder wash cytology, intravenous urography, cystoscopy, bladder biopsy, urethral biopsy, and bilateral retrograde pyelography. The upper tract cytologic result is positive for the right and negative for the left. What is the next step in management?

    a. Repeat upper tract cytology in 6 months
    b. Ureteropyeloscopy
    c. Right nephroureterectomy
    d. Intravesical bacille Calmette-Guérin (BCG)
    e. Right nephrostomy and infusion of BCG

19. After radical nephroureterectomy for a stage T3 transitional cell carcinoma (TCC) of the renal pelvis, which of the following is true?

    a. Local relapse is the main limitation to survival.
    b. Adjuvant radiation decreases local relapse.
    c. Adjuvant chemotherapy increases survival.
    d. Adjuvant radiation does not improve survival.
    e. Adjuvant radiation plus chemotherapy increases survival.

20. Which of the following statements is true regarding metastatic TCC of the upper urinary tract?

    a. It is not chemosensitive.
    b. It responds to the same chemotherapy as that used for bladder cancer.
    c. It is uniquely sensitive to taxanes.
    d. It is uniquely sensitive to interleukin-2.
    e. It responds best to debulking surgery plus chemotherapy.

21. A 46-year-old man is diagnosed with a 2-cm grade 3 tumor of the left renal pelvis. He is otherwise healthy. Acceptable treatment options include which of the following?

    a. Ureteroscopic ablation of the tumor
    b. Percutaneous resection of the tumor followed by BCG therapy
    c. Laparoscopic nephroureterectomy
    d. Open nephroureterectomy
    e. Both c and d.

22. After a total laparoscopic nephroureterectomy, surveillance of the ipsilateral ureteral orifice is done by which modality?

    a. Interval cystoscopy and ureteroscopy of the stump
    b. Cystoscopy with retrograde pyelography
    c. Cystoscopy and urine cytology
    d. Radiographic imaging with CT
    e. No specific surveillance of the distal ureter required

23. When endoscopic treatment of TCC of the upper urinary tract is used, ureteroscopy is generally preferred for which type of tumors?

    a. Small papillary tumors of the renal pelvis or ureter
    b. Large-volume tumors of the renal pelvis
    c. Small papillary tumors in the upper tracts of patients with previous urinary diversion
    d. Large bulky tumors of the lower pole of the kidney
    e. Large parenchymal invasive tumors of the renal pelvis

24. Which of the following is NOT a distinct advantage of the ureteroscopic approach?

    a. Decreased morbidity rate when compared with percutaneous renal surgery
    b. Maintenance of a closed system without exposure of nonurothelial surfaces to tumor cells
    c. Higher risk of tumor implantation outside the urinary tract
    d. Ease of access to the entire urinary tract without extensive dilatation of the ureteral orifice
    e. Usually can be done on an outpatient basis

25. A 60-year-old man who had undergone prior urinary diversion and a right nephroureterectomy is diagnosed with a grade 1 tumor of the lower pole collecting system of his solitary kidney. What is the optimal approach for this patient?

    a. Ureteroscopy with laser therapy of the lower pole tumor
    b. Nephroureterectomy
    c. Open lower pole partial nephrectomy
    d. Placement of a nephrostomy tube and BCG therapy
    e. Percutaneous access and resection of the lower pole tumor

26. Which of the following statements regarding adjuvant therapy for upper tract TCC is the most accurate?

    a. Adjuvant therapy with BCG has shown a definite advantage with regard to survival and tumor recurrence rates.
    b. Adjuvant therapy with mitomycin has shown a definite improvement with regard to survival and tumor recurrence rates.
    c. Although many studies have shown responses to instillation therapy, no significant improvement in survival or recurrence rate has been demonstrated.

d. The most common complication of instillation therapy is systemic absorption of the agent.
e. Granulomatous disease of the kidney is rare after upper tract BCG therapy.

27. An otherwise healthy 50-year-old man presents with a grade 1 tumor of the intramural ureter. The endoscopic approach or approaches that are acceptable options are which of the following?
   a. Ureteroscopic treatment
   b. Transurethral resection of the ureteral orifice and distal ureter
   c. Percutaneous antegrade ureteroscopy
   d. Placement of a ureteral stent and BCG therapy
   e. Both a and b.

28. Which of the following statements is not true regarding follow-up after treatment of upper urinary tract TCC?
   a. Patients undergoing conservative (organ-sparing) therapy need interval endoscopy of the ipsilateral urinary tract for tumor recurrence.
   b. Follow-up should be identical for all patients regardless of tumor stage or grade.
   c. Efficient and cost-effective follow-up should be based on tumor grade and stage.
   d. Cross-sectional imaging with CT or MRI is necessary with high-grade and high-stage tumors to assess for local recurrence and metastatic spread.
   e. All patients need interval evaluation of the contralateral urinary tract to assess for bilateral disease.

29. A 67-year-old patient with a solitary kidney has a large tumor of the renal pelvis. His urinary cytologic result is negative, and CT shows no evidence of invasive disease. What is the best course of action?
   a. Radical nephroureterectomy and hemodialysis
   b. Single-stage percutaneous access and resection of the entire tumor
   c. Single-stage ureteroscopic treatment of the entire tumor
   d. Endoscopic evaluation and biopsy with continued endoscopic therapy only if the pathologic evaluation shows a low potential for tumor progression
   e. Laparoscopic nephroureterectomy and hemodialysis

30. All of the following statements regarding the percutaneous approach to upper tract TCCs are true except which one?
   a. The nephrostomy tract can be maintained for immediate postoperative surveillance nephroscopy.
   b. Tumor seeding of the nephrostomy tract is a common complication.
   c. Adjuvant therapy with BCG can be given through the established nephrostomy.
   d. The larger endoscopes used for percutaneous removal of TCC allow for tumor staging as well as grading.
   e. Percutaneous tumor resection has a higher morbidity rate when compared with a ureteroscopic approach.

Answers

1. **c. Stage and grade.** Treatment may be based primarily on the risk the tumor poses and the efficacy of specific treatment rather than on other considerations. [p 2845]

2. **d. Dysuria and hematuria.** The common symptoms of localized disease (hematuria and dysuria) and advanced upper tract tumors (weight loss, fatigue, anemia, and bone pain) are similar in type and frequency to those of bladder cancer. [p 2846]

3. **e. None of the above.** Flank pain caused by obstruction by tumor or clot is more prevalent in upper tract tumors, being reported in 10% to 40% of cases. Flank pain in patients with upper tract tumors does not correlate with either locally advanced tumor stage or worse prognosis, as is the case with bladder cancer. [p 2846]

4. **b. A filling defect.** A filling defect is the most common finding on imaging studies. [p 2846]

5. **a. Papillary and invasive.** Approximately 85% of renal pelvis tumors are papillary; the remainder are sessile. In contrast to the majority of bladder tumors' being noninvasive, 50% to 60% of renal pelvis tumors are invasive. [p 2846]

6. **c. low grade and noninvasive.** Although invasion is still more common among ureteral tumors than among bladder tumors, 55% to 75% of ureteral tumors are low grade and low stage. [p 2846]

7. **d. Distal.** Ureteral tumors occur in the distal, middle, or proximal segment in 70%, 25%, and 5% of cases, respectively. [p 2846]

8. **a. Ipsilateral recurrence is common.** After conservative treatment, ipsilateral upper tract tumor recurrence is common in a proximal to distal direction and is seen in 33% to 55% of cases. [p 2846]

9. **b. Multifocal field change.** The high rate of ipsilateral recurrence is due in part to a multifocal field change. [p 2846]

10. **a. Determined mainly by stage.** Tumor multifocality per se does not lessen patient survival independent of stage. [p 2846]

11. **b. Stage.** The single most important determinant of outcome is tumor stage. [p 2847]

12. **e. Para-aortic nodes.** Renal pelvis and upper ureteral tumors spread initially to para-aortic and paracaval nodes, whereas distal ureteral tumors spread to pelvic nodes. [p 2847]

13. **b. Unreliable follow-up.** Reasons to consider nephron sparing include the presence of a tumor in a solitary kidney, synchronous bilateral tumors, or a predisposition to form multiple recurrences, as in endemic Balkan nephropathy. [p 2847]

14. **d. Radical nephroureterectomy.** Radical nephroureterectomy with excision of a bladder cuff is recommended for large, high-grade, invasive tumors of the renal pelvis and proximal ureter. [p 2849]

15. **d. Complete distal ureterectomy with a bladder cuff.** The role of complete distal ureterectomy with excision of a bladder cuff in radical nephroureterectomy for upper tract tumors is well established. The risk of tumor recurrence in a remaining ureteral stump is 30% to 75%. [pp 2849–2850]

16. **b. It is helpful for determining prognosis.** The rationale for continuing regional lymphadenectomy is that it adds little time or morbidity to the surgery, is important for prognosis, and may occasionally have therapeutic value. [p 2851]

17. **a. Segmental ureterectomy.** Segmental ureterectomy and

ureteroureterostomy are indicated for noninvasive grade 1 and 2 tumors of the proximal ureter or midureter that are too large for complete endoscopic ablation, and for grade 3 or invasive tumors when nephron sparing for preservation of renal function is a factor. Repeated endoscopic ablation of the tumor is not categorically incorrect. However, the rapid and large tumor recurrence is a matter of concern and favors segmental ureterectomy. [pp 2855–2856]

18. **b. Ureteropyeloscopy.** Occasionally, one is faced with a patient who has an isolated positive cytologic result from the upper urinary tract. By definition the patient should have negative results from intravenous urography and retrograde pyelography, cystoscopy, and biopsy from the bladder and urethra. Ureteropyeloscopy is indicated in such cases, as the yield for direct visualization of small lesions is superior to that of retrograde pyelography. [pp 2867–2868]

19. **d. Adjuvant radiation does not improve survival.** In one series of patients with tumor stages of T2, T3, or N+, all patients with local relapse also had distant relapse, leading the authors of the report to conclude that adjuvant radiation is not beneficial. Another retrospective review of patients with stage T3 disease with or without adjuvant radiation found that radical nephroureterectomy alone provides a high rate of local control. Adjuvant radiation for high-stage disease does not decrease local relapse or protect against a high rate of distant failure. [p 2870]

20. **b. It responds to the same chemotherapy as that used for bladder cancer.** The systemic chemotherapy regimens offered for treatment of patients with metastatic urothelial tumors of the upper urinary tract are the same as those used for transitional cell carcinoma of the bladder. [pp 2872–2873]

21. **e. Both c and d.** Percutaneous management is acceptable in patients with low-grade (grade 1) disease regardless of the status of the contralateral kidney. Patients with grade 3 disease do poorly regardless of the modality chosen but should probably undergo nephroureterectomy to maximize cancer therapy (provided that they are medically fit). Radical nephroureterectomy with excision of a bladder cuff is recommended for large, high-grade invasive tumors of the renal pelvis and proximal ureter. Nephroureterectomy can be performed either completely laparoscopically or assisted with an open incision in the lower abdomen. The indications for laparoscopic nephroureterectomy are the same as those for open nephroureterectomy. [pp 2849, 2851]

22. **e. No specific surveillance of the distal ureter required.** No surveillance is needed because the ureter has been removed in identical manner to the open surgical counterpart. [p 2850]

23. **a. Small papillary tumors of the renal pelvis or ureter.** The ureteroscopic approach to tumors is generally favored for ureteral and smaller renal tumors. Tumors of the upper urinary tract can be approached in a retrograde or antegrade manner. The approach chosen depends largely on the tumor location and size. In general, a retrograde ureteroscopic approach is used for low-volume ureteral and renal tumors. An antegrade percutaneous approach is preferred for larger tumors of the upper ureter or kidney, or those that cannot be adequately manipulated in a retrograde approach because of location (i.e., lower pole calyx) or previous urinary diversion. [p 2861]

24. **c. Higher risk of tumor implantation outside the urinary tract.** The advantages of a ureteroscopic approach are lower morbidity than the percutaneous and open surgical counterparts and the maintenance of a closed system. With a closed system, nonurothelial surfaces are not exposed to the possibility of tumor seeding. [p 2861]

25. **e. Percutaneous access and resection of the lower pole tumor.** A percutaneous approach may avoid the limitations of flexible ureteroscopy, especially when working in complicated calyceal systems or areas that are difficult to access such as the lower pole calyx or the upper urinary tract of patients with urinary diversion. [p 2865]

26. **c. Although many studies have shown responses to instillation therapy, no significant improvement in survival or recurrence rate has been demonstrated.** Many studies have described small retrospective uncontrolled series of patients undergoing therapy with thiotepa, mitomycin, and BCG. Although the cumulative experience appears encouraging, no individual study has shown statistical improvement with relation to survival and recurrence rates. [p 2869]

27. **e. Both a and b.** When a tumor protrudes from the ureteral orifice, complete ureteroscopic ablation of the tumor or aggressive transurethral resection of the entire most distal ureter can be performed with acceptable results. [pp 2862, 2863]

28. **b. Follow-up should be identical for all patients regardless of tumor stage or grade.** All patients should be assessed at 3-month intervals the first year after they are rendered tumor-free by endoscopic or open surgical approaches. If an organ-sparing approach is chosen, the ipsilateral urinary tract must be assessed as well as the remainder of the urinary tract. The frequency and duration of the follow-up depend largely on the grade and stage of the lesion but are usually every 6 months for several years and then annually. Metastatic restaging is required in all patients at significant risk for disease progression to local or distant sites. This group includes those with high-grade and/or high-stage disease, who should be assessed by use of cross-sectional imaging, chest radiography, liver function tests, and selective use of bone scanning. [pp 2670–2672]

29. **d. Endoscopic evaluation and biopsy with continued endoscopic therapy only if the pathologic evaluation shows a low potential for tumor progression.** Endoscopic management is completed only after the pathologic evaluation shows that the patient is an acceptable candidate for continued minimally invasive endoscopic management. If the tumor is high grade or invasive, the patient should proceed to nephroureterectomy and dialysis, provided that he or she is medically fit. [pp 2849, 2851, 2861]

30. **b. Tumor seeding of the nephrostomy tract is a common complication.** A major concern of the percutaneous approach is potential seeding of nonurothelial surfaces with tumor cells. Although there have been several reported cases of nephrostomy tract infiltration with high-grade tumors, there were no reported occurrences in the three largest series. Tract seeding is a possibility but appears to be an uncommon event. [p 2866]

Chapter 81

Neoplasms of the Testis

Jerome P. Richie • Graeme S. Steele

Questions

1. A young adult man presents with a right testicular mass after having undergone bilateral orchiopexy as a child. He undergoes right inguinal orchiectomy and left testis biopsy. The testicular mass is a mixed nonseminomatous germ cell tumor (NSGCT) containing embryonal carcinoma with vascular invasion—clinical stage T2N0M0 (chest radiograph and abdominal CT scan were normal). Biopsy of the left testis reveals intratubular germ cell neoplasia (carcinoma in situ [CIS]). Appropriate management of this patient includes which of the following?

    a. Three cycles of chemotherapy (BEP) and left radical inguinal orchiectomy
    b. Four cycles of chemotherapy (EP) with another transscrotal biopsy of the left testis in 6 months
    c. Left radical inguinal orchiectomy, androgen replacement therapy, and surveillance protocol for mixed germ cell tumors
    d. Modified (template) right-sided retroperitoneal lymph node dissection (RPLND)
    e. Modified (template) right-sided RPLND with low-dose external beam radiotherapy to the left testis

2. A young adult man presents with a 7-cm left testis tumor; the serum α-fetoprotein (AFP) value is elevated (220 ng/ml); the clinical stage of disease is T2N1M0S1. He undergoes radical inguinal orchiectomy. Pathologic study reveals an anaplastic seminoma with vascular invasion. The serum AFP value normalizes after orchiectomy. Further management of this patient should include which of the following?

    a. Low-dose external beam radiotherapy to abdominal and pelvic lymph nodes
    b. Low-dose external beam radiotherapy to abdominal, pelvic, and mediastinal lymph nodes
    c. Bilateral RPLND with adjuvant radiotherapy
    d. Bilateral RPLND
    e. Two cycles of chemotherapy (BEP)

3. A young adult man who lost his right testis at a young age because of torsion undergoes left radical inguinal orchiectomy for a testis tumor. Pathology reports a 3-cm mixed NSGCT, no vascular invasion, and embryonal component 10%. Serum tumor markers reveal persistently elevated β-human chorionic gonadotropin (βHCG) levels. The clinical stage is T1N0M0. What is the best management of this tumor?

    a. Adjuvant cisplatin-based chemotherapy
    b. Bilateral RPLND with excision of the left spermatic cord
    c. Modified left RPLND with excision of both right and left spermatic cords
    d. Androgen replacement therapy and surveillance protocol for germ cell tumor if the serum βHCG level normalizes
    e. Androgen replacement therapy and low-dose external beam radiotherapy to abdominal and pelvic lymph nodes

4. A 40-year-old man undergoes bilateral RPLND for clinical stage IIB mixed NSGCT. With respect to adjuvant therapy in this setting, cisplatin-based chemotherapy should be administered to which group of patients?

    a. All patients regardless of the pathologic stage of disease
    b. Only those patients with tumor recurrence outside of the retroperitoneum
    c. Patients with microscopic evidence of disease in two lymph nodes
    d. Patients with more than six positive lymph nodes
    e. Any patient with a single involved retroperitoneal lymph node measuring 1 cm in diameter

5. A patient presents with a 6-cm right-sided testis tumor and abdominal discomfort. He undergoes right radical inguinal orchiectomy; pathologic study reveals mixed germ cell tumor. Serum tumor markers are elevated (AFP, 800 ng/ml; βHCG, 2500 mIU/ml). An abdominal CT scan reveals a 10-cm retroperitoneal mass. The patient undergoes cisplatin-based chemotherapy with resultant 75% resolution of the retroperitoneal mass and normalization of serum tumor markers. What is the best management at this stage?

    a. Observation with physical examinations every 4 months, serum tumor markers, chest radiograph, and abdominal CT scan
    b. Fine-needle aspiration of the residual retroperitoneal mass followed by salvage radiotherapy for persistent germ cell tumor
    c. Abdominal exploration, tumorectomy, and bilateral RPLND
    d. Abdominal exploration and tumorectomy
    e. Ifosfamide-based salvage chemotherapy

6. A young adult man undergoes cisplatin-based chemotherapy for a mixed germ cell tumor, with complete response. Two years later, he presents with shortness of breath; recurrent disease is detected in both the retroperitoneum and the mediastinum. He then undergoes high-dose cisplatin-based chemotherapy with 80% resolution of all disease. Abdominal and thoracic exploration is planned. Which of the following statements is correct?

    a. The incidence of viable tumor in a partially resolved mass after salvage chemotherapy is lower than it is after primary adjuvant chemotherapy.
    b. During abdominal exploration, frozen section analysis of the residual mass detects only fibrous tissue and necrosis; thoracic exploration can therefore safely be omitted.
    c. Laparoscopic surgery in this scenario has clearly been shown to be of both diagnostic and therapeutic benefit.
    d. External beam radiotherapy is appropriate after surgical exploration if teratoma is detected.
    e. Neither abdominal nor thoracic exploration is warranted in this patient.

7. A 45-year-old man is found to have a well-delineated 4-cm retroperitoneal mass after cisplatin-based chemotherapy for clinical stage III seminoma. Which of the following statements is correct?

    a. This mass is likely unresectable and therefore best left alone.
    b. Only diffuse desmoplastic retroperitoneal masses should be resected after chemotherapy in patients with advanced seminoma.
    c. Salvage chemotherapy is the best option at this stage.
    d. Surgical resection with bilateral RPLND is the best management at this stage.
    e. There is no possibility that this mass contains embryonal carcinoma.

8. A 72-year-old man with benign prostatic hyperplasia and bothersome symptoms of bladder outlet obstruction presents with a 6-cm painless right-sided testicular mass with an associated hydrocele confirmed by scrotal ultrasonography. Which of the following statements is true?

    a. This mass is likely a spermatocytic seminoma and should therefore be left well alone.
    b. The hydrocele should be aspirated and sclerosed with tetracycline and the fluid sent for cytologic study.
    c. Radical inguinal orchiectomy is indicated to exclude the possibility of a hematologic malignancy.
    d. The testicular mass is most likely metastatic disease from either lung or prostate tumor.
    e. Despite the ultrasonographic findings, chronic epididymitis is the most likely cause of this clinical picture.

9. A young adult man presents with a 7-cm right testicular tumor that is found to be invading the scrotal wall and epididymis on that side. Possible sites of lymph node involvement in this patient include which of the following?

    a. Inguinal lymph nodes
    b. Pelvic lymph nodes
    c. Interaortocaval lymph nodes
    d. Left para-aortic lymph nodes
    e. All of the above

10. The incidence of syncytiotrophoblastic elements in seminoma corresponds to which of the following?

    a. The degree of tumor anaplasia
    b. βHCG production
    c. The presence of testicular lymphoma
    d. The presence and extent of retroperitoneal metastases
    e. AFP production by the tumor

11. With respect to anaplastic seminoma, which of the following statements is false?

    a. Morphologically, histiocytic lymphoma and embryonal carcinoma may closely resemble anaplastic seminoma.
    b. Anaplastic seminomas are more aggressive than spermatocytic seminomas.
    c. Anaplastic seminomas have an increased rate of metastatic spread compared with classic seminomas.
    d. Anaplastic seminomas are more likely to elaborate βHCG than are classic seminomas.
    e. Anaplastic seminomas have greater mitotic activity than do spermatocytic seminomas.

12. With respect to choriocarcinoma, which of the following statements is false?

    a. Patients with pure choriocarcinoma may present with evidence of advanced distant metastasis.
    b. Choriocarcinoma may be associated with very elevated serum βHCG values.
    c. Choriocarcinomas are best managed by RPLND.
    d. Choriocarcinomas occur in a younger adult age group.
    e. Choriocarcinomas rarely occur in African males.

13. Which of the following choices regarding mixed germ cell tumors is correct?

    a. Mixed germ cell tumors represent approximately 15% of NSGCTs.
    b. The most frequent combination is seminoma and embryonal cell carcinoma.
    c. Mixed germ cell tumors represent approximately 15% of germ cell tumors.
    d. Mixed germ cell tumors can sometimes be classified as seminomas.
    e. The most frequent combination is embryonal carcinoma, yolk sac tumor, teratoma, and syncytiotrophoblasts.

14. Which of the following choices regarding CIS (intratubular germ cell neoplasia) of the testis is false?

    a. The incidence of CIS in the male population is 0.8%.
    b. The prevalence of CIS in the contralateral testis in a patient with a germ cell tumor is 5%.
    c. Testicular CIS develops from fetal gonocytes.
    d. Tumor markers for CIS have not been described.
    e. CIS is not evenly distributed throughout the testis, making diagnosis with a single biopsy difficult.

15. With respect to the epidemiology of testicular tumors, which of the following statements is false?

    a. The age-adjusted incidence in Denmark rose from 3.4 to 6.4 per 100,000 between 1945 and 1970.
    b. Overall, the highest incidence is noted in young adults, which makes these neoplasms the most common solid tumors of men between 20 and 34 years of age.
    c. Spermatocytic seminoma occurs most often in patients between the ages of 45 and 55 years.
    d. The incidence of testicular tumors in black African men is higher than that among African-American men.
    e. Approximately 2% to 3% of testicular tumors are bilateral.

16. With respect to the lymphatic drainage of the testis, which one of the following statements is correct?

    a. The primary drainage of the right testis is usually located within the group of lymph nodes in the left para-aortic region.
    b. The spermatic cord contains four to eight lymphatic channels that traverse the inguinal canal and peritoneal space.
    c. The spermatic vessels cross dorsal to the ureter, whereas the testicular lymphatics cross ventrally.
    d. Lymphatic drainage has been shown to cross over from right to left, and therefore cross-metastases occur more commonly in patients with right-sided tumors.
    e. Suprahilar lymph node spread is invariable in stage N1 disease.

17. What is the most common clinical symptom or sign in a young adult man with a germ cell tumor of the testis?

    a. Testicular pain
    b. Testicular swelling on the side of the tumor
    c. Reactive hydrocele, which transilluminates in a darkened room
    d. Bilateral gynecomastia
    e. Chronic cough with hemoptysis

18. With respect to ultrasonography of the testis, which of the following statements is incorrect?

    a. Any hypoechoic area within the tunica albuginea is markedly suspicious for testicular cancer.

b. Ultrasonography avoids the delay in diagnosis previously attributed to confusion with epididymitis.
c. Intrascrotal fluid collections make adequate visualization of the testis impossible.
d. In patients with palpably normal genitalia and evidence of extragonadal germ cell malignancy, sonography has been reported to be successful in identifying occult testicular neoplasms.
e. Trans-scrotal ultrasonography has the ability to detect testicular microlithiasis.

19. With respect to clinical staging of germ cell tumors of the testis, which of the following statements is incorrect?

    a. Modern staging techniques have reduced the false-negative staging error in clinical stage T1N0M0 to approximately 20%.
    b. Approximately 10% to 15% of patients with clinical stage T1N0M0 seminoma harbor occult retroperitoneal metastases.
    c. In general, 5% of patients with clinical stage I germ cell tumors harbor occult disease in extranodal sites.
    d. Abdominal and pelvic MRI scans have a significant advantage over CT scans with respect to diagnosing micrometastatic disease.
    e. Spermatic cord involvement increases the likelihood of metastatic disease.

20. Which of the following statements concerning tumor markers in germ cell tumors is incorrect?

    a. Serum AFP elevations do not occur in pure seminomas.
    b. The metabolic half-life of AFP is between 5 and 7 days.
    c. Syncytiotrophoblastic cells are responsible for the production of βHCG.
    d. Approximately 5% to 10% of seminoma patients have detectable levels of βHCG.
    e. Placental alkaline phosphatase (PLAP) is elevated in 40% of patients with testicular CIS.

21. What percentage of patients with advanced NSGCTs have normal tumor markers?

    a. 2%
    b. 5%
    c. 10%
    d. 20%
    e. 30%

22. Approximately what percentage of patients presenting with seminoma have disease confined to the testis?

    a. 35%
    b. 55%
    c. 75%
    d. 95%
    e. 99%

23. The overall cure rate for all stages of seminoma approximates what percentage?

    a. 50%
    b. 60%
    c. 70%
    d. 80%
    e. 90%

24. Management options for clinical stage I seminoma after radical inguinal orchiectomy include all of the following except which one?

    a. Surveillance protocol
    b. Para-aortic and pelvic radiotherapy
    c. Modified RPLND
    d. Single-agent chemotherapy
    e. Para-aortic radiotherapy

25. Reliable prognostic factors for pure seminoma include all the following except which one?

    a. Tumor size
    b. Lymphatic invasion
    c. Serum βHCG level
    d. The patient's age
    e. Vascular invasion

26. The 5-year disease-free survival rate for patients with clinical stage T1N2M0 seminoma approximates what percentage?

    a. 50%
    b. 60%
    c. 70%
    d. 80%
    e. 90%

27. Approximately what percentage of patients with clinical stage T1N3M0 seminoma treated with radiotherapy alone will develop metastatic disease?

    a. 50%
    b. 60%
    c. 70%
    d. 80%
    e. 90%

28. In patients with pure seminoma, combination cisplatin-based chemotherapy is most appropriate treatment for which of the following clinical stages?

    a. T1N0M0
    b. T2N0M0
    c. T1N2M0
    d. T1N3M0
    e. T2N1M0

29. In NSGCTs, all the following prognostic factors are used to determine risk of metastatic disease except which one?

    a. T stage
    b. Embryonal cell carcinoma (>40%)
    c. Teratoma (>50%)
    d. Vascular invasion
    e. Absence of yolk sac elements

30. Surveillance in low-risk (absence of prognostic factors) NSGCT is appropriate in all of the following patients except which one?

    a. A motivated and reliable patient
    b. A patient with an allergy to radiographic contrast agents
    c. A diabetic patient
    d. A patient in whom tumor markers persist after orchiectomy
    e. A patient who underwent scrotal orchiectomy

31. A young adult male with clinical stage T1N2M0 NSGCT undergoes induction chemotherapy with near resolution of a 5-cm left para-aortic mass. At this stage, what is the appropriate management?

    a. Salvage chemotherapy
    b. Tumorectomy and bilateral RPLND
    c. Modified RPLND
    d. Radiotherapy
    e. Surveillance

32. What is the incidence of viable germ cell elements in resected specimens after primary chemotherapy for NSGCT?

    a. 0% to 9%
    b. 10% to 19%

c. 20% to 29%
d. 30% to 39%
e. 40% to 49%

33. The most common sites of origin of extragonadal tumors are all of the following except which one?

    a. Mediastinum
    b. Retroperitoneum
    c. Sacrococcygeal region
    d. Liver
    e. Pineal gland

34. With respect to Leydig cell tumors, all the following statements are correct except which one?

    a. Approximately 10% are benign.
    b. Undescended testis is an important predisposing factor.
    c. Characteristic intracytoplasmic inclusion bodies (Reinke crystals) are often seen.
    d. There are no consistent reliable histologic features of malignancy.
    e. The clinical presentation may be confused with virilizing type of adrenogenital syndrome.

35. Which of the following statements regarding patterns of spread of germ cell tumors is false?

    a. The primary drainage of the right testis is usually located within the group of lymph nodes in the interaortocaval region at the level of the second vertebral body.
    b. Lymphatic drainage has not been shown to cross over from right to left.
    c. Suprahilar lymph node spread has been shown to be rare in stage N1 disease.
    d. Lymphatics of the epididymis drain primarily into the obturator lymph nodes.
    e. The distant failure rate despite surgical excision of negative retroperitoneal lymph nodes is approximately 5%.

36. Modified RPLND preserves fertility in most patients by sparing which of the following structures?

    a. Internal iliac arteries
    b. Genitofemoral nerve
    c. Postganglionic sympathetic nerve fibers
    d. Seminal vesicles
    e. Pelvic parasympathetic plexus

37. With respect to the International Germ Cell Classification of advanced disease, which of the following statements is false?

    a. The response of poor-risk disease to chemotherapy is approximately 50%.
    b. The response of good-risk disease to chemotherapy is approximately 90%.
    c. Pretreatment tumor markers are an integral part of this classification.
    d. Pretreatment pulmonary metastases are an integral part of this classification.
    e. Early use of chemotherapy in poor-risk disease is advisable.

Answers

1. **d. Modified (template) right-sided retroperitoneal lymph node dissection (RPLND).** The management of testicular CIS depends on a variety of factors such as patient age, whether the patient has bilateral or unilateral CIS, associated testicular atrophy, and the philosophy of the treating physician. In germ cell tumors, CIS of the contralateral testis is present in 5% of patients and with time probably evolves into invasive cancer in the majority of these patients. Although CIS can easily be cured by radiation therapy, this therapy may have undesirable side effects on both fertility and androgen production. Furthermore, the incidence of CIS in the general population is low and therefore screening programs are generally not recommended. [p 2880]

2. **d. Bilateral RPLND.** The potential advantages of RPLND in the treatment of testis cancer stem from the fact that retroperitoneal deposits are usually the first and frequently the sole evidence of extragonadal spread. Such therapy is capable of eradicating resectable disease in the majority of patients with stage N1-2 tumors. Thorough excision of the retroperitoneal lymph nodes therefore remains the epitome or gold standard of staging. Although noninvasive staging techniques are somewhat accurate, 20% to 25% of patients with clinical stage T1-3N0M0 disease are understaged by all available modalities of nonsurgical staging. The cure rate for patients with pathologically confirmed stage I disease is roughly 95% with surgery alone. The 5% to 10% of patients who may relapse after negative RPLND for low-stage disease have a high cure rate with chemotherapy. [pp 2894, 2896]

3. **d. Androgen replacement therapy and surveillance protocol for germ cell tumor if the serum βHCG level normalizes.** There are nonmalignant causes of persistent elevated levels of both AFP and βHCG. Liver damage secondary to drugs (chemotherapy, anesthetics, or antiepileptics), viral hepatitis, and alcohol abuse may all lead to an elevated AFP level. Furthermore, nonmalignant causes of persistent βHCG elevations include hypogonadism and marijuana use. Clearly, every effort should be made to exclude all false-positive causes of tumor marker elevation before subjecting patients to adjuvant therapy. [p 2889]

4. **d. Patients with more than six positive lymph nodes.** In a review of 39 patients who underwent RPLND at the Brigham and Women's Hospital for pathologic stage T1-3N1-2M0 disease, with fewer than six positive nodes and no node larger than 2 cm, only 3 of 39 patients relapsed at a median follow-up of 3.5 years. Thus, for patients with minimal retroperitoneal disease, resected completely, careful follow-up is recommended. For patients with more extensive disease, adjuvant chemotherapy with two cycles can be initiated relatively shortly after RPLND and almost always prevents relapse. [p 2900]

5. **c. Abdominal exploration, tumorectomy, and bilateral RPLND.** RPLND after chemotherapy involves both resection of residual disease and full bilateral node dissection. In the best of hands, this procedure is associated with an 18% complication rate, which is contributed to by both the technically demanding nature of the surgery and other factors such as reduced pulmonary reserve due to bleomycin. [p 2903]

6. **b. During abdominal exploration, frozen section analysis of the residual mass detects only fibrous tissue and necrosis; thoracic exploration can therefore safely be omitted.** Herr showed that, at the time of RPLND, if frozen section analysis shows only necrosis, then surgical resection of

residual masses followed by only limited RPLND is safe, as opposed to residual mass resection and complete RPLND, which is considered the standard of care. In addition, the histologic finding of necrosis plus fibrosis was shown to be strongly predictive of necrosis-fibrosis in patients with concomitant pulmonary disease; this information can then be used to avoid thoracic exploration in some patients. [p 2903]

7. **d. Surgical resection with bilateral RPLND is the best management at this stage.** Residual disease may be well delineated and distinct from surrounding structures and thus usually resectable. According to the Memorial Sloan-Kettering group, surgery is justifiable in this setting because these masses often represent residual seminoma. [p 2894]

8. **c. Radical inguinal orchiectomy is indicated to exclude the possibility of a hematologic malignancy.** Accounting for about 5% of all testis tumors, lymphomas constitute the most common secondary neoplasms of the testis and the most frequent of all testis tumors in patients older than 50 years of age. The median age at occurrence is approximately 60 years. Primary lymphoma of the testis may occur in children; eight cases in patients ranging from 2 to 12 years of age were reviewed in one study. [p 2909]

9. **e. All of the above.** Involvement of the epididymis or cord may lead to pelvic and inguinal lymph node metastasis, whereas tumors confined to the testis proper usually spread to retroperitoneal nodes. [p 2882]

10. **b. βHCG production.** Syncytiotrophoblastic elements occur in 10% to 15% of seminomas, and lymphocytic infiltration in approximately 20%. The incidence of syncytiotrophoblastic elements corresponds to the frequency of βHCG production. [p 2878]

11. **a. Morphologically, histiocytic lymphoma and embryonal carcinoma may closely resemble anaplastic seminoma.** Morphologically, histiocytic lymphoma, and embryonal carcinoma may closely resemble anaplastic seminoma. [p 2878]

12. **c. Choriocarcinomas are best managed by RPLND.** Choriocarcinoma may occur as a palpable nodule, the size depending on the extent of local hemorrhage. Patients with pure choriocarcinoma may present with evidence of advanced distant metastasis and what seems a paradoxically small intratesticular lesion that may not distort the normal testicular size or shape. [p 2878]

13. **e. The most frequent combination is embryonal carcinoma, yolk sac tumor, teratoma, and syncytiotrophoblasts.** In classifying more than 6000 testis tumors, one study found that in roughly 60%, more than one histologic pattern was identified. The most frequent combination is embryonal carcinoma, yolk sac tumor, teratoma, and syncytiotrophoblasts. [p 2879]

14. **e. CIS is not evenly distributed throughout the testis, making diagnosis with a single biopsy difficult.** CIS is usually evenly distributed throughout the testis; therefore, open surgical biopsy (3 × 3 × 3 mm) will generally be positive in cases in which CIS exists. [p 2880]

15. **d. The incidence of testicular tumors in black African men is higher than that among African-American men.** Variable incidence rates are noted between different ethnic groups within a given geographic region. The incidence of testicular tumors in American black men is approximately one third that in American whites but 10 times that in African black men. [p 2881]

16. **d. Lymphatic drainage has been shown to cross over from right to left, and therefore cross-metastases occur more commonly in patients with right-sided tumors.** Cross-metastases were reported to occur more commonly in patients with right-sided tumors, because of lymphatic drainage from right to left. These observations obviously have important implications for the surgical management of testis cancer. [p 2883]

17. **b. Testicular swelling on the side of the tumor.** The usual presentation of a testicular tumor is a nodule or painless swelling of one gonad. This may be noted incidentally by the patient or by his sexual partner. The classic description is that of a lump, swelling, or hardness of the testis. Approximately 30% to 40% of patients may complain of a dull ache or a heavy sensation in the lower abdomen, anal area, or scrotum. In approximately 10% of patients, acute pain is the presenting symptom. Occasionally, patients with a previously small atrophic testis note enlargement. On rare occasions, infertility may be the presenting complaint. Acute onset of pain is rare unless there is associated epididymitis or bleeding within the tumor. [p 2884]

18. **c. Intrascrotal fluid collections make adequate visualization of the testis impossible.** Ultrasonography of the scrotum is basically an extension of the physical examination. Any hypoechoic area within the tunica albuginea is markedly suspicious for testicular cancer. With the advent of scrotal ultrasonography and its general availability throughout the United States, the delay in diagnosis from confusion with epididymitis should be markedly reduced. Intrascrotal fluid collections are no barrier to the examination of the underlying testicular parenchyma by ultrasonography. In patients with palpably normal genitalia and evidence of extragonadal germ cell malignancy, sonography has been reported to be successful in identifying occult testicular neoplasms. [p 2884]

19. **d. Abdominal and pelvic MRI scans have a significant advantage over CT scans with respect to diagnosing micrometastatic disease.** MRI offers no advantage over CT for imaging and staging the retroperitoneum in patients with testis cancer. [p 2887]

20. **e. Placental alkaline phosphatase (PLAP) is elevated in 40% of patients with testicular CIS.** Small studies using enzyme-linked immunoabsorbent assays indicate that as many as 40% of patients with advanced disease have elevated levels of PLAP. [p 2888]

21. **c. 10%.** The overall sensitivity of any test or marker varies with the amount of tumor burden. Determinations of AFP and HCG, in concert with other staging modalities, have helped reduce the understaging error in germ cell tumors to a level of 10% to 15%. Expressed another way, approximately 10% to 15% of patients with nonseminomatous germ cell tumors can be expected to have normal marker levels even at advanced stages of disease. [p 2888]

22. **c. 75%.** Seminomas account for 30% to 60% of all germ cell tumors of the testis, depending on the hospital population from which the statistics are being reported. Approximately 75% of seminomas are confined to the testis at the time of clinical presentation. Between 10% and 15% of patients harbor metastatic disease in regional retroperitoneal lymph nodes, and no more than 5% to 10% have advanced to juxtaregional lymph node or visceral metastases, which represents a smaller percentage than among patients with NSGCTs, in whom the incidence of occult metastatic retroperitoneal disease is significantly higher. [p 2890]

23. **e. 90%.** The established treatment for low-stage seminoma has been inguinal orchiectomy followed by therapeutic or adjuvant radiation therapy (see Fig. 81–1). This treatment represents a highly effective method of treating low-stage

disease with minimal morbidity; with the advent of multidrug chemotherapy for cure of patients with more disseminated disease, the overall cure rate for all stages exceeds 90%. [p 2890]

24. **c. modified RPLND.** In patients with clinically localized disease, treatment options after orchiectomy include adjuvant radiation therapy to retroperitoneal lymph nodes, single-agent chemotherapy, and surveillance. Currently, adjuvant radiotherapy remains the treatment of choice; however, the success of surveillance protocols for low-stage NSGCT has encouraged the use of surveillance protocols in stage I seminoma patients as well. [p 2890]

25. **d. The patient's age.** The surveillance series with the most data on recurrence after surgery is the nationwide Danish study involving 261 patients. Univariate analysis showed tumor size, histologic subtype, presence of necrosis, and invasion of rete testis to be predictive of recurrence, but only tumor size was a statistically significant predictor on multivariate analysis. The 4-year relapse-free survival rate was 6% for tumors smaller than 3 cm, 18% for tumors 3 to 6 cm, and 36% for tumors larger than 6 cm. In this study, tumors larger than 6 cm accounted for approximately 25% of the study population. Other studies have reported that vascular invasion increases the risk for failure in stage I seminoma patients. Therefore, although reliable prognostic factors for seminoma have not been developed, it seems appropriate for patients with tumors smaller than 6 cm in diameter, absence of vascular invasion, and normal βHCG levels to be given the option of surveillance. [p 2892]

26. **e. 90%.** Patients with stage II (N1) disease have enjoyed survival rates above 90%, which statistically does not differ from the rates for patients with stage I disease. [p 2893]

27. **a. 50%.** For patients with stage II (N3) disease treated by radiation therapy alone, approximately one half of patients develop metastatic disease outside the treated fields. One study reported an 11% versus 56% relapse rate when comparing patients with N1-2 and N3 disease who received adjuvant irradiation in a nonrandomized trial. [p 2893]

28. **d. T1N3M0.** Seminoma patients with bulky retroperitoneal disease have traditionally received adjuvant irradiation. More recently, however, adjuvant chemotherapy has been preferred to retroperitoneal irradiation for retroperitoneal tumors greater than 5 cm in diameter. At Brigham and Women's Hospital and Dana Farber Cancer Institute, patients with N1 and N2 disease receive 30 and 35 Gy of radiation, respectively, whereas patients with N3 disease are treated with primary cisplatin-based chemotherapy. [p 2893]

29. **c. Teratoma (>50%).** Six factors have been analyzed in many of these studies and include stage of the primary tumor (pT $\leq$ 2); vascular (including lymphatic) invasion; presence of embryonal carcinoma; absence of yolk sac elements; and elevated preorchiectomy markers. In the Medical Research Council series, four features were independently predictive of relapse: invasion of testicular veins or lymphatics, absence of yolk sac elements, and presence of embryonal cell carcinoma. Of the 259 patients, 55 patients had three or four factors and a relapse rate of 58%; 89 patients had two factors and a relapse rate of 24%; 81 patients had one factor and a relapse rate of 10%; and 8 patients had no factors and no relapses. [pp 2897–2898]

30. **d. A patient in whom tumor markers persist after orchiectomy.** Surveillance is appropriate only for patients with clinical stage T1-3N0M0 disease, without any risk factors for relapse, who are motivated to rigidly adhere to a surveillance protocol and who fully understand the risks of failure to comply with the follow-up schedule. These patients require meticulous evaluation before entering a well-designed and well-managed surveillance protocol. Tumor staging should be carried out compulsively in this selected group of patients with no evidence of suspicious nodes or pulmonary masses. [p 2899]

31. **b. Tumorectomy and bilateral RPLND.** The recognition of teratoma within surgically excised residual masses after combination chemotherapy for advanced disease is a relatively recent phenomenon. The rationale to resect residual teratoma is multifactorial. Indolent teratoma growth known as the growing teratoma syndrome may compromise vital organ function; malignant transformation of mature teratoma to sarcoma and adenocarcinoma, which is resistant to chemotherapy, has been well described; chemotherapy and radiotherapy are relatively ineffective against benign or malignant teratoma; and expansion of benign solid and cystic teratomatous elements may compromise vital organ function. [p 2903]

32. **b. 10% to 20%.** Early retrospective studies revealed that RPLND defines three subsets of patients based on histopathologic analysis of the resected specimen: 40%, necrosis/fibrosis; 40%, adult teratoma; 20%, residual NSGCT. Therefore, approximately 60% of patients with evidence of a residual mass on postchemotherapy imaging studies will have either viable cancer or teratoma. More recently, however, the Memorial Sloan-Kettering group reported that the likelihood of malignancy in postchemotherapy resected tumor was 13%, with the remainder of tumor specimens containing teratoma or necrosis. In addition, the Indiana group reported that of 417 patients who underwent postchemotherapy RPLND for residual disease, only 10% were found to have viable germ cell tumor in their pathologic specimens. [p 2903]

33. **d. Liver.** The most common sites of origin are, in decreasing order of frequency, the mediastinum, retroperitoneum, sacrococcygeal region, and pineal gland, although many unusual sources have also been reported. [p 2904]

34. **b. Undescended testis is an important predisposing factor.** The etiology of Leydig cell tumors is unknown. In contrast to germ cell tumors, there appears to be no association with cryptorchidism. The experimental production of Leydig cell tumors in mice after chronic estrogen administration or after intrasplenic testicular autografting is consistent with a hormonal basis. The lesions are generally small, yellow to brown, and well circumscribed and rarely exhibit hemorrhage or necrosis. Microscopically, the tumors consist of relatively uniform, polyhedral, closely packed cells with round, slightly eccentric nuclei and eosinophilic granular cytoplasm with lipid vacuoles, brownish pigmentation, and occasional characteristic inclusions known as Reinke crystals. Pleomorphism with large and bizarre cell forms may occur, and mitotic figures may or may not be identified. None of these features appears to be consistently related to malignant potential. Virilizing types of congenital adrenocortical hyperplasia may also produce the endocrine signs and symptoms of interstitial cell tumors, so differential tests must be carried out to clarify the diagnosis. [pp 2905–2906]

35. **b. Lymphatic drainage has not been shown to cross over from right to left.** Lymphatics of the epididymis drain into the external iliac chain, affording locally extensive testicular tumors access to pelvic lymph nodes. Inguinal node metastasis may result from scrotal involvement by the primary tumor, prior inguinal or scrotal surgery, or retrograde lymphatic spread secondary to massive retroperitoneal lymph node deposits. [p 2883]

36. **c. Postganglionic sympathetic nerve fibers.** Modified (tem-

plate) RPLND has significant advantages. By use of this technique, a complete dissection can be performed in the area most likely to be involved with retroperitoneal nodal disease, yet modification in a less likely area can spare some of the ejaculatory consequences. Two studies reported excellent return of ejaculation with nerve-sparing RPLND. These techniques involve removal of nodal-bearing tissue from around the postganglionic fibers, are somewhat more time-consuming, and may require a steeper learning curve as well. Nonetheless, ejaculation can be preserved in 100% of patients and fertility noted in 75% of patients undergoing this procedure. [p 2896]

37. **d. Pretreatment pulmonary metastases are an integral part of this classification.** In 1997, an international consensus was convened to address the multiplicity of prognostic systems. As a result of this meeting, a new prognostic classification was published: the International Germ Cell Consensus Classification (see Table 81–13). This validated model facilitates collaboration of clinical trials as well as providing a means of comparison of clinical results across studies. This collaboration provided agreement on the use of pretreatment serum tumor marker levels (AFP, βHCG, and lactate dehydrogenase) and metastases to organs other than the lung as poor-risk prognostic factors. The classification contains three subclassifications of good-, intermediate-, and poor-prognosis disease, but for clinical purposes patients are classified as having either good-risk (good and intermediate prognosis) disease or poor-risk (poor prognosis) disease. Chemotherapy is tailored according to this classification. For those patients predicted to have a more favorable outcome (i.e., good risk), the goals have been to maintain high cure rates while reducing treatment-related toxicity. Patients with minimal or moderate disease do well with standard chemotherapy, with response rates in the 91% to 95% category. Patients with advanced disease, however, had only a 53% therapeutic response. Therefore, more aggressive chemotherapy should be used in patients with advanced extent disease according to this category. [pp 2901–2902]

Chapter 82

Surgery of Testicular Tumors

Joel Sheinfeld • James McKiernan • George J. Bosl

Questions

1. A 23-year-old male patient presents after undergoing transscrotal orchiectomy after presumed hydrocele surgery. Pathologic studies reveal embryonal carcinoma with vascular invasion. Serum tumor markers and results of the physical examination and CT of the chest, abdomen, and pelvis are normal. Which of the following is appropriate?
   a. Observation
   b. Retroperitoneal lymph node dissection (RPLND)
   c. RPLND plus excision of the scrotal scar
   d. RPLND plus scrotectomy and inguinal lymph node dissection
   e. RPLND plus scrotal and inguinal radiation

2. A 23-year-old male patient undergoes right orchiectomy for seminoma and chemotherapy for a 10-cm retroperitoneal mass. His tumor markers are normal both before and after treatment. Following treatment, his mass measures 5 cm. Which of the following statements is true?
   a. Residual retroperitoneal disease can usually be resected completely.
   b. The probability of viable disease in the retroperitoneum is approximately 25%.
   c. Postchemotherapy RPLND is associated with low rate of morbidity.
   d. Postchemotherapy radiation is warranted.
   e. Percutaneous biopsy is accurate.

3. Which of the following statements is true regarding testicular anatomy?
   a. The right testicular vein drains to the right renal vein.
   b. The left testicular artery arises from the left renal artery.
   c. The left testis lymphatic drainage is to the interaortocaval and paracaval nodes.
   d. The right testis lymphatic drainage is to paracaval, interaortocaval, and para-aortic nodes.
   e. The right testicular artery arises from the right renal artery.

4. A 19-year-old male patient presents after undergoing four cycles of etoposide and platinum chemotherapy for a nonseminomatous germ cell tumor (NSGCT) diagnosed by needle biopsy of a left 5-cm para-aortic mass. The left testis, which before treatment had a 2-cm mass, is now without any abnormality on a sonogram and by physical examination, and the patient's tumor markers are normal. Which of the following is appropriate treatment of this patient's testicles?
   a. Observation
   b. Radiation
   c. Left radical inguinal orchiectomy
   d. Testes biopsy and orchiectomy if viable disease remains
   e. Bilateral orchiectomy

5. Which of the following is the most common site for late recurrence of NSGCT?
   a. Retroperitoneum
   b. Lung
   c. Liver
   d. Brain
   e. Mediastinum

6. Which of the following associations is correct when describing the events of ejaculation?
   a. Lumbar sympathetics and bulbourethral muscle contraction
   b. Bladder neck contraction and pudendal somatic nerves
   c. Sympathetic fibers and bladder neck contraction

d. Pelvic parasympathetics and emission
e. Lumbar sympathetics and erection

7. During postchemotherapy RPLND, each of the following structures can be ligated without attendant morbidity except which one?

   a. Inferior mesenteric vein
   b. Inferior mesenteric artery
   c. Right and left testicular arteries
   d. Right renal vein
   e. Lumbar arteries

8. Which of the following is NOT true regarding laparoscopic RPLND?

   a. It is feasible when performed by experienced laparoscopists.
   b. It has well-established therapeutic efficacy.
   c. It is associated with shorter recovery times than open RPLND.
   d. It has fewer postoperative analgesic requirements than open RPLND.
   e. It is associated with lower rate of morbidity in the primary setting than following chemotherapy.

9. A 23-year-old male patient undergoes right orchiectomy for a mixed NSGCT without vascular invasion. Results of the physical examination and CT of the chest, abdomen, and pelvis are normal, and the patient's preoperative beta human chorionic gonadotropin level is elevated and remains elevated after orchiectomy. Which of the following treatments is the most appropriate?

   a. Surveillance
   b. Two cycles of platinum-based chemotherapy
   c. Four cycles of etoposide and platinum, or three cycles of bleomycin, etoposide, and platinum
   d. RPLND
   e. Radiation to the retroperitoneum

10. A 33-year-old man undergoes left orchiectomy for NSGCT, and his serum tumor markers normalize. Imaging reveals a 2-cm mass in the para-aortic region, and he undergoes primary RPLND. During the operation, excessive bleeding leads to an incomplete resection. Pathologic studies reveal four positive lymph nodes, the largest of which measures 3.5 cm with extranodal extension. Which of the following treatments is the most appropriate?

    a. Observation
    b. Redo RPLND
    c. Two cycles of platinum-based chemotherapy
    d. Four cycles of etoposide and platinum or three cycles of bleomycin, etoposide, and platinum
    e. Salvage chemotherapy

11. Abnormal fertility in testicular cancer patients is associated with all of the following except which one?

    a. Chemotherapy
    b. Primary germ cell defect
    c. Nerve-sparing RPLND
    d. Circulating levels of beta human chorionic gonadotropin
    e. Radiation to the scrotum

12. Which of the following is the strongest risk factor for postoperative pulmonary complications in bleomycin-treated patients?

    a. Preoperative pulmonary function test results
    b. Concentration of inspired oxygen during operation
    c. Total fluid administered in the perioperative period
    d. History of acute bleomycin toxicity
    e. Age

13. A 25-year-old male patient undergoes four cycles of etoposide and platinum for stage IIb NSGCT. Postchemotherapy CT scans of the chest, abdomen, and pelvis are normal. There was no teratoma in the primary tumor. What is the probability of residual teratoma or viable cancer in the retroperitoneum?

    a. 0%
    b. 0% to 5%
    c. 20% to 30%
    d. 40% to 50%
    e. 60% to 70%

14. What is the most common adjunctive procedure performed during postchemotherapy RPLND?

    a. Splenectomy
    b. Left nephrectomy
    c. Right nephrectomy
    d. Vena caval resection
    e. Bowel resection

15. Which of the following statements is true regarding resection of residual thoracic disease after chemotherapy for NSGCT?

    a. It is unsafe to perform in conjunction with RPLND.
    b. It is unnecessary if retroperitoneal specimens reveal fibrosis.
    c. It is more likely to reveal fibrosis in the setting of a solitary pulmonary mass and fibrosis in the retroperitoneum.
    d. It is not necessary to remove a right lung nodule if a left lung nodule reveals fibrosis.
    e. It is safely performed via the same incision as that used for the RPLND.

16. A 21-year-old patient undergoes four cycles of etoposide and platinum after right-sided orchiectomy for mixed NSGCT. During postchemotherapy RPLND, frozen section of the para-aortic lymph nodes above the inferior mesenteric artery reveals viable germ cell tumor. What should the remainder of the dissection include?

    a. Paracaval and interaortocaval tissue
    b. Interaortocaval tissue
    c. Paracaval, interaortocaval, and para-aortic tissue below the inferior mesenteric artery
    d. No further dissection warranted
    e. Right suprahilar tissue

17. Malignant transformation, that is, into non–germ cell elements, is a feature associated with which of the following?

    a. Seminoma
    b. Yolk sac tumors
    c. Embryonal carcinoma
    d. Teratoma
    e. Choriocarcinoma

18. A 32-year-old patient with bulky retroperitoneal NSGCT has completed induction primary chemotherapy with partial regression of a 10-cm interaortocaval mass. His α-fetoprotein level remains elevated. What is the appropriate management in this setting?

    a. Radiation therapy to the retroperitoneum
    b. Bilateral RPLND
    c. Modified RPLND
    d. Second-line chemotherapy
    e. Nerve-sparing RPLND

19. Late relapse is a feature most commonly associated with which of the following?

    a. Seminoma
    b. Yolk sac tumor

c. Embryonal carcinoma
d. Choriocarcinoma
e. Teratoma

20. A 24-year-old patient with stage IIC NSGCT completes induction chemotherapy with complete resolution of a 6-cm para-aortic mass. His α-fetoprotein level has normalized, but his human chorionic gonadotropin level is markedly elevated. What is the appropriate therapy at this point?

    a. Radiation therapy to the retroperitoneum
    b. Salvage chemotherapy
    c. Full RPLND
    d. Exploratory laparotomy
    e. Modified RPLND

21. A 25-year-old patient with stage IIC NSGCT has completed primary platinum-based chemotherapy. Tumor markers have normalized according to appropriate half-life, and he underwent bilateral postchemotherapy RPLND. Final pathologic studies revealed a focus of yolk sac tumor. What is the appropriate therapy at this point?

    a. Careful observation
    b. Radiation therapy
    c. Two additional cycles of platinum-based chemotherapy
    d. Four additional cycles of platinum-based chemotherapy
    e. Re-exploration in 6 weeks

Answers

1. **c. RPLND plus excision of the scrotal scar.** In the setting of scrotal contamination and clinical stage I disease, the patient is best managed with RPLND and wide excision of the scrotal scar. Observation is not suitable because of the presence of vascular invasion and scrotal contamination. [p 2922]

2. **b. The probability of viable disease in the retroperitoneum is approximately 25%.** Postchemotherapy residual masses in the setting of pure seminoma are difficult problems to manage. The morbidity associated with complete RPLND is great because of the severe desmoplastic reaction surrounding the tumor. Complete RPLND is rare. In a study from Memorial Sloan-Kettering Cancer Center, residual masses larger than 3 cm were associated with a 27% chance of harboring viable malignancy. [p 2939]

3. **d. The right testis lymphatic drainage is to paracaval, interaortocaval, and para-aortic nodes.** Lymphatic drainage is crucial to the understanding of metastatic spread of testicular cancer. The left testis drains mainly to the para-aortic and interaortic lymph nodes. However, crossover drainage from right to left is more common, and therefore the right testis drains to paracaval, interaortocaval, preaortic, and para-aortic lymph nodes. The right testicular vein drains directly into the vena cava and the left vein into the left renal vein. Both testicular arteries arise from the aorta between the renal and inferior mesenteric arteries. [p 2923]

4. **c. Radical inguinal orchiectomy.** Delayed orchiectomy after chemotherapy is indicated, as the testis represents a privileged site and is often refractory to chemotherapy. Up to 50% of testes removed in this setting will contain either viable germ cell tumor or teratoma. [p 2922]

5. **a. Retroperitoneum.** The most common site of late recurrence for both teratoma and viable NSGCT is the retroperitoneum, and, when associated with viable germ cell tumor, it is associated with a mortality rate of 75%. [p 2925]

6. **c. Sympathetic fibers and bladder neck contraction.** Lumbar sympathetic fibers innervating the seminal vesicles, vas deferens, and prostate control the act of emission. Bladder neck contraction is also controlled via sympathetic nerves and is necessary for antegrade ejaculation. Pudendal somatic innervation from S2-S4 controls the relaxation of the external urethral sphincter and rhythmic contractions of the perineal muscles and bulbourethral muscle. [p 2925]

7. **d. Right renal vein.** The inferior mesenteric artery can be ligated in younger patients without ischemic injury to the colon provided that the marginal arterial supply is intact. Lumbar arteries are routinely divided to expose the tissue behind the great vessels. The right renal vein has limited anastomotic flow, and ligation will lead to renal vein hypertension and loss of kidney function. Additional exposure of the distal left para-aortic and left parailiac space can be accomplished by further extending the incision in the left leaf of the parietal peritoneum inferiorly and, if necessary, sacrificing the inferior mesenteric artery. The testicular arteries can be ligated at their origin as needed, with collateral circulation provided by the arterial supply of the vas deferens. [p 2928]

8. **b. It has well-established therapeutic efficacy.** Although no randomized trial has been conducted, multiple studies describing the feasibility of laparoscopic RPLND have been reported. In general, the postoperative pain and recovery times are shorter than those for open RPLND. However, because of the short median follow-up and the frequent use of adjuvant chemotherapy, no statement can yet be made regarding therapeutic efficacy. [p 2931]

9. **c. four cycles of etoposide and platinum, or three cycles of bleomycin, etoposide, and platinum.** This patient has stage I-S disease, and RPLND alone in this setting is associated postoperatively with a high incidence of persistently elevated tumor markers. Full induction chemotherapy is warranted, with four cycles of platinum and etoposide or three cycles of platinum, etoposide, and bleomycin. [p 2932]

10. **d. Four cycles of etoposide and platinum or three cycles of bleomycin, etoposide, and platinum.** Because of the findings of viable disease, extranodal extension, and nodes larger than 2 cm, this patient is not a good candidate for observation. The operation described is incomplete, and no interaortocaval dissection was performed. It therefore cannot be assumed that this patient is without evidence of disease, and adjuvant chemotherapy with two cycles is not possible. Reoperation in this setting is not warranted unless there is a persistent mass after full induction chemotherapy. Salvage chemotherapy refers to high-dose chemotherapy administered to patients in whom primary chemotherapy has failed, and this patient has not yet received primary chemotherapy. [p 2933]

11. **c. Nerve-sparing RPLND.** Patients undergoing primary prospective nerve-sparing RPLND have paternity rates similar to those of testicular cancer patients undergoing surveillance. The other choices are all either reversible or permanent causes of subnormal fertility in testicular cancer patients. [p 2933]

12. **c. Total fluid administered in the perioperative period.**

The single most important risk factor for postoperative pulmonary complications in patients previously treated with bleomycin is the overall fluid and blood transfusion requirements. [p 2934]

13. **c. 20% to 30%.** The interpretation of postchemotherapy CT scans as normal or abnormal is subject to variability. However, in the three large series of RPLND in the setting of a "normal" CT scan, the findings of teratoma or viable germ cell tumor ranged from 20% to 30%. [p 2936]

14. **b. Left nephrectomy.** The left kidney is the most common organ removed in most series of postchemotherapy RPLND. In the series of Nash and colleagues, 20% of patients required nephrectomy, and these patients usually presented with hilar or suprahilar left-sided residual masses. [p 2937]

15. **c. It is more likely to reveal fibrosis in the setting of a solitary pulmonary mass and fibrosis in the retroperitoneum.** The predictors of fibrosis in thoracic specimens include fibrosis in the retroperitoneum, a solitary mass, and pretreatment tumor markers. In the setting of fibrosis in the retroperitoneum, there is a 30% chance of finding discordant histologic results in the chest. Even in the presence of benign results from pathologic studies in one lung, there can still be teratoma or viable germ cell tumor in the contralateral lung. [p 2938]

16. **c. Paracaval, interaortocaval, and para-aortic tissue below the inferior mesenteric artery.** The presence of left-sided viable disease makes full bilateral dissection mandatory. Prospective nerve-sparing techniques can be employed in this setting in select candidates to preserve antegrade ejaculation. [p 2937]

17. **d. Teratoma.** Despite the histologically benign nature of teratoma, there is a risk of malignant transformation, that is, the development of non–germ cell malignant elements such as sarcoma or carcinoma. The overall incidence is approximately 6% to 8% in the postchemotherapy setting, and the most common histologic subtypes include rhabdomyosarcoma and carcinoma. [p 2935]

18. **d. Second-line chemotherapy.** Increased serum concentrations of α-fetoprotein and human chorionic gonadotropin after primary cisplatin-based chemotherapy are often characterized by unresectable, viable germ cell tumor, and second-line salvage chemotherapy is usually recommended for these nonresponders. [pp 2934, 2936]

19. **e. Teratoma.** Late relapse of germ cell tumor following definitive therapy is defined as recurrence occurring more than 2 years after completion of therapy and being without evidence of disease. Teratoma is the most common histologic subtype involved in cases of late relapse. This is likely due to its combination of prolonged doubling time and chemotherapy resistance. [p 2935]

20. **b. Salvage chemotherapy.** Increased serum concentrations of α-fetoprotein and human chorionic gonadotropin after primary cisplatin-based chemotherapy are often characterized by unresectable, viable germ cell tumor, and second-line salvage chemotherapy is usually recommended for these nonresponders. If the complete resolution of radiographic abnormalities following chemotherapy seen in this patient were accompanied by normalization of tumor markers, then therapeutic options include observation versus postchemotherapy RPLND. In this setting, 20% to 30% of patients will have either viable germ cell tumor or teratoma at the time of RPLND. [pp 2934, 2936–2937]

21. **c. Two additional cycles of platinum-based chemotherapy.** The patient's prognosis is related to serum tumor marker level at the time of RPLND, prior treatment burden, and the pathologic findings for the resected specimen. If viable germ cell tumor is present at any site but all disease is completely resected, two additional cycles provide survival benefit in this subset of patients. Einhorn reported only 2 long-term survivors of 22 patients (9%) with completely resected viable germ cell tumor after cisplatin, bleomycin, and vinblastine chemotherapy if additional postoperative chemotherapy was not given. Fox and colleagues reported that 70% of patients with completely resected viable germ cell tumor after primary chemotherapy followed by two cycles of postoperative chemotherapy remained disease-free compared with zero of seven patients without additional chemotherapy. [pp 2936–2937]

Chapter 83

Tumors of the Penis

Donald F. Lynch, Jr. • Curtis A. Pettaway

Questions

1. Which of the following penile lesions does NOT have malignant potential?

    a. Balanitis xerotica obliterans
    b. Condyloma acuminata
    c. Coronal papillae
    d. Bowen's disease
    e. Leukoplakia

2. Which of the following infections is associated with cervical dysplasia?

    a. HIV infection
    b. Herpesvirus infection
    c. Gonorrhea
    d. Human papillomavirus (HPV) infection
    e. Lymphogranuloma venereum

3. What is the major difference between Bowen's disease and erythroplasia of Queyrat?

    a. Loss of rete pegs
    b. Difference in keratin staining
    c. Different viral etiologic agents
    d. Location
    e. Potential for metastasis

4. Kaposi's sarcoma of the AIDS-related (epidemic)

type is associated with which of the following etiologic agents?

   a. HPV type 16
   b. Human herpesvirus (HHV) type 8
   c. HPV type 32
   d. *Haemophilus ducreyi* (chancroid [soft chancre])
   e. Coxsackievirus type 23

5. Where do penile cancers most commonly arise?

   a. Glans
   b. Shaft
   c. Frenulum
   d. Coronal sulcus
   e. Scrotum

6. Which of the following is not considered a risk factor for the development of squamous penile cancer?

   a. Cigarette smoke
   b. HPV infection
   c. Phimosis
   d. Gonorrhea
   e. Chewing tobacco

7. All of the following are preventive strategies to decrease the incidence of penile cancer except which one?

   a. Circumcision after 21 years of age
   b. Avoiding sexual promiscuity
   c. Daily genital hygiene
   d. Avoiding cigarette smoke
   e. Circumcision before puberty

8. Which of the following statements regarding penile cancer is NOT true?

   a. Cancer may develop anywhere on the penis.
   b. Because of the associated discomfort, patients usually present to physicians within the first month of noting the lesion.
   c. Phimosis may obscure the nature of the lesion.
   d. Penetration of Buck's fascia and the tunica albuginea by the tumor permits invasion of the vascular corpora.
   e. Cancer cells reach the contralateral inguinal region because of lymphatic cross-communications at the base of the penis.

9. Before a treatment plan for penile cancer is initiated, which of the following statements is true?

   a. Adequate biopsies to determine stage are unimportant, as all patients should be treated with amputation.
   b. Radiologic studies play no role in decision making.
   c. DNA flow cytometry should be performed on virtually all specimens, as it provides crucial information.
   d. Tumor stage and grade and vascular invasion status all provide prognostically important information.
   e. No disfiguring therapy is indicated, as spontaneous remissions have been noted in approximately 10% of cases.

10. Which of the following statements is true regarding the natural history of penile cancer?

    a. Metastasis from the primary tumor often involves lung, liver, and bone as initial sites.
    b. Lymphatic drainage from the primary tumor is ipsilateral alone in most cases.
    c. The initial pattern of metastasis often involves spread from the corpora cavernosa to the pelvic lymph nodes.
    d. The initial pattern of metastasis involves inguinal lymph nodes beneath the fascia lata.
    e. The initial pattern of metastasis involves inguinal lymph nodes above the fascia lata.

11. Which of the following statements concerning hypercalcemia in patients with penile cancer is true?

    a. It is more commonly due to massive bone metastases than bulky soft tissue metastases.
    b. It is often related to uremia because of ureteral obstruction.
    c. It may be due to the action of parathyroid hormone–like substances released from the tumor.
    d. It is related to the action of osteoblasts on bone formation.
    e. It is managed with aggressive diuretic administration as first-line therapy.

12. The following statements are true regarding imaging tests in patients with penile cancer except which one?

    a. Both ultrasonography and MRI lack sensitivity for the detection of corpus cavernosum involvement.
    b. CT is not an appropriate test for determining primary tumor stage.
    c. CT may be beneficial for detecting enlarged inguinal nodes in obese patients or those who have had prior inguinal therapy.
    d. Lymphangiography can detect abnormal architecture in normal-sized lymph nodes.
    e. Inguinal palpation is preferred to CT and lymphangiography for determining inguinal nodal status.

13. According to the current 1997 version of the International Union Against Cancer/TNM staging system for penile cancer, which of the following statements is true?

    a. Primary tumor stage is based on the size of the primary lesion.
    b. Lymph node stage is based on the resectability of involved nodes.
    c. Stage T2 tumors are based on biopsy and involve corpora cavernosa only.
    d. Large verrucous carcinomas are considered stage Ta.
    e. Stage T1 tumors may involve the urethra at the meatus.

14. What is the strongest prognostic factor for survival in penile cancer?

    a. The presence of lymph node metastasis
    b. The grade of the primary tumor
    c. The stage of the primary tumor
    d. Vascular invasion present in the primary tumor
    e. The extent of lymph node metastasis

15. Criteria for curative surgical resection (>70% 5-year survival) in patients treated for lymph node metastasis include all of the following except which one?

    a. No more than two positive inguinal lymph nodes
    b. No positive pelvic lymph nodes
    c. Absence of extranodal extension of cancer
    d. Unilateral metastasis
    e. A single metastasis of only 6 cm in size

16. Surgical staging of the inguinal region is strongly considered under all of the following conditions except which one?

    a. Palpable adenopathy
    b. Stage T2 or greater primary tumor
    c. Presence of vascular invasion in primary tumor
    d. Presence of predominantly high-grade cancer in primary tumor
    e. Stage Ta tumors

17. A watchful waiting strategy toward the management of the inguinal region in patients with no palpable adenopathy is recommended for all of the following situations except which one?

a. Primary tumor stage Tis
b. Primary tumor stage Ta
c. Primary tumor stage T1, grade I
d. Primary tumor stage T1, grade II
e. Noncompliant patients

18. Strategies to minimize the morbidity of inguinal staging in patients with no palpable adenopathy include all the following except which one?

    a. Superficial inguinal lymph node dissection
    b. Modified complete inguinal dissection
    c. Standard ilioinguinal dissection
    d. Sentinel lymph node biopsy
    e. Intraoperative lymphatic mapping

19. All of the following inguinal procedures have been associated with false-negative findings and inguinal recurrence except which one?

    a. Inguinal node biopsy
    b. Superficial inguinal dissection
    c. Sentinel lymph node dissection
    d. Fine needle aspiration cytology
    e. Sentinel lymph node biopsy

20. For patients with proven unilateral metastasis, all of the following surgical considerations are true except which one?

    a. Ipsilateral ilioinguinal lymphadenectomy should be performed.
    b. A contralateral staging procedure is not indicated.
    c. A contralateral staging procedure is indicated.
    d. Both a superficial dissection and deep ipsilateral dissection are performed.
    e. Ipsilateral pelvic dissection provides useful prognostic information.

21. Adjuvant or neoadjuvant chemotherapy should be given in addition to surgery for all of the following cases except which one?

    a. A single pelvic nodal metastasis
    b. Extranodal extension of cancer
    c. Fixed inguinal masses
    d. Two unilateral inguinal nodes with focal metastases
    e. A single 6-cm inguinal lymph node

22. The majority of penile cancers are of which of the following histologic types?

    a. Melanoma
    b. Bowenoid papulosis
    c. Squamous cell carcinoma
    d. Epidemic Kaposi's sarcoma
    e. Verrucous carcinoma

23. Which of the following chemotherapeutic agents have been used in combination therapy for penile cancer?

    a. Bleomycin
    b. Methotrexate
    c. Cisplatin
    d. 5-Fluorouracil (5-FU)
    e. All of the above

24. Indications for radiation therapy as primary treatment for penile cancer include which of the following?

    a. Young, sexually active patient with a small lesion
    b. Patient who refuses surgery
    c. Patients with inoperable tumor who need local treatment but desire to retain the penis
    d. None of the above
    e. a, b, and c

25. Penile reconstruction is most often done using which material?

    a. Inflatable penile prosthesis
    b. A radial forearm flap
    c. Abdominal tube graft
    d. Strip graft from the upper thigh
    e. None of the above

26. Primary penile melanoma is thought to be rare for what reason?

    a. Penile skin is protected from exposure to the sun.
    b. The keratin content in penile skin is decreased.
    c. Penile blood supply precludes such tumor development.
    d. Effective topical chemotherapy exists.
    e. None of the above.

27. Lymphomatous infiltration of the penis is most likely secondary to which condition?

    a. An autoimmune disorder
    b. Diffuse disease
    c. Metastasis from a distant primary tumor
    d. Chronic infection
    e. Previous venereal infection

28. What is the most frequently encountered sign of metastatic involvement of the penis?

    a. Pain
    b. Urethral discharge
    c. Ecchymoses
    d. Priapism
    e. Preputial swelling

29. Which of the following features of Buschke-Löwenstein tumor characterizes it as different from condyloma acuminatum?

    a. Propensity for early distant metastasis
    b. Disruption of the rete pegs
    c. Loss of pigmentation
    d. Autoamputation as a frequent feature
    e. Invasion and destruction of adjacent tissues by compression

30. Which of the following statements about how verrucous carcinoma of the penis differs from classic Buschke-Löwenstein tumor is true?

    a. The terms describe the same disease.
    b. Verrucous carcinoma will sometimes exhibit spontaneous regression.
    c. The proportion of melanin pigment in verrucous carcinoma is higher than in Buschke-Löwenstein tumor.
    d. Simultaneous bilateral inguinal metastases occur commonly with Buschke-Löwenstein tumor.
    e. Circumcision is not protective for verrucous carcinoma.

31. Small lesions of erythroplasia of Queyrat may be successfully treated by which of the following?

    a. Topical 5% 5-FU
    b. Neodymium:yttrium-aluminum-garnet (Nd:YAG) laser
    c. Local excision
    d. External beam radiation therapy
    e. All of the above

32. The majority of wound problems in inguinal node dissection are due to which of the following?

    a. Infection
    b. Recurrent or residual cancer
    c. Loss of skin at the wound edge
    d. Use of permanent suture material
    e. Improper placement of incision

Answers

1. **c. Coronal papillae.** Coronal papillae present as linear, curved, or irregular rows of conical or globular excrescences, varying from white to yellow to red, arranged along the coronal sulcus. They are considered acral angiofibromas. These lesions have not been associated with malignancy. [p 2946]

2. **d. Human papillomavirus (HPV) infection.** HPV is recognized as the principal etiologic agent in cervical dysplasia and cervical cancer. [p 2947]

3. **d. Location.** Carcinoma in situ of the penis is referred to by urologists and dermatologists as erythroplasia of Queyrat if it involves the glans penis, prepuce, or penile shaft, and as Bowen's disease if it involves the remainder of the genitalia or perineal region. [p 2950]

4. **b. Human herpesvirus (HHV) type 8.** HHV type 8—also known as KSHV (Kaposi's sarcoma-associated herpesvirus)—is strongly suspected to be the etiologic agent of epidemic (AIDS-related) Kaposi's sarcoma. [p 2947]

5. **a. Glans.** Penile tumors may present anywhere on the penis but occur most commonly on the glans (48%) and prepuce (21%). [p 2953]

6. **d. Gonorrhea.** No convincing evidence has been found linking penile cancer to other factors such as occupation, other venereal diseases (gonorrhea, syphilis, herpes), marijuana use, or alcohol intake. [p 2952]

7. **a. Circumcision after 21 years of age.** Adult circumcision appears to offer little or no protection from subsequent development of the disease. These data suggest that the crucial period of exposure to certain etiologic agents may have already occurred at puberty and certainly by adult age, rendering later circumcision relatively ineffective as a prophylactic tool for penile cancer. [p 2951]

8. **b. Because of the associated discomfort, patients usually present to physicians within the first month of noting the lesion.** Patients with cancer of the penis, more than patients with other types of cancer, seem to delay seeking medical attention. In large series, from 15% to 50% of patients have been noted to delay medical care for more than a year. [p 2953]

9. **d. Tumor stage and grade and vascular invasion status all provide prognostically important information.** Confirmation of the diagnosis of carcinoma of the penis and assessment of the depth of invasion, the presence of vascular invasion, and histologic grade of the lesion by microscopic examination of a biopsy specimen are mandatory before the initiation of any therapy. [p 2953]

10. **e. The initial pattern of metastasis involves inguinal lymph nodes above the fascia lata.** The lymphatics of the prepuce form a connecting network that joins with the lymphatics from the skin of the shaft. These tributaries drain into the superficial inguinal nodes (the nodes external to the fascia lata). [p 2952]

11. **c. It may be due to the action of parathyroid hormone–like substances released from the tumor.** Parathyroid hormone and related substances may be produced by both tumor and metastases that activate osteoclastic bone resorption. [p 2954]

12. **a. Both ultrasonography and MRI lack sensitivity for the detection of corpus cavernosum involvement.** The sensitivity of ultrasonography for detecting cavernosum invasion was 100% in one study. This study confirmed the value of ultrasonography in assessing the primary tumor also reported by other investigators. For lesions suspected of invading the corpus cavernosum, both ultrasonography and contrast-enhanced MRI may provide unique information, especially when organ-sparing surgery is considered. [p 2955]

13. **d. Large verrucous carcinomas are considered stage Ta.** According to this staging system, designations for primary tumors are as follows: Tx indicates that the primary tumor cannot be assessed; T0 indicates no evidence of tumor; Tis indicates carcinoma in situ; Ta indicates noninvasive verrucous carcinoma, T1 indicates tumor invading subepithelial connective tissue; T2 indicates tumor invading corpus spongiosum or cavernosum; T3 indicates tumor invading urethra or prostate; and T4 indicates tumor invading other adjacent structures. [p 2956]

14. **e. The extent of lymph node metastasis.** The presence and extent of metastasis to the inguinal region are the most important prognostic factors for survival in patients with squamous penile cancer. [p 2957]

15. **e. A single metastasis of only 6 cm in size.** Taken together, these data suggest that the pathologic criteria associated with long-term survival after attempted curative surgical resection of inguinal metastases (i.e., 80% 5-year survival) include (1) minimal nodal disease (up to two involved nodes in most series), (2) unilateral involvement, (3) no evidence of extranodal extension of cancer, and (4) the absence of pelvic nodal metastases. [p 2959]

16. **e. Stage Ta tumors.** Tumor histologic type associated with little or no risk for metastasis includes those patients with primary tumors exhibiting (1) carcinoma in situ or (2) verrucous carcinoma. [p 2962]

17. **e. Noncompliant patients.** Noncompliant patients should be in the high-risk category. [p 2963]

18. **c. Standard ilioinguinal dissection.** In patients with no evidence of palpable adenopathy who are selected to undergo inguinal procedures by virtue of adverse prognostic factors within the primary tumor, the goal is to define whether metastases exist with minimal morbidity for the patient. A variety of treatment options for this purpose have been reported and include (1) fine needle aspiration cytology, (2) node biopsy, (3) sentinel lymph node biopsy, (3) extended sentinel lymph node dissection, (4) intraoperative lymphatic mapping, (5) superficial dissection, and (6) modified complete dissection. [p 2963]

19. **b. Superficial inguinal dissection.** One series found that the sensitivity of fine needle aspiration cytology was approximately 71% in 18 patients with clinically negative lymph nodes. This finding and the technical difficulty with lymphangiography make aspiration less practical as a staging technique for patients with no palpable lymph nodes. Biopsies directed to a specific anatomic area can be unreliable in identifying microscopic metastasis and are no longer recommended. [pp 2963–2964]

20. **b. A contralateral staging procedure is not indicated.** Clinical support for a bilateral procedure is based on the finding of contralateral metastases in more than 50% of patients so treated, even if the contralateral nodal region was negative to palpation. [pp 2964–2965]

21. **d. Two unilateral inguinal nodes with focal metastases.** For patients requiring ilioinguinal lymphadenectomy because

of the presence of metastases, adjuvant chemotherapy should be considered for those exhibiting more than two positive lymph nodes, extranodal extension of cancer, or pelvic nodal metastasis. Reports from one center further confirmed the value of adjuvant chemotherapy. Of 25 node-positive patients treated with adjuvant combination vincristine, bleomycin, and methotrexate (VBM), 82% survived 5 years, compared with 37% of 31 patients treated with surgery alone. [pp 2967, 2970]

22. **c. Squamous cell carcinoma.** The majority of tumors of the penis are squamous cell carcinomas demonstrating keratinization, epithelial pearl formation, and various degrees of mitotic activity. [p 2953]

23. **e. All of the above.** 5-FU has been used as a continuous intravenous infusion in combination with cisplatin in a limited number of patients. VBM was administered in 12 weekly treatments to 17 patients as either a neoadjuvant (5 patients) or a postoperative (12 patients) treatment program at the Milan National Tumor Institute. [pp 2969–2970]

24. **e. a, b, and c.** Radiation therapy may be considered in a select group of patients: (1) young individuals presenting with small (2 to 4 cm), superficial, exophytic, noninvasive lesions on the glans or coronal sulcus; (2) patients refusing surgery as an initial form of treatment; and (3) patients with inoperable tumor or distant metastases who require local therapy to the primary tumor but who express a desire to retain the penis. [p 2967]

25. **b. A radial forearm flap.** Modifications of the forearm flap have enhanced the versatility of microvascular free transfer reconstruction of the penis. [p 2971]

26. **a. Penile skin is protected from exposure to the sun.** Melanoma and basal cell carcinoma rarely occur on the penis, presumably because the organ's skin is protected from exposure to the sun. [p 2973]

27. **b. Diffuse disease.** When lymphomatous infiltration of the penis is diagnosed, a thorough search for systemic disease is necessary. [p 2974]

28. **d. Priapism.** The most frequent sign of penile metastasis is priapism; penile swelling, nodularity, and ulceration have also been reported. [p 2974]

29. **e. Invasion and destruction of adjacent tissues by compression.** The Buschke-Löwenstein tumor differs from condyloma acuminatum in that condylomata, regardless of size, always remain superficial and never invade adjacent tissue. Buschke-Löwenstein tumor displaces, invades, and destroys adjacent structures by compression. Aside from this unrestrained local growth, it demonstrates no signs of malignant change on histologic examination and does not metastasize. [p 2949]

30. **a. The terms describe the same disease.** Buschke-Löwenstein tumor is synonymous with verrucous carcinoma and giant condyloma acuminatum. [p 2949]

31. **e. All of the above.** When lesions are small and noninvasive, local excision, which spares penile anatomy and function, is satisfactory. Circumcision will adequately treat preputial lesions. Fulguration may be successful but often results in recurrences. Radiation therapy has successfully eradicated these tumors, and well-planned, appropriately delivered radiation results in minimal morbidity. Topical 5-FU as the 5% base causes denudation of malignant and premalignant areas while preserving normal skin. There are also reports of successful treatment with Nd:YAG laser. [p 2950]

32. **c. Loss of skin at the wound edge.** The majority of wound problems are secondary to the loss of skin at the edge of the wound. [p 2972]

Chapter 84

Surgery of Penile and Urethral Carcinoma

S. Machele Donat • Paul Cozzi • Harry W. Herr

Questions

1. Biopsy of a penile lesion provides all of the following information except:
   a. confirmation of the histologic diagnosis.
   b. assessment of normal appearing adjacent tissue for invasion.
   c. depth of invasion or clinical stage.
   d. assessment of urethral involvement.

2. Laser therapy may provide effective treatment for all but which one of the following lesions?
   a. Invasive stage T2 lesions
   b. Carcinoma in situ
   c. Bowenoid papulosis
   d. Superficial stage Ta penile cancers

3. Mohs' micrographic surgery provides which of the following?
   a. Compromise of local control
   b. Effective therapy for invasive tumors (greater than stage T2)
   c. Retention of function and anatomic integrity of the penis
   d. Effective therapy for large lesions

4. Successful local control by partial penectomy depends on which of the following?
   a. Division of the penis at least 2 cm proximal to the gross tumor
   b. Cleanliness of the patient
   c. Use of adjuvant chemotherapy
   d. Status of inguinal nodes

5. Patients who should undergo surgical dissection of the ilioinguinal lymph nodes bilaterally include all of the following except which group?

   a. Those with invasive primary tumors and clinically negative nodes
   b. Those with palpable nodes that persist following excision of the primary lesion at any stage
   c. Those with superficial primary tumors and clinically negative nodes
   d. Those with biopsy-proven node-positive disease (N+)

6. When compared with the standard groin dissection, the modified groin dissection has all of the following features except which one?

   a. The node dissection is limited, excluding regions lateral to the femoral artery and caudad to the fossa ovalis.
   b. The saphenous veins are preserved.
   c. Transposition of the sartorius muscles is eliminated.
   d. The required incision is much longer.

7. A pelvic node dissection for male penile cancer should include all of the following areas except which one?

   a. Distal common iliac nodes
   b. Para-aortic and paracaval node dissection
   c. External iliac nodes
   d. Obturator groups of nodes

8. Which of the following measures may help prevent lymphedema following a radical ilioinguinal node dissection?

   a. Preservation of Colles' fascia in the flap dissection
   b. Low-dose heparin in the perioperative period
   c. A 6-week delay between treatment of the primary tumor and the node dissection
   d. Postoperative bed rest and elastic stockings

9. What is the most frequent site of both stricture disease and urethral cancer in the male?

   a. Pendulous urethra
   b. Fossa navicularis
   c. Bulbomembranous urethra
   d. Prostatic urethra

10. Which of the following is true concerning distal urethral carcinoma in the male?

    a. Prognosis depends on histologic cell type.
    b. It has a better prognosis than invasive prostatic urethral cancer.
    c. It has a worse prognosis than bulbomembranous urethral cancer.
    d. It cannot be treated effectively with conservative surgical therapy.

11. When a delayed urethrectomy is performed in male patients after radical cystectomy, which of the following is necessary to ensure a complete dissection and decrease the risk of a local recurrence?

    a. Removal of the fossa navicularis and urethral meatus
    b. Bilateral groin dissections
    c. A total penectomy
    d. Removal of the urethral meatus

12. Possible causes for female urethral carcinoma include all of the following except which one?

    a. Childhood urinary tract infections
    b. Leukoplakia
    c. Chronic irritation or urinary tract infections
    d. Proliferative lesions such as caruncles

13. What is the most common histologic type of proximal urethral cancer in women?

    a. Adenocarcinoma
    b. Squamous cell carcinoma
    c. Melanoma
    d. Transitional cell carcinoma

14. What is the most significant prognostic factor for local control and survival in female urethral cancer?

    a. Anatomic location and extent of the tumor
    b. Age at presentation
    c. Histologic type of the tumor
    d. Hematuria

15. Radiation therapy for female urethral carcinoma is most successful:

    a. as a single modality for proximal invasive tumors.
    b. used in conjunction with chemotherapy for low-stage distal urethral tumors.
    c. at controlling distant metastatic disease.
    d. at controlling small lesions in the distal urethra.

Answers

1. **d. assessment of urethral involvement.** Before the administration of therapy, a biopsy is required to provide histologic confirmation of the diagnosis of penile cancer and staging information by assessing the depth of microscopic invasion. Adjacent normal tissue should be included to evaluate invasion, a crucial differential point with regard to planning definitive surgery. [p 2983]

2. **a. Invasive stage T2 lesions.** Laser therapy has gained popularity in recent years for the treatment of premalignant lesions and carcinoma in situ (Bowen's disease, erythroplasia of Queyrat, bowenoid papulosis) and some stage Ta and T1 penile cancers. [p 2983]

3. **c. Retention of function and anatomic integrity of the penis.** Mohs' micrographic surgery allows retention of function and anatomic integrity of the penis without compromising local control rates in small (<1 to 2 cm) superficial noninvasive tumors and is contraindicated for larger or invasive lesions. [pp 2984–2985]

4. **a. Division of the penis at least 2 cm proximal to the gross tumor.** Successful local control by partial penectomy depends on division of the penis at least 2 cm proximal to the gross tumor extent. [p 2985]

5. **c. Those with superficial primary tumors and clinically negative nodes.** Patients with invasive primary tumors and clinically negative nodes, those with palpable nodes that persist following excision of the primary lesion (any stage), or those with biopsy-proven node-positive disease (N+) should undergo surgical dissection of the ilioinguinal lymph nodes bilaterally. Those with superficial primary tumors and clinically normal nodes or those with initially enlarged nodes that regress with antibiotic therapy following excision of a superficial primary tumor may be followed expectantly. [p 2986]

6. **d. The required incision is much longer.** The modified groin dissection (see Fig. 84–6) differs from the standard dissection in that (1) the skin incision is shorter; (2) the node dissection is limited, excluding regions lateral to the femoral artery and caudad to the fossa ovalis; (3) the saphenous veins are preserved; and (4) the transposition of the sartorius muscles is eliminated. [p 2988]

7. **b. Para-aortic and paracaval node dissection.** The pelvic lymphadenectomy includes the distal common iliac, external iliac, and obturator groups of nodes. No further therapeutic benefit is gained from proximal iliac or para-aortic node dissection. [p 2990]

8. **d. Postoperative bed rest and elastic stockings.** Efforts to minimize lymphedema during the initial postoperative period include applying thigh-high elastic wraps or stockings and elevating the foot of the bed. [p 2991]

9. **c. Bulbomembranous urethra.** The incidence of urethral stricture in men later developing a carcinoma of the urethra ranges from 24% to 76% and most frequently involves the bulbomembranous urethra, which is also the portion of the urethra most commonly involved by tumor. [p 2991]

10. **b. It has a better prognosis than invasive prostatic urethral cancer.** In general, anterior urethral carcinoma is more amenable to surgical control, and its prognosis is better than that for posterior urethral carcinoma, which is often associated with extensive local invasion and distant metastasis. [p 2992]

11. **a. Removal of the fossa navicularis and urethral meatus.** It is important that the fossa navicularis and meatus are also taken in the dissection because of the high incidence of involvement of the squamous epithelium. [p 2994]

12. **a. Childhood urinary tract infections.** Causes associated with subsequent development of malignancy include chronic irritation or urinary tract infections; proliferative lesions such as caruncles, papillomas, adenomas, and polyps; and leukoplakia of the urethra. [p 2996]

13. **b. Squamous cell carcinoma.** Carcinomas of the proximal or entire urethra tend to be high grade and locally advanced, with squamous cell carcinoma accounting for 60%; transitional cell carcinoma, 20%; adenocarcinoma, 10%; undifferentiated tumor and sarcomas, 8%; and melanoma, 2%. [p 2997]

14. **a. Anatomic location and extent of the tumor.** The most significant prognostic factor for local control and survival is the anatomic location and extent of the tumor (see Tables 84–2 and 84–3), with low-stage distal urethral tumors having a better prognosis than high-stage proximal urethral tumors. [p 2997]

15. **d. at controlling small lesions in the distal urethra.** Radiation therapy alone, as with surgical excision, is often sufficient to control small lesions in the distal urethra. [p 2998]

SECTION XI

CARCINOMA OF THE PROSTATE

Chapter 85

Epidemiology, Etiology, and Prevention of Prostate Cancer

Robert E. Reiter • Jean B. DeKernion

Questions

1. What is the prostate cancer incidence in the United States currently doing?
   a. Increasing
   b. Decreasing
   c. Stabilizing
   d. Fluctuating dramatically

2. Which of the following is true of prostate cancer worldwide?
   a. It is the leading cancer diagnosis in men.
   b. It is the leading cause of cancer-related mortality.
   c. It is more common in northern European countries than in southern European ones.
   d. It is entirely genetic in origin.

3. The rise and fall of prostate cancer incidence and the switch of newly diagnosed cancers from late to early stages are caused by which of the following?
   a. An increase in the prevalence of prostate cancer
   b. Widespread prostate cancer screening
   c. Changes in the aggressiveness of prostate cancers
   d. An increase in the treatment of prostate cancer

4. Men with one first-degree relative who has prostate cancer have which risk for prostate cancer themselves?
   a. A decreased chance of developing prostate cancer compared with average men
   b. A twofold increased risk of developing prostate cancer
   c. An 11-fold increased risk of developing prostate cancer
   d. The same risk of developing prostate cancer as average men.

5. Hereditary prostate cancer is believed to be transmitted primarily in what manner?
   a. Autosomal dominant with high penetrance
   b. Autosomal recessive
   c. X-linked
   d. Autosomal dominant with low penetrance

6. Shorter numbers of CAG repeats in exon 1 of the androgen receptor are believed to be associated with:
   a. a higher risk of prostate cancer.
   b. African-American race.
   c. a higher transactivation potential.
   d. all of the above.

7. Elevated serum levels of insulin-like growth factor (IGF) have been associated with which of the following?
   a. A higher risk of developing prostate cancer
   b. A lower risk of developing prostate cancer
   c. Short stature
   d. Premature aging

8. Which of the following statements is true about the carotenoid lycopene?
   a. It has antioxidant activity.
   b. It is found in tomatoes.
   c. Its bioavailability is improved by cooking.
   d. Higher consumption of it is associated with a lower risk of prostate cancer.

9. Men who inherit the HPC1 gene are more likely to develop which of the following?
   a. Very aggressive prostate cancers
   b. Prostate cancer at an early age
   c. Latent prostate cancer
   d. Lung cancer

10. Chromosomal regions with a high frequency of loss of heterozygosity in prostate cancer are believed to:
    a. harbor prostate cancer tumor suppressor genes.
    b. be associated with an improved clinical outcome for patients with prostate cancer.
    c. play no role in prostate cancer development.
    d. be inherited.

11. What is the most common site of loss of heterozygosity in prostate cancer?
    a. Chromosome 8q
    b. Chromosome 4q
    c. Chromosome 10p
    d. Chromosome 8p

12. Which of the following statements about Nkx3.1 is true?
    a. It is a homeobox gene.
    b. It involved in ductal morphogenesis.
    c. It is a potential prostate cancer tumor suppressor gene.
    d. All of the above

13. Loss or mutation of the PTEN tumor suppressor gene promotes prostate cancer progression by:

a. leading to constitutive expression of the *Akt* oncogene.
b. leading to loss of the *Akt* oncogene.
c. causing loss of heterozygosity on chromosome 10.
d. activating the epidermal growth factor receptor.

14. Which of the following statements is true regarding loss of the p27 tumor suppressor gene?

    a. It is associated with a worse prognosis for men undergoing radical prostatectomy.
    b. It is associated with a better prognosis in men undergoing radical prostatectomy.
    c. It causes cells to stop cycling.
    d. It causes prostate cancer.

15. Genes that are amplified in prostate cancer include which of the following?

    a. PTEN
    b. MYC
    c. *Bcl-2*
    d. E-cadherin

16. Vascular endothelial growth factor (VEGF) may promote prostate cancer by what mechanism?

    a. Blocking metalloproteinase expression
    b. Stimulating new blood vessel formation
    c. Starving tumors of oxygen
    d. Causing new gene mutations

17. Potential prevention strategies for prostate cancer include which of the following?

    a. Screening for high-risk individuals
    b. Blocking dihydrotestosterone production
    c. Dietary intervention
    d. Taking retinoic acid

18. What is the key component in soy that is thought to protect from cancer?

    a. Genistein
    b. Lycopene
    c. Selenium
    d. Vitamin E

19. Finasteride is a controversial chemoprevention agent for what reason?

    a. It blocks androgen receptor activity
    b. It leads to increased intraprostatic levels of testosterone
    c. It leads to lower levels of dihydrotestosterone
    d. Clinical trials with the agent have shown toxicity

20. Retinoic acid and vitamin D belong to what class of chemoprevention agents?

    a. Antiandrogens
    b. Polyamine inhibitors
    c. Differentiation agents
    d. Proliferation agents

Answers

1. **c. Stabilizing.** Recent studies suggest that incidence rates may now be leveling off. [p 3003]

2. **c. It is more common in northern European countries than southern European ones.** Prostate cancer is the fourth most common male malignancy worldwide. Scandinavian countries have a particularly high rate of prostate cancer diagnosis and death when compared with southern European countries. [p 3004]

3. **b. Widespread prostate cancer screening.** One study examined the Surveillance, Epidemiology, and End Results (SEER) statistics to see whether there was evidence of a "screening" effect. It was concluded that the rise and fall in prostate cancer incidence and the migration from late to early stages of disease could largely be attributed to screening. [p 3006]

4. **b. A twofold increased risk of developing prostate cancer.** Men with one first-degree relative with prostate cancer had a twofold risk of developing prostate cancer, whereas men with two or three affected first-degree relatives had a 5- to 11-fold risk, respectively. [p 3006]

5. **a. Autosomal dominant with high penetrance.** Segregation analyses suggested that familial clustering was most likely explained by autosomal dominant inheritance of a rare allele (population frequency = 0.003). [p 3006]

6. **d. all of the above.** The length of the polymorphic repeat is inversely related to the transcriptional activity of the androgen receptor (AR) gene (i.e., it modulates the response of AR to androgens). For example, long CAG repeats are associated with androgen insensitivity in patients with spinobulbar muscular atrophy (Kennedy's disease). Short CAG repeat lengths are hypothesized to result in enhanced AR-mediated androgen activity and increased susceptibility to benign prostatic hyperplasia and prostate cancer. One study reported that men with CAG repeat lengths less than 18 had a 1.5-fold relative risk of prostate cancer compared with those with CAG repeat lengths higher than 26. The prevalence of short CAG repeat lengths was highest in African Americans. [p 3008]

7. **a. A higher risk of developing prostate cancer.** Three studies have correlated plasma IGF-1 levels with an increased risk of prostate cancer. Men with IGF levels in the highest quartile had a 4.3-fold higher risk of prostate cancer compared with men in the lowest quartile. [p 3009]

8. **a. It has antioxidant activity.** Lycopene is a carotenoid present at high concentrations in tomatoes. Lycopene is a potent antioxidant. It has been suggested that lycopene bioavailability is increased by cooking. [p 3010]

9. **b. Prostate cancer at an early age.** Individuals linked to this locus tend to develop prostate cancer at an early age. [p 3012]

10. **a. harbor prostate cancer tumor suppressor genes.** The existence of a tumor suppressor locus is suggested by the loss of specific chromosomal regions identified by loss of heterozygosity and comparative genomic hybridization studies. [p 3013]

11. **d. Chromosome 8p.** Analyses of sporadic prostate cancers have revealed a number of potential tumor suppressor sites, the most common of which is located on chromosome 8p. [p 3013]

12. **d. All of the above.** Nkx3.1, an androgen-regulated and prostate-specific gene, belongs to a larger family of homeobox genes. One group of researchers demonstrated that mice deficient in Nkx3.1 (via gene targeting) have significant de-

fects in prostate ductal morphogenesis and secretory protein production. Most intriguingly, aging Nkx3.1-deficient mice developed dysplastic changes and even cancer. [p 3013]

13. **a. leading to constitutive expression of the *Akt* oncogene.** Activation of phosphoinositide-3 kinase (PI3 kinase) via these and other signals leads to activation of *Akt*, a known oncogene, which then can lead to cancer cell proliferation and/or inhibition of apoptosis. Loss of PTEN in prostate cancer leads to constitutive activation of PI3 kinase, and, in turn, *Akt* and its downstream signals. [p 3015]

14. **a. It is associated with a worse prognosis for men undergoing radical prostatectomy.** Studies of patients undergoing radical prostatectomy have found an association between loss of p27 expression and an increased risk of biochemical recurrence. [p 3015]

15. **b. MYC.** MYC is amplified and overexpressed in many locally advanced and metastatic tumors. Amplification of this oncogene in locally advanced tumors predicts for systemic progression and death secondary to prostate cancer. [p 3015]

16. **b. Stimulating new blood vessel formation.** VEGF is one of the best described and most active proangiogenic genes expressed by cancers. [p 3016]

17. **a. Screening for high-risk individuals.** Findings suggest that genetic or serum testing may play a role in prostate cancer prevention strategies. [p 3017]

18. **a. Genistein.** Genistein, the most abundant isoflavone in soy products, is of particular interest because it is a natural inhibitor of tyrosine kinase receptors such as EGFR and Her-2/neu, all implicated in prostate carcinogenesis. Genistein has been shown to inhibit the proliferation of cancer cells, including prostate cancer, both in vitro and in vivo. [pp 3017–3018]

19. **b. It leads to increased intraprostatic levels of testosterone.** Because of limitations with other drugs, interest has focused on inhibitors of 5α-reductase activity, such as finasteride. The National Cancer Institute is currently studying the use of finasteride for prostate cancer prevention in the Prostate Cancer Prevention Trial. The use of finasteride to prevent prostate cancer is controversial. Inhibition of 5α-reductase leads to increases in prostatic testosterone. [p 3018]

20. **c. Differentiation agents** Because retinoids are able to induce terminal differentiation in cultured cancer cell lines, there has been a longstanding interest in their use for cancer prevention. Vitamin D has potent growth inhibitory and differentiating effects on various normal and malignant tissues and cells. [p 3019]

Chapter 86

Pathology of Prostatic Neoplasia

Jonathan I. Epstein

Questions

1. Which of the following statements regarding prostatic intraepithelial neoplasia (PIN) is NOT true?
    a. Low-grade PIN should not be commented on in diagnostic reports.
    b. PIN2 and PIN3 are considered high-grade PIN.
    c. High-grade PIN predominates in the transition zone.
    d. The incidence of high-grade PIN in needle biopsy specimens averages 5% to 10%.
    e. High-grade PIN is thought to be a precursor of many prostate cancers.

2. According to the largest studies, when high-grade PIN is found by needle biopsy, what is the approximate probability of finding carcinoma on subsequent biopsy?
    a. 5%
    b. 10%
    c. 30%
    d. 50%
    e. 70%

3. What percentage of stage T1c cancers are located predominantly in the transition zone?
    a. 5%
    b. 15%
    c. 30%
    d. 50%
    e. 70%

4. What percentage of prostate cancers are multifocal?
    a. 15%
    b. 25%
    c. 40%
    d. 60%
    e. 85%

5. What does the Gleason grade factor in?
    a. The two highest grade architectural patterns
    b. The most prevalent and second most prevalent architectural patterns
    c. The highest and lowest grade architectural patterns
    d. The highest architectural pattern and highest cytologic grade
    e. The most prevalent architectural pattern and cytologic grade

6. Which of the following statements is NOT true regarding a needle biopsy showing a small focus of atypical glands?
    a. The average incidence of atypical glands on biopsy is less than 10%.
    b. Repeated biopsies that have negative results do not rule out cancer.
    c. Repeated biopsy should increase the sampling of the initial atypical site.
    d. The chance of finding cancer by subsequent biopsy is 40% to 50%.

e. The level of serum prostate-specific antigen (PSA) correlates with the chance of finding cancer on subsequent biopsy.

7. What percentage of tumors with positive margins progress after radical prostatectomy?

    a. 10%
    b. 30%
    c. 50%
    d. 70%
    e. 90%

8. Which of the following is least crucial to note in every radical prostatectomy pathology report?

    a. Margin status
    b. Gleason score
    c. Organ-confined status
    d. DNA ploidy status
    e. Seminal vesicle invasion status

9. Which of the following subtypes of prostate cancer is associated with a worse prognosis compared with ordinary acinar carcinoma?

    a. Mucinous carcinoma
    b. Ductal adenocarcinoma
    c. Small cell carcinoma
    d. Squamous cell carcinoma
    e. All of the above

10. Which of the following immunohistochemical markers is least useful in distinguishing between prostate adenocarcinoma and transitional cell carcinoma?

    a. PSA
    b. Prostate-specific acid phosphatase
    c. CK7
    d. High-molecular-weight cytokeratin 34βE12
    e. Uroplakin

Answers

1. **c. High-grade PIN predominates in the transition zone.** Several studies have noted an increase of high-grade PIN in the peripheral zone of the prostate, corresponding to the site of origin for most adenocarcinomas of the prostate. [p 3025]

2. **c. 30%.** The largest studies published to date on this issue report a 23% to 35% probability of cancer found on subsequent biopsy. [p 3026]

3. **b. 15%.** In clinical stage T2 carcinomas and in 85% of nonpalpable tumors diagnosed on needle biopsy (stage T1c), the major tumor mass is peripheral in location. [p 3026]

4. **e. 85%.** Adenocarcinoma of the prostate is multifocal in more than 85% of cases. [p 3026]

5. **b. The most prevalent and second most prevalent architectural patterns.** In the Gleason grading system, both the primary (predominant) and the secondary (second most prevalent) architectural patterns are identified and assigned a grade from 1 to 5, with 1 the most differentiated and 5 the least undifferentiated. [p 3027]

6. **e. The level of serum prostate-specific antigen (PSA) correlates with the chance of finding cancer on subsequent biopsy.** Surprisingly, in men with a prior atypical biopsy, the level of serum PSA elevation or results of digital rectal examination do not correlate with the risk of a subsequent biopsy showing carcinoma. [p 3030]

7. **c. 50%.** In only approximately 50% of men with positive margins does the disease progress after radical prostatectomy (see Table 86–1). [p 3031]

8. **d. DNA ploidy status.** The evaluation of ploidy on radical prostatectomy specimens is controversial for the same reasons as is ploidy on needle biopsy specimens. The strongest data to support the prognostic importance of ploidy are in patients with pelvic node metastases who are undergoing radical prostatectomy. [pp 3031–3032]

9. **e. All of the above.** Mucinous adenocarcinoma of the prostate gland is one of the least common morphologic variants of prostatic carcinoma (see Fig. 86–3A). It has an aggressive biologic behavior and, like nonmucinous prostate carcinoma, has a propensity to produce bone metastases and increased serum acid phosphatase and PSA levels with advanced disease. The average survival time of patients with small cell carcinoma of the prostate is less than 1 year. Most prostatic duct adenocarcinomas are of advanced stage at presentation and have an aggressive course. Pure primary squamous carcinoma of the prostate is rare and is associated with a poor survival. [pp 3032–3033]

10. **c. CK7.** CK7 and CK20 positivities in transitional cell carcinoma are 70% to 100% and 15% to 71%, respectively. The problem with these markers is that they are not specific. [p 3034]

Chapter 87

Ultrasonography and Biopsy of the Prostate

Martha K. Terris

Questions

1. Before transrectal ultrasonographically guided prostate biopsy is done, all patients should follow all of the following preparations except which one?

    a. They should receive antibiotic prophylaxis.
    b. They should provide informed consent.
    c. They should discontinue all aspirin or nonsteroidal anti-inflammatory medications.
    d. They should receive an enema.
    e. They should receive emergency contact information in case they experience problems after the procedure.

2. Which of the following statements about transrectal ultrasonographic imaging is NOT true?

    a. It should be performed in the transverse and sagittal planes.
    b. It is a powerful tool for prostate cancer screening.
    c. It should be interpreted at the time of the examination from real-time images.
    d. It has gained popularity as a means of guiding prostate biopsies.
    e. It is limited by the high incidence of isoechoic prostate tumors.

3. Which of the following statements about transrectal sonography after radical prostatectomy is NOT true?

    a. It should show a smooth tapering of the bladder neck to the urethra.
    b. It often reveals a hypoechoic mass anterior to the anastomosis, which usually represents recurrent cancer.
    c. It should have an intact fat plane between the bladder neck/urethra and the rectum.
    d. It should be accompanied by biopsies of the perianastomotic area and bladder neck in patients suspected of having a local recurrence, even if the ultrasonographic image is normal.
    e. It often demonstrates a blunted, nontapered appearance of the vesicourethral anastomosis in incontinent patients.

4. Which of the following statements about transrectal ultrasonographic images of the seminal vesicles is NOT true?

    a. Images often appear normal even if the vesicles are involved with prostate cancer.
    b. Images can reveal cystic dilatation of the seminal vesicles caused by prostate cancer involving the ejaculatory ducts.
    c. If seminal vesicles exhibit hyperechogenicity, they are likely to be involved with cancer.
    d. If seminal vesicles exhibit anterior displacement or loss of the "beak sign," they are likely to be involved with prostate cancer.
    e. If seminal vesicles exhibit asymmetry alone, they are probably involved with prostate cancer.

5. Which of the following statements about repeated transrectal ultrasonographically guided biopsies is NOT true?

    a. They should be performed if prostatic intraepithelial neoplasia is apparent on the initial biopsy samples.
    b. They should not consist of only sextant biopsies.
    c. They are increasingly common.
    d. They reveal cancer in approximately 30% of patients.
    e. If they are free of cancer, ensure that the patient does not have prostate malignancy.

6. Which of the following is NOT a component of extended field biopsies?

    a. Sextant biopsies
    b. Trapezoid area biopsies
    c. Transition zone biopsies
    d. Lateral biopsies
    e. Anterior horn biopsies

7. Which of the following statements concerning ultrasonographic estimates of prostate volume is true?

    a. They are extremely accurate.
    b. They increase initially because of edema after external beam irradiation.
    c. They decrease more with androgen deprivation therapy in patients with malignancy than in those with benign disease.
    d. They decrease more with androgen deprivation therapy in patients with large glands than in those with small prostates.
    e. They decrease more with radiation therapy in patients with low-grade prostate cancer than in those with high-grade cancer.

8. Which of the following tumors can be isoechoic with the peripheral zone during prostate ultrasonographic imaging?

    a. Adenocarcinoma
    b. Chronic myelogenous leukemia
    c. Rhabdomyosarcoma
    d. Both a and c
    e. All of the above.

9. Which of the following statements is true concerning complications of prostate biopsy?

    a. Complications are uncommon.
    b. Complications rarely include hematuria.
    c. Complications can be life-threatening because of bacterial sepsis.
    d. Complications include the same risk for urinary retention in men with obstructive voiding symptoms as in those without obstructive voiding symptoms.
    e. Complications include the same risk for discomfort in young men as in old men.

Answers

1. **c. They should discontinue all aspirin or nonsteroidal anti-inflammatory medications.** Patients should be discouraged from taking aspirin or nonsteroidal anti-inflammatory drugs for 10 days before the procedure, but recent use should not be considered an absolute contraindication to biopsy. [p 3040]

2. **b. It is a powerful tool for prostate cancer screening.** Because of the limited sensitivity of ultrasonography, coupled with the expense, enthusiasm for transrectal ultrasonographic screening has dissipated. [p 3038]

3. **b. It often reveals a hypoechoic mass anterior to the anastomosis, which usually represents recurrent cancer.** Many patients will demonstrate a nodule of tissue anterior to the anastomosis, representing the ligated dorsal vein complex. [p 3047]

4. **e. If seminal vesicles exhibit asymmetry alone, they are probably involved with prostate cancer.** Asymmetry of the lobulations of the seminal vesicles is very common in normal men and of no clinical significance in the absence of other suspicious features. [p 3051]

5. **e. If they are free of cancer, ensure that the patient does not have prostate malignancy.** Many patients undergoing repeated biopsies may require an additional biopsy session because the rate of cancer detection on the third set of biopsies is up to 30%. [p 3050]

6. **b. Trapezoid area biopsies.** These extended field methods all involve a combination of sextant, lateral, anterior, and, in some protocols, midline prostatic sampling. [p 3049]

7. **d. They decrease more with androgen deprivation therapy in patients with large glands than in those with small prostates.** The volume can decrease as much as 60% in large glands and as little as 10% in small glands. [p 3047]

8. **e. All of the above.** The echogenicity of rhabdomyosarcoma is similar to that of the normal prostate. Hematolymphoid malignancies involving the prostate are generally inapparent with transrectal ultrasonographic imaging. [p 3048]

9. **c. Complications can be life-threatening because of bacterial sepsis.** The most serious complication of transrectal ultrasonographically guided prostatic biopsies is bacterial sepsis. [p 3043]

Chapter 88

Diagnosis and Staging of Prostate Cancer

H. Ballentine Carter • Alan W. Partin

Questions

1. What is the most useful first-line test for diagnosis of prostate cancer?

   a. Digital rectal examination (DRE)
   b. Prostate-specific antigen (PSA) assay
   c. Prostatic acid phosphatase (PAP) assay
   d. Transrectal ultrasonography (TRUS)
   e. Combination of DRE and PSA.

2. Most detectable PSA in sera is bound to which of the following?

   a. Albumin
   b. α_1-Antichymotrypsin (ACT)
   c. α_2-Macroglobulin (MG)
   d. Human kallikrein
   e. ACT and MG

3. Serum PSA levels vary with which factor?

   a. Age
   b. Race
   c. Prostate volume
   d. ACT concentration
   e. Age, race, and prostate volume

4. Serum PSA elevations are specific for which of the following?

   a. The presence of prostate disease
   b. The presence of prostate cancer
   c. The presence of prostate enlargement
   d. The presence of prostate inflammation
   e. None of the above

5. A 60-year-old man taking finasteride (Proscar) for 2 years with a PSA value of 4 ng/ml would most likely, if he were not taking finasteride, have which PSA value?

   a. 2 ng/ml
   b. 6 ng/ml
   c. 8 ng/ml
   d. 12 ng/ml
   e. 4 ng/ml

6. Which of the following tests has the highest positive predictive value for prostate cancer?

   a. PSA
   b. DRE
   c. TRUS
   d. Combination of DRE and TRUS
   e. human glandular kallikrein (hK2)

7. The goals of staging for prostate cancer include all of the following except which one?

a. To predict the prognosis
   b. To select rational therapy on the basis of predicted extent of disease
   c. To select radical retropubic or perineal prostatectomy
   d. Both a and b
   e. To predict the pathologic extent of disease

8. The currently available modalities for assessing disease extent in men with prostate cancer include which of the following?

   a. DRE
   b. Serum PSA
   c. Histologic grade
   d. Bone scan
   e. All of the above

9. Pathologic staging is superior to clinical staging because all of the following factors are known except which one?

   a. PSA
   b. Surgical margin status
   c. Seminal vesicle involvement
   d. Tumor volume
   e. Presence of capsular penetration

10. What pathologic finding or findings at radical prostatectomy are highly predictive of the presence of occult metastatic disease?

    a. Positive surgical margins
    b. Seminal vesicle involvement
    c. Lymph node involvement
    d. Both b and c
    e. Both a and b

11. The finding of pathologic perineural invasion of cancer (PNI) on a prostate biopsy specimen suggests:

    a. organ-confined disease.
    b. 20% likelihood of capsular penetration.
    c. 75% likelihood of capsular penetration.
    d. pelvic lymph node involvement.
    e. a bilateral nerve-sparing prostatectomy should not be considered.

12. Which staging modality provides the highest degree of understaging?

    a. Bone scan
    b. Immunoscintigraphy
    c. PSA
    d. PAP
    e. DRE

13. As general guidelines regarding PSA levels and pathologic stage, which of the following statements is true?

    a. Twenty-five percent of men with a PSA value less than 4.0 ng/ml have organ-confined disease.
    b. One hundred percent of men with a PSA value greater than 50 ng/ml have pelvic lymph node involvement.
    c. Ten percent of men with a PSA value greater than 10 ng/ml have extraprostatic extension.
    d. Serum PSA has no predictive value for staging.
    e. Sixty-seven percent of men with a PSA value between 4.0 and 10.0 ng/ml have organ-confined disease.

14. With respect to the Gleason primary and secondary grade, all of the following statements are true except which one?

    a. Primary grade ranges from 1 to 5.
    b. Secondary grade ranges from 1 to 5.
    c. Secondary grade and primary grade are summed to provide a Gleason score (2–10).
    d. The primary grade represents the second largest area of cancer on the biopsy specimen.
    e. The presence of a Gleason primary or secondary grade 4 or 5 on any biopsy specimen is predictive of poor prognosis.

15. On the basis of the Partin tables, a man with a PSA value of 7.4 before biopsy, a Gleason score of $3 + 4 = 7$ on a biopsy specimen, and a nonsuspicious (T1c) DRE before biopsy has all of the following except:

    a. 49% likelihood of organ-confined disease.
    b. 40% likelihood of isolated capsular penetration.
    c. 22% likelihood of pelvic lymph node involvement.
    d. 97% likelihood of regionally confined disease.
    e. 8% likelihood of seminal vesicle invasion.

Answers

1. **e. Combination of DRE and PSA.** The DRE and serum PSA are the most useful first-line tests for assessing the risk that prostate cancer is present in an individual. [p 3056]

2. **b. α_1-Antichymotrypsin (ACT).** Most detectable PSA in sera (65% to 90%) is bound to ACT. [p 3057]

3. **e. Age, race, and prostate volume.** In the absence of prostate cancer, serum PSA levels vary with age, race, and prostate volume. [p 3057]

4. **e. None of the above.** Serum PSA elevations may occur as a result of disruption of the normal prostatic architecture that allows PSA to diffuse into the prostatic tissue and gain access to the circulation. This can occur in the setting of prostate disease (benign prostatic hyperplasia [BPH], prostatitis, prostate cancer) and with prostate manipulation (prostate massage, prostate biopsy). The presence of prostate disease (prostate cancer, benign prostatic hyperplasia, and prostatitis) is the most important factor affecting serum levels of PSA. PSA elevations may indicate the presence of prostate disease, but not all men with prostate disease have elevated PSA levels. Furthermore, PSA elevations are not specific for cancer. [pp 3057–3058]

5. **c. 8 ng/ml.** Finasteride (a 5α-reductase inhibitor for treatment of BPH) at 5 mg has been shown to lower PSA levels by 50% after 12 months of treatment. Thus, one can multiply the PSA level by 2 to obtain the "true" PSA level of a patient who has been taking finasteride for 12 months or more. Men who are to be treated with finasteride should have a baseline PSA measurement before initiation of treatment and should be followed with serial PSA measurements. If the PSA value does not decrease by 50%, or if there is a rise in the PSA value when the patient is taking finasteride, these men should be suspected of having an occult prostate cancer. [p 3058]

6. **a. PSA.** PSA is the single test with the highest positive predictive value for cancer. [p 3058]

7. **d. Both a and b.** The goals in staging of prostate cancer are twofold: (1) to predict prognosis and (2) to rationally select therapy on the basis of predicted extent of disease. [p 3064]

8. **e. All of the above.** The currently available modalities for assessing disease extent in men with prostate cancer are DRE, serum tumor markers, histologic grade, radiographic imaging, and pelvic lymphadenectomy. [p 3064]

9. **a. PSA.** Pathologic staging is more useful than clinical staging in the prediction of prognosis because tumor volume, surgical margin status, extent of extracapsular spread, and involvement of seminal vesicles and pelvic lymph nodes can be determined. [p 3066]

10. **d. Both b and c.** The finding of seminal vesicle invasion or lymph node metastases on pathologic evaluation after radical prostatectomy is associated with a very low probability of total eradication of tumor and a high probability of distant disease. [p 3066]

11. **c. 75% likelihood of capsular penetration.** PNI in a prostatectomy specimen has little independent prognostic staging value as initially reported by Byar. However, in biopsy cores, its presence is associated with a higher chance of non-organ-confined disease at prostatectomy. De la Taille and colleagues demonstrated that the presence of PNI on a biopsy specimen was closely associated with high PSA values, poorly differentiated tumor, and involvement of multiple cores with cancer, and thus a higher pathologic stage. Seventy-five percent of men with PNI on a biopsy specimen will have capsular penetration on examination of the prostatectomy specimen. [p 3067]

12. **e. DRE.** Histologic evaluation of surgical specimens after radical prostatectomy for presumed organ-confined disease demonstrates a significant degree of understaging by DRE. Table 88–5 summarizes several large radical prostatectomy series in which understaging, or false-negative prediction of organ-confined status by DRE, could be determined. In these series, understaging of disease increases with increasing clinical stage. [p 3067]

13. **e. Sixty-seven percent of men with a PSA value between 4.0 and 10.0 ng/ml have organ-confined disease.** As a general guideline, the majority of men (80%) with PSA values less than 4.0 ng/ml have pathologically organ-confined disease, two thirds of men with PSA levels between 4.0 and 10.0 ng/ml have organ-confined cancer, and more than 50% of men with PSA levels more than 10.0 ng/ml have disease beyond the prostate. Pelvic lymph node involvement is found in nearly 20% of men with PSA levels greater than 20 ng/ml and in most men (75%) with serum PSA levels greater than 50 ng/ml. [p 3068]

14. **d. The primary grade represents the second largest area of cancer on the biopsy specimen.** The pathologic criteria and method for determining the Gleason grade of a prostatic tumor are discussed in Chapter 86. The Gleason grading system is based on a low-power microscopic description of the architectural criteria of the cancer. A Gleason grade (or pattern) of 1 to 5 is assigned as a primary grade (the pattern occupying the greatest area of the specimen) and a secondary grade (the pattern occupying the second largest area of the specimen). A Gleason sum (2–10) is determined by adding the primary grade and the secondary grade. The presence of Gleason pattern 4 or greater (primary or secondary) or a Gleason sum of 7 or greater is predictive of a poorer prognosis. [p 3069]

15. **c. 22% likelihood of pelvic lymph node involvement.** Probability tables, based on the parameters of preoperative clinical stage, serum PSA level, and Gleason sum, have been constructed based on large numbers of men who have undergone radical prostatectomy with precise determination of the pathologic stage. In Table 88–7, numbers within the nomogram represent the percent probability of having a given final pathologic stage based on logistic regression analyses for all three variables combined; dashes represent data categories in which insufficient data existed to calculate a probability. This information is useful in counseling men with newly diagnosed prostate cancer with respect to treatment alternatives and probability of complete eradication of tumor, keeping in mind that men with organ-confined, high-grade cancers are often not cured of prostate cancer with surgery because of early microscopic spread of disease. [pp 3069–3071]

Chapter 89

Radical Prostatectomy

James A. Eastham • Peter T. Scardino

Questions

1. What is the lifetime risk of developing a clinically detected prostate cancer?
   a. 5% to 10%
   b. 15% to 20%
   c. 30% to 35%
   d. 50% to 55%
   e. >75%

2. Which clinical features identify a patient as potentially having an indolent prostate cancer?
   a. Clinical stage T1c-T2, serum prostate-specific antigen (PSA) result of 10 ng/ml or less, Gleason grade of 4 or 5 in one biopsy core only, no more than three biopsy cores involved
   b. Clinical stage T1c-T2, serum PSA result of 4 ng/ml or less, PSA density of 0.3 or less, Gleason score of 4 or 5 in less than 50% of the biopsy specimens
   c. Clinical stage T1c-T3, serum PSA result less than 20 ng/ml
   d. Clinical stage T1c, PSA density of 0.1 or less, no Gleason grade 4 or 5 in the biopsy specimen, fewer than three biopsy cores involved, and no core with more than 50% involvement with cancer
   e. Clinical stage T1c, serum PSA result less than 10 ng/ml, no Gleason grade 5 in the biopsy specimen

3. Which clinical feature is most often associated with a poor outcome in men with clinically localized prostate cancer managed conservatively (watchful waiting)?

   a. Serum PSA value of 20 ng/ml or less at the time of diagnosis
   b. Bilaterally palpable disease
   c. More than 50% of the biopsy specimen involved with cancer
   d. Poorly differentiated tumors
   e. Age at diagnosis younger than 70 years

4. What is the actuarial probability of freedom from serum PSA recurrence 5 years after radical prostatectomy for clinically localized prostate cancer from most recent series?

   a. 0% to 10%
   b. 20% to 30%
   c. 40% to 50%
   d. 60% to 70%
   e. 70% to 80%

5. Which of the following clinical prognostic factors have been associated with freedom from serum PSA progression after radical prostatectomy?

   a. Patient's age at diagnosis, serum PSA, biopsy Gleason grade
   b. Patient's age at diagnosis, PSA density, clinical stage
   c. Serum PSA level, Gleason grade in the biopsy specimen, clinical stage
   d. PSA density, number of positive biopsy cores, prostate volume on ultrasonography
   e. Ethnicity, PSA density, prostate volume on ultrasonography

6. In a multivariate analysis of clinical and pathologic factors, which of the following factors were associated with clinical outcome after radical prostatectomy?

   a. Preoperative serum PSA value, pathologic stage, Gleason grade in the radical prostatectomy specimen, and surgical margin status
   b. Preoperative serum PSA level, clinical stage, biopsy Gleason score
   c. Patient's age at diagnosis, clinical stage, PSA density
   d. Preoperative serum PSA value, clinical stage, biopsy Gleason score
   e. Patient's age at diagnosis, PSA density, pathologic stage

7. Factors that have been associated with the development of an anastomotic stricture after radical prostatectomy include which of the following?

   a. Prior transurethral resection of the prostate
   b. Excessive intraoperative blood loss
   c. Urinary extravasation at the anastomotic site
   d. All of the above
   e. None of the above

8. What is the reported incidence of urinary incontinence from most centers with a broad experience in performing radical prostatectomy?

   a. 0% to 10%
   b. 20% to 30%
   c. 40% to 50%
   d. 60% to 70%
   e. 80% to 90%

9. Which factors are associated with the recovery of continence after radical prostatectomy?

   a. Younger patient age, palpable tumor at the prostatic apex, no prior transurethral resection of the prostate
   b. Younger patient age, neurovascular bundle preservation, absence of an anastomotic stricture
   c. Clinical stage T1c cancer, pathologic stage, negative surgical margins
   d. Age younger than 50 years at surgery, preoperative serum PSA value less than 10 ng/ml, pathologic stage T2 cancer
   e. Operative time, operative blood loss

10. Intraoperative videotaping suggested that which of the following factors can have an impact on the recovery of potency after radical prostatectomy?

    a. Division of the striated sphincter when placing urethral sutures
    b. Degree of hemostasis at the end of the surgical procedure
    c. Division of the posterior striated sphincter
    d. Oversewing back-bleeding on the anterior surface of the prostate after division of the dorsal venous complex
    e. All of the above

11. Neoadjuvant hormonal therapy before radical prostatectomy results in which of the following?

    a. Reduction in the preoperative serum PSA value
    b. Reduction in the biochemical failure rate after radical prostatectomy
    c. Reduction in the rate of positive surgical margins
    d. All of the above
    e. a and c only.

12. For men who develop biochemical recurrence after radical prostatectomy, factors associated with local recurrence rather than systemic recurrence include which of the following?

    a. First detectable serum PSA within 6 months of surgery, Gleason score of 7 or greater, pathologic stage T3
    b. Age younger than 70 years at the time of recurrence, first detectable serum PSA result less than 2 ng/ml, Gleason score of 5 or less
    c. Histologically normal pelvic lymph nodes and seminal vesicles, Gleason score of 5 or less, first detectable serum PSA level more than 1 year after surgery, PSA doubling time of more than 6 months
    d. Pathologic stage T2, Gleason score 8 to 10, negative bone scan
    e. First detectable serum PSA more than 4 months after surgery, negative biopsy of the prostatic fossa, PSA doubling time of less than 3 months

13. What is the most common complication after salvage radical prostatectomy?

    a. Urinary incontinence
    b. Rectal injury
    c. Ureteral transection
    d. Deep venous thrombosis
    e. Wound infection

14. Which of the following clinical factors had a positive correlation with pathologic stage after salvage radical prostatectomy?

    a. Time since completion of radiation therapy
    b. Biopsy Gleason grade
    c. Serum PSA value less than 10 ng/ml at the time of salvage surgery
    d. Patient's age at the time of initial diagnosis of prostate cancer
    e. Serum PSA doubling time

15. What is the current rate of pelvic lymph node metastasis in men undergoing radical prostatectomy?

    a. Less than 10%
    b. 10% to 15%
    c. 20% to 25%
    d. 30% to 35%
    e. 40% to 45%

Answers

1. **b. 15% to 20%.** The lifetime risk of developing a clinically detected prostate cancer is about 16%. [p 3080]

2. **d. Clinical stage T1c, PSA density of 0.1 or less, no Gleason grade 4 or 5 in the biopsy specimen, fewer than three biopsy cores involved, and no core with more than 50% involvement with cancer.** In a study of preoperative clinical and pathologic features in 157 men with stage T1c prostate cancer who underwent radical prostatectomy, those findings were correlated with the pathologic features of the tumor specimen. The model reported in the study for predicting "an insignificant" tumor included (1) PSA density of 0.1, no Gleason grade of 4 or 5 in the biopsy specimen, fewer than three biopsy cores involved (minimum of six cores obtained) and no core with more than 50% involvement with cancer, or (2) PSA density of 0.15, no Gleason grade of 4 or 5 in the biopsy sample, and less than 3 mm cancer on only one prostate biopsy sample (minimum of six cores obtained). [p 3081]

3. **d. Poorly differentiated tumors.** The cancer-specific mortality rate at 10 years was 9% for well-differentiated tumors, 24% for moderately differentiated cancers, and 46% for poorly differentiated cancers. [pp 3082–3083]

4. **e. 70% to 80%.** The actuarial probability of freedom from PSA recurrence after radical retropubic prostatectomy from several recent series, summarized in Table 89–5, showed remarkably similar 5-year, progression-free values of 77% to 80% for patients treated between 1966 and 1998. [p 3084]

5. **c. Serum PSA level, Gleason grade in the biopsy specimen, clinical stage.** Freedom from progression after radical prostatectomy is related to several well-established clinical prognostic factors, including clinical stage, Gleason grade in the biopsy specimen, and serum PSA levels. [p 3084]

6. **a. Preoperative serum PSA value, pathologic stage, Gleason grade in the radical prostatectomy specimen, and surgical margin status.** In a multivariate analysis of clinical and pathologic prognostic factors, preoperative serum PSA level, pathologic stage, Gleason grade in the radical prostatectomy specimen, and surgical margin status were each independently associated with outcome after radical prostatectomy. [p 3086]

7. **d. All of the above.** Prior transurethral resection of the prostate, excessive intraoperative blood loss, and urinary extravasation at the anastomotic site may contribute to stricture development. [p 3088]

8. **a. 0% to 10%.** Most centers with broad expertise in radical prostatectomy report that fewer than 10% of patients are incontinent after surgery. [p 3089]

9. **b. Younger patient age, neurovascular bundle preservation, absence of an anastomotic stricture.** Factors associated with an increased chance of regaining continence were younger age, preservation of both neurovascular bundles, a modification in the technique of anastomosis (introduced in 1990), and the absence of an anastomotic stricture. [p 3089]

10. **e. All of the above.** Four steps in the procedure seemed to correlate with recovery of sexual function: (1) oversewing back-bleeders from the proximal dorsal vein on the anterior surface of the prostate, (2) dividing the striated sphincter when placing urethral sutures, (3) dividing the posterior striated sphincter, and (4) hemostasis at the end of the operation. [p 3092]

11. **e. a and c only.** In randomized, prospective, controlled clinical trials, neoadjuvant hormonal therapy reduced the rate of positive surgical margins from an average of 47% to an average of 22%, reduced the preoperative serum PSA levels by 96% (range, 90% to 99%), and reduced prostate volume by 34%. Preliminary results indicated no difference in the progression rate between treated and untreated patients. [p 3096]

12. **c. Histologically normal pelvic lymph nodes and seminal vesicles, Gleason score of 5 or less, first detectable serum PSA level more than 1 year after surgery, PSA doubling time of more than 6 months.** Local recurrence is more likely in men with histologically normal lymph nodes and seminal vesicles, a Gleason score of 5 or less, the first detectable PSA level more than 1 year after surgery, and a PSA doubling time of more than 6 months. [p 3101]

13. **a. Urinary incontinence.** In a series of more than 80 salvage radical prostatectomies, although morbidity of the operation has changed over the years, urinary incontinence remains high. An estimated 58% of patients have persistent leakage requiring two or more pads a day and 20% have required an artificial urinary sphincter. [p 3101]

14. **c. Serum PSA value less than 10 ng/ml at the time of salvage surgery.** Preoperative serum PSA levels, but not clinical stage or biopsy grade, had a positive correlation with pathologic stage. If the preoperative PSA value was less than 10 ng/ml, only 15% of the patients had advanced pathologic features, compared with 86% of patients with such features if the PSA level was greater than 10 ng/ml. [p 3101]

15. **a. Less than 10%.** Before the widespread use of serum PSA, the incidence of pelvic lymph node metastases at the time of radical prostatectomy for clinically localized prostate cancer was in excess of 20%. In more recent series, however, the incidence of pelvic lymph node metastases was 2% to 7%. [p 3097]

Chapter 90

Anatomic Radical Retropubic Prostatectomy

Patrick C. Walsh

Questions

1. What is the arterial blood supply to the prostate?
   a. The pudendal artery
   b. The superior vesical artery
   c. The inferior vesical artery
   d. The external iliac artery

2. What vessels are located in the neurovascular bundle?
   a. Capsular arteries and veins
   b. Pudendal artery and vein
   c. Hemorrhoidal artery and vein
   d. Santorini's plexus

3. A radical prostatectomy may compromise the arterial blood supply to the penis by injuring the aberrant blood supply from which artery?
   a. The obturator artery
   b. The inferior vesical artery
   c. The superior vesical artery
   d. All of the above

4. The main parasympathetic efferent innervation to the pelvic plexus arises from:
   a. S1.
   b. S2-S4.
   c. T11-L2.
   d. L3-S1.

5. What is the relationship of the neurovascular bundle to the prostatic fascia?
   a. Inside Denonvilliers' fascia
   b. Outside the lateral pelvic fascia
   c. Inside the prostatic fascia
   d. Between the layers of the prostatic fascia and the levator fascia

6. Why is there less blood loss during radical perineal prostatectomy?
   a. It is easier to ligate the dorsal vein complex through the perineal approach than through the retropubic approach.
   b. There is no need to divide the puboprostatic ligaments.
   c. The dorsal vein complex is not divided because the dissection occurs beneath the lateral fascia and anterior pelvic fascia.
   d. Because the perineum is elevated, there is lower venous pressure.

7. What anatomic structure is responsible for the maintenance of passive urinary control after radical prostatectomy?
   a. The bladder neck
   b. Levator ani musculature
   c. The preprostatic sphincter
   d. The striated urethral sphincter

8. What is the major nerve supply to the striated sphincter and levator ani?
   a. The neurovascular bundle
   b. Sympathetic fibers from T11 to L2
   c. The pudendal nerve
   d. The obturator nerve

9. What is the posterior extent of the pelvic lymph node dissection?
   a. The external iliac vein
   b. The obturator nerve
   c. The obturator vessels
   d. The sacral foramen

10. In opening the endopelvic fascia, there are often small branches traveling from the prostate to the pelvic sidewall. What are these branches?
    a. Tributaries from the obturator artery
    b. Tributaries from the external iliac artery
    c. Tributaries from the inferior vesical artery
    d. Tributaries from the pudendal artery and veins

11. How extensively should the puboprostatic ligaments be divided?
    a. Superficially, with just enough excised to expose the junction between the anterior apex of the prostate and the dorsal vein complex
    b. Extensively, down to the pelvic floor, including the pubourethral component
    c. Not at all; the puboprostatic ligaments should be left intact
    d. Widely enough to permit a right angle to be placed around the dorsal vein complex

12. When the dorsal vein complex is divided anteriorly, what is the most common major structure that can be damaged, and what is the most common adverse outcome?
    a. Aberrant pudendal arteries; impotence
    b. Neurovascular bundle; impotence
    c. Striated urethral sphincter; incontinence
    d. Levator ani musculature; incontinence

13. What is the most common site for a positive surgical margin, and when does this occur?
    a. Posterolateral; during release of the neurovascular bundle
    b. Posterior; when the prostate is dissected from the rectum
    c. Apex; during division of the striated urethral sphincter-dorsal vein complex

d. Bladder neck; during separation of the prostate from the bladder

14. How should the back-bleeders from the dorsal vein complex on the anterior surface of the prostate be oversewn, and why?
    a. The edges should be pulled together in the midline to avoid bleeding.
    b. Bunching sutures should be used to avoid excising too much striated sphincter.
    c. The edges should be oversewn in the shape of a V to avoid advancing the neurovascular bundles too far anteriorly on the prostate.
    d. They should be oversewn horizontally to avoid a positive surgical margin.

15. After the dorsal vein complex has been ligated and the urethra has been divided, what posterior structure, other than the neurovascular bundles, attaches the prostate to the pelvic floor?
    a. Rectourethralis
    b. Denonvilliers' fascia
    c. Rectal fascia
    d. Posterior portion of the striated sphincter complex

16. Once the apex of the prostate has been released, what is the best way to retract the prostate for exposure of the neurovascular bundle?
    a. Traction on the catheter, producing upward rotation of the apex of the prostate
    b. Use of a sponge stick to roll the prostate on its side
    c. Downward displacement of the prostate with a sponge stick
    d. Use of finger dissection to release the prostate posteriorly

17. To avoid a positive surgical margin, what is the best way to release the neurovascular bundle?
    a. Right-angle dissection beginning on the posterior surface of the prostate and dissecting anterolaterally
    b. Using sharp dissection, laterally dissecting toward the rectum
    c. Using finger dissection to fracture the neurovascular bundle from the prostate
    d. Using electrocautery to separate the neurovascular bundle from the prostate

18. What is the latest point at which a decision can be made regarding preservation or excision of the neurovascular bundle?
    a. When perineural invasion is identified on the needle biopsy specimen
    b. When the neurovascular bundle is being released from the prostate and fixation is identified
    c. When the prostate has been removed and tissue covering the posterolateral surface of the prostate is thought to be inadequate
    d. When the patient is found to have a positive biopsy result at the apex

19. Before the lateral pedicles are divided, what is the last major branch of the neurovascular bundle that must be identified and released?
    a. Apical branch
    b. Posterior branch, traveling over the seminal vesicles to the base of the prostate
    c. Capsular branch
    d. Bladder neck branch

20. When the vesicourethral anastomosis sutures are being tied, if tension is found, what is the best way to release it?
    a. Creating an anterior bladder neck flap
    b. Placing the Foley catheter on traction postoperatively
    c. Releasing attachments of the bladder to the peritoneum
    d. Using Vest sutures

21. If there is excessive bleeding from the dorsal vein complex while it is being divided, what should the surgeon do?
    a. Abandon the operation and close the incision
    b. Ligate the hypogastric arteries
    c. Inflate a Foley balloon and place traction on it
    d. Divide the dorsal vein complex completely over the urethra and oversew the end

22. If a rectal injury occurs during the operation, what is the most certain way to avoid the development of a fistula with the fewest side effects?
    a. Loop colostomy
    b. End colostomy
    c. Hartman's pouch
    d. Interposition of omentum

23. In postoperative patients who require transfusions of blood for hypotension, what is the correct approach and why?
    a. Avoid re-exploration because it might damage the anastomosis
    b. Perform re-exploration of the patient to evacuate the hematoma in an effort to decrease the likelihood of bladder contracture
    c. Place the Foley catheter on traction
    d. Administer fresh frozen plasma

24. What is the most common cause of incontinence after radical prostatectomy?
    a. Intrinsic sphincter deficiency
    b. Detrusor instability
    c. Failure to reconstruct the bladder neck
    d. Injury to the neurovascular bundles

Answers

1. **c. The inferior vesical artery.** The prostate receives arterial blood supply from the inferior vesical artery. [p 3107]

2. **a. Capsular arteries and veins.** The capsular branches run along the pelvic sidewall in the lateral pelvic fascia posterolateral to the prostate, providing branches that course ventrally and dorsally to supply the outer portion of the prostate. Histologically, the capsular arteries and veins are surrounded by an extensive network of nerves. These capsular vessels provide the macroscopic landmark that aids in the identification of the microscopic branches of the pelvic plexus that innervate the corpora cavernosa. [p 3108]

3. **d. All of the above.** The major arterial supply to the corpora cavernosa is derived from the internal pudendal artery. However, pudendal arteries can arise from the obturator, inferior vesical, and superior vesical arteries. Because these aberrant branches travel along the lower part of the bladder

and anterolateral surface of the prostate, they are divided during radical prostatectomy. This may compromise arterial supply to the penis, especially in older patients with borderline penile blood flow. [p 3108]

4. **b. S2-S4.** The autonomic innervation of the pelvic organs and external genitalia arises from the pelvic plexus, which is formed by parasympathetic visceral efferent preganglionic fibers that arise from the sacral center (S2 to S4). [pp 3108-3109]

5. **d. Between the layers of the prostatic fascia and the levator fascia.** The neurovascular bundles are located in the lateral pelvic fascia *between* the prostatic and levator fasciae (see Fig. 90-4). [pp 3109-3110]

6. **c. The dorsal vein complex is not divided because the dissection occurs beneath the lateral fascia and anterior pelvic fascia.** In an effort to avoid injury to the dorsal vein of the penis and Santorini's plexus during radical perineal prostatectomy, the lateral fascia and anterior pelvic fascia are reflected off the prostate. This accounts for the reduced blood loss associated with radical perineal prostatectomy. [p 3109]

7. **d. The striated urethral sphincter.** The striated sphincter contains fatigue-resistant, slow-twitch fibers that are responsible for passive urinary control. [p 3111]

8. **c. The pudendal nerve.** The pudendal nerve provides the major nerve supply to the striated sphincter and levator ani. [p 3111]

9. **c. The obturator vessels.** The obturator artery and vein are skeletonized but are usually left undisturbed and are not ligated unless excessive bleeding occurs. At the completion of the dissection, the vasculature in the hypogastric and obturator fossa should be neatly skeletonized. [p 3112]

10. **d. Tributaries from the pudendal artery and veins.** The incision in the endopelvic fascia is carefully extended in an anteromedial direction toward the puboprostatic ligaments. At this point, one often encounters small arterial and venous branches from the pudendal vessels, which perforate the pelvic musculature to supply the prostate. These vessels should be ligated with clips to avoid coagulation injury to the pudendal artery and nerve, which are located just deep to this muscle as they travel along the pubic ramus. [p 3113]

11. **a. Superficially, with just enough excised to expose the junction between the anterior apex of the prostate and the dorsal vein complex.** The dissection should continue down far enough to expose the juncture between the apex of the prostate and the anterior surface of the dorsal vein complex at the point where it will be divided. The pubourethral component of the complex must remain intact to preserve the anterior fixation of the striated urethral sphincter to the pubis. [pp 3113-3114]

12. **c. Striated urethral sphincter; incontinence.** The goal is to divide the complex with minimal blood loss while avoiding damage to the striated sphincter. [p 3114]

13. **c. Apex; during division of the striated urethral sphincter-dorsal vein complex.** The exact plane on the anterior surface of the prostate can be visualized, avoiding inadvertent entry into the anterior prostate and ensuring minimal excision of the striated sphincter musculature. This is the most common site for positive surgical margins, because it can be difficult to identify the anterior apical surface of the prostate. [pp 3114-3115]

14. **c. The edges should be oversewn in the shape of a V to avoid advancing the neurovascular bundles too far anteriorly on the prostate.** To avoid back-bleeding from the anterior surface of the prostate, the edges of the proximal dorsal vein complex on the anterior surface of the prostate are sewn in the shape of a V with a running 2-0 chromic suture (see Fig. 90-11). If one tries to pull these edges together in the midline, the neurovascular bundles can be advanced too far anteriorly on the prostate. [pp 3115-3116]

15. **d. Posterior portion of the striated sphincter complex.** The posterior band of urethra is now divided to expose the posterior portion of the striated urethral sphincter complex. The posterior sphincter complex is composed of skeletal muscle and fibrous tissue. [p 3117]

16. **b. Use of a sponge stick to roll the prostate on its side.** When the surgeon releases the neurovascular bundle, there should be no upward traction on the prostate. Rather, the prostate should be rolled from side to side. [p 3118]

17. **a. Right-angle dissection beginning on the posterior surface of the prostate and dissecting anterolaterally.** After the plane between the rectum and prostate in the midline has been developed, it is possible to release the neurovascular bundle from the prostate, beginning at the apex and moving toward the base, by using the sponge stick to roll the prostate over on its side. Beginning on the rectal surface, the bundle is released from the prostate by spreading a right angle gently. With use of this plane, Denonvilliers' fascia and the prostatic fascia remain on the prostate; only the residual fragments of the levator fascia are released from the prostate laterally. [p 3118]

18. **c. When the prostate has been removed and tissue covering the posterolateral surface of the prostate is thought to be inadequate.** Clues that indicate that wide excision of the neurovascular bundle is necessary include inadequate tissue covering the posterolateral surface of the prostate once the prostate had been removed, leading to secondary wide excision of the neurovascular bundle. This last point is very important to understand. You do not have to make the decision about whether to excise or preserve the neurovascular bundle until the prostate is removed, and, if there is not enough soft tissue covering the prostate, you can excise the neurovascular bundle then. [p 3120]

19. **b. Posterior branch, traveling over the seminal vesicles to the base of the prostate.** The surgeon should look for a prominent arterial branch traveling from the neurovascular bundle over the seminal vesicles to supply the base of the prostate. This posterior vessel should be ligated on each side and divided. By this method, the neurovascular bundles are no longer tethered to the prostate and fall posteriorly. [p 3121]

20. **c. Releasing attachments of the bladder to the peritoneum.** The anterior suture is tied initially. There should be no tension. If there is, the bladder should be released from the peritoneum. [p 3125]

21. **d. Divide the dorsal vein complex completely over the urethra and oversew the end.** If there is troublesome bleeding from the dorsal vein complex at any point, the surgeon should completely divide the dorsal vein complex over the urethra and oversew the end. This is the single best means to control bleeding from the dorsal vein complex. Any maneuver short of this will only worsen the bleeding. To gain exposure for the prostatectomy, one must put traction on the prostate. If the dorsal vein is not completely divided, traction opens the partially transected veins and usually worsens the bleeding. [p 3126]

22. **d. Interposition of omentum.** It is wise to interpose omentum between the rectal closure and the vesicourethral anasto-

mosis to reduce the possibility of a rectourethral fistula. [p 3126]

23. **b. Perform re-exploration of the patient to evacuate the hematoma in an effort to decrease the likelihood of bladder contracture.** These results suggest that patients requiring acute transfusions for hypotension after radical prostatectomy should undergo exploration to evacuate the pelvic hematoma in an effort to decrease the likelihood of bladder neck contracture and incontinence. [p 3127]

24. **a. Intrinsic sphincter deficiency.** After radical prostatectomy, incontinence is usually secondary to intrinsic sphincter deficiency. [p 3127]

Chapter 91

Radical Perineal Prostatectomy

Robert P. Gibbons

Questions

1. How do outcomes after radical perineal prostatectomy compare with those after radical retropubic prostatectomy?
   a. They are comparable with regard to potency, pathologic outcomes, and cancer control rates.
   b. They are comparable with regard to cancer control rates, but pathologic outcomes and potency are not as good.
   c. They are comparable with regard to pathologic outcomes, but cancer control rates and potency are not as good.
   d. They are comparable with regard to potency, but pathologic outcomes and cancer control rates are not as good.
   e. They are not comparable with regard to potency, pathologic outcomes, and cancer control rates.

2. Compared with laparoscopic radical prostatectomy, radical perineal prostatectomy is:
   a. associated with more morbidity.
   b. associated with a longer hospital stay.
   c. technically demanding, with a steep learning curve.
   d. as easy to learn as retropubic prostatectomy.
   e. associated with a higher transfusion rate.

3. Technical advantages of radical perineal prostatectomy include which of the following?
   a. Dorsal vein complex transected under direct vision
   b. Clear exposure and access to pelvic lymph nodes
   c. Clear exposure and access to the apex of the prostate
   d. Avoidance of the need to perform a water-tight closure
   e. Can be performed without an assistant familiar with the procedure

4. Which of the following statements is true regarding pelvic lymphadenectomy?
   a. It is advised as a separate procedure to be performed before radical perineal prostatectomy.
   b. It is advised as a separate procedure to be performed at the same time as radical perineal prostatectomy.
   c. It is not advised to be performed with radical perineal prostatectomy.
   d. It can rarely be omitted because of the high incidence of positive lymph nodes in patients who are candidates for radical prostatectomy.
   e. It can often be omitted because of the low incidence of positive lymph nodes in patients who are candidates for radical prostatectomy.

5. Which of the following statements is true regarding a nerve-sparing radical perineal prostatectomy?
   a. It should not increase the risk of an iatrogenic positive margin.
   b. It is difficult because the neurovascular bundles are usually not visualized.
   c. It is necessary to preserve libido and the sensation of orgasm.
   d. It should be offered to only highly selected patients.
   e. It is necessary for any effective treatment program for erectile dysfunction.

6. Prehospital preparation for radical perineal prostatectomy includes which of the following?
   a. Admission to the hospital on the day of surgery after at-home "modified" bowel preparation
   b. Admission to the hospital the day before surgery for a full mechanical bowel preparation and intravenous fluids
   c. Routine collection of 2 units of autologous blood
   d. Discussion of an anticipated 5-day hospital course
   e. Initiation of low-molecular-weight heparin prophylaxis for deep venous thrombosis

7. Positioning and preparation of the patient for radical perineal prostatectomy include which of the following?
   a. Placement of sequential pneumatic compression devices
   b. Arm abducted at least 90 degrees for access by the anesthesiologist
   c. All pressure points well padded
   d. Shaving of the lower abdomen, the genitalia, and perineum
   e. Liberal use of the Trendelenburg position to maintain exposure

8. Initial steps of radical perineal prostatectomy include which of the following?
   a. Use of the Lowsley retractor to locate the placement of the incision
   b. Extending the initial skin incision through the superficial central tendon
   c. Incising the external rectal sphincter muscle fibers to improve exposure
   d. Incising the levator ani muscles laterally to improve exposure
   e. Keeping a moist, folded sponge placed over the exposed rectum for the duration of the procedure

9. The prostate is exposed:
   a. by using Deaver's retractors to stabilize the prostate.
   b. in the middle of the gland by retraction of rectourethralis muscle fibers.
   c. at its base adjacent to the bladder neck.
   d. at its apex adjacent to the urethra.
   e. by following the seminal vesicles to Denonvilliers' fascia.

10. In an extended wide-field radical perineal prostatectomy, which of the following statements is true?
    a. The anterior layer of Denonvilliers' fascia is left attached to the prostate.
    b. The posterior layer of Denonvilliers' fascia is left attached to the rectum.
    c. Both layers of Denonvilliers' fascia are left attached to the prostate.
    d. Both layers of Denonvilliers' fascia are left attached to the rectum.
    e. The neurovascular bundles are lateral to Denonvilliers' fascia at this stage of the procedure and are not susceptible to damage.

11. Which of the following statements is true regarding the neurovascular bundles?
    a. They are best identified after transection of the urethra.
    b. They are best identified while the apex of the prostate is being exposed.
    c. They are best identified while the lateral pedicles are being exposed.
    d. They are protected by both layers of Denonvilliers' fascia and are difficult to damage during the dissection of the rectum from this fascia.
    e. They are best preserved by transverse dissection of the plane between the two layers of Denonvilliers' fascia.

12. Exposure of the urethra is facilitated by:
    a. encircling the urethra with umbilical tape.
    b. the presence of the Lowsley retractor.
    c. division of the puboprostatic ligaments.
    d. division of the dorsal vein complex.
    e. retracting the neurovascular bundles medially.

13. Exposure of the anterior bladder neck is facilitated by:
    a. transection of the striated urethral sphincter.
    b. sharp dissection along the surface of the anterior prostate capsule.
    c. division of the dorsal vein complex.
    d. not dividing the puboprostatic ligaments.
    e. vertical orientation of the blades of the Lowsley retractor.

14. How is the prostate separated from the bladder neck?
    a. Sharply or with the cautery after the anterior bladder neck is opened
    b. Sharply or with the cautery after division of the trigone and placement of a ureteral catheter
    c. Sharply or with the cautery after exposure of the ampullae of the vas
    d. Sharply or with the cautery after mobilization of the seminal vesicles
    e. Bluntly without opening the bladder

15. How is the bladder reanastomosed to the urethra?
    a. Using a figure-of-eight suture placed in the manner of Jewett
    b. With interrupted sutures placed in a "tennis racquet" manner
    c. With interrupted sutures, beginning at the anterior bladder neck
    d. With a running suture, beginning at the posterior bladder neck
    e. Using the curved Lowsley retractor as a needle guide

16. A rectal injury that occurs during a radical perineal prostatectomy should:
    a. be repaired after completion of the bladder/urethral reanastomosis.
    b. be repaired at the time of injury.
    c. be repaired with a single layer of nonabsorbable suture.
    d. have the repair reinforced with omentum.
    e. have the repair followed by a diverting colostomy.

Answers

1. **a. They are comparable with regard to potency, pathologic outcomes, and cancer control rates.** One study described modifications to the perineal approach incorporating many of these observations, so that the two procedures are virtually identical with regard to potency and pathologic outcomes. Cancer control rates are likewise comparable. [p 3131]

2. **d. as easy to learn as retropubic prostatectomy.** Skillful laparoscopic surgeons note that laparoscopic radical prostatectomy is technically demanding, with a steep learning curve. Conversely, radical perineal prostatectomy can be learned at least as easily as retropubic prostatectomy. [p 3131]

3. **c. Clear exposure and access to the apex of the prostate.** Technical advantages include (1) clear exposure and access to the apex of the prostate to optimize the complete removal of this crucial margin and allow precise transection of the urethra; (2) generally less blood loss because it is not necessary to transect the dorsal vein complex; and (3) the vesicle-urethral anastomotic sutures can be tied under direct vision to perform a water-tight closure that is without tension and dependent. [p 3131]

4. **e. It can often be omitted because of the low incidence of positive lymph nodes in patients who are candidates for radical prostatectomy.** Most patients who are candidates for radical prostatectomy (clinically organ-confined disease) have a very low incidence of lymph node involvement. Tables that are based on clinical stage, grade, and prostate-specific antigen value are used to select the majority of these patients who do not "routinely" need a preliminary pelvic lymph node dissection. [p 3132]

5. **d. It should be offered to only highly selected patients.** In one pathologic analysis of 200 patients undergoing radical perineal prostatectomy, 15% had tumors completely penetrating the capsule but still confined to the specimen (an extended dissection including the adjacent posterolateral periprostatic fascia and enclosed neurovascular bundle was performed). In addition, 7% of the nerve-sparing dissections resulted in solitary, positive posterolateral margins. On the basis of this experience, these authors recommended an extended dissection, sacrificing the neurovascular bundle on each side, unless *all* of the following criteria are present: good potency with a strong desire by the patient to preserve it; acceptance by the patient of the discretionary risk of an iatrogenic positive margin; little or no clinically recognized

adjacent tumor (and none with a Gleason score of 7); and a neurovascular bundle that could be easily and cleanly dissected off the prostate. With these criteria, potency returned by 24 months in 70% of men who were fully potent before surgery. [p 3132]

6. **a. Admission to the hospital on the day of surgery after at-home "modified" bowel preparation.** Patients can have a regular diet up until midnight of the day before surgery. They take neomycin, 1.0 g orally, at 12:00, 14:00, 16:00, 18:00, and 20:00 hours on the day before surgery and give themselves a Fleet enema at 21:00 hours. This "modified" bowel preparation, along with the parenteral preoperative antibiotics and wound irrigation, has effectively prevented perineal wound infections even if fecal contamination occurs or a rectal repair is required. Patients are admitted to the hospital on the morning of surgery after this at-home preparation. [p 3133]

7. **c. All pressure points well padded.** Care is taken to be sure that any pressure points are well padded. Three-inch tape stretching between the stirrups and posterior to the rectum secures the position. [p 3133]

8. **e. Keeping a moist, folded sponge placed over the exposed rectum for the duration of the procedure.** An index finger is bluntly tunneled beneath the superficial central tendon and above the ventral wall of the rectum and the central tendon is transected (see Fig. 91–5C). A moist, folded sponge is placed over the exposed rectum for protection for the duration of the procedure. [pp 3134, 3138]

9. **d. at its apex adjacent to the urethra.** At this point, the handle of the Lowsley retractor is depressed and the prostate is rotated toward the incision until the apex of the prostate can be palpated as well as the adjacent urethra. With the Lowsley retractor stabilizing the prostate, the rectourethralis muscle is transected with scissors to the apex of the prostate (see Fig. 91–6). [pp 3134, 3138]

10. **c. Both layers of Denonvilliers' fascia are left attached to the prostate.** An extended wide-field radical dissection leaves both Denonvilliers' layers attached to the prostate. [p 3134]

11. **b. They are best identified while the apex of the prostate is being exposed.** The space between the lateral edge of the prostate and the adjacent fibers of the levator ani is bluntly exposed as an avascular plane and developed to the junction of the apex of the prostate and urethra on both sides (see Fig. 91–11). The neurovascular bundles are prominently seen at this point and are ligated and transected if this is an extended wide-field procedure. If this is a nerve-sparing procedure, the neurovascular bundles can be followed into the plane between the two layers of Denonvilliers' fascia, where they can be dissected out along their vertical course. [pp 3134, 3139]

12. **b. the presence of the Lowsley retractor.** The apex of the prostate and adjacent urethra can be readily palpated because of the presence of the Lowsley retractor. [pp 3136, 3140]

13. **e. vertical orientation of the blades of the Lowsley retractor.** The curved Lowsley retractor is replaced with the straight Lowsley retractor, which is placed into the transected urethra and rotated so that the bladder blades are in a vertical plane. [pp 3136, 3141]

14. **a. Sharply or with the cautery after the anterior bladder neck is opened.** The opening in the anterior bladder neck should be widened sufficiently to accept the middle finger. Then the lateral attachments of the prostate with the bladder neck can be safely incised, either sharply or with the cautery (see Fig. 91–16). This will ensure an optimal surgical margin at the bladder neck. [pp 3136, 3141]

15. **c. With interrupted sutures, beginning at the anterior bladder neck.** The urethra is anastomosed to the anterior bladder neck at the 12-, 1-, and 11-o'clock positions with interrupted sutures of 2-0 braided absorbable suture material with the knot tied on the outside of the lumen. [pp 3138, 3143]

16. **b. be repaired at the time of injury.** Rectal injuries are generally not a problem if the patient has had bowel preparation and the injury was noted and corrected intraoperatively. Injury is most likely to occur when the rectourethralis muscle is divided or the plane established between the rectum and prostate/seminal vesicles, and should be repaired immediately rather than delaying the repair until later in the procedure. [p 3142]

Chapter 92

Radiation Therapy for Prostate Cancer

Anthony V. D'Amico • Juanita Crook • Clair J. Beard • Theodore L. DeWeese • Mark Hurwitz
Irving Kaplan

Questions

1. An advance in the radiotherapeutic management of prostate cancer includes which of the following?
   a. Three-dimensional conformal technique and image guidance for radioactive source placement in the prostate gland
   b. The ability to deliver doses greater than 90 Gy
   c. Prostate immobilization techniques
   d. The ability to visualize and target microscopic disease by using optical imaging
   e. The ability to remove all uncertainty related to patient set-up

2. What are the three most important predictors of prostate-spe-

cific antigen (PSA) failure-free survival after external beam radiation therapy?

a. Patient's age, performance status, and weight
b. Patient's age, PSA level, and weight
c. PSA value, biopsy Gleason score, and clinical T stage
d. PSA value, biopsy Gleason score, and age
e. Biopsy Gleason score, age, and weight

3. The percentage of positive prostate biopsies is:

a. not an important predictor of PSA failure-free survival after external beam radiation therapy.
b. equal to the number of cores sampled divided by 100.
c. not an important predictor of PSA failure-free survival after radical prostatectomy.
d. able to identify the majority of patients at high risk or low risk for PSA failure after external beam radiation therapy who otherwise would be in an intermediate-risk group.
e. equal to the PSA value divided by the biopsy Gleason score.

4. Two years after definitive radiotherapy for prostate cancer, what should the serum PSA level be?

a. Undetectable
b. <0.5 ng/ml
c. Stable and not rising
d. Normal
e. None of the above

5. One year after radiotherapy, the serum PSA value has fallen to within the "normal range" (2.5 ng/ml) but then starts to rise, with subsequent readings of 3.5 and 5.1 ng/ml over a 6-month period. What would appropriate management be?

a. Tell the patient that radiotherapy has not worked and discuss salvage prostatectomy and cryosurgery.
b. Tell the patient that his PSA value is still normal and not to worry.
c. Tell the patient that he likely has a recurrence and that his rising PSA may indicate a distant component to the failure.
d. None of the above.
e. Both a and b.

6. With regard to the PSA nadir after radiotherapy, which of the following statements is true?

a. An early nadir is good.
b. Patients showing distant failure reach a nadir later.
c. Patients who are cured may take 24 to 30 months to reach a nadir.
d. A nadir greater than 0.5 ng/ml means that treatment has failed.
e. None of the above.

7. Prostate biopsy samples should be negative for disease by what time after radiotherapy?

a. 6 months
b. 12 months
c. 18 months
d. 30 months
e. None of the above

8. Which of the following statements is true regarding local control after radiation therapy for prostate cancer?

a. It is an unimportant end point because it does not predict for survival.
b. It is lower in patients with early disease because they receive lower doses of radiation.
c. It is equal for all types of radiation treatment.
d. It is associated with treatment technique and dose of radiation.
e. None of the above.

9. Which of the following statements is true regarding conformal radiation therapy?

a. It is available in almost all radiation centers.
b. It is more accurate than conventional radiation.
c. It is unassociated with improved outcomes in prostate cancer patients.
d. It is a form of particle therapy.
e. None of the above.

10. Which of the following statements is true regarding complications after radiation therapy?

a. They are related to treatment technique, type of radiation used, and total dose given.
b. They are identifiable in the majority of treated patients.
c. They are higher with dose escalation protocols.
d. They are lower with particle beam therapy.
e. None of the above.

11. Dose escalation trials using conformal radiation show improved outcomes at which of the following doses?

a. 60 Gy
b. 66 Gy
c. 70 Gy
d. Above 75 Gy
e. None of the above

12. Dose escalation trials show a benefit for all of the following groups except which one?

a. Patients with favorable tumors (T1 or T2, Gleason score of <7) and PSA levels of less than 10
b. Patients with favorable tumors (T1 or T2, Gleason score of <7) and PSA levels of greater than 20
c. Patients with unfavorable tumors (T2b or T3, Gleason score of >7) and PSA levels of less than 10
d. Patients with unfavorable tumors (T2b or T3, Gleason score of ≥7) and PSA levels of greater than 4
e. None of the above

13. Which of the following statements is true regarding particle beam therapy?

a. It has a theoretical advantage over photon therapy.
b. It has been shown to be more effective than photon therapy.
c. It is less expensive than photon therapy.
d. It is less toxic than photon therapy.
e. None of the above.

14. Which of the following statements is true regarding intensity-modulated radiation therapy?

a. It is a form of particle therapy.
b. It has been proved to improve treatment outcome.
c. It gives equal emphasis to the target tissue (prostate) and normal tissue (bladder and rectum) during treatment planning.
d. It can be delivered inexpensively because of software improvements.
e. None of the above.

15. With regard to complications of permanent implant brachytherapy, which of the following statements is true?

a. There is a higher rate of urinary toxicity than with external beam irradiation.
b. There is a higher rate of rectal toxicity than with external beam irradiation.

c. This therapy is associated with a higher rate of impotence than is radical prostatectomy.
d. This therapy is associated with a higher rate of impotence than is external beam irradiation.
e. None of the above.

16. Which of the following statements is true regarding high-dose-rate brachytherapy?

    a. It is usually delivered as monotherapy for advanced prostate cancer.
    b. It uses high-activity iodine-103 or paladium-103 (^{103}Pd) as the source.
    c. It does not require a surgical procedure.
    d. It is generally delivered in several fractions as a boost to external beam irradiation.
    e. None of the above.

17. When comparing iodine 125 (^{125}I) to ^{103}Pd, which of the following statements is true?

    a. ^{125}I has a shorter half-life than ^{103}Pd.
    b. ^{125}I delivers a significantly higher dose to the rectum when compared with ^{103}Pd.
    c. ^{125}I delivers a significantly higher dose to the urethra when compared with ^{103}Pd.
    d. The dose prescribed for a ^{125}I implant is higher than the dose for a ^{103}Pd implant.
    e. None of the above.

18. When prostate brachytherapy monotherapy is compared with a brachytherapy boost, which of the following statements is true?

    a. A higher implant dose is used with monotherapy than with the boost.
    b. Brachytherapy monotherapy is associated with a higher rate of rectal complications than is brachytherapy boost.
    c. Brachytherapy monotherapy is preferred for patients with preexisting urinary outlet obstruction.
    d. Brachytherapy monotherapy is preferred for larger glands.
    e. None of the above.

19. Prostate brachytherapy monotherapy is appropriate for which group of patients?

    a. Patients with T3 cancer
    b. All patients with T1c prostate cancer
    c. Patients with a high probability of having organ-confined disease
    d. Patients with a high probability of having organ-confined disease, prostates weighing less than 60 g, and low American Urological Association (AUA) symptom scores
    e. None of the above

20. MRI-guided prostate brachytherapy is able to provide optimal placement of the radioactive sources within the prostate gland for what reason?

    a. A real-time imaging mechanism permits the physician to verify that the trajectory of the catheter containing the radioactive sources is in the ideal location when compared with the pre-plan.
    b. The magnetic field aligns the sources perfectly.
    c. The procedure can be done under local anesthesia.
    d. A Foley catheter is not needed.
    e. Both a and b.

21. With MRI-guided prostate brachytherapy, patients with large prostate glands (>60 g) can have implants and still have very low acute urinary retention rates (4%) for what reason?

    a. MRI guidance allows for urethral sparing.
    b. With MRI guidance, one can put in fewer sources.
    c. A Foley catheter is not needed with MRI-guided brachytherapy.
    d. A cystoscopy is not performed with MRI-guided brachytherapy.
    e. The procedure can be performed with local anesthesia.

22. What is the principal reason for neoadjuvant androgen suppression before initiation of radiation therapy?

    a. To prevent early development of metastatic disease
    b. To reduce prostate size, thus minimizing the field size and side effects of external beam treatment
    c. To reduce the tumor burden requiring eradication with radiation
    d. To delay the need for radiation
    e. Because this approach has been shown to improve overall survival

23. For a patient with a Gleason score of 8, which of the following statements is best supported by the findings of phase III studies?

    a. Androgen suppression should always be used with radiation.
    b. Androgen suppression improves overall survival when used with radiation.
    c. Androgen suppression improves biochemical freedom from failure (bNED) survival when given in addition to standard dose radiation.
    d. Androgen suppression has no role in treatment based on this factor alone.
    e. Androgen suppression should be given for 4 months before radiation.

24. The findings of RTOG 92–02 indicate that when given in combination with radiation for T3 Gleason score 7 disease:

    a. prolonged adjuvant androgen deprivation provides added benefit as compared with neoadjuvant therapy alone.
    b. the optimal duration of androgen suppression with radiation is now defined.
    c. prolonged androgen deprivation results in improved overall survival.
    d. neoadjuvant androgen deprivation is sufficient.
    e. radiation alone is suboptimal therapy.

25. A patient has a history of hormone-refractory metastatic prostate cancer. He now has a new painful lesion of his upper femoral shaft. What is a typical course of palliative radiation therapy for this man?

    a. One fraction of radiation at 3000 cGy
    b. 7 weeks of daily radiation to 7000 cGy
    c. 10 fractions of daily radiation to 3000 cGy
    d. One fraction of radiation at 7000 cGy
    e. None of the above

26. A patient with a history of metastatic prostate cancer, under treatment with a luteinizing hormone-releasing hormone agonist and a nonsteroidal antiandrogen, presents to your office with a 3-week history of increasing middle to low back pain and 2 days of leg weakness. What is the most appropriate first step at this point?

    a. Increasing the dose of nonsteroidal antiandrogen
    b. MRI of the thoracic and lumbar spine
    c. Radiation therapy with a systemic radionuclide such as strontium-89
    d. Treatment with a selective COX-2 inhibitor for 5 to 7 days and re-evaluation
    e. None of the above

27. What is the most common toxicity of systemic radionuclide therapy with strontium-89 and samarium-153?

a. Hematologic toxicity, particularly with a decrement in the platelet count
b. Neurologic toxicity, including tinnitus
c. Genitourinary toxicity, particularly azotemia
d. Hepatic toxicity associated with an elevation of transaminase levels
e. None of the above

28. What would be an attractive gene therapy approach that could be combined with radiation for the treatment of prostate cancer?
a. One that requires prolonged transgene expression
b. One that kills cells by a mechanism that complements and does not overlap with radiation-induced cell death
c. One that requires all prostate cancer cells to be transduced
d. Both a and c
e. None of the above

Answers

1. **a. Three-dimensional conformal technique and image guidance for radioactive source placement in the prostate gland.** The first advance has been the generation of linear accelerators and conformal techniques capable of delivering high doses of radiation deep within the pelvis while simultaneously respecting the normal tissue tolerance of the anterior rectal wall, prostatic urethra, femoral heads, and bladder neck. The second advance was made when image-guided techniques were introduced for use during the insertion of radioactive sources directly into the prostate gland. [p 3147]

2. **c. PSA value, biopsy Gleason score, and clinical T stage.** The pretreatment prognostic factors that have established roles in predicting recurrence include the PSA value, biopsy Gleason score, and the 1992 American Joint Committee on Cancer Staging (AJCC) clinical stage. [p 3148]

3. **d. able to identify the majority of patients at high risk or low risk for PSA failure after external beam radiation therapy who otherwise would be in an intermediate-risk group.** Of particular importance is that the majority of patients (158/207 [76%]) in the intermediate-risk group could be classified into either a 30% or an 85% 5-year PSA control high- or low-risk cohort, respectively, by using the preoperative prostate biopsy data. [p 3149]

4. **c. Stable and not rising.** It is clear that there is no distinct PSA threshold that defines successful treatment, but that PSA stability after the nadir is important. [p 3149]

5. **c. Tell the patient that he likely has a recurrence and that his rising PSA may indicate a distant component to the failure.** The level of PSA nadir achieved to some extent reflects the type of failure. The median PSA nadir for patients exhibiting local failure is 2 to 3 ng/ml and for those exhibiting distant failure is 5 to 10 ng/ml. The postnadir doubling time of the PSA value also correlates with the type of failure, with distant failures having shorter PSA doubling times of 3 to 6 months and local failures having longer PSA doubling times of 11 to 13 months. [p 3150]

6. **c. Patients who are cured may take 24 to 30 months to reach a nadir.** The time to nadir has been shown to be inversely proportional to disease-free survival. The median time to nadir in patients who remain free from failure is 22 to 33 months, with 92% of men whose PSA value reached a nadir at 36 months or longer remaining disease free. [pp 3149–3150]

7. **d. 30 months.** In a series of 498 men followed with sequential systematic postradiotherapy biopsies, biopsy samples cleared at a mean time of 30 months after radiotherapy. [p 3151]

8. **d. It is associated with treatment technique and dose of radiation.** Tumor control was better in patients who received higher doses of radiation to larger fields, at the expense of increased complications. [p 3151]

9. **b. It is more accurate than conventional radiation.** The result is loosely described as *conformal* radiation therapy because the radiation beams conform to the shape of the treatment target. [p 3151]

10. **a. They are related to treatment technique, type of radiation used, and total dose given.** The percentage of patients who experience side effects and the severity of the side effects differ somewhat from series to series depending on the morbidity scale used and also on whether the assessment is physician or patient based (see Table 92–2). [pp 3152–3153]

11. **d. Above 75 Gy.** Dose escalation therapy, to doses greater than 75 Gy, is still experimental, but the early data appear to be highly favorable. [p 3154]

12. **a. Patients with favorable tumors (T1 or T2, Gleason score of <7) and PSA levels of less than 10.** Patients with favorable tumors (Gleason score of <6, T1 or T2a) who also had a PSA level of less than 10 ng/ml derived no benefit from dose escalation because all patients in this group did well. Patients with unfavorable tumors (Gleason score of 7 to 10, and T2b or T3) who also had a PSA level of greater than 20 ng/ml also derived no benefit from dose escalation. [p 3154]

13. **a. It has a theoretical advantage over photon therapy.** The heavy particle beams are difficult to produce and to control but have certain theoretical advantages over conventional x-ray and electron beams. [p 3156]

14. **c. It gives equal emphasis to the target tissue (prostate) and normal tissue (bladder and rectum) during treatment planning.** The goal of this method of treatment planning and delivery is to maximize treatment to the target, for example, the prostate, while minimizing treatment to the surrounding tissues to a degree that is not possible with conformal therapy. [p 3155]

15. **a. There is a higher rate of urinary toxicity than with external beam irradiation.** One study showed that 37% of patients report grade I urinary toxicity (symptoms not requiring medical intervention) within the first 60 days after implantation. Grade II urinary toxicity (requiring medical intervention), with a mean duration of 19 months after implantation and with a likelihood of resolution of 68% at 36 months, has been reported. Significant continued obstruction requiring self-catheterization occurs in 1% to 5% of patients. [pp 3161–3162]

16. **d. It is generally delivered in several fractions as a boost to external beam irradiation.** This therapy is delivered as a boost in two to four applications, either before or after external beam irradiation. [p 3162]

17. **d. The dose prescribed for a ^{125}I implant is higher than the dose for a ^{103}Pd implant.** Higher activity seeds are re-

quired for ^{103}Pd versus ^{125}I to deliver a similar tumoricidal dose (i.e., 1.3 mCi per palladium seed versus 0.4 mCi per iodine seed). [p 3158]

18. **b. Brachytherapy monotherapy is associated with a higher rate of rectal complications than is brachytherapy boost.** There is relatively little radiation delivered to the rectum with brachytherapy alone. However, the prostatic urethra receives a full dose. When an implant is combined with external beam therapy the dosage to the urethra is less, but increased radiation is received by the rectum. [p 3161]

19. **d. Patients with a high probability of having organ-confined disease, prostates weighing less than 60 g, and low American Urological Association (AUA) symptom scores.** Larger prostatic volumes—specifically, glands larger than 60.0 g—were associated with urinary toxicities. Other investigators reported that transurethral prostatic resection in the distant past is not a contraindication to implantation. Patients with a pretreatment AUA score higher than 20 demonstrated a 29% risk of developing urinary retention, whereas a pretreatment score of less than 10 was associated with a 2% risk. [p 3162]

20. **a. A real-time imaging mechanism permits the physician to verify that the trajectory of the catheter containing the radioactive sources is in the ideal location when compared with the pre-plan.** By using this technique, the three-dimensional trajectory that the catheter containing the radioactive sources traverses can be checked intraoperatively and compared, within a few seconds, with the ideal location based on the pre-plan using real-time MRI. [p 3159]

21. **a. MRI guidance allows for urethral sparing.** Therefore, despite implanting 45 men with glands greater than 60 g, the acute urinary retention rate was 4% and the need for prolonged use of oral α_{1a}-blockers was 5%, consistent with a urethral sparing technique. [pp 3160–3161]

22. **c. To reduce the tumor burden requiring eradication with radiation.** Short-duration neoadjuvant androgen suppression therapy may be used with the goal of reducing the local tumor burden requiring eradication by subsequent radiation. [p 3163]

23. **c. Androgen suppression improves biochemical freedom from failure (bNED) survival when given in addition to standard dose radiation.** Among strategies to improve outcome for patients with locally advanced prostate cancer, hormonal manipulation in combination with radiation therapy has consistently demonstrated improvement in treatment outcome as compared with standard-dose radiation alone. A meta-analysis of both retrospective and prospective trials of androgen deprivation in combination with radiation therapy demonstrated near-universal benefit in regard to local/regional control, disease-free survival, and bNED survival. [p 3163]

24. **a. prolonged adjuvant androgen deprivation provides added benefit as compared with neoadjuvant therapy alone.** The optimal type, timing, and duration of androgen suppression in combination with radiation therapy remains to be defined. In RTOG 92–02, patients with T2c-T4, N0-1, M0 disease were randomized to receive a total of 4 months of total androgen suppression with radiation administered after 2 months or the same regimen followed by an additional 2 years of goserelin. Subgroup analysis revealed significant improvement in overall survival for patients with Gleason scores 8 to 10. [p 3164]

25. **c. 10 fractions of daily radiation to 3000 cGy.** A frequently used regimen in the United States is to give 3000 cGy in 10 divided fractions. [p 3164]

26. **b. MRI of the thoracic and lumbar spine.** The diagnostic tool of choice to evaluate a spinal cord compression is MRI. [p 3165]

27. **a. Hematologic toxicity, particularly with a decrement in the platelet count.** Toxicity of strontium-89 is mainly hematologic. Platelet depression is dose dependent. [p 3165]

28. **b. One that kills cells by a mechanism that complements and does not overlap with radiation-induced cell death.** A rational combination of one these approaches with a more standard cytotoxic therapy such as radiation may provide superior cell killing as a result of nonoverlapping modes of cell death. [p 3166]

Chapter 93

Cryotherapy for Prostate Cancer

Katsuto Shinohara • Peter R. Carroll

Questions

1. Contemporary cryotherapy of the prostate gland has been most facilitated by which of the following?
   a. The availability of liquid nitrogen
   b. Transrectal ultrasonography (TRUS)
   c. Temperature monitoring of the prostate
   d. Androgen deprivation therapy
   e. Fluoroscopy

2. Which of the following statements concerning open cryosurgery of the prostate performed in the 1970s is true?
   a. It was performed through the retropubic approach.
   b. It resulted in low a complication rate.
   c. It achieved favorable results in terms of survival.
   d. It used thermosensors to monitor the freezing process.
   e. It was later reported to have a local recurrence rate of 15%.

3. What is the characteristic appearance of frozen tissue on ultrasonography?

   a. A hyperechoic area
   b. A hyperechoic rim with an acoustic shadow
   c. A hypoechoic area
   d. A mixed echogenic area
   e. An anechoic area

4. What is the most clinically important parameter of tissue ablation other than lowest temperature achieved by cryotherapy?

   a. The diameter of the probe
   b. The velocity of tissue freezing
   c. The velocity of tissue thawing
   d. The number of freeze/thaw cycles
   e. The duration of freezing

5. Prostate cell death is unlikely to occur completely until tissue temperature reaches what temperature?

   a. 0°C
   b. −20°C
   c. −40°C
   d. −60°C
   e. −80°C

6. A patient with Gleason's grade 3+3, clinical stage T1c prostate cancer associated with a serum prostate-specific antigen (PSA) value of 6.8 ng/ml is noted to have a prostate gland volume of 70 ml. Which of the following statements is accurate?

   a. This patient is best treated with cryosurgery.
   b. This patient requires transurethral resection of the prostate before cryosurgery.
   c. This patient requires neoadjuvant hormone therapy to downsize the gland before cryosurgery.
   d. This patient is likely to develop urinary tract obstruction after cryosurgery.
   e. This patient cannot undergo cryosurgery.

7. One year after cryosurgery for clinical stage T2a, PSA 7.0, Gleason's grade 3+3 cancer, a patient is found to have benign glands on a prostate biopsy specimen from the right apex. No malignancy is detected. His PSA level is detectable at 0.1 ng/ml. What is the next step in management?

   a. Repeat cryoablation of the right lobe
   b. Radiation therapy
   c. Surveillance
   d. Repeat the biopsy
   e. Androgen deprivation

8. Which parameter most accurately predicts for cancer control after cryotherapy?

   a. A PSA nadir less than 0.1 ng/ml
   b. Preoperative T stage
   c. A preoperative serum PSA value less than 15 ng/ml
   d. A preoperative Gleason score less than 6
   e. A prostate volume less than 40 ml

9. What is the likelihood of impotence after complete cryoablation of the prostate in men who were previously potent?

   a. 0% to 10%
   b. 20% to 30%
   c. 40% to 50%
   d. 60% to 70%
   e. 80% to 90%

10. Three months after cryotherapy, a patient complains of urinary frequency and dysuria. Urinalysis reveals pyuria. What is the most likely diagnosis?

    a. Pelvic abscess
    b. Bladder neck contracture
    c. Tissue sloughing
    d. Rectourethral fistula
    e. Extravasation of urine

Answers

1. **b. Transrectal ultrasonography (TRUS).** Use of TRUS for real-time monitoring of the freezing process, improved cryoprobes, and better understanding of cryobiology have all contributed to the resurgence of interest in cryosurgery. [p 3171]

2. **c. It achieved favorable results in terms of survival.** In an early report on the open transperineal approach to treat patients with various stages of prostate cancer, approximately 41% of patients eventually had evidence of persistent or recurrent disease. Although the technique compared favorably with other treatment modalities with respect to survival, morbidity was significant. Sloughing of urethral tissue was common. Urethrorectal or urethrocutaneous fistulas developed in 13% of patients, bladder neck obstruction in 2.3%, and urinary incontinence in 6.5%. This early experience was reviewed more recently: cancer recurrence was documented in 78.4% of the men, and 47.1% died of prostate cancer. Local recurrence was documented in at least 67% of those undergoing the procedure. [p 3172]

3. **b. A hyperechoic rim with an acoustic shadow.** The frozen area could be seen as a well-marginated hyperechoic rim with acoustic shadowing by ultrasonography. [p 3172]

4. **d. The number of freeze/thaw cycles.** In a clinical setting, the number of freezing cycles, the lowest temperature achieved, and the existence of any regional "heat sinks" may be more important factors relating to cancer destruction. Repeating a freeze/thaw cycle results in more extensive tissue damage compared with a single cycle. [p 3173]

5. **c. −40°C.** Complete cell death is unlikely to occur at temperatures higher than −20°C, and temperatures lower than −40°C are required to completely destroy cells. [p 3172]

6. **c. This patient requires neoadjuvant hormone therapy to downsize the gland before cryosurgery.** A gland in excess of 50 ml may be treated best with neoadjuvant androgen deprivation to reduce target volume and allow for more effective cryoablation. [p 3174]

7. **c. Surveillance.** Benign epithelium, often very focal, has been seen in up to 71% of patients after cryotherapy. The significance of benign epithelium is unknown, and such findings may represent areas of the prostate not frozen to low temperatures, perhaps in the area of the urethral warmer. [p 3177]

8. **a. A PSA nadir less than 0.1 ng/ml.** Biochemical failure (subsequent rise in PSA > 0.2 ng/ml) was lowest in those who achieved PSA nadirs less than 0.1 ng/ml (21%) but

was common in those with higher nadir values. Biopsy failure was lowest in those with nadirs less than 0.1 ng/ml (1.5%), followed by those with nadirs less than 0.4 ng/ml (10%). [p 3178]

9. **e. 80% to 90%.** More contemporary series report higher impotence rates of 80% or more. This is probably because of the use of multiple freeze/thaw cycles and extension of the ice ball beyond the prostate into the area of the neurovascular bundles. [p 3178]

10. **c. Tissue sloughing.** Tissue sloughing is manifested by irritative and obstructive voiding symptoms. Pyuria is noted as well. Urinary retention is not uncommon. This condition typically occurs 3 to 8 weeks after the procedure. [p 3179]

Chapter 94

Hormonal Therapy of Prostate Cancer

Fritz H. Schröder

Questions

1. Endocrine independence of prostate cancer is most likely caused by which of the following?
   a. A changing endocrine environment
   b. Genetic instability
   c. A preexisting population of independent cells
   d. A Western diet

2. Which of the following statements concerning prognostic factors is true?
   a. They have to be repeatedly evaluable.
   b. They have surrogate value in predicting survival.
   c. They are based on the pretreatment prostate-specific antigen (PSA) value.
   d. They correlate with outcome parameters.

3. Which of the following statements concerning survival of patients with metastatic prostate cancer is true?
   a. Survival is prolonged by endocrine treatment.
   b. Survival is longer if endocrine treatment is immediate.
   c. Survival amounts to 2.5 to 3.5 years.
   d. Survival is irrelevant as an end point because quality of life is decisive.

4. Which of the following statements concerning early endocrine treatment is true?
   a. It should be routinely applied to men with a rising PSA value.
   b. It has not been shown to be advantageous in men with a rising PSA value.
   c. It is not useful in conjunction with radiotherapy of T3 disease.
   d. It is the treatment of choice in all noncurable cases.

5. Which of the following statements concerning loss of libido and potency with endocrine treatment is true?
   a. It is inevitable in most men undergoing endocrine treatment.
   b. It is acceptable because most men at risk are inactive anyway.
   c. It is less pronounced with luteinizing hormone-releasing hormone (LHRH) agonists.
   d. It does not occur in 30% of men after castration.

6. Which of the following statements concerning side effects of endocrine treatment is true?
   a. They are usually mild and acceptable to patients.
   b. They always include gynecomastia.
   c. They depend on age at initiation of treatment and increase with duration of treatment.
   d. They are independent of the type of treatment used.

7. Castration is considered the "gold standard" of hormonal therapy for what reason?
   a. Its effect on plasma testosterone is immediate.
   b. It is cheap and easy to do.
   c. It has the least mental impact.
   d. No other treatment has been shown to produce longer survival.

8. What is the dosage of diethylstilbestrol (DES) that suppresses plasma testosterone to a castration level?
   a. 1 mg/day
   b. Less than 1 mg/day
   c. More than 1 mg/day
   d. It has never been studied.

9. Which of the following statements concerning side effects of estrogen treatment is true?
   a. They occur only after prolonged treatment (>1 year).
   b. They decrease with parenteral use.
   c. They differ from castration only with respect to cardiovascular problems.
   d. They are troublesome but usually not lethal.

10. LHRH agonist depots have become standard treatment for what reason?
    a. They avoid the mutilating effect of castration.
    b. They are cheap and easy to apply.
    c. They were shown to be superior to castration with respect to major end points.
    d. They have a more favorable profile of side effects than castration does.

11. The mechanism of action of pure and steroidal antiandrogens is different. Which of the following applies?

a. Steroidal antiandrogens are more potent than nonsteroidal ones.
b. Nonsteroidal antiandrogens raise luteinizing hormone (LH) and plasma testosterone levels and in this way preserve potency.
c. Steroidal antiandrogens are more toxic in recent comparative studies.
d. Steroidal antiandrogens are antigonadotropic (decrease LH + testosterone production).

12. Antiandrogens may be useful as monotherapy for what reason?
    a. They produce castration levels of testicular and adrenal androgens.
    b. They have been shown to be equally effective as castration.
    c. They have a more favorable profile of side effects during long-term use.
    d. They preserve potency.

13. "Antiandrogen rebound," or clinical or biochemical progression caused by the antiandrogen used, may be due to which of the following factors?
    a. The inherent androgenic activity of nonsteroidal antiandrogens
    b. Point mutations in the androgen receptor
    c. Amplification of the androgen receptor
    d. All of the above

14. Prostate cancer progression under antiandrogen treatment necessitates which of the following?
    a. A study of liver function tests
    b. An increase in the dosage
    c. A switch to another antiandrogen
    d. Discontinuation of the antiandrogen

15. The addition of an antiandrogen to castration in the treatment of metastatic prostate cancer is useful for what purpose?
    a. To prolong survival
    b. To prevent biochemical and clinical flares
    c. To prolong time to disease progression
    d. To prevent the progression to hormone-independent growth

16. Patients with M+ prostate cancer progress and die under endocrine treatment after median times of:
    a. 12 to 18 and 24 months, respectively.
    b. 24 and 48 months, respectively.
    c. 18 to 24 and 30 to 36 months, respectively.
    d. 24 to 30 and 36 to 42 months, respectively.

17. It does not make much sense to delay endocrine treatment in patients with bone metastases of prostate cancer for what reason?
    a. Benefit is limited because of a short time to disease progression.
    b. Side effects are minimal in such patients.
    c. It has been shown that early treatment prolongs survival.
    d. Cardiovascular side effects are seen only with longer treatment periods.

18. Clinical data indicate that early endocrine treatment may, if at all, prolong survival in which group of patients?
    a. Those with N+ and T3 disease
    b. Those with soft tissue metastases
    c. Those with rising PSA value after radiotherapy
    d. Those assigned to watchful waiting with first signs of progression

19. Which of the following statements concerning neoadjuvant endocrine treatment is true?
    a. It was shown to prolong the time to clinical progression after radical prostatectomy.
    b. It leads to a decrease of prostate volume of 30% to 40%.
    c. It improves overall survival in combination with radiotherapy.
    d. It has not been evaluated in randomized studies.

20. Future development of endocrine therapy must be directed toward which of the following?
    a. Improving maximal androgen blockade
    b. The implementation of early treatment whenever biochemical progression occurs
    c. Minimizing side effects in groups of patients requiring long-term treatment
    d. Patients with large primary tumors (because the prostate will shrink by 40%)

Answers

1. **c. A preexisting population of independent cells.** The observation that a favorable response to endocrine treatment is temporary was subsequently confirmed in every single clinical trial. Clinical observations and findings in experimental model systems that imitate human prostate cancer are compatible with the presence in the same tumor of hormone-dependent and hormone-independent populations of cells. [p 3182]

2. **d. They correlate with outcome parameters.** Both prognostic factors and criteria of response and progression are expected to show strong correlations with outcome, especially survival. [p 3185]

3. **c. Survival amounts to 2.5 to 3.5 years.** Endocrine treatment periods in cases of metastatic disease are compatible with the duration of survival of these patients and amount to 2.5 to 3.5 years. [p 3188]

4. **b. It has not been shown to be advantageous in men with a rising PSA value.** Randomized trials of endocrine treatment of locally confined, nonmetastatic disease or in patients with rising PSA values after potentially curative management are not available. These trials will be difficult to conduct because of the very long natural history and the absence of surrogate end points to replace overall survival. The question of whether early or delayed endocrine treatment is preferable in these cases is one of the debated open questions in this field. [p 3188]

5. **a. It is inevitable in most men undergoing endocrine treatment.** All types of endocrine treatment that decrease plasma testosterone to castration levels or interact with the androgen receptor at the target cell level have been shown to be associated with loss of libido and potency. [pp 3189–3190]

6. **c. They depend on age at initiation of treatment and increase with duration of treatment.** There is an increasing volume of evidence showing that osteoporosis is a phenome-

non of andropause and is strongly accentuated by castration. One study has shown a significant loss of bone mineral density (BMD) in men after orchiectomy for prostate cancer. The authors also showed that BMD loss increases beyond the period of 36 months. [p 3190]

7. **d. No other treatment has been shown to produce longer survival.** No other form of endocrine treatment was ever conclusively shown to be more effective than castration. [p 3191]

8. **c. More than 1 mg/day.** This finding was supported by observations of authors who found that DES at 1 mg/day would not suppress the diurnal variation of plasma testosterone when compared with a 3 mg/day regimen. [p 3193]

9. **b. They decrease with parenteral use.** It is believed that the cardiovascular side effects seen with the oral application of DES can be avoided by eliminating the necessity of the initial passage through the portal system and through the liver. [p 3193]

10. **a. They avoid the mutilating effect of castration.** The depot preparations obviously avoid the mutilating effect of castration. LHRH agonists have become standard forms of treatment for prostate cancer. [p 3194]

11. **d. Steroidal antiandrogens are antigonadotropic (decrease LH + testosterone production).** With steroidal antiandrogens, LH is suppressed and plasma testosterone levels fall with the use of pure antiandrogens. The rise of plasma testosterone is self-limiting at a level of about 1.5 times the normal plasma testosterone levels in intact males. [p 3195]

12. **c. They have a more favorable profile of side effects during long-term use.** With antiandrogens as monotherapy, osteoporosis, muscle wasting, and anemia may be expected to be absent or less pronounced than after castration or the use of LHRH agonists, which bring plasma testosterone to castration levels. [p 3196]

13. **b. Point mutations in the androgen receptor.** The mechanism of this paradoxical androgenic effect of flutamide and other antiandrogens is most likely due to proliferation of tumor cells with a mutated androgen receptor. [p 3199]

14. **d. Discontinuation of the antiandrogen.** Advice: If progression under maximal androgen blockade occurs, the antiandrogen, especially flutamide, should be discontinued. [p 3199]

15. **b. To prevent biochemical and clinical flares.** Antiandrogens in combination with LHRH analogues prevent the clinical signs of flare during initial use. [p 3199]

16. **c. 18 to 24 and 30 to 36 months, respectively.** EORTC studies 30805 and 30843 show that about half of the patients with metastatic disease progress after 18 to 24 months and die after 30 to 36 months. [p 3201]

17. **a. Benefit is limited because of a short time to disease progression.** Because of these short periods of median times, the question of early versus delayed treatment is of little relevance in this particular group of patients. [p 3201]

18. **a. Those with N+ and T3 disease.** The issue of early versus delayed endocrine treatment in locally extensive and lymph node–positive prostate cancer seems unresolved in spite of increasing evidence from one randomized study that early treatment may be advantageous in terms of survival. There is no question that early endocrine treatment delays disease progression. [pp 3202, 3203]

19. **b. It leads to a decrease of prostate volume of 30% to 40%.** The possibility of improving results of radical prostatectomy and radiotherapy by pretreating eligible patients by endocrine means (neoadjuvant treatment) is attractive and based on early observations that prostates containing cancer will shrink by about 40% within 3 to 6 months after castration. [p 3203]

20. **c. Minimizing side effects in groups of patients requiring long-term treatment.** Future developments and study efforts should concentrate on minimizing side effects in patients requiring long-term treatment. [pp 3203–3204]

Chapter 95

Management of Hormone-Resistant Prostate Cancer

Mario A. Eisenberger • Michael Carducci

Questions

1. The diagnosis of hormone-refractory prostate cancer is best characterized by which of the following?

   a. Clinically, by demonstration of disease progression after various sequential hormonal manipulations
   b. Evidence of a rising prostate-specific antigen (PSA) value after gonadal suppression
   c. Special molecular characterization of metastatic sites
   d. Slow and incomplete response to androgen deprivation treatment
   e. The extent of metastatic involvement and magnitude of PSA elevation

2. The most adequate approach for asymptomatic patients with evidence of disease progression after "combined androgen blockade" regimens (gonadal androgen suppression + nonsteroidal antiandrogen) is:

   a. discontinue the antiandrogen and wait 4 to 8 weeks for evidence of response; if the patient remains asymptomatic and his PSA continues to rise, restart the same antiandrogen.

b. restage (via bone scanning, computed tomography), identify the baseline PSA value, and discontinue antiandrogen; consider sequential endocrine manipulations (especially if the patient remains asymptomatic) before giving chemotherapy; monitor disease activity carefully by employing serial evaluations with scans and PSA assays.

c. restage as above and start chemotherapy.

d. discontinue antiandrogen and treat with a steroidal antiandrogen; treat with chemotherapy when the patient develops symptoms.

e. restage as above, discontinue antiandrogen, monitor PSA values, and treat with ketoconazole + prednisone until the patient becomes symptomatic.

3. The most adequate statement about antiandrogen withdrawal syndrome is:

   a. it has been reported only with nonsteroidal antiandrogens.
   b. typically, responses to antiandrogen withdrawal reflect symptomatic improvements after discontinuation of all androgen deprivation treatment.
   c. it represents evidence of a PSA decline and less frequently objective improvements (on physical examination, x-ray films, and scans) and/or symptomatic benefit. When it occurs, it is usually seen between 4 and 8 weeks after the discontinuation of steroidal and nonsteroidal antiandrogens.
   d. it is defined as major responses that occur in the majority of patients after discontinuation of steroidal and nonsteroidal antiandrogens.
   e. the median duration of the syndrome is 12 months.

4. Epidural cord compression represents one of the most devastating oncologic complications of solid tumors, particularly of metastatic prostate cancer. Which of the following statements reflects most accurately this clinical problem?

   a. It is always characterized by evidence of neuromotor dysfunction (in addition to pain).
   b. Radiation is given to symptomatic areas based on clinical findings.
   c. The presence of persistent back pain (of any character and nature) should raise the suspicion of neurologic compromise.
   d. If the pain is completely relieved by corticosteroids, radiation may not be necessary unless there is recurrence of symptoms.
   e. Narcotics should not be given because they may mask signs and symptoms.

5. Patients presenting with severe back pain, paraplegia, and neurogenic bowel or bladder symptoms of recent onset are best approached as follows:

   a. intravenous corticosteroids, external beam radiation therapy.
   b. oral corticosteroids, magnetic resonance imaging (MRI) of the spine, radiation therapy.
   c. intravenous corticosteroids, MRI of the entire spine, radiation to all involved areas.
   d. MRI of the entire spine, plain x-ray studies of the spine to assess bone stability, and intravenous corticosteroids, with consideration of immediate neurosurgical decompression of epidural masses or unstable vertebral bodies followed by postoperative radiotherapy.
   e. MRI of the entire spine, plain x-ray films of the spine, intravenous corticosteroids, immediate radiation therapy followed by surgical decompression or stabilization of epidural masses or fractured unstable vertebral bodies.

6. Which of the following considerations reflects most accurately the extent of metastasis in patients with hormone-refractory disease?

   a. Pulmonary involvement is fairly common and is usually associated with involvement of other visceral sites.
   b. Retroperitoneal nodal involvement is seen in approximately 20% of cases, and less than 10% have visceral (liver and lung) involvement. Visceral involvement is unlikely to be of major prognostic significance.
   c. Performance status, hemoglobin level, and extent of disease involvement are the stronger predictors of survival.
   d. The pretreatment PSA level is the most important prognostic factor for survival, and it always correlates well with the extent of disease.
   e. Neurologic problems are primarily due to brain metastasis.

7. Adequate pain control is a major management challenge in metastatic prostate cancer. Which approach is most likely to address this problem adequately?

   a. Aggressive management should be employed in cases of severe bone pain only.
   b. Aggressive pharmacologic regimens involving narcotic analgesics should always be used.
   c. The problem should be addressed in a stepwise fashion starting with non-narcotic drugs and changing to narcotics depending on the severity of symptoms.
   d. Pain is a multidisciplinary problem requiring a series of steps, including definition of the pain syndrome, assessment of the pattern and severity of symptoms using validated scales, and consideration of all available therapeutic options such as radiation, surgery, and pharmacologic treatment.
   e. Narcotics should be reserved for extreme cases only.

8. Adequate pain control can be accomplished with one or several combined approaches. Which is the least effective option in terms of risk-benefit ratio?

   a. systemic chemotherapy.
   b. "spot" radiotherapy to painful areas.
   c. high-dose systemic corticosteroids.
   d. systemic radiopharmaceuticals.
   e. whole body radiotherapy.

9. Taxane-based regimens have consistently shown activity in patients with metastatic disease. Which of the following is the least likely toxicity associated with these regimens?

   a. Neurotoxicity (usually cumulative).
   b. Hypersensitivity reactions, myalgias, hypotension (associated with the drug vehicle Cremophor).
   c. Nephrotoxicity.
   d. Myelotoxicity.
   e. Alopecia.

10. Given below are supportive measures employed to prevent or ameliorate toxicities related to chemotherapy except for:

    a. hematopoietic growth factors (granulocyte/macrophage colony-stimulating factor) shorten the duration of chemotherapy-induced neutropenia and may reduce the incidence of neutropenic fever.
    b. prophylactic use of corticosteroids, antihistamines, and H_2 receptor antagonists significantly reduces the incidence and severity of taxane- or Cremophor-induced hypersensitivity reactions.
    c. serotonin antagonists and corticosteroids are extremely effective in the prophylaxis and control of platinum-induced nausea and vomiting.
    d. hematopoietic growth factors reduce the severity of thrombocytopenia and bleeding episodes.

e. aggressive oral care with antiseptic mouthwash preparations, local anesthetics, or systemic analgesics for odynophagia and topical or systemic antifungal preparations represent the method of choice to control moderately severe mucositis.

11. Which of the following clinical pictures most adequately illustrates a partial clinical response (benefit) to chemotherapy?

    a. Reduction of a liver metastasis by 30%
    b. Complete relief of pain
    c. Reduction of the rate of rise of PSA value (decrease in the PSA velocity by 50% or more), stabilization of bone scan, and soft tissue visceral metastasis
    d. A 50% decline in the PSA value for 2 weeks, with some improvements in nonmeasurable soft tissue lesions and bone scan findings compared with the baseline
    e. Significant pain relief; some improvement in the bone scan; 60% decline of the PSA value for longer than 8 weeks; and no appearance of new lesions on the physical examination, x-ray films, and scans

12. Which of the following statements best describes the utility of PSA as a marker in the assessment of therapeutic benefits to chemotherapy?

    a. A 50% decline in PSA during chemotherapy has been shown to represent a surrogate for survival.
    b. PSA is considered the best outcome measure for randomized trials.
    c. PSA can be used as a surrogate for response in phase II trials, but the ultimate benefit is measured by survival impact in phase III studies.
    d. Changes correlate with any type of benefit, and a rise equals progression.
    e. PSA secretion always accurately reflects disease activity and is not affected by drugs.

13. The combination of mitoxantrone + prednisone has shown the following benefits in patients with hormone-refractory prostate cancer:

    a. prolonged survival compared with prednisone alone.
    b. higher measurable response rates than prednisone.
    c. higher PSA response rates and better pain control than prednisone alone.
    d. higher PSA response than mitoxantrone alone.
    e. severe toxicities.

14. Target-oriented treatment is represented by all of the following except:

    a. treatment approaches aimed at specific molecular pathways involved in tumor cell proliferation and apoptosis.
    b. inhibition of tumor angiogenesis can be accomplished by agents targeted at various molecular and cellular elements, including drugs and antibodies that interfere with the signal transduction of growth factors such as vascular endothelial growth factor (VEGF), platelet-derived growth factor (PDGF), basic fibroblast growth factor (FGF), and endothelial cell structure and function.
    c. tumor-specific antigens with gene-based vaccines and antibodies.
    d. differentiation therapy that interferes with specific proliferation of molecular targets such as butyrates, retinoids, and vitamin D analogues, among others.
    e. sophisticated tumor embolization approaches based on imaging techniques.

Answers

1. **a. clinically, by demonstration of disease progression after various sequential hormonal manipulations.** There is an increasing body of data on the experience of second-line endocrine manipulations in patients with evidence of disease progression after initial androgen deprivation, which suggests that there may be a role for this approach before institution of chemotherapy. [p 3212]

2. **b. restage (via bone scanning, computed tomography), identify the baseline PSA value, and discontinue antiandrogen; consider sequential endocrine manipulations (especially if the patient remains asymptomatic) before giving chemotherapy; monitor disease activity carefully by employing serial evaluations with scans and PSA assays.** The first step should involve the discontinuation of these agents and careful observation including serial monitoring of PSA levels for a period of 4 to 8 weeks before embarking on the next therapeutic maneuver. [p 3212]

3. **c. it represents evidence of a PSA decline and less frequently objective improvements (on physical examination, x-ray films, and scans) and/or symptomatic benefit. When it occurs, it is usually seen between 4 and 8 weeks after the discontinuation of steroidal and nonsteroidal antiandrogens.** The interpretation of some studies is confounded by the previously unrecognized antiandrogen withdrawal syndrome. This syndrome is characterized by a decrease in PSA value and less frequently objective reductions of measurable tumors, after the discontinuation of the antiandrogens (steroidal and nonsteroidal), and this may have contributed to some of the clinical responses reported with some of the chemotherapeutic regimens developed in the early 1990s. Typically, after discontinuation of the antiandrogen, there may be a decline in PSA value, and less commonly other symptomatic and/or objective evidence of disease improvement, which typically has a short median duration (approximately 3 months). A prospective evaluation of patients with stage D_2 disease treated with flutamide suggests that the actual incidence of flutamide withdrawal response is lower (15%) than previously reported retrospectively and that it may be enhanced by the use of corticosteroids. [pp 3215–3216]

4. **c. the presence of persistent back pain (of any character and nature) should raise the suspicion of neurologic compromise.** Among the most important complications in oncology is the development of epidural cord compression. Because of the frequent involvement of vertebral bodies by prostate cancer, the incidence of cord compression is particularly prominent. The spectrum of clinical manifestations in epidural cord compression includes pain, sensory abnormalities, and progressive motor changes including the devastating development of loss of sphincter control of the bladder and bowel, which may result in stool and urinary incontinence. The presence of significant back pain in patients with extensive vertebral bone involvement is frequently the first sign. [p 3211]

5. **d. MRI of the entire spine, plain x-ray studies of the spine to assess bone stability, and intravenous corticosteroids, with consideration of immediate neurosurgical decompression of epidural masses or unstable vertebral bodies followed by postoperative radiotherapy.** Early rec-

ognition and an aggressive therapeutic posture coupled with the widespread availability of noninvasive procedures such as MRI provide the opportunity for a more effective management of this potentially hazardous complication. The emergency management of these patients includes the administration of high-dose parenteral corticosteroids, external beam radiation, and surgical decompression with spinal stabilization. [p 3211]

6. **c. performance status, hemoglobin level, and extent of disease involvement are the stronger predictors of survival.** Clinical involvement of visceral sites is relatively uncommon even in patients with widespread hormone-resistant disease. Table 95–1 illustrates the distribution of metastatic sites reported in different series included in chemotherapy phase II trials. These figures suggest that clinical evidence of visceral metastasis is observed in less than 10% of patients, whereas about 20% have demonstrable soft tissue nodal disease. Because patients with visceral involvement usually have a less satisfactory clinical outcome than those with soft tissue nodal disease, separation of these two groups (visceral versus nodal involvement) may be important for the evaluation of treatment responses in patients with measurable disease sites. [pp 3210–3211]

7. **d. pain is a multidisciplinary problem requiring a series of steps, including definition of the pain syndrome, assessment of the pattern and severity of symptoms using validated scales, and consideration of all available therapeutic options such as radiation, surgery, and pharmacologic treatment.** Cancer-related pain is undoubtedly the most debilitating symptom associated with metastatic prostatic carcinoma. Prompt recognition of the various pain syndromes associated with this disease is crucial to accomplish effective control of this devastating symptom. Table 95–9 describes the most common pain syndromes and their respective therapeutic considerations. [pp 3219–3220]

8. **e. whole body radiotherapy.** Initial management strategies of various pain syndromes include pharmacologic treatment, localized radiotherapy, "multispot" or wide field radiotherapy, radiopharmaceuticals, high-dose corticosteroids, surgery, and neurolytic procedures. [p 3220]

9. **c. nephrotoxicity.** Corticosteroids are used with taxanes to prevent and minimize the incidence of anaphylactic reactions (Tables 95–6 and 95–7). Toxicities associated with these regimens include hematologic effects, mucositis, nausea and vomiting, edema, deep venous thrombosis, fatigue, and diarrhea. [pp 3214, 3216, 3217]

10. **d. hematopoietic growth factors reduce the severity of thrombocytopenia and bleeding episodes.** Studies referenced in Tables 95–6 and 95–7 describe the use of hematopoietic growth factors; the prophylactic use of corticosteroids, antihistamines, and H_2 receptor antagonists; the use of serotonin antagonists and corticosteroids; and aggressive oral care. [p 3214]

11. **e. significant pain relief; some improvement in the bone scan; 60% decline of the PSA value for longer than 8 weeks; and no appearance of new lesions on the physical examination, x-ray films, and scans.** Consensus guidelines include the following: patient eligibility: an increase in measurable sites, new bone scan lesions, a PSA value of 5 ng/ml or greater for patients with no measurable disease, two consecutive rises in PSA values at least 1 week apart, progression after antiandrogen withdrawal, and evidence of castrate testosterone levels; responses: objective (measurable responses), and PSA level decline by 50% or more confirmed 4 weeks later; progression: one or more new lesions on a bone scan, an increase or new measurable lesions, an increase in PSA level by 25% over the baseline or by 50% over the nadir. [p 3213]

12. **c. can be used as a surrogate for response in phase II trials, but the ultimate benefit is measured by survival impact in phase III studies.** Table 95–3 illustrates selected phase III trials reported in patients with hormone-resistant disease. These data demonstrate that none of the chemotherapeutic regimens tested on these trials was shown to be superior to another with regard to survival despite the fact that the incidence of PSA responses (defined as 50% or more decline in PSA for longer than 4 weeks), subjective benefits, and time to progression have been shown to be significantly improved in favor of some treatment arms. [p 3218]

13. **c. higher PSA response rates and better pain control than prednisone alone.** Significant palliative benefits could be attributed to the corticosteroid alone. However, in a prospective randomized comparison of mitoxantrone plus prednisone versus prednisone alone, the combination resulted in significant improvements of various quality of life issues. Interestingly, however, survival was not significantly different between the treatment arms. This study represents the first randomized comparison designed specifically for the evaluation of an end point that has been a major focus of attention over the past decade. However, the significance and impact of such assessments obviously require additional scrutiny in carefully designed clinical trials. [p 3216]

14. **e. sophisticated tumor embolization approaches based on imaging techniques.** The increased understanding of molecular mechanisms involved in the complexities of cancer cell proliferation and differentiation has resulted in several new compounds targeting important molecular steps, which are in active clinical development at the present time. The process of tumor angiogenesis may be inhibited by various mechanisms and some compounds are in active stages of development, such as TNP-470, CM-101, thalidomide, tecogalan, angiostatin, endostatin, anti-VEGF antibodies, small molecules designed to block important signal transduction steps of various growth factors such as VEGF, FGF, and PDGF, and anti-integrin therapies (small molecules or humanized antibodies) are actively undergoing preclinical and clinical testing. Suramin, which has known activity against prostate cancer, has been shown to inhibit binding of basic FGF and also significant antiangiogenesis properties. Tumor vaccines acting as tumor-specific immune stimulants or designed to replace critical molecularly altered genes or gene products identified under the umbrella of gene therapy have been shown to be feasible treatments, which are in active development in patients with various malignancies including prostate cancer. Differentiation therapy involves the use of different drugs that are able to affect the proliferation of tumor cells. Among agents with significant differentiating activity in vitro are the retinoids, vitamin D derivatives, and butyrates. [pp 3221–3222]

SECTION XII

URINARY LITHIASIS AND ENDOUROLOGY

Chapter 96

Urinary Lithiasis: Etiology, Diagnosis, and Medical Management

Mani Menon • Martin I. Resnick

Questions

1. Which pattern of inheritance has been postulated for kidney stones?

   a. Autosomal dominant
   b. Polygenic with partial penetrance
   c. Sex-linked recessive
   d. None
   e. Autosomal recessive

2. The evidence of urinary lithiasis peaks at which of the following age ranges?

   a. 10 to 30 years
   b. 20 to 40 years
   c. 30 to 50 years
   d. 40 to 60 years
   e. 50 to 70 years

3. Calcium oxalate stones predominate in which region of the United States?

   a. Northeast
   b. Midwest
   c. West
   d. Southwest
   e. Southeast

4. Which factor is involved with water intake and urolithiasis?

   a. Volume ingested
   b. Mineral content
   c. Trace element content
   d. All of the above
   e. None of the above

5. What is the point at which nucleation occurs in pure solutions?

   a. Formation product
   b. Concentration product
   c. Solubility product
   d. Saturation ratio
   e. Concentration product ratio

6. What is the process by which nucleation occurs in pure solutions?

   a. Homogeneous nucleation
   b. Heterogeneous nucleation
   c. Epitaxy
   d. Aggregation
   e. Agglomeration

7. The theory of stone formation called the fixed particle hypothesis refers to which process?

   a. Adherence of crystals to glomeruli
   b. Adherence of crystals to the renal tubule
   c. Adherence of crystals to calyces
   d. Adherence of crystals to the renal pelvis
   e. Adherence of crystals to the ureter

8. Inhibitors of calcium oxalate crystal formation present in urine include which of the following?

   a. Citrate
   b. Pyrophosphate
   c. RNA fragments
   d. Glucosamine
   e. All of the above

9. What is the proteinaceous component of stones called?

   a. Concentric lamination
   b. Protein-crystal complex
   c. Matrix
   d. Nephrocalcin
   e. Osteocalcin

10. Approximately what percentage of dietary calcium is absorbed?

    a. 10% to 25%
    b. 20% to 35%
    c. 30% to 45%
    d. 40% to 55%
    e. 50% to 65%

11. Calcium is maximally absorbed in which portion of the gastrointestinal tract?

    a. Stomach
    b. Jejunum
    c. Jejunum and proximal ileum
    d. Ileum
    e. Ascending colon

12. Which vitamin D metabolite stimulates intestinal calcium absorption?

    a. 1,25-dihydroxyvitamin D
    b. 1,25-dihydroxyvitamin D_1
    c. 1,25-dihydroxyvitamin D_2
    d. 1,25-dihydroxyvitamin D_3
    e. 1,25-dihydroxyvitamin D_4

13. Which hormone is responsible for regulating renal phosphate reabsorption?

    a. Parathyroid hormone
    b. Thyroxine
    c. Cortisol
    d. Nephrocalcin
    e. Calcitrol

14. What percentage of urinary oxalate is derived from endogenous production in the liver?

    a. 40%
    b. 50%
    c. 60%
    d. 70%
    e. 80%

15. Metabolic acidosis can result from a defect in which of the following?

    a. Acid excretion
    b. Bicarbonate excretion
    c. Acid or bicarbonate excretion
    d. Acid reabsorption
    e. Acid or bicarbonate reabsorption

16. What effect does metabolic acidosis have on citrate metabolism?

    a. It reduces citrate excretion.
    b. It increases citrate excretion.
    c. It reduces citrate reabsorption.
    d. It increases citrate reabsorption.
    e. It has no effect.

17. What is normal urinary cystine excretion?

    a. Less than 10 mg/day
    b. Less than 20 mg/day
    c. Less than 30 mg/day
    d. Less than 40 mg/day
    e. Less than 50 mg/day

18. What are the types of hypercalciuria?

    a. Resorptive and absorptive
    b. Absorptive and renal
    c. Renal and resorptive
    d. Resorptive, absorptive, and renal
    e. None of the above

19. What is the underlying abnormality of renal hypercalciuria?

    a. Enhanced calcium filtration
    b. Enhanced calcium secretion
    c. Enhanced calcium reabsorption
    d. Primary renal wasting of calcium
    e. Primary renal storage of calcium

20. What is the prevalence of stone disease in patients with hyperparathyroidism?

    a. 1%
    b. 5%
    c. 10%
    d. 15%
    e. 20%

21. In the inpatient setting, what is the most common cause of hypercalciuria?

    a. Injection
    b. Immobilization
    c. Malignancy
    d. Endocrine disorder
    e. Medical induction

22. Sarcoidosis is associated with hypercalciuria for which of the following reasons?

    a. Absorptive hypercalciuria
    b. Renal hypercalciuria
    c. Resorptive hypercalciuria
    d. Acidosis
    e. Medical induction

23. Varied conditions can result in hypercalcemia; these include which of the following?

    a. Hyperthyroidism
    b. Glucocorticoid excess
    c. Pheochromocytoma
    d. Immobilization
    e. All of the above

24. What are the hereditary characteristics of primary hyperoxaluria?

    a. Autosomal dominant
    b. Autosomal recessive
    c. Sex-linked recessive
    d. Polygenic with full penetrance
    e. Polygenic with partial penetrance

25. What is the primary cause of enteric hyperoxaluria?

    a. Excessive intake of oxalate
    b. Reduced excretion of oxalate
    c. Increased fat in the diet
    d. Decreased fat in the diet
    e. Malabsorption

26. Postulated causes of increased oxalate excretion include which of the following?

    a. Increased filtration of oxalate
    b. Increased secretion of oxalate
    c. Increased dietary protein intake
    d. Decreased dietary protein intake
    e. Decreased dietary carbohydrate intake

27. Hyperuricosuria has been reported to occur in what percentage of calcium oxalate stone formers?

    a. 5% to 30%
    b. 10% to 40%
    c. 20% to 50%
    d. 30% to 60%
    e. 40% to 70%

28. What is the primary mechanism of action of citrate in preventing stones?

    a. Reducing the excretion of calcium
    b. Reducing the excretion of oxalate
    c. As a complexing agent of calcium

d. As a complexing agent of oxalate
e. As a complexing agent of phosphate

29. Typically, hypomagnesuria is associated with what other abnormality?

    a. Hypercalciuria
    b. Hyperoxaluria
    c. Hyperuricosuria
    d. Hypocitraturia
    e. Renal tubular acidosis

30. Type I (distal) renal tubular acidosis (RTA) is characterized by which abnormality?

    a. Hyperkalemia
    b. Hypochloremia
    c. Alkalosis
    d. Hypercitraturia
    e. None of the above

31. What is the primary defect of type II (proximal) RTA?

    a. Failure of bicarbonate reabsorption in the glomerulus
    b. Failure of bicarbonate reabsorption in the proximal tubule
    c. Failure of bicarbonate reabsorption in the loop of Henle
    d. Failure of bicarbonate reabsorption in the distal tubule
    e. Failure of bicarbonate reabsorption in the collecting duct

32. The most common abnormality identified in patients with uric acid stones is:

    a. acidic urine.
    b. alkaline urine.
    c. low uric acid concentration.
    d. high uric acid concentration.
    e. RTA.

33. The factors influencing uric acid stone formation include which of the following?

    a. Urinary pH
    b. Urinary concentration of uric acid
    c. Uric acid excretion
    d. All of the above
    e. None of the above

34. Approximately what percentage of patients with gout form uric acid stones?

    a. 5%
    b. 10%
    c. 15%
    d. 20%
    e. 25%

35. Urease-producing bacteria hydrolyze urea to which of the following?

    a. Uric acid
    b. Carbon monoxide
    c. Carbon dioxide
    d. Ammonium
    e. Carbon dioxide and ammonium

36. Antibiotics are ineffective in treating struvite stones for what reason?

    a. Resistant bacteria
    b. Poor excretion of antibiotics
    c. Ineffective antibiotics
    d. Bacteria inaccessible to antibiotics
    e. Antibiotics inactivated by the stone

37. Acetohydroxamic acid, a urease inhibitor, has been used to treat patients with struvite stones. Side effects include which of the following?

    a. Deep venous thrombosis
    b. Hypertension
    c. Hypotension
    d. Visual disturbance
    e. Cardiac toxicity

38. What is the occurrence of homozygous cystinuria in the United States?

    a. 1 per 5000 population
    b. 1 per 10,000 population
    c. 1 per 15,000 population
    d. 1 per 20,000 population
    e. 1 per 25,000 population

39. Adverse reactions to D-penicillamine include which of the following?

    a. Constipation
    b. Diarrhea
    c. Melena
    d. Visual disturbance
    e. Liver toxicity

40. Indinavir stones result from treating which of the following diseases?

    a. Coronary artery insufficiency
    b. Crohn's disease
    c. Ulcerative colitis
    d. HIV-1 infection
    e. Emphysema

41. Stones generally do not pass spontaneously if they are larger than what size?

    a. 2 mm
    b. 3 mm
    c. 4 mm
    d. 5 mm
    e. 6 mm

42. Which of the following studies is replacing intravenous urography in the initial evaluation of patients presenting with renal colic?

    a. Kidney, ureter, and bladder study
    b. Renal tomography
    c. Ultrasonography
    d. CT
    e. MRI

43. Acute obstruction secondary to a ureteral stone results in which of the following?

    a. Decreased renal function
    b. Increased citrate excretion
    c. Increased calcium excretion
    d. Increased phosphate excretion
    e. Increased uric acid excretion

44. Which of the following is the least accurate method of stone analysis?

    a. Chemical analysis
    b. X-ray diffraction
    c. Polarizing microscopy
    d. Infrared spectroscopy
    e. Magnetic resonance spectroscopy

45. A diet high in meat results in all but which of the following?

    a. Increased calcium excretion
    b. Increased uric acid excretion
    c. Decreased citrate excretion
    d. Increased oxalate excretion
    e. Increased urinary pH

46. What is the most common renal structural abnormality identified in patients with calcium-containing stones?
    a. Ureteropelvic junction obstruction
    b. Infundibular obstruction
    c. Calyceal obstruction
    d. Medullary sponge kidney
    e. Proximal tubule obstruction

47. Twenty-four-hour analysis of urine to identify causative factors in calcium stone formation should include at a minimum all but which of the following?
    a. Calcium
    b. Phosphorus
    c. Uric acid
    d. Oxalate
    e. Sulfate

48. What is the reported recurrence rate for patients with untreated calcium stones?
    a. 2% per year
    b. 7% per year
    c. 12% per year
    d. 15% per year
    e. 18% per year

49. Patients with urolithiasis should preferably increase urinary output to what volume?
    a. 500 ml/day
    b. 1 L/day
    c. 2 L/day
    d. 3 L/day
    e. 4 L/day

50. Potential effects of severe dietary restriction of calcium include which of the following?
    a. Osteoporosis
    b. Decreased oxalate excretion
    c. Increased uric acid excretion
    d. Decreased uric acid excretion
    e. Increased citrate excretion

51. What percentage of urinary oxalate comes from dietary sources?
    a. 5%
    b. 10%
    c. 15%
    d. 20%
    e. 25%

52. Thiazide diuretics exert their effect by:
    a. reducing sodium resorption in the proximal tubule.
    b. reducing phosphate resorption in the distal tubule.
    c. enhancing phosphate resorption in the proximal tubule.
    d. enhancing calcium resorption in the distal tubule.
    e. reducing calcium resorption in the proximal tubule.

53. Which excretory change results from neutral or alkaline phosphate therapy?
    a. Decreased citrate excretion
    b. Increased calcium excretion
    c. Increased pyrophosphate excretion
    d. Increased uric acid excretion
    e. Decreased urinary pH

54. Allopurinol inhibits which of the following enzymes?
    a. Ribonuclease
    b. Urease
    c. Xanthine oxidase
    d. Ornithine decarboxylase
    e. Calcium phosphatase

55. Potassium citrate is commonly used in preference to sodium citrate in the treatment of patients with calcium stones and hypocitraturia for what reason?
    a. Sodium citrate enhances uric acid excretion.
    b. Sodium citrate increases oxalate excretion.
    c. Sodium citrate does not affect citrate excretion.
    d. Sodium citrate does not lower urinary calcium excretion.
    e. Sodium citrate increases phosphorus excretion.

56. What is the most common composition of vesical calculi in noninfected urine?
    a. Calcium oxalate
    b. Calcium phosphate
    c. Struvite
    d. Cystine
    e. Uric acid

57. Prostate calculi are most commonly composed of which of the following?
    a. Calcium oxalate
    b. Calcium phosphate
    c. Struvite
    d. Cystine
    e. Uric acid

58. Typically, stone formation in very low birth weight infants is attributed to which of the following?
    a. Dehydration
    b. Infection
    c. Furosemide
    d. High oxygen levels
    e. Antibiotics

59. What is the most common anatomic abnormality in children that is believed to be responsible for stone formation?
    a. Calyceal obstruction
    b. Infundibular obstruction
    c. Ureteropelvic obstruction
    d. Ureteral obstruction
    e. Ureterovesical obstruction

60. What is the rate of stone passage of pregnant women with ureteral colic?
    a. 18% to 22%
    b. 25% to 36%
    c. 43% to 55%
    d. 52% to 60%
    e. 66% to 85%

Answers

1. **b. Polygenic with partial penetrance.** Genetic studies have concluded that urolithiasis may be the result of a polygenic defect with partial penetrance. [p 3231]

2. **b. 20 to 40 years.** The peak incidence of urinary calculi occurs from the 20s to the 40s. [p 3231]

3. **e. Southeast.** Hospitals in the southeastern United States showed an increased discharge rate but only for calcium oxalate stones. [p 3232]

4. **d. All of the above.** Factors involved in the relationship between water intake and urolithiasis are (1) the volume of water ingested as opposed to that lost by perspiration and respiration and (2) the mineral or trace element content of the water supply of the region. [p 3233]

5. **c. Solubility product.** The point at which saturation is reached and crystallization begins is referred to as the thermodynamic solubility product (K_{sp}). [p 3234]

6. **a. Homogeneous nucleation.** The process by which nuclei form in pure solutions is called homogeneous nucleation. [p 3235]

7. **b. Adherence of crystals to the renal tubule.** One study calculated that free-particle stone formation was mathematically impossible and that stone disease requires the adherence of crystals to the renal epithelium—the fixed particle hypothesis. [p 3236]

8. **e. All of the above.** Inhibitors of calcium oxalate crystal formation present in urine include citrate, pyrophosphate, glycosaminoglycans, RNA fragments, and nephrocalcin. [p 3237]

9. **c. Matrix.** Depending on their type, kidney stones contain between 10% and 65% of noncrystalline material or matrix. Extensive investigations have characterized matrix as a derivative of several of the mucoproteins of urine and serum. [p 3238]

10. **b. 20% to 35%.** Of the calcium content of the average Western adult diet, about 30% to 45% (300 to 400 mg) is absorbed. [p 3239]

11. **c. Jejunum and proximal ileum.** Calcium is probably maximally absorbed in the jejunum and the proximal portion of the ileum. [p 3239]

12. **d. 1,25-dihydroxyvitamin D_3.** It is generally accepted that 1,25-dihydroxyvitamin D_3 is the vitamin D metabolite that is the most potent stimulator of intestinal calcium absorption. [pp 3239–3240]

13. **a. Parathyroid hormone.** Parathyroid hormone is the major hormonal regulator of renal phosphate reabsorption. [p 3240]

14. **e. 80%.** Eighty percent of the oxalate found in urine comes from endogenous production in the liver. [p 3241]

15. **a. Acid excretion.** A defect in either acid excretion or bicarbonate reabsorption can lead to metabolic acidosis. [p 3241]

16. **a. It reduces citrate excretion.** Metabolic acidosis reduces citrate excretion by augmenting citrate reabsorption and mitochondrial oxidation. [p 3242]

17. **b. Less than 20 mg/day.** In normal individuals, filtered cystine is almost completely reabsorbed in the proximal nephron. Urinary cystine excretion is less than 20 mg/day. [p 3243]

18. **d. Resorptive, absorptive, and renal.** One study suggested that hypercalciuria was heterogeneous in origin and that three types exist: (1) absorptive hypercalciuria, in which the primary abnormality was an increased intestinal absorption of calcium; (2) renal hypercalciuria, characterized by a primary renal leak of calcium; and (3) resorptive hypercalciuria, characterized by increased bone demineralization. [p 3243]

19. **d. Primary renal wasting of calcium.** In this condition, the underlying abnormality is a primary renal wasting of calcium. [p 3244]

20. **a. 1%.** The prevalence of stone disease in hyperparathyroidism is only about 1%. [p 3246]

21. **c. Malignancy.** In an inpatient setting, the most common cause of hypercalcemia is a malignancy. [p 3247]

22. **a. Absorptive hypercalciuria.** The sarcoid granuloma produces 1,25-dihydroxyvitamin D_3, causing increased intestinal calcium absorption, hypercalcemia, and hypercalciuria. [p 3248]

23. **e. All of the above.** In hyperthyroidism, hypercalcemia and hypercalciuria result from a stimulation of bone resorption mediated by thyroxine and triiodothyronine. Glucocorticoids affect calcium metabolism through three mechanisms: their action on bone, intestine, and parathyroid glands. Of these, their action on bone is the most important. Glucocorticoid excess leads to increased bone resorption, decreased bone formation, and osteopenia. Hypercalcemia, when seen in patients with pheochromocytoma, occurs most often in patients with multiple endocrine neoplasia type 2, in which primary hyperparathyroidism, medullary carcinoma of the thyroid, and adrenal gland tumor coexist. Islet cell tumors of the pancreas secrete vasoactive intestinal polypeptide, which can also cause hypercalcemia. Prolonged bed rest can lead to hypercalcemia as the result of increased bone turnover. [pp 3248–3249]

24. **b. Autosomal recessive.** Primary hyperoxaluria type I is an autosomal recessive inborn error of metabolism characterized by nephrocalcinosis, tissue deposition of oxalate (oxalosis), and death from renal failure before the age of 20 years in untreated patients. [pp 3249–3250]

25. **e. Malabsorption.** Malabsorption from any cause, including small bowel resection, intrinsic disease, or jejunoileal bypass, increases the colonic permeability of oxalate as the result of exposure of the colonic epithelium to bile salts. [p 3251]

26. **c. Increased dietary protein intake.** Increased dietary protein intake and altered renal excretion of oxalate have been postulated as causes by some investigators. [p 3251]

27. **b. 10% to 40%.** Hyperuricosuria was seen in 277 of 1117 (24%) calcium stone formers evaluated in one study and in 10% of patients seen in another study in Dallas. In Dallas, it coexisted with other abnormalities in 40% of patients. Of the stones analyzed by the first group, 12% contained a mixture of calcium oxalate and uric acid. [p 3252]

28. **c. As a complexing agent of calcium.** The primary mechanism of action of citrate is as a complexing agent for calcium. [p 3253]

29. **d. Hypocitraturia.** Most patients with hypomagnesuria also have hypocitraturia. [p 3253]

30. **e. None of the above.** Distal RTA is characterized by hypokalemic, hyperchloremic, non-anion gap metabolic acidosis, and a urinary pH consistently above 6.0. [p 3255]

31. **b. Failure of bicarbonate reabsorption in the proximal tubule.** The primary defect here is a failure of bicarbonate reabsorption in the proximal tubule, leading to urinary bicarbonate excretion. [p 3256]

32. **a. acidic urine.** Patients with uric acid stones often have prolonged periods of acidity in the urine. [p 3258]

33. **d. All of the above.** Three factors are involved in uric acid urolithiasis. First, patients tend to excrete excessively acid urine at a relatively fixed, low urinary pH. Second, they may absorb, produce, or excrete more uric acid than patients without gout or uric acid stones. Third, urinary volume is diminished in these patients. [p 3258]

34. **d. 20%.** The frequency of uric acid stones in patients with gout is about 20%. [p 3259]

35. **e. Carbon dioxide and ammonium.** Urease-producing bacteria hydrolyze urea to carbon dioxide and ammonium molecules. [p 3260]

36. **d. Bacteria inaccessible to antibiotics.** Struvite calculi harbor infective bacteria within their interstices. [p 3261]

37. **a. Deep venous thrombosis.** The side effects of therapy with acetohydroxamic acid in patients with infection stones included deep venous thrombosis, tremor, headache, palpitations, edema, nausea, vomiting, diarrhea, loss of taste, hallucinations, rash, alopecia, abdominal pain, and anemia. [p 3263]

38. **d. 1 per 20,000 population.** Heterozygous cystinuria occurs in 1 of 20 to 1 of 200 individuals, whereas homozygous cystinuria occurs in about 1 per 20,000 persons in the United States. [p 3264]

39. **b. Diarrhea.** Side effects include gastrointestinal complications, such as nausea, vomiting, diarrhea, and impairment in taste and smell; dermatologic complications, such as urticaria and pemphigus; hypersensitivity reactions; fevers; chills; and arthralgia. [p 3265]

40. **d. HIV-1 infection.** Nephrolithiasis has been reported to occur in 4% to 13% of patients administered the protease inhibitor for the treatment of HIV-1 infection. [p 3267]

41. **c. 4 mm.** If the smaller diameter is less than 4 mm, spontaneous stone passage is likely. [p 3267]

42. **d. CT.** CT has been used clinically with increasing frequency since 1972. Helical or spiral CT has greatly enhanced the application of this relatively new imaging technology. The scans are rapidly performed, do not require contrast agents, and, because of the high cost of intravenous contrast agents and the rapid nature of the study, are very cost-effective when compared with intravenous urography. [p 3271]

43. **a. Decreased renal function.** Ureteral obstruction, whether partial or complete, produces a progressive decrease in renal excretory function. [p 3273]

44. **a. Chemical analysis.** Chemical analysis of renal calculi has been all but abandoned. [p 3273]

45. **e. Increased urinary pH.** Ten ounces of meat ingested daily causes a 156% increase in urinary calcium excretion. The other effects of meat intake are believed to be the result of the high content of sulfur-containing amino acids found in animal protein. Increased acidity of the urine may diminish the inhibitory action of urinary glycosaminoglycans, potent inhibitors of calcium oxalate crystal growth and aggregation. It has been estimated that roughly half the increased levels of urinary calcium, oxalate, and uric acid seen in stone-forming patients may be attributed to a diet rich in animal protein. [p 3274]

46. **d. Medullary sponge kidney.** Medullary sponge kidney is the most common renal structural abnormality seen in patients with calcium-containing stones; up to 2% of patients have this. [p 3275]

47. **e. Sulfate.** Calcium, oxalate, magnesium, and phosphorus should be analyzed in the acidified sample; uric acid in the alkaline sample; and creatinine in untreated aliquots. [p 3275]

48. **b. 7% per year.** It can be estimated that the recurrence rate will be about 7% per year, with 50% of patients having recurrences within 10 years, in an unselected urologic practice. [p 3276]

49. **d. 3 L/day.** Patients should measure their 24-hour urinary output once a week and adjust the fluid intake to maintain an output of 3 L/day or more. [p 3278]

50. **a. Osteoporosis.** Severe dietary calcium restriction results in a markedly negative calcium balance as a result of continued gastrointestinal calcium losses and increased bone resorption. This loss of bone calcium may lead to osteoporosis, particularly in older women. [p 3279]

51. **b. 10%.** About 40% of the oxalate present in urine comes from metabolic production in the liver, 40% comes from the conversion of ascorbate, and less than 10% comes from dietary sources. [p 3280]

52. **d. enhancing calcium resorption in the distal tubule.** Thiazides directly stimulate calcium resorption in the distal nephron while promoting excretion of sodium. [p 3280]

53. **c. Increased pyrophosphate excretion.** Urinary phosphorus excretion is markedly increased during therapy with neutral or alkaline phosphate, which results in an increase in the inhibitor activity of urine, perhaps because of increased renal excretion of pyrophosphate and citrate. [p 3281]

54. **c. Xanthine oxidase.** Allopurinol inhibits xanthine oxidase and decreases the production of uric acid. [p 3283]

55. **d. Sodium citrate does not lower urinary calcium excretion.** Sodium citrate does not lower urinary calcium excretion, perhaps because of the increased sodium load associated with therapy. [p 3284]

56. **e. Uric acid.** In contrast to renal stones, bladder stones are usually composed of uric acid (in noninfected urine) or struvite (in infected urine). [p 3286]

57. **b. Calcium phosphate.** Inorganic salts (calcium phosphate and calcium carbonate) impregnate the corpora amylacea, converting them into calculi. [p 3287]

58. **c. Furosemide.** Initially, stone formation was attributed exclusively to furosemide-induced hypercalciuria; however, it has become apparent that renal calcifications can occur in infants who have not received furosemide. [p 3290]

59. **c. Ureteropelvic obstruction.** In those series that provide a breakdown of anatomic lesions responsible for stone formation, ureteropelvic junction obstruction is the most common lesion. [p 3290]

60. **e. 66% to 85%.** Approximately 66% to 85% of pregnant women with ureteric colic spontaneously pass the calculi when treated conservatively with hydration, analgesics, and, if infected, antibiotics. [p 3292]

Chapter 97

Ureteroscopy and Retrograde Ureteral Access

Li-Ming Su • R. Ernest Sosa

Questions

1. In a male patient with a large median lobe, difficulty in the introduction of a guide wire into the ureter can be overcome by:

   a. giving the patient indigo carmine intravenously.
   b. decreasing the hip flexure of the ipsilateral leg.
   c. inducing a diuretic state.
   d. changing to a 70-degree lens.
   e. rotating the cystoscope 180 degrees.

2. Passage of a ureteroscope can be frustrated by all of the following conditions except which one?

   a. A full bladder
   b. An inadequately dilated distal ureter
   c. A large prostatic middle lobe
   d. Poor bowel preparation
   e. Prior ureteral reimplant

3. A ureteral filling defect found by retrograde pyelography can be most accurately characterized by which method?

   a. A ureteroscopically directed biopsy
   b. Ureteral brushings
   c. Ureteral barbotage with glycine for cytology
   d. Interval follow-up retrograde pyelography
   e. A trial of alkalinization of the urine with follow-up studies

4. A partially obstructed distal ureter with proximal tortuosity could best be accessed with which of the following?

   a. A super-stiff guide wire
   b. An angle-tipped hydrophilic guide wire and an open-ended stent
   c. Antegrade passage of a guide wire
   d. Direct ureteroscopic access
   e. Cystoscopic resection of the distal ureter

5. Which of the following statements regarding balloon dilation of the distal ureter is true?

   a. It does not always require fluoroscopy.
   b. It is unnecessary when using a miniature ureteroscope.
   c. It is preceded by passage of a safety guide wire.
   d. It can be safely performed to a 24 Fr size.
   e. It can be performed with a Fogarty balloon.

6. To sample a lesion on a pedicle in the ureter, all the following tools may be used except which one?

   a. A safety guide wire
   b. A stone basket
   c. A cold cup forceps
   d. A ureteral brush
   e. A ureteral resectoscope

7. Which of the following statements regarding indwelling ureteral stents is true?

   a. They can be introduced without fluoroscopy if the upper extent of the guide wire is known.
   b. They can be left in place for periods longer than 6 months.
   c. They can be used to passively dilate a small ureter.
   d. They allow stone fragments to pass through their lumens.
   e. They are made of a radiolucent material to be biocompatible.

8. Difficulties in passing a flexible ureteroscope can be lessened by all but which one of the following maneuvers?

   a. Removing the safety guide wire
   b. Emptying the bladder
   c. Dilating the ureteral orifice
   d. Rotating the ureteroscope so that the guide wire is at the 12-o'clock position
   e. Monitoring with fluoroscopy

9. In a previously operated ureterovesicle junction, identification of the orifice can be helped by which of the following?

   a. Using a small guide wire
   b. Using a hydrophilic stent
   c. Overdistention of the bladder
   d. Giving the patient intravenous indigo carmine
   e. Rotating the ipsilateral side up

10. During a ureteroscopy, a lesion is encountered in the distal ureter. What should the surgeon do?

    a. Perform a biopsy of the lesion as it is identified
    b. Continue the ureteroscopy and perform a biopsy of the lesion later
    c. Use a laser to ablate the lesion to prevent spread
    d. Place an indwelling stent and plan an interval procedure
    e. Get a washing sample for cytology and fulgurate the lesion but discontinue the endoscopic procedure.

Answers

1. **e. rotating the cystoscope 180 degrees.** Rotation of the cystoscope 180 degrees allows retraction of the median lobe by the blunt beak of the cystoscope, thus exposing the orifice (see Fig. 97–3B). This configuration also provides a more direct angle for passage of the guide wire into the distal ureter. [pp 3315–3316]

2. **d. Poor bowel preparation.** Difficulty in passing the ureteroscope can be due to the presence of an overdistended bladder, inadequate dilatation of the distal ureter, or anatomic abnormalities such as the presence of a large prostatic median lobe, ureteral stricture, or a prior ureteral reimplantation. [p 3314]

3. **a. A ureteroscopically directed biopsy.** Integral to the evaluation and diagnosis of any upper tract filling defect is the use of ureteroscopy to perform a biopsy of suspicious lesions. [p 3317]

4. **b. An angle-tipped hydrophilic guide wire and an open-ended stent.** To access a J-shaped ureter, as in patients with prostatic enlargement, or for a ureter obstructed by an impacted stone, an angled guide wire can help steer past the critical point. Alternatively, a hydrophilic guide wire can be used in such situations. For this, an open-ended ureteral stent is first introduced through the cystoscope to intubate the ureteral orifice. The selected guide wire is passed through the stent into the orifice and advanced up the ureteral lumen. [pp 3307–3308]

5. **c. It is preceded by passage of a safety guide wire.** The first step in balloon dilatation of the ureter is to have a radiologic image of the ureter. An excretory urogram or a retrograde ureterogram can outline the course of the ureter and the point of narrowing. Once the anatomy is known, a guide wire is placed. The balloon dilator is advanced over a guide wire to the point of narrowing or obstruction. [p 3310]

6. **a. A safety guide wire.** To obtain tissue from a lesion, a biopsy sample can be obtained using different devices. These include the cold cup biopsy forceps, a ureteral resectoscope, a stone basket, and an endoscopic brush. [p 3317]

7. **c. They can be used to passively dilate a small ureter.** If ureteral dilatation must be performed, this can be accomplished by one of two means: passive or active dilatation. Passive dilatation entails placement of either an open-ended or an indwelling double pigtail stent for 24 to 48 hours before interval ureteroscopy or stone extraction. [p 3316]

8. **a. Removing the safety guide wire.** The ureteroscope should be passed into the ureter under fluoroscopic guidance before any ancillary equipment is attached to the ureteroscope. Moreover, the ureteroscope should be aligned to have the working wire at the 12-o'clock position to prevent the ureteroscope lens from snagging the roof of the ureteral orifice and "telescoping" the distal ureter during passage (see Fig. 97–2A and B). Last, before passage of a flexible ureteroscope, one should ensure that the bladder is empty and that the distal ureter is adequately dilated. [p 3312]

9. **d. Giving the patient intravenous indigo carmine.** In cases in which the orifices are obscured by inflammation and edema or scarring from prior surgery, use of intravenous indigo carmine or methylene blue will result in the efflux of blue urine, delineating the location of the hidden orifices. [p 3315]

10. **a. Perform a biopsy of the lesion as it is identified.** Biopsy should be attempted at the initial pass of the ureteroscope to minimize the need for multiple passes of the endoscope with increased risk of bleeding and poor visualization. [p 3317]

Chapter 98

Percutaneous Approaches to the Upper Urinary Tract

Elspeth M. McDougall • Evangelos N. Liatsikos • Caner Z. Dinlenc • Arthur D. Smith

Questions

1. What is the established total maximum dose equivalent limit for personnel exposed to fluoroscopic procedures?

    a. 5 rem
    b. 10 rem
    c. 15 rem
    d. 20 rem
    e. 25 rem

2. What is the main source of radiation exposure to the endourologist?

    a. Radiation leakage from the fluoroscopic unit
    b. Scattered radiation from beams deflected off the patient
    c. The metal instruments
    d. The image intensifier
    e. The x-ray monitors

3. Which of the following technical features is most important for a fluoroscopic C-arm unit?

    a. Rotation of 90 degrees
    b. Digital imaging

c. Last-image-hold, fluoroscopic beam under the table
d. Large memory capacity
e. Collimation

4. In which of the following situations is the scattered radiation to the operator greatest?
    a. Use of multiple short pulses of radiation for positioning the needle
    b. Patients weighing less than 60 kg
    c. Image intensifier in a lateral position
    d. Emission tube below the table
    e. Emission tube above the table

5. In which of the following situations is arterial bleeding most likely?
    a. Direct posterolateral puncture
    b. Direct posteromedial puncture
    c. Superior pole puncture
    d. Midzone puncture
    e. Inferior pole puncture

6. When bleeding occurs during the dilatation of the tract, what should one do?
    a. Take out the dilator
    b. Continue and place a bigger dilator to tamponade the bleeding
    c. Continue with a smaller dilator
    d. Insert a tamponade catheter and stop the procedure
    e. Perform angiography and embolization

7. The bull's-eye sign is observed on the fluoroscopic screen when:
    a. the needle hub is superimposed on the needle shaft, and the plane of the needle is in line with the x-ray beam.
    b. a calix is depicted end-on.
    c. the needle is 90 degrees to the x-ray beam.
    d. a stone is superimposed on the calix.
    e. the needle hub is superimposed on the needle shaft, and the plane of the needle is vertical to the x-ray beam.

8. How is the depth of needle penetration monitored?
    a. By layers of resistance
    b. By maintaining the bull's-eye sign
    c. By aspiration of blood
    d. By rotation of the C-arm back to the vertical position
    e. By injection of contrast medium through the needle

9. Triangulation is the preferred technique for gaining access to which structure?
    a. The renal pelvis
    b. An upper calix
    c. A lower calix full of stones
    d. A horseshoe kidney
    e. A transplant kidney

10. At the end of the percutaneous procedure, there is oozing from the nephrostomy tract. What should the urologist do?
    a. Clamp the nephrostomy catheter and allow tamponade
    b. Take out the nephrostomy tube
    c. Redilate and explore endoscopically
    d. Observe
    e. Use a tamponade balloon

11. The dilatation should always be performed:
    a. before placement of the second guide wire.
    b. over the longest distance possible.
    c. to confirm the position of the wire.
    d. with the fluoroscopic unit off.
    e. over the stiff portion of the guide wire.

12. The insertion of the second safety guide wire must be performed:
    a. through a double-lumen catheter.
    b. at the end of the procedure.
    c. only if a perforation is seen in the collecting system.
    d. if a long procedure is planned.
    e. to prevent excessive bleeding.

13. Which untoward event can happen if excessive force is exerted during dilatation with fascial dilators?
    a. Displacement of the guide wire
    b. Dislocation of stones to the upper ureter
    c. Kinking of the wire
    d. Avulsion of the pedicle
    e. Perforation of the renal pelvis

14. A pregnant woman needs to have percutaneous drainage of her upper urinary system because of obstruction. Which approach must be used?
    a. Percutaneous nephrostomy under CT guidance
    b. Antegrade percutaneous nephrostomy
    c. Percutaneous nephrostomy under ultrasonographic guidance
    d. Puncture with general anesthesia
    e. Retrograde percutaneous nephrostomy

15. Tract dilatation with the Amplatz dilators should always be performed:
    a. in a stepwise fashion at 2 Fr intervals.
    b. over a floppy guide wire.
    c. over the 8 Fr Teflon catheter.
    d. with the fluoroscopic unit off.
    e. up to 34 Fr.

16. The 8 Fr catheter that is included in the Amplatz set has what role?
    a. It prevents kinking of the wire.
    b. It facilitates introduction of a second wire.
    c. It enables aspiration of fluid to confirm correct position.
    d. It prevents excessive bleeding.
    e. It helps establish a tract to the bladder.

17. What should the dilatation catheters reach?
    a. The renal hilum
    b. The calices just as far as the lumen
    c. The renal capsule
    d. The target object (stone or tumor)
    e. The ureteropelvic junction

18. The final diameter of the tract should exceed the tube or instrument that is finally going to be inserted by how much?
    a. 1 to 2 Fr
    b. 2 to 4 Fr
    c. 6 to 8 Fr
    d. 9 to 10 Fr
    e. 10 to 12 Fr

19. A characteristic "waist" is evident fluoroscopically when which of the following devices is used for tract dilatation?
    a. Amplatz dilators
    b. Balloon catheter
    c. 8 Fr catheter
    d. 22-gauge "skinny" needle
    e. 30 Fr dilator

20. What is the main disadvantage of the Cope catheter?
    a. It needs to be removed under fluoroscopic control.
    b. It cannot be used to regain access.
    c. It is small and causes leakage from the skin.
    d. It is too costly.
    e. Tight loop formation and encrustation at the end hole may make removal difficult.

21. Which nephrostomy tube would be advisable for an obese patient?
    a. The Councill catheter
    b. The Cope loop
    c. The re-entry tube
    d. The endopyelotomy tube
    e. The Foley catheter

22. The balloon of the nephrostomy catheters should always be inflated with water or saline for what reason?
    a. Other materials erode the balloon.
    b. The balloon should be radiolucent.
    c. Such inflation decreases the chances of infection.
    d. They should not be inflated with water or saline.
    e. Contrast materials have a higher viscosity and can occlude the balloon port.

23. What percentage of patients require angiography and embolization after percutaneous procedures?
    a. 9% to 10%
    b. 5% to 7%
    c. 0.8% to 1.5%
    d. 1% to 2%
    e. 2% to 3%

24. What percentage of patients suffer injuries to the colon during percutaneous procedures?
    a. >1%
    b. 5%
    c. 10%
    d. <1%
    e. >2%

25. When there is colonic perforation, open surgical correction is necessary:
    a. after urinary extravasation.
    b. before tract dilatation.
    c. after tract dilatation.
    d. if there is intraperitoneal perforation.
    e. after the percutaneous tract to the kidney matures.

26. What percentage of patients have sepsis after percutaneous stone removal?
    a. 0.25% to 1.5%
    b. 2.5% to 3%
    c. 3% to 4.5%
    d. 5% to 6%
    e. 10%

27. Three days after a percutaneous procedure and during the re-entry tube retrieval, there is secondary bleeding from the nephrostomy tract. What is the best treatment for this condition?
    a. Angiography and embolization
    b. Observation
    c. Removal of the re-entry tube
    d. Open surgical exploration
    e. Exchange to a larger catheter

28. What is the most common medical problem associated with fungal bezoars?
    a. Urinary tract catheter
    b. Chronic antibiotic use
    c. Diabetes mellitus
    d. Immunosuppression
    e. Age greater than 70 years

29. Which technique has the best success rate for treatment of a stone-bearing calyceal diverticulum?
    a. The indirect percutaneous approach
    b. The direct percutaneous approach
    c. The ureteroscopic intrarenal approach
    d. Extracorporeal shock wave lithotripsy
    e. Open partial nephrectomy

30. At which pressure is the Whitaker test positive?
    a. 10 cm H_2O
    b. 13 cm H_2O
    c. 15 cm H_2O
    d. 22 cm H_2O
    e. 25 cm H_2O

31. In dealing percutaneously with a renal cyst, what is the most effective form of therapy?
    a. Percutaneous drainage alone
    b. Percutaneous drainage and sclerotherapy
    c. Percutaneous resection of the cyst wall
    d. Intrarenal incision and drainage of the cyst
    e. Intrarenal drainage of the cyst

32. Which organism is most commonly responsible for a renal abscess?
    a. *Escherichia coli*
    b. *Proteus mirabilis*
    c. *Klebsiella*
    d. *Serratia*
    e. *Candida*

33. For treatment of a simple renal or perirenal abscess, what is the frequency with which a percutaneous approach will be successful?
    a. 10%
    b. 20%
    c. 50%
    d. 80%
    e. 95%

34. In patients with a perinephric abscess, which characteristic is best suited to a percutaneous approach and drainage?
    a. Calcified debris
    b. Thick purulent drainage
    c. A multiloculated cavity
    d. A single cavity with an isodense appearance on a CT scan
    e. A cyst in a nonfunctioning kidney

35. Which of the following is the distinguishing characteristic of lymphocele fluid?
    a. Electrolytes similar to those in serum
    b. Cholesterol level higher than that in serum
    c. Protein level higher than that in serum
    d. Absence of lymphocytes
    e. All of the above

Answers

1. **a. 5 rem.** The National Council on Radiation Protection has established the total radiation effective dose equivalent limit for occupational exposure as 5 rem. [p 3321]

2. **b. Scattered radiation from beams deflected off the patient.** The major source of the radiation dose received by the endourologist is scattered radiation from the patient. [p 3321]

3. **c. Last-image-hold, fluoroscopic beam under the table.** Use of a last-image-hold feature is of great importance in reducing the overall irradiation time. [p 3321]

4. **e. Emission tube above the table.** When the tube is above the operating table, there is a combination of leakage and scattered radiation. However, when the image intensifier is placed superiorly, radiation leakage is minimized, as the emission tube is shielded by an additional layer of material. The scattered radiation to the operator is also reduced. [p 3321]

5. **b. Direct posteromedial puncture.** In more than 50% of kidneys, the posterior segmental artery is located in the middle or upper half of the posterior renal surface, and it may be damaged with an excessively medial needle puncture of an upper calyx. A direct posterior puncture that is too medial risks injury to the posterior segmental artery, which is the artery most commonly injured in endourologic procedures. [pp 3322–3323]

6. **b. Continue and place a bigger dilator to tamponade the bleeding.** The working sheath can be used to limit bleeding from the percutaneous tract. [p 3337]

7. **a. the needle hub is superimposed on the needle shaft, and the plane of the needle is in line with the x-ray beam.** An 18-gauge translumbar angiography needle is advanced in the plane of the fluoroscope beam with the C-arm in the 30-degree position (see Fig. 98–7). The appropriate direction for needle advancement is determined by obtaining a bull's-eye sign on the fluoroscopic screen. This effect can be observed only when the needle hub is superimposed on the needle shaft and is evident when the plane of the needle is the same as that of the x-ray beam. [pp 3324–3325]

8. **d. By rotation of the C-arm back to the vertical position.** The depth of needle penetration is monitored by rotating the C-arm back to the vertical position. [p 3325]

9. **b. An upper calix.** One of the more frequently used techniques for access to a superior calix is triangulation. [p 3327]

10. **a. Clamp the nephrostomy catheter and allow tamponade.** The tube is clamped, allowing tamponade to be used for the pelvicaliceal system. [p 3337]

11. **e. over the stiff portion of the guide wire.** The main principle of dilatation is that it should always be performed over a guide wire. The wire must be stiff enough to support the dilatation. Ideally, it will reach down the ureter into the bladder to avoid dislodgment during use of the fascial dilators. [p 3331]

12. **a. through a double-lumen catheter.** The insertion of the safety guide wire requires the use of a double-lumen catheter or a coaxial system to accommodate two wires. [p 3331]

13. **e. Perforation of the renal pelvis.** Caution must be exercised not to exert unnecessary force when introducing the dilators because their tips can perforate the renal pelvis medially, causing excessive blood loss or extravasation of irrigating fluid into the retroperitoneum. [p 3332]

14. **c. Percutaneous nephrostomy under ultrasonographic guidance.** Ultrasonographically guided nephrostomy puncture is preferred for patients in whom retrograde ureteral catheterization is unsuccessful and in pregnant women in whom there is a need for decompression of an obstructed kidney. [p 3330]

15. **c. over the 8 Fr Teflon catheter.** The tract is initially dilated until the curved 8 Fr Teflon catheter can be inserted over the wire. The larger dilators are tapered to fit over this catheter. The use of the tapered catheter facilitates the entire dilatation process. [p 3332]

16. **a. It prevents the kinking of the wire.** Because of its flexibility, the 8 Fr catheter can pass easily into the ureter, sliding over the guide wire and protecting and stabilizing the guide wire to prevent kinking during progressive dilatation. In addition, this catheter allows larger dilators to slide easily over it. [p 3332]

17. **b. The calices just as far as the lumen.** Dilators must be advanced over the working guide wire until they enter the caliceal lumen. However, further insertion may damage the integrity of the pelvicaliceal system and should be avoided. [p 3332]

18. **b. 2 to 4 Fr.** The final diameter of the tract should exceed the tube or instrument size by 2 Fr to 4 Fr, to allow adequate flow of fluid around the instrument. [p 3333]

19. **b. Balloon catheter.** As the balloon is inflated, a characteristic "waist" appears in areas of high resistance, such as the renal capsule or a previous operative scar. [pp 3333–3334]

20. **e. Tight loop formation and encrustation at the end hole may make removal difficult.** The main problem is that if a tight loop forms and the end hole becomes encrusted, the catheter becomes very difficult to remove. [p 3335]

21. **a. The Councill catheter.** In obese and hypermobile patients, nephrostomy tubes can easily be pulled out. The balloon on the Councill catheter holds it more firmly in place. [p 3335]

22. **e. Contrast materials have a higher viscosity and can occlude the balloon port.** Balloons should always be inflated with water or saline. The use of contrast agents should be avoided. [p 3336]

23. **c. 0.8% to 1.5%.** Of patients undergoing percutaneous renal procedures, 0.8% to 1.5% required angiography and embolization for uncontrolled bleeding. [p 3337]

24. **d. <1%.** Colonic perforation is a rare complication of the percutaneous procedures, being reported in less than 1% of cases. [p 3339]

25. **d. if there is intraperitoneal perforation.** Surgical correction is considered only in cases of intraperitoneal perforation of the colon or in the presence of peritonitis or sepsis. [p 3339]

26. **a. 0.25% to 1.5%.** Sepsis has been reported in 0.25% to 1.5% of patients undergoing percutaneous stone removal. [p 3340]

27. **a. Angiography and embolization.** The source of bleeding

is embolized under angiographic control, and hemorrhage ceases. [p 3338]

28. **c. Diabetes mellitus.** About half the reported cases of fungal concretions are in diabetic patients. [p 3338]

29. **b. The direct percutaneous approach.** In percutaneous treatment of a stone-bearing calyceal diverticulum, it is most important to enter the calyceal diverticulum *directly* to remove the calculus and deliver therapy. An indirect approach is associated with a higher incidence of failure. [pp 3354–3355]

30. **d. 22 cm H$_2$O.** If the difference in pressure between the renal pelvis and the bladder is less than 13 to 15 cm H$_2$O, the system is unobstructed. In contrast, a renal pelvis/bladder pressure differential greater than 22 cm H$_2$O indicates obstruction. A pressure difference of 15 to 22 cm H$_2$O is considered equivocal. [pp 3347–3348]

31. **b. Percutaneous drainage and sclerotherapy.** Percutaneous drainage of renal cysts unaccompanied by sclerotherapy is of little therapeutic value. Sclerotherapy with ethanol or with bismuth phosphate generally results in a satisfactory outcome in 75% to 100% of patients. Given the simultaneous diagnostic and therapeutic aspects of cyst drainage and sclerotherapy, it is the obvious route of first-line treatment. [p 3342]

32. **a. *Escherichia coli*.** The responsible organism is most commonly a gram-negative bacterium such as *Escherichia coli* or, less commonly, *Proteus mirabilis* or *Klebsiella pneumoniae*. [p 3342]

33. **d. 80%.** In the simple abscess case, percutaneous drainage yields success rates greater than 80%. [p 3344]

34. **d. A single cavity with an isodense appearance on a CT scan.** Unfavorable factors for a percutaneous approach include fungal infection, calcification of the wall of the mass, calcified debris within the mass, thick purulent drainage, multiloculated cavity, markedly diseased nonfunctioning kidney (an indication for nephrectomy), and an infected hematoma. [p 3346]

35. **a. Electrolytes similar to those in serum.** The values of creatinine and other electrolytes reflect values found in serum. In lymphocele fluid from the pelvis, the levels of cholesterol and protein are often lower than those in serum. In the drained pale yellow or clear fluid, lymphocytes can usually be detected. [p 3346]

Chapter 99

Surgical Management of Urinary Lithiasis

James E. Lingeman • David A. Lifshitz • Andrew P. Evan

Questions

1. What percentage of renal calculi can be successfully managed with extracorporeal shock wave lithotripsy (ESWL)?

   a. 90% to 95%
   b. 80% to 85%
   c. 70% to 75%
   d. 60% to 65%
   e. 50% to 55%

2. What is the risk of mortality from an untreated struvite staghorn stone?

   a. Less than 10%
   b. 10% to 30%
   c. 30% to 50%
   d. 50% to 70%
   e. Greater than 70%

3. What is the single most important factor when choosing among ESWL, ureteroscopic stone removal (URS), and percutaneous nephrolithotomy (PNL) for renal calculi?

   a. Stone composition
   b. Stone location
   c. Anatomic abnormalities
   d. Stone burden
   e. Body habitus

4. What is the preferred treatment for renal calculi 10 to 20 mm in diameter?

   a. ESWL
   b. ESWL with ureteral stenting
   c. Flexible ureteroscopy with holmium laser lithotripsy
   d. PNL
   e. Laparoscopic pyelolithotomy

5. What is the preferred treatment for renal calculi 20 to 30 mm in diameter?

   a. ESWL with ureteral stenting
   b. PNL
   c. URS
   d. Laparoscopic pyelolithotomy
   e. Open surgery

6. What is the preferred initial treatment for staghorn calculi?

   a. ESWL with ureteral stenting
   b. Flexible URS with holmium laser lithotripsy
   c. PNL
   d. Extended pyelolithotomy with multiple radial nephrotomies
   e. Anatrophic nephrolithotomy

7. ESWL monotherapy (with ureteral stenting) may be considered for staghorn calculi of what size?

   a. Less than 250 mm^2
   b. Less than 500 mm^2
   c. Less than 1000 mm^2

d. Less than 1500 mm^2
e. Less than 2500 mm^2

8. What is the most difficult stone composition to fragment with ESWL?

   a. Calcium oxalate dihydrate
   b. Calcium oxalate monohydrate
   c. Struvite
   d. Hydroxyapatite
   e. Uric acid

9. What is the preferred treatment approach for a symptomatic 1.5 cm stone in a calyceal diverticulum in the lower pole?

   a. ESWL
   b. Flexible ureteroscopy
   c. PNL
   d. PNL plus fulguration of the diverticulum
   e. Laparoscopic diverticulectomy

10. What is the preferred initial treatment for a 12 mm stone in the renal pelvis of a horseshoe kidney with minimal hydronephrosis?

    a. ESWL
    b. Flexible ureteroscopy
    c. PNL
    d. Laparoscopic pyelolithotomy
    e. Symphysiotomy with pyelolithotomy

11. Factors affecting stone-free rates for lower pole calculi include all of the following except which one?

    a. Infundibulopelvic angle
    b. Stone size
    c. Infundibular width
    d. Stone composition
    e. Infundibular length

12. What is the preferred treatment approach for a 1.5 cm renal calculus in a patient who weighs 375 pounds?

    a. ESWL
    b. Flexible ureteroscopy
    c. PNL
    d. ESWL using the "blast path"
    e. Open surgery

13. What is the preferred treatment option in a patient with a symptomatic 1.5 cm renal calculus and a coagulopathy?

    a. ESWL
    b. ESWL after administration of fresh frozen plasma
    c. Indwelling ureteral stent
    d. Flexible ureteroscopy
    e. PNL

14. Residual fragments after ESWL have been associated with which of the following?

    a. Hypertension
    b. An increased rate of recurrent stones
    c. A decreased rate of recurrent stones
    d. Perinephric hematomas
    e. Hematuria

15. What is the most sensitive test for identifying residual fragments after PNL?

    a. Nephrotomograms
    b. MRI
    c. Ultrasonography
    d. Noncontrast CT
    e. Contrast-enhanced CT

16. Factors affecting the probability of spontaneous passage of ureteral calculi include all of the following except which one?

    a. Stone size
    b. Stone location at presentation
    c. Stone composition
    d. Side
    e. Duration of symptoms

17. Irreversible loss of renal function can occur within what time period with a completely obstructing ureteral stone?

    a. 1 week
    b. 2 to 4 weeks
    c. 4 to 6 weeks
    d. More than 6 weeks
    e. 3 months

18. What is the stone-free rate for patients with ureteral stones less than 1 cm located in the proximal ureter and treated primarily with ESWL?

    a. Between 90% and 100%
    b. Between 80% and 90%
    c. Between 70% and 80%
    d. Between 60% and 70%
    e. Between 50% and 60%

19. Ureteral stenting when ESWL is performed for ureteral stones is appropriate for all of the following reasons except which one?

    a. Solitary kidney
    b. Relief of severe symptoms (colic, nausea, vomiting)
    c. Enhancement of stone fragmentation
    d. Relief of obstruction
    e. Aid in location of difficult-to-visualize stones

20. What is the stone-free rate for patients with ureteral stones less than 1 cm located in the proximal ureter and treated with flexible ureteroscopy?

    a. Between 90% and 100%
    b. Between 80% and 90%
    c. Between 70% and 80%
    d. Between 60% and 70%
    e. Between 50% and 60%

21. What is the stone-free rate for patients with ureteral stones less than 1 cm located in the distal ureter and treated with rigid ureteroscopy?

    a. Between 90% and 100%
    b. Between 80% and 90%
    c. Between 70% and 80%
    d. Between 60% and 70%
    e. Between 50% and 60%

22. For a patient with an 0.8 cm stone in the proximal ureter requiring intervention, flexible ureteroscopy would be preferred in all of the following circumstances except which one?

    a. Morbid obesity
    b. Bleeding diathesis
    c. Cystinuria
    d. Impacted stone (present in the same location for more than 2 months)
    e. Age greater than 60 years

23. Appropriate treatment options for bladder calculi include all of the following except which one?

    a. Irrigation with Suby's G solution
    b. ESWL
    c. Electrohydraulic lithotripsy (EHL)
    d. Ultrasonic lithotripsy
    e. Holmium laser lithotripsy

24. What is the most common stone composition in patients with urinary diversions?

a. Calcium oxalate monohydrate
b. Uric acid
c. Ammonium acid urate
d. Calcium oxalate dihydrate
e. Struvite

25. Risk factors for the formation of stones in patients with urinary diversions include all of the following except which one?

    a. Hyperchloremic metabolic acidosis
    b. Hypocitraturia
    c. Hyperoxaluria
    d. Urinary tract infection
    e. Hypercalciuria

26. Which continent diversion has the highest risk of stone formation?

    a. Kock pouch
    b. Mainz pouch
    c. Indiana pouch
    d. Orthotopic hemi-Kock pouch
    e. Cecal reservoir

27. Metabolic changes associated with pregnancy relevant to urolithiasis include all of the following except which one?

    a. Absorptive hypercalciuria
    b. Hypercalcemia
    c. Hyperuricosuria
    d. Increased citrate excretion
    e. Increased magnesium excretion

28. What is the preferred initial diagnostic study for suspected urolithiasis in pregnant patients?

    a. Kidney, ureter, and bladder (KUB)
    b. Tailored intravenous pyelography (i.e., two or three films)
    c. Renal ultrasonography
    d. Spiral CT
    e. MRI

29. The risk of retrograde stone propulsion is greatest with which of the following intracorporeal lithotripsy technologies?

    a. EHL
    b. Holmium laser
    c. Pulsed dye laser
    d. Ultrasonic lithotripsy
    e. Ballistic lithotripsy

30. The coumarin dye wave length (540 nm) of the pulsed dye laser is not absorbed by which of the following?

    a. Calcium oxalate dihydrate
    b. Calcium oxalate monohydrate
    c. Cystine
    d. Struvite
    e. Uric acid

31. What are the preferred initial power settings for holmium laser lithotripsy of ureteral stones?

    a. 0.6 J, 6 Hz
    b. 0.6 J, 10 Hz
    c. 1.0 J, 10 Hz
    d. 1.2 J, 10 Hz
    e. 1.0 J, 15 Hz

32. Which intracorporeal lithotripsy technology will fragment the highest percentage of stones?

    a. Ultrasound
    b. Ballistic lithotripsy
    c. Coumarin dye laser
    d. Holmium laser
    e. Electrokinetic lithotripsy

33. Which intracorporeal lithotripsy technology has the least risk of ureteral perforation?

    a. Ultrasound
    b. Ballistic
    c. Holmium laser
    d. EHL
    e. Erbium laser

34. Energy sources for ESWL include all of the following except which one?

    a. Electrohydraulic
    b. Holmium laser
    c. Piezoelectric
    d. Electromagnetic
    e. Microexplosive

35. What is a major disadvantage of ultrasonographic imaging for ESWL?

    a. Inability to visualize ureteropelvic junction (UPJ) stones
    b. Exposure to ionizing radiation
    c. Inability to visualize radiolucent stones
    d. Expense of ultrasonography systems
    e. Inability to visualize ureteral stones

36. Factors influencing the amount of pain during ESWL include all but which of the following?

    a. Power level applied
    b. Body habitus
    c. Type of shock wave generator
    d. Shock wave energy density at the point of skin penetration
    e. Stone location

37. Which lithotriptor produces the highest stone-free rates?

    a. Wolf Piezolith 2300
    b. Siemens Lithostar
    c. Modified Dornier HM3
    d. Unmodified Dornier HM3
    e. EDAP LT 01

38. Possible mechanisms producing stone fragmentation during ESWL include all of the following except which one?

    a. Compression fracture
    b. Spallation
    c. Acoustic cavitation
    d. Dynamic fatigue
    e. Vaporization

39. What percentage of kidneys experience trauma during ESWL?

    a. 0% to 20%
    b. 20% to 40%
    c. 40% to 60%
    d. 60% to 80%
    e. 80% to 100%

40. Risk factors for enhanced bioeffects of shock waves include all of the following except which one?

    a. Patient's age greater than 60 years
    b. Pediatric age
    c. Stone burden
    d. Preexisting hypertension
    e. Reduced renal mass

41. The primary insult to the kidney exposed to shock waves occurs in which of the following tissues?

a. Blood vessels
b. Proximal tubule
c. Renal papillae
d. Glomerulus
e. Renal capsule

42. What is the most common secondarily infecting organism after percutaneous stone removal?

    a. *Proteus mirabilis*
    b. *Klebsiella oxytoca*
    c. *Pseudomonas aeruginosa*
    d. *Staphylococcus epidermidis*
    e. *Enterococcus (Streptococcus) faecalis*

43. What is the initial step in performing PNL?

    a. Percutaneous puncture of the renal collecting system
    b. Placement of a double J stent
    c. Insertion of a ureteral catheter
    d. Administration of intravenous contrast material
    e. Antegrade placement of a guide wire into the ureter

44. What is the preferred site of puncture into the renal collecting system during access for PNL?

    a. Upper pole infundibulum
    b. Anterior lower pole calyx
    c. Posterior lower pole calyx
    d. Upper pole calyx
    e. Renal pelvis

45. Risk factors for colon injury during PNL include all of the following except which one?

    a. Horseshoe kidney
    b. Kyphoscoliosis
    c. Access lateral to the posterior axillary line
    d. Previous jejunoileal bypass for obesity
    e. Upper pole puncture

46. To minimize the risk of lung and pleura injury during supracostal upper pole access for PNL:

    a. the puncture should be performed during full expiration.
    b. the puncture should be performed during full inspiration.
    c. CO_2 should be injected through the ureteral catheter to identify the upper pole calyx.
    d. the puncture should be done with local anesthesia.
    e. the puncture should be performed by a radiologist.

47. Indications for supracostal access during PNL include all of the following except which one?

    a. Predominant stone distribution in the upper pole
    b. Access to the UPJ or proximal ureter required
    c. Cystine stones
    d. Multiple lower pole infundibula and calyces containing stone material
    e. Horseshoe kidneys

48. During access for PNL, what is the preferred initial wire?

    a. Amplatz super stiff
    b. Benson
    c. Glide wire
    d. Lunderquist
    e. J-tipped movable core

49. What is the most common serious error in PNL access?

    a. Not using an Amplatz sheath
    b. Overadvancement of the dilator/sheath
    c. Anterior calyceal puncture
    d. Ultrasonographically guided puncture
    e. The use of telescoping metal dilators

50. What is the appropriate irrigating solution for PNL?

    a. 3% sorbitol
    b. Sterile water
    c. Glycine
    d. Dilute contrast material
    e. 0.9% saline

51. Middle or upper pole access for PNL in horseshoe kidneys is preferred for all of the following reasons except which one?

    a. A higher incidence of retrorenal colon
    b. Malrotation of the renal collecting system
    c. Incomplete ascent of horseshoe kidneys
    d. Anterior medial location of lower pole calyces
    e. Facilitated access to the UPJ or upper ureter

52. What is the most significant complication of PNL?

    a. Hemorrhage
    b. Extravasation of irrigation fluid
    c. Incomplete stone removal
    d. Urinary tract infection
    e. Pleural effusion

53. What is the risk of arteriovenous fistula formation after PNL?

    a. 1 in 10
    b. 1 in 100
    c. 1 in 200
    d. 1 in 500
    e. 1 in 1000

54. If uncontrolled bleeding persists following nephrostomy tube placement after PNL, what would the preferred approach be?

    a. Insertion of a double-J stent
    b. Administration of furosemide (Lasix) to promote a diuresis
    c. Surgical exploration
    d. Immediate angiography
    e. Insertion of a Kaye tamponade balloon

55. If a retroperitoneal injury to the colon is diagnosed after PNL, what is the preferred management, usually?

    a. Surgical exploration and repair
    b. Diverting colostomy with later definitive repair
    c. Leaving the nephrostomy tube in for 2 weeks to allow the tract to mature
    d. Insertion of a double-J stent and withdrawal of the nephrostomy tube into the colon
    e. Immediate removal of the nephrostomy tube

56. The use of double-J stents to reduce the risk of steinstrasse after ESWL has been demonstrated to be beneficial for what size of stones?

    a. Greater than 5 mm
    b. Greater than 10 mm
    c. Greater than 15 mm
    d. Greater than 20 mm
    e. Greater than 25 mm

57. Indications for flexible ureteroscopy for the management of renal calculi include all of the following except which one?

    a. Failed ESWL
    b. Morbid obesity
    c. Cystine calculi
    d. Patients receiving anticoagulants
    e. Staghorn stones

Answers

1. **b. 80% to 85%.** The majority of "simple" renal calculi (about 80% to 85%) can be treated satisfactorily with ESWL. [p 3365]

2. **b. 10% to 30%.** The 10-year mortality rate of untreated staghorn stones was 28%, versus 7.2% in patients treated conservatively or by surgery. [p 3366]

3. **d. Stone burden.** Stone burden (size and number) is perhaps the single most important factor in deciding the appropriate treatment modality for a patient with kidney calculi. [p 3367]

4. **a. ESWL.** Calculi between 10 and 20 mm are still largely treated with ESWL as the first-line management. [p 3368]

5. **b. PNL.** High retreatment rates and the need for auxiliary procedures were the basis for the National Institutes of Health consensus conference recommendation in 1988 that patients with stones larger than 2 cm, infected or not, should be approached with PNL initially, followed, if needed, by ESWL. [p 3368]

6. **c. PNL.** The management of staghorn stones with a combined approach must be viewed as primarily percutaneous in nature, with ESWL being used only as adjunct to minimize the number of accesses required. [p 3370]

7. **b. Less than 500 mm^2.** ESWL monotherapy was successful (stone-free rate of 92%) in only a small group of patients with 500 mm^2 or smaller stone burden in nondilated collecting systems. [p 3370]

8. **b. Calcium oxalate monohydrate.** Cystine and brushite are the stones most resistant to ESWL, followed by calcium oxalate monohydrate. Next, in descending order, are hydroxyapatite, struvite, calcium oxalate dihydrate, and uric acid stones. [p 3370]

9. **c. PNL.** [p 3373]

10. **a. ESWL.** ESWL can achieve satisfactory results in properly selected patients, such as those with small stones (<1.5 cm) in the presence of normal urinary drainage. For larger stones or when there is evidence of poor urinary drainage, PNL should be used as the primary approach. [p 3373]

11. **d. Stone composition.** Stone size affects the results of ESWL treatment for lower pole stones more than it does the results for stones in other calyceal locations. When stratified by stone size, the results of meta-analysis showed stone-free rates of 74%, 56%, and 33% for stones less than 10 mm, 11 to 20 mm, and larger than 20 mm, respectively. Three anatomic features that may play a role in stone clearance were described in one study: the angle between the lower pole infundibulum and the renal pelvis, the diameter of the lower pole infundibulum, and the spatial distribution of the calyces. Another study noted that the infundibular width plays a significant role in stone clearance after ESWL and added infundibular length as an additional significant predictive factor. [p 3374]

12. **b. Flexible ureteroscopy.** Retrograde ureteroscopic intrarenal surgery may be the preferred modality of treatment for morbidly obese patients when the stone burden is not excessively large. [p 3376]

13. **d. Flexible ureteroscopy.** When anticoagulation cannot be temporarily discontinued, the use of ureteroscopy in combination with holmium laser lithotripsy is preferred. One study reported that even when patients' coagulopathies were not fully corrected, stones could be successfully treated with no increase in complications from bleeding. [p 3376]

14. **b. An increased rate of recurrent stones.** At follow-up (1.6 to 85.4 months), 43% of the patients had a significant symptomatic episode or required intervention. [p 3377]

15. **d. Noncontrast CT.** Although flexible nephroscopy is often considered the "gold standard" for assessing residual stones after PNL, the routine use of flexible nephroscopy has been challenged by studies showing the high sensitivity of noncontrast CT in detecting residual stones. Noncontrast CT had 100% sensitivity for detecting residual stones after PNL in 36 patients evaluated by both CT and flexible nephroscopy. [p 3378]

16. **c. Stone composition.** One study analyzed 75 patients with ureteral calculi and found that the interval to stone passage was highly variable and dependent on stone size, location, and side. Stones that were smaller, more distal, and on the right side were more likely to pass spontaneously. In another study, duration of symptoms before presentation was the most influential factor, followed by the degree of hydronephrosis. [p 3379]

17. **b. 2 to 4 weeks.** Even with complete ureteral obstruction, irreversible loss of renal function does not occur for more than 2 weeks but can progress to total renal unit loss at up to 6 weeks. [p 3380]

18. **b. Between 80% and 90%.** For stones smaller than 1 cm, the stone-free rate for ESWL was 84%. [p 3382]

19. **c. Enhancement of stone fragmentation.** Although early reports supported the routine use of a ureteral stent to bypass ureteral stones before ESWL, data analyzed by the American Urological Association ureteral calculi guidelines panel showed no improvement in fragmentation with stenting, and therefore routine stent placement before ESWL was discouraged. However, ureteral stenting is appropriate for other indications, such as management of pain, relief of obstruction, and stones that are difficult to visualize, and is mandatory in a patient who has a solitary obstructed kidney. [p 3382]

20. **a. Between 90% and 100%.** A review of the current literature shows excellent results for flexible ureteroscopic lithotripsy utilizing the holmium laser for proximal ureteral calculi, with a mean stone-free rate of 95% associated with a low perforation and stricture rate of about 1% (see Table 99–4). [p 3382]

21. **a. Between 90% and 100%.** A review of the current literature shows excellent results for rigid ureteroscopic lithotripsy utilizing the holmium laser for distal ureteral calculi, with a mean stone-free rate of 95% associated with a low perforation and stricture rate of about 1% (see Table 99–4). [p 3382]

22. **e. Age greater than 60 years.** Despite the improved results of ureteroscopic treatment for proximal ureteral stones, at present most urologists still favor ESWL as the initial approach for stones less than 1 cm in the proximal ureter. However, flexible ureteroscopy may be the treatment of choice for patients in whom ESWL has failed, for patients with a history of cystine stones, in the presence of distal ob-

struction, for impacted stones, for obese patients, for patients with bleeding diathesis, and when ESWL is not readily available. [p 3382]

23. **a. Irrigation with Suby's G solution.** Conservative management attempting stone dissolution with the use of Suby's G or M solution is protracted and now rarely, if ever, appropriate. Several modalities exist for the treatment of bladder calculi, including cystolitholapaxy; cystolithotripsy with electrohydraulic, ultrasonic, laser, or pneumatic lithotripsy; percutaneous cystolithotomy; and open cystolithotomy. Shock-wave lithotripsy may be another option. [p 3384]

24. **e. Struvite.** Stones are a well-known complication of urinary diversion, with the majority of calculi being composed of struvite and/or carbonate/apatite. [p 3386]

25. **c. Hyperoxaluria.** Risk factors for calculi in these patients include hyperchloremic metabolic acidosis with resultant hypercalciuria and hypocitraturia, urinary tract infection with a urea-splitting organism, incomplete diversion emptying, foreign bodies such as staples and nonabsorbable sutures, and mucus production by the diversion. [p 3386]

26. **a. Kock pouch.** Continent diversions seem particularly at risk. The Indiana pouch has a reported rate of 3% to 13%; the Kock pouch, 4% to 43%; the orthotopic hemi-Kock pouch, 3%; the Mainz pouch, 8%; and the cecal reservoir, 20%. The Kock pouch has been singled out as particularly lithogenic because of its construction with nonabsorbable staples and previously utilized Marlex mesh collars in the construction of the afferent nipple valve. [p 3386]

27. **b. Hypercalcemia.** Pregnancy induces a state of absorptive hypercalciuria and mild hyperuricosuria that is offset by increased excretion of urinary inhibitors such as citrate and magnesium, as well as increased urinary output. The metabolic changes in pregnancy do not influence the rate of new stone occurrence. However, paradoxically, it has been suggested that metabolic alterations in urine may contribute to accelerated encrustation of stents during pregnancy. [p 3389]

28. **c. Renal ultrasonography.** To avoid the small risk of radiation, ultrasonography has become the first-line diagnostic study for urolithiasis in pregnancy. [p 3389]

29. **e. Ballistic lithotripsy.** Ballistic lithotripsy is accompanied by a relatively high rate of stone propulsion of between 2% and 17% when ureteral stones are treated (see Table 99–7). The holmium laser has been associated with a reduced potential for causing retropulsion owing to the weak shock wave that is typically induced during holmium laser lithotripsy. [pp 3394, 3396]

30. **c. Cystine.** The coumarin wave length was chosen because it is absorbed by all stone materials other than cystine but not by surrounding tissues. Cystine calculi do not absorb the 504 nm laser light and, hence, are not fragmented with the coumarin-pulsed dye laser. [pp 3392–3393]

31. **a. 0.6 J, 6 Hz.** It is recommended to commence treatment using low-pulse energy (i.e., 0.6 J) with a pulse rate of 6 Hz and increase the pulse frequency (in preference to increasing the pulse energy) as needed to speed fragmentation. [pp 3394–3395]

32. **d. Holmium laser.** The ability of the holmium laser to fragment all stones regardless of composition is a clear advantage over the coumarin-pulsed dye laser. Successful fragmentation of ureteral stones of all compositions is reported in 91% to 100% of the cases with a mean stone-free rate of 95%. Currently, the holmium laser is the most effective and versatile intracorporeal lithotriptor with a good margin of safety. [p 3393]

33. **b. Ballistic.** When compared with EHL or ultrasonic or laser lithotripsy, ballistic devices have a significantly lower risk of ureteral perforation. [p 3396]

34. **b. Holmium laser.** There are three primary types of shock wave generators: electrohydraulic (Spark Gap), electromagnetic, and piezoelectric. Microexplosive generators have also been produced but have not gained mainstream acceptance. [pp 3398, 3402]

35. **e. Inability to visualize ureteral stones.** Sonographic localization of a kidney stone requires a highly trained operator. Furthermore, localization of stones in the ureter is difficult or impossible. [p 3403]

36. **b. Body habitus.** Thin patients have more pain during ESWL because the converging shock wave is more concentrated at the point of skin penetration. [pp 3403–3404]

37. **d. Unmodified Dornier HM3.** To date, despite the proliferation of lithotriptors and the variety of solutions devised for stone targeting and shock wave delivery, no other lithotriptor system has convincingly equaled or surpassed the results produced by the unmodified Dornier HM3 device. [p 3404]

38. **e. Vaporization.** Four potential mechanisms for ESWL stone breakage have been described: (1) compression fracture, (2) spallation, (3) acoustic cavitation, and (4) dynamic fatigue. [p 3406]

39. **e. 80% to 100%.** ESWL is now known to induce acute structural changes in the treated kidney in a majority, if not all, treated patients. Morphologic studies using both MRI and quantitative radionuclide renography have suggested that 63% to 85% of all ESWL patients treated with an unmodified HM3 lithotriptor exhibit one or more forms of renal injury within 24 hours of treatment. [p 3410]

40. **c. Stone burden.** Patients with existing hypertension are at increased risk for the development of perinephric hematomas as a consequence of ESWL. Age is a factor on both ends of the scale in that children and the elderly both appear to be at a greater risk for structural and functional changes after exposure to shock waves. These responses are probably related to a reduction in the large renal reserve present in most healthy adult patients. [p 3411]

41. **a. Blood vessels.** Macroscopically, the acute changes noted in dog and pig kidneys treated with a clinical dose of shock waves are strikingly similar to those described for patients. This lesion is predictable in size, is focal in location, and is unique in the types of injuries (primarily vascular insult) induced. Regions of damage reveal rupture of nearby thin-walled veins, walls of small arteries, and glomerular and peritubular capillaries (see Fig. 99–20), which correlates with the vasoconstriction measured in both treated and untreated kidneys. These observations show that both the microvasculature and the nephron are susceptible to shock wave damage; however, the primary injury appears to be a vascular insult. [pp 3413, 3414]

42. **d. *Staphylococcus epidermidis*.** Cephalosporins are the most appropriately used antibiotics for prophylaxis of surgical procedures in noninfected stone cases, as the most common secondarily infecting organism is *S. epidermidis*. [p 3416]

43. **c. Insertion of a ureteral catheter.** When performed as a single-stage procedure, PNL is initiated by the cystoscopic placement of a ureteral catheter. [p 3417]

44. **c. Posterior lower pole calyx.** Because the posterior calyces

are generally oriented so that the long axis points to the avascular area of the renal cortex, a posterolateral puncture directed at a posterior calyx would be expected to traverse through the avascular zone. [p 3418]

45. **e. Upper pole puncture.** A puncture placed too laterally may injure the colon. The position of the retroperitoneal colon is usually anterior or anterolateral to the lateral renal border. Therefore, risk of colon injury is usually only with a very lateral (lateral to the posterior axillary line) puncture. Posterior colonic displacement is more likely in thin female patients with very little retroperitoneal fat, and/or elderly patients, as well as in patients with jejunoileal bypass resulting in an enlarged colon. Other factors increasing the risk of colon injury include anterior calyceal puncture, previous extensive renal operation, horseshoe kidney, and kyphoscoliosis. A retrorenal colon is more frequently noted on the left side. [pp 3418–3419]

46. **a. the puncture should be performed during full expiration.** A supracostal puncture should be performed only during full expiration. [p 3420]

47. **c. Cystine stones.** A supracostal puncture is indicated when the predominant distribution of stone material is in the upper calyces; when there is an associated UPJ stricture requiring endopyelotomy; in cases of multiple lower pole infundibula and calyces containing stone material or an associated ureteral stone; in staghorn calculi with substantial upper pole stone burden; and in horseshoe kidneys. [p 3421]

48. **c. Glide wire.** The glide wire is preferred for entering the collecting system, as it is the most flexible and maneuverable wire available. [p 3422]

49. **b. Overadvancement of the dilator/sheath.** Overadvancement of the dilator/sheath is the most common serious error in access for PNL and may result in significant trauma to the renal collecting system and/or excessive hemorrhage. [p 3424]

50. **e. 0.9% saline.** Physiologic solutions should be used for irrigation during PNL to minimize the risk of dilutional hyponatremia in the event of large volume extravasation. [p 3425]

51. **a. A higher incidence of retrorenal colon.** The abnormal location of the horseshoe kidney may be associated with a retrorenal colon. [p 3429]

52. **a. Hemorrhage.** Bleeding is the most significant complication of PNL, with transfusion rates varying from less than 1% to 10%. [p 3430]

53. **c. 1 in 200.** Bleeding from an arteriovenous fistula or pseudoaneurysm requiring emergency embolization is seen in less than 0.5% of patients. [p 3430]

54. **e. Insertion of a Kaye tamponade balloon.** If bleeding is not controlled by nephrostomy tube placement and clamping, a Kaye nephrostomy tamponade balloon catheter should be placed (Cook Urological, Spencer, IN). The Kaye nephrostomy tube incorporates a low-pressure 12 mm balloon that may be left inflated for prolonged periods to tamponade bleeding from the nephrostomy tract. [p 3431]

55. **d. Insertion of a double-J stent and withdrawal of the nephrostomy tube into the colon.** Colonic injury is an unusual complication often diagnosed on a postoperative nephrostogram. Typically, the injury is retroperitoneal; thus, signs and symptoms of peritonitis are infrequent. If the perforation is extraperitoneal, management may be expectant with placement of a ureteral catheter or double-J stent to decompress the collecting system and by withdrawing the nephrostomy tube from an intrarenal position to an intracolonic position, thus serving as a colostomy tube. The colostomy tube is left in place for a minimum of 7 days and is removed after a nephrostogram or a retrograde pyelogram showing no communication between the colon and the kidney. [p 3432]

56. **d. Greater than 20 mm.** Stents may be particularly advantageous with stones larger than 20 mm. [p 3433]

57. **e. Staghorn stones.** One study reported the first large series (208 patients) of renal calculi treated by retrograde intrarenal surgery using a flexible deflectable ureteroscope after 1 to 2 weeks of ureteral stenting. The indications for the procedure included patients in whom ESWL had failed (single stone of <1 cm or up to 5 particles of <5 mm), radiolucent stones (<1.5 cm), concomitant ureteral and renal stones, renal stones associated with intrarenal stenosis, nephrocalcinosis or urinary diversion, patients with a need for complete stone removal (e.g., pilots), and patients with bleeding disorders. Treatment of staghorn stones with retrograde intrarenal surgery has been described although not widely accepted. [p 3435]

SECTION XIII

UROLOGIC SURGERY

Chapter 100

Basics of Laparoscopic Urologic Surgery

Inderbir S. Gill • Kurt Kerbl • Anoop M. Meraney • Ralph V. Clayman

Questions

1. Before Gaur's 1991 description of the balloon dilator, attempts at retroperitoneal laparoscopy encountered technical difficulties that were primarily associated with which one of the following?

   a. An increased incidence of vascular injuries
   b. Retroperitoneal adhesions
   c. Inadvertent bowel injuries
   d. An inadequate working space
   e. Dilated lymphatic channels

2. During retroperitoneal renal laparoscopy, balloon dilatation should be performed in which one of the following compartments?

   a. Anterior pararenal space
   b. Posterior pararenal space
   c. Lateral pararenal space
   d. Medial pararenal space
   e. All of the above

3. After balloon dilatation of the pelvic extraperitoneal space, the anatomic landmarks that may be identified include all the following except which one?

   a. Pulsations of the external iliac artery
   b. The intact bladder, containing the inflated Foley balloon
   c. The pubic symphysis
   d. Cooper's ligaments
   e. The median umbilical ligament

4. Advantages of commercially available, trocar-mounted, silicone balloon dilators include all the following except which one?

   a. The facility to perform laparoscopically controlled dilatation of the retroperitoneum
   b. Greater tensile strength than self-made latex balloons
   c. Availability in round and oblong shapes for precise retroperitoneal or pelvic extraperitoneal dilatation, respectively
   d. Cost-effectiveness compared with the self-made balloons
   e. None of the above

5. Which one of the following is true regarding gasless retroperitoneal laparoscopy?

   a. The risk of hypercarbia associated with CO_2 insufflation is increased.
   b. Routine open surgical instruments cannot be employed in conjunction with laparoscopic instruments.
   c. Valveless, reusable trocars cannot be utilized.
   d. Usually a smaller working space is available compared with conventional retroperitoneal laparoscopy.
   e. All of the above.

6. A 60-year-old woman weighing 256 lb is undergoing retroperitoneal laparoscopic radical nephrectomy for a 7 cm right renal mass. After the initial retroperitoneal open Hasson access and balloon dilatation with 800 ml of air, three reusable 10 mm ports are introduced. Despite the CO_2 insufflation pressure being set at 20 mm Hg, the working space is inadequate, and laparoscopic visualization is inadequate for laparoscopic dissection. A constant hissing sound is audible and the insufflator reads a pressure of 7 mm Hg, and a flow rate of 4 L/min. Which one of the following would best correct the problem?

   a. Increasing the insufflation pressure to 25 mm Hg
   b. Performing an additional balloon dilatation
   c. Replacing the primary port with a Bluntport (U.S. Surgical, Norwalk, Conn.) device
   d. Replacing all the reusable ports with disposable ports
   e. None of the above

7. Increased CO_2 build-up during laparoscopy may be related to all the following except which one?

   a. Severe chronic respiratory disease
   b. Subcutaneous emphysema
   c. Increased insufflation pressures
   d. Prolonged operative time
   e. Radical nephrectomy.

8. Perceived advantages of retroperitoneal laparoscopy compared with transperitoneal laparoscopy include all the following except which one?

   a. It is associated with a decreased incidence of bowel injury.
   b. It is associated with a decreased incidence of paralytic ileus.
   c. It is associated with a decreased incidence of port-site hernias.
   d. It provides direct and rapid access to the renal hilum.
   e. It is technically easier to learn.

9. After a retroperitoneal laparoscopic radical nephrectomy for renal cell cancer, significant difficulty is encountered in entrapping the specimen because of the restricted space available. What would the best maneuver at this time be?

   a. Convert to an open procedure
   b. Break the specimen in the retroperitoneum and then entrap it
   c. Introduce a tissue morcellator
   d. Create a peritoneotomy, and entrap the specimen in the peritoneal cavity
   e. Any of the above

10. After extraperitoneal pelvic lymph node dissection, the incidence of which one of the following is higher than with transperitoneal pelvic node dissection?

    a. Urinoma
    b. Lymphocele
    c. Bowel injury
    d. Hematoma
    e. Shoulder-tip pain

Answers

1. **d. An inadequate working space.** Similar to the early experiences with pelvic extraperitoneoscopy, difficulty was encountered in obtaining an adequate working space, as well as in achieving satisfactory pneumoretroperitoneum. [p 3495]

2. **b. Posterior pararenal space.** The space dorsolateral to Gerota's fascia is the posterior pararenal space; this is the space dilated during retroperitoneoscopy. [p 3496]

3. **e. The median umbilical ligament.** Pelvic anatomic landmarks identified in the preperitoneal space after balloon dilatation include the decompressed bladder containing the Foley balloon, the pubic symphysis in the midline, and the superior pubic ramus, Cooper's ligaments, and pulsations of the external iliac artery on either side. [p 3496]

4. **d. Cost-effectiveness compared with the self-made balloons.** Although economically advantageous, a drawback of the self-styled balloons is the lack of the stiff shaft, and thus the inability to manually direct the balloon into a specific location for precise dilatation, as well as the inability to insert a laparoscope within the balloon for visualization. [p 3500]

5. **d. Usually a smaller working space is available compared with conventional retroperitoneal laparoscopy.** Valveless trocars can be utilized, and the use of conventional open surgical instruments can be resorted to, if necessary. However, compared with conventional laparoscopy, this technique provides a limited exposure, especially in obese patients. [p 3500]

6. **c. Replacing the primary port with a Bluntport device.** Utilization of the Bluntport device minimizes CO_2 leakage around the 1.5 cm primary port incision, thus reducing the incidence of air leak and subcutaneous emphysema. [p 3501]

7. **e. Radical nephrectomy.** The potential for developing hypercarbia exists during both transperitoneal and preperitoneal laparoscopic procedures. Conceivably, this assumes greater importance in patients with preexisting airway and cardiovascular compromise. Vigilant perioperative anesthetic management is essential to prevent the development of potential complications related to CO_2 build-up. A rise in end-tidal CO_2 should prompt the anesthesiologist to adjust the respiratory rate and tidal volume to enhance CO_2 elimination. Simultaneously, the insufflation pressure of CO_2 should be decreased by the surgeon. [p 3502]

8. **e. It is technically easier to learn.** Retroperitoneoscopy is associated with unique anatomic orientation and a relatively restricted initial working area compared with transperitoneal laparoscopy. This results in a steeper learning curve with the former technique. [p 3503]

9. **d. Create a peritoneotomy, and entrap the specimen in the peritoneal cavity.** Retroperitoneoscopic entrapment of these larger specimens may be difficult. This problem is overcome by laparoscopically creating an intentional peritoneotomy at the end of the procedure to allow entrapment of the specimen within the larger peritoneal cavity. [p 3504]

10. **b. Lymphocele.** Absence of the peritoneal absorptive surface after extraperitoneoscopic lymphadenectomy may increase the risk of development of postoperative lymphocele. [p 3504]

Chapter 101

The Adrenals

E. Darracott Vaughan, Jr. • Jon D. Blumenfeld • Joseph Del Pizzo • Steven J. Schichman
R. Ernest Sosa

Questions

1. Why are the adrenals quite large at the time of birth?

    a. Because of a large fetal adrenal cortex
    b. Because of a large fetal adrenal medulla
    c. Because of an ectopic gonadal tissue
    d. Because of fusion to the kidney
    e. Because of an adrenal hemorrhage

2. What is the best imaging study to diagnose adrenal hemorrhage in the newborn?

    a. CT
    b. Ultrasonography
    c. MRI
    d. Intravenous pyelography (IVP)
    e. Adrenal venography

3. Why is it important to identify the left inferior phrenic vein during left adrenalectomy?

    a. To avoid renal vein injury
    b. To avoid diaphragmatic injury
    c. Because it is the main adrenal venous drainage
    d. As a guide to the aorta
    e. Because troublesome bleeding results if it is damaged

4. What are the principal androgens from the adrenal?

    a. Dehydroepiandrosterone (DHEA) and androstenedione
    b. DHEA and cortisol
    c. Androstenedione and cortisol
    d. DHEA and aldosterone
    e. Aldosterone and androstenedione

5. What stimulates the cascade leading to cortisol secretion?

    a. Enkephalins
    b. Melanocyte-stimulating hormone
    c. Antidiuretic hormone
    d. Corticotropin (ACTH)
    e. Angiotensin II

6. What is the major control mechanism for aldosterone secretion?

    a. ACTH
    b. Angiotensin II
    c. High potassium level
    d. High sodium level
    e. Low potassium level

7. What is the hallmark of the presence of adrenal tumors in women who present with hirsutism?

    a. Testosterone and DHEA
    b. DHEA and cortisol
    c. Testosterone and cortisol
    d. DHEA and aldosterone
    e. Testosterone and aldosterone

8. What is the primary metabolite of adrenal medullary catecholamines?

    a. Metanephrine
    b. Dopamine
    c. Norepinephrine
    d. Epinephrine
    e. Vanillylmandelic acid

9. What is the most common cause of Cushing's syndrome?

    a. Adrenal carcinoma
    b. Adrenal adenoma
    c. Cushing's disease
    d. Ectopic ACTH
    e. Ectopic corticotropin-releasing factor

10. What is one cause of Cushing's syndrome that is often forgotten?

    a. Exogenous steroid use
    b. Adrenal carcinoma
    c. Adrenal adenoma
    d. Ectopic ACTH
    e. Pituitary adenoma

11. What is a cause of pseudo-Cushing's syndrome?

    a. Obesity
    b. Hypertension
    c. Diabetes
    d. Depression
    e. Congestive heart failure

12. What is the most direct way to determine the presence of Cushing's syndrome?

    a. Plasma ACTH assay
    b. Three 24-hour urinary cortisol determinations
    c. Measurement of diurnal variations of cortisol
    d. Plasma cortisol assay
    e. High-dose dexamethasone administration

13. What is the most common reason that dexamethasone suppression tests are now utilized?

    a. To identify adrenal carcinoma
    b. To identify pseudo-Cushing's syndrome
    c. To identify adrenal adenoma
    d. To identify pituitary adenoma
    e. To identify ectopic ACTH

14. Currently, what is the ideal way to determine whether a patient has ACTH-dependent or ACTH-independent hypercortisolism?

    a. 24-hour cortisone excretion assay
    b. Concurrent measurement of ACTH and cortisone
    c. Measurement of diurnal variation of plasma cortisone

d. Low-dose dexamethasone test
e. High-dose dexamethasone test

15. What is the most direct way to demonstrate pituitary hypersecretion of ACTH?

    a. Plasma ACTH assay
    b. Brain MRI
    c. Brain CT
    d. Plasma cortisol assay
    e. Petrosal venous sinus sampling of ACTH

16. What characterizes Nelson's syndrome?

    a. Ectopic ACTH secretion
    b. Ectopic corticotropin-releasing hormone secretion
    c. Multiple endocrine tumors
    d. Pituitary tumor after bilateral adrenalectomy
    e. Recurrent cortical tissue after bilateral adrenalectomy

17. What is the best test to identify an adrenal cause of Cushing's syndrome during pregnancy?

    a. IVP
    b. Sonography
    c. MRI
    d. CT
    e. Adrenal venography

18. What is the size that best delineates adrenal benign tumors from adrenal malignancies?

    a. 5 cm
    b. 6 cm
    c. 3 cm
    d. 7 cm
    e. 4 cm

19. Which adrenal pathologic diagnoses are characterized by signal intensity ratio on a T2-weighted MR image?

    a. Neural tumors, carcinoma, metastatic lesions
    b. Neural tumors, adenoma, myelolipoma
    c. Carcinoma, adenoma, incidentaloma
    d. Metastatic lesions, adenoma, carcinoma
    e. Neural tumors, adenoma, carcinoma

20. What is a useful pathologic method for delineating large benign adrenal adenomas from adrenal carcinoma?

    a. Electron microscopy
    b. Transforming growth factor-β assay
    c. Masson's trichrome stain
    d. Hematoxylin-eosin stain
    e. Flow cytometry

21. What is the 5-year survival rate for patients with adrenocortical carcinoma?

    a. 15%
    b. 25%
    c. 35%
    d. 45%
    e. 55%

22. What unrecognized adrenal disorder should be considered in a cancer patient who is critically ill?

    a. Addison's disease
    b. Conn's syndrome
    c. Cushing's disease
    d. Nelson's syndrome
    e. Carney's syndrome

23. What are the primary biochemical characteristics of primary hyperaldosteronism?

    a. Hypokalemia, high plasma renin activity (PRA), high aldosterone level
    b. Hypokalemia, low PRA, high aldosterone level
    c. Hyperkalemia, low PRA, high aldosterone level
    d. Hyperkalemia, high PRA, high aldosterone level
    e. Normokalemia, high PRA, high aldosterone level

24. What is the important dietary control that must be utilized before one can rule out hypokalemia in a patient with hyperaldosteronism?

    a. Low sodium diet
    b. Low potassium diet
    c. High potassium diet
    d. Normal sodium intake
    e. Low calcium diet

25. What is the response to a postural stimulation test in a patient with hyperaldosteronism caused by an adenoma?

    a. Rise in PRA, rise in aldosterone
    b. Rise in PRA, fall in aldosterone
    c. Fall in PRA, fall in aldosterone
    d. Fall in PRA, rise in aldosterone
    e. Stable PRA, rise in aldosterone

26. What is the best methodology for lateralizing aldosterone secretion in a patient with primary hyperaldosteronism?

    a. 19-iodocholesterol scan
    b. Adrenal venography
    c. MRI
    d. Ultrasonography
    e. Adrenal vein sampling

27. In a patient with primary hyperaldosteronism resulting from a solitary adenoma, what preparation should be used to determine that the patient is ready for unilateral adrenalectomy?

    a. Blood pressure control and sodium repletion
    b. Sodium and potassium repletion
    c. Blood pressure control and potassium repletion
    d. Thiazide diuretic for blood pressure control
    e. Blood volume repletion

28. What is the appropriate treatment of the patient with primary hyperaldosteronism resulting from bilateral hyperplasia when there is no lateralization of aldosterone secretion?

    a. Spironolactone
    b. A β-blocker
    c. An angiotensin-converting enzyme inhibitor
    d. Hydrochlorothiazide
    e. Phenoxybenzamine

29. What are the cure and improvement rates in patients with primary hyperaldosteronism resulting from an adrenal adenoma after adrenalectomy?

    a. 60%
    b. 70%
    c. 80%
    d. 90%
    e. 100%

30. What percentage of patients with a pheochromocytoma present without hypertension?

    a. 5%
    b. 10%
    c. 15%
    d. 20%
    e. 25%

31. What characterizes catechol-induced myocardiopathy?

    a. Low cardiac ejection fraction
    b. Hepatic dysfunction
    c. Irreversible cardiac disease

d. Malignant hypertension
e. Encephalopathy

32. In what groups are multiple pheochromocytomas or ectopic catecholamine-secreting paragangliomas found?
    a. Children, those with multiple endocrine adenoma (MEA), familial groups
    b. Children, those with MEA, women
    c. Children, those with MEA, elderly
    d. Those with MEA, women, elderly
    e. Familial groups, children, women

33. What radiologic test is of most value in localizing a pheochromocytoma in a patient with the biochemical characteristics of the disease?
    a. Angiography
    b. CT
    c. MRI
    d. Sonography
    e. IVP

34. What is the appropriate preoperative preparation for a patient with a pheochromocytoma?
    a. β-Blockade alone
    b. Hydrochlorothiazide
    c. Angiotensin-converting enzyme inhibitor
    d. α-Blockade with phenoxybenzamine
    e. Spironolactone

35. What is the advantage of a modified posterior approach to the right adrenal gland?
    a. Early exposure of the adrenal vein
    b. Avoidance of the pleura
    c. Early control of the adrenal artery
    d. Less renal damage than other approaches
    e. Less hepatic injury than other approaches

36. During any open adrenalectomy, which portion of the gland should be freed initially?
    a. Cephalad and lateral
    b. Medial and lateral
    c. Renal and medial
    d. Inferior and medial
    e. Inferior and lateral

37. How does the adrenal dissection differ in a patient with a pheochromocytoma?
    a. It allows early separation from the kidney.
    b. It gains early ligation of the adrenal vein.
    c. It gains early ligation of the adrenal arteries.
    d. Early dissection from the liver on the spleen is used.
    e. A thoracoabdominal approach is used.

38. When is open adrenalectomy preferred?
    a. For pheochromocytoma
    b. For adrenal adenoma
    c. In Conn's syndrome
    d. For adrenal cyst
    e. For adrenal carcinoma

39. What is the primary use of partial adrenalectomy?
    a. For pheochromocytoma
    b. For patients with bilateral tumor
    c. For adrenal adenoma
    d. For adrenal carcinoma
    e. For myelolipoma

40. What is the approach of choice for most adrenal tumors?
    a. Posterior
    b. Modified posterior
    c. Laparoscopic
    d. Transabdominal
    e. Thoracoabdominal

41. What is one relative contraindication to laparoscopic adrenalectomy?
    a. Pheochromocytoma
    b. Obesity
    c. Adrenal adenoma
    d. Conn's syndrome
    e. Cushing's syndrome

42. Which of the following is a technical difference in transperitoneal laparoscopic adrenalectomy?
    a. Early separation of liver and spleen
    b. Careful control of the adrenal vein
    c. Avoidance of renal vascular injury
    d. Maintaining lateral and cephalad attachments
    e. Careful control of adrenal arteries

Answers

1. **a. Because of a large fetal adrenal cortex.** The adrenal weight at birth is quite large (5 to 10 g) because of the fetal adrenal cortex, which may play a major role in fetal embryogenesis and homeostasis. [p 3508]

2. **c. MRI.** Adrenal hemorrhage at the time of birth is a condition now readily diagnosed by MRI. [pp 3508–3509]

3. **e. Because troublesome bleeding results if it is damaged.** Not well recognized is the left inferior phrenic vein, which typically communicates with the adrenal vein but then courses medially and can be injured during dissection of the medial edge of the gland. [p 3509]

4. **a. Dehydroepiandrosterone (DHEA) and androstenedione.** The principal androgens are DHEA, dehydroepiandrosterone sulfate (DHEAS), and androstenedione. [p 3511]

5. **d. Corticotropin (ACTH).** ACTH is produced from a large protein (290 amino acids) termed pro-opiomelanocortin (POMC). Other POMC-derived peptides include β-lipotropin, α- and β-melanocyte-stimulating hormone, β-endorphin, and methionine-enkephalin (see Fig. 101–9). ACTH secretion is characterized by an inherent diurnal rhythm leading to parallel changes in cortisol and ACTH. ACTH secretion is reciprocally related to the circulating cortisol level. [p 3512]

6. **b. Angiotensin II.** In contrast to glucocorticoids and adrenal androgens, the primary physiologic control of aldosterone secretion is angiotensin II. [p 3512]

7. **a. Testosterone and DHEA.** Elevated serum concentrations of testosterone and DHEA are the hallmark of the presence of adrenal tumors in women who present with hirsutism. [p 3514]

8. **e. Vanillylmandelic acid.** The primary metabolite in the urine is vanillylmandelic acid, with metanephrine, normetanephrine, and their derivatives contributing to total metabolic products. [p 3515]

9. **c. Cushing's disease.** Cushing's disease accounts for 75% to

85% of patients with endogenous Cushing's syndrome. [p 3515]

10. **a. Exogenous steroid use.** An exogenous source of Cushing's syndrome should always first be excluded because therapeutic steroids are the most common cause. Often the patient does not even realize that he or she is using a steroid-containing preparation, especially creams or lotions. [p 3515]

11. **d. Depression.** Patients with nonendocrine disorders that mimic the clinical and sometimes biochemical manifestations of Cushing's syndrome must be separated from those patients with true Cushing's syndrome; these patients have been said to have pseudo-Cushing's syndrome. Abnormally regulated cortical secretion, albeit mild, may exist in as many as 80% of patients with major depression. [pp 3517–3518]

12. **b. Three 24-hour urinary cortisol determinations.** At the present time, the determination of 24-hour excretion of cortisol in the urine is the most direct and reliable index of cortisol secretion. One study recommended that urinary cortisol should be measured in two and preferably three consecutive 24-hour urine specimens collected on an outpatient basis. [p 3518]

13. **b. To identify pseudo-Cushing's syndrome.** These low-dose suppression tests are now reserved primarily for patients with equivocal 24-hour urinary cortisol excretion and are especially useful for identifying patients with pseudo-Cushing's syndrome. [p 3519]

14. **b. Concurrent measurement of ACTH and cortisone.** The ideal way to determine whether a patient has ACTH-dependent or ACTH-independent hypercortisolism is the concurrent measurement of both plasma ACTH (corticotropin) and cortisol. [p 3519]

15. **e. Petrosal venous sinus sampling of ACTH.** The most direct way to demonstrate pituitary hypersecretion of ACTH is to measure its level in the petrosal venous sinus and compare that level to the peripheral level. [p 3520]

16. **d. Pituitary tumor after bilateral adrenalectomy.** Generally, patients with severe Cushing's disease did well after bilateral adrenalectomy through a bilateral posterior approach with resolution of the disease. Ten percent to 20% of patients, however, subsequently developed pituitary tumors, usually chromophobe adenomas, perhaps caused by the lack of hypothalamic/pituitary feedback and high ACTH and related compounds. This entity, termed Nelson's syndrome, may arise many years after bilateral adrenalectomy. [p 3522]

17. **c. MRI.** The authors have used MRI to identify an adenoma in a pregnant patient with Cushing's syndrome. [p 3523]

18. **a. 5 cm.** CT may underestimate the size of an adrenal lesion, and one study suggested that exploration be performed when the lesion is more than 5 cm on CT or MRI scans. [p 3524]

19. **a. Neural tumors, carcinoma, metastatic lesions.** There are a number of entities other than adrenal carcinoma, however, that can cause high intensity, including neural tumors, metastatic tumors to the adrenal, and hemorrhage into a variety of adrenal lesions. [p 3525]

20. **e. Flow cytometry.** One study reported that flow cytometry accurately demonstrated aneuploid stem lines in four cases classified histologically as carcinoma. [p 3526]

21. **c. 35%.** Except for testosterone-secreting tumors, adrenocortical carcinomas are highly malignant, with both local and hematogenous spread and a 5-year survival rate of about 35%. [p 3528]

22. **a. Addison's disease.** Adrenal insufficiency may be an important aspect of the care of a patient with cancer and may be due to replacement of the adrenals with metastases, infiltration with lymphoma, hemorrhagic necrosis in association with anticoagulation, or sepsis as well as impaired adrenal steroidogenesis in patients receiving aminoglutethimide, ketoconazole, mitotane, or suramin. Addison's disease is rare, the death rate being approximately 0.3 per 100,000, with the most common cause being either tuberculosis or adrenal atrophy. Other causes include malignant infiltration. [p 3529]

23. **b. Hypokalemia, low PRA, high aldosterone level.** The syndrome of primary hyperaldosteronism is now identified by the combined findings of hypokalemia, suppressed PRA, and high urinary and plasma aldosterone levels in hypertensive patients. [p 3532]

24. **d. Normal sodium intake.** Because severe hypokalemia occurs less frequently in patients with restricted dietary sodium intake, certain authors do not recommend screening patients for this syndrome unless they are adequately salt loaded. [p 3536]

25. **b. Rise in PRA, fall in aldosterone.** In patients with primary aldosteronism with highly autonomous aldosterone production, plasma aldosterone levels decrease during this test, reflecting the influence of the diurnal fall in ACTH, which is normally a relatively minor stimulus for aldosterone production. The PRA level rises. [p 3537]

26. **e. Adrenal vein sampling.** Adrenal vein sampling of aldosterone remains the cornerstone for localization of aldosterone production. [p 3538]

27. **c. Blood pressure control and potassium repletion.** Adrenalectomy should be preceded by several weeks of adequate control of hypertension and correction of hypokalemia and other metabolic abnormalities. [p 3539]

28. **a. Spironolactone.** The cornerstone of medical therapy in primary aldosteronism caused by bilateral hyperplasia is spironolactone (Aldactone), a competitive antagonist of the aldosterone receptor. [p 3539]

29. **d. 90%.** Hypertension was either cured or improved to an acceptable target in more than 90% of the patients with an adenoma. [p 3539]

30. **b. 10%.** About 10% of pheochromocytomas are found in normotensive patients. [p 3540]

31. **a. Low cardiac ejection fraction.** One specific entity that has gained more recognition is catecholamine-induced cardiomyopathy. Experimentally injected catecholamines can cause foci of myocardial necrosis, with inflammation and fibrosis. These patients may have a reduction in blood pressure because of a global reduction in myocardial pump functions, considered to be due to both a down-regulation of β-receptors and a decrease of viable myofibrils. [pp 3541–3542]

32. **a. Children, those with multiple endocrine adenoma (MEA), familial groups.** Familial pheochromocytomas may be divided into different types of genetic abnormalities. Pheochromocytomas occur in MEA 2, a triad including pheochromocytoma, medullary carcinoma of the thyroid, and parathyroid adenomas. Pheochromocytoma may also be a part of multiple endocrine neoplasia 3. In contrast to adults, children manifest a higher incidence of familial pheochromocytomas (10%) and bilaterality (24%). [pp 3543–3544]

33. **c. MRI.** There are multiple uses of MRI in patients with pheochromocytoma. The test appears to be as accurate as CT in identifying lesions, while having a characteristically bright, "light bulb" image on T2-weighted study (see Figs.

101–41 and 101–42). In addition, sagittal and coronal imaging can give excellent anatomic information about the relationship between the tumor and the surrounding vasculature as well as the draining venous channels (see Figs. 101–42 and 101–43). The authors believe that MRI should be the initial scanning procedure in patients with biochemical findings of a pheochromocytoma. [pp 3545–3547]

34. **d. α-Blockade with phenoxybenzamine.** Phenoxybenzamine hydrochloride (Dibenzyline), a long-acting α-adrenergic blocker, controls blood pressure in patients with pheochromocytoma. [p 3547]

35. **a. Early exposure of the adrenal vein.** The major advantage of this approach is that the adrenal vein is identified without difficulty because it emerges from the segment of the inferior vena cava exposed and courses up to the adrenal, which now rises toward the operating surgeon. [p 3550]

36. **a. Cephalad and lateral.** On the right side, the liver within the peritoneum is lifted off the anterior surface of the adrenal (see Fig. 101–46A). Quite often, the adrenal gland cannot be identified precisely until these maneuvers are performed. One should not attempt to dissect into the body of the adrenal or to dissect the inferior surface of the adrenal off the kidney. The kidney is useful for retraction. The dissection should continue from lateral to medial along the posterior abdominal and diaphragmatic musculature with precise ligation or clipping of the small but multiple adrenal arteries. [pp 3550–3552]

37. **b. It gains early ligation of the adrenal vein.** A major deviation from this technique is used in patients with pheochromocytoma, in whom the initial dissection should be aimed toward early control and division of the main adrenal vein on either side. [p 3551]

38. **e. For adrenal carcinoma.** The transabdominal approach is commonly chosen for patients with pheochromocytomas, for pediatric patients, and for some patients with adrenal carcinomas. [p 3553]

39. **b. For patients with bilateral tumor.** A major use of partial adrenalectomy is in patients at risk for multiple adrenal tumors such as von Hippel-Lindau type 2 patients. [p 3554]

40. **c. Laparoscopic.** Laparoscopy offers a shorter length of hospital stay, a decrease in postoperative pain, a shorter time to return to preoperative activity level, improved cosmesis, and reduced morbidity in the fragile patient afflicted with Cushing's disease. [p 3554]

41. **b. Obesity.** Few absolute contraindications to laparoscopic adrenalectomy exist. Relative contraindications include prior intra-abdominal trauma or surgery, morbid obesity, uncorrected coagulopathies, and large pheochromocytomas. Prior trauma or surgery involving the spleen, liver, kidney, or tail of the pancreas may preclude a safe laparoscopic procedure. Dense adhesions can limit the surgeon's ability to obtain adequate exposure, vascular control, and safe dissection and removal of the adrenal gland. [p 3555]

42. **d. Maintaining lateral and cephalad attachments.** We do not recommend releasing the lateral attachments of the adrenal gland at this time. [p 3557]

Chapter 102

Surgery of the Kidney

Andrew C. Novick

Questions

1. What is the maximum period of unprotected warm renal ischemia that can be tolerated with no permanent loss of renal function?

   a. 10 minutes
   b. 20 minutes
   c. 30 minutes
   d. 45 minutes
   e. 60 minutes

2. What is the single most effective and commonly employed method of protecting the kidney from warm ischemic damage?

   a. Mannitol
   b. Inosine
   c. Calcium channel blockers
   d. Surface hypothermia
   e. Perfusion hypothermia

3. Renal ischemia is most damaging to which of the following parts of the nephron?

   a. Proximal tubule
   b. Descending limb of Henle's loop
   c. Ascending limb of Henle's loop
   d. Distal tubule
   e. Renal medulla

4. Renal ischemic damage from temporary renal vascular occlusion during surgery can be minimized by which of the following?

   a. Leaving the kidney covered with ice slush for 10 minutes before beginning the renal operation.
   b. Occlusion of both the renal artery and the renal vein.
   c. Intermittent unclamping and reclamping of the renal artery.
   d. Intermittent unclamping and reclamping of the renal artery and vein.
   e. Adjunctive intra-arterial injection of mannitol.

5. The thoracoabdominal approach for radical nephrectomy is most advantageous in which of the following settings?

   a. Large upper pole left renal tumor
   b. Large upper pole right renal tumor
   c. Large central (hilar) renal tumor
   d. Renal tumor with extensive lymphadenopathy
   e. Renal tumor with level I vena caval thrombus

6. What is the most important surgical aspect of radical nephrectomy with respect to prevention of recurrent malignancy postoperatively?
   a. Removal of the ipsilateral adrenal gland
   b. Preliminary ligation of the renal artery
   c. Preliminary ligation of the renal artery and vein
   d. Removal of the kidney outside Gerota's fascia
   e. Performance of complete regional lymphadenectomy

7. The least common location of vena caval hemorrhage during retroperitoneal surgery is at the level of the:
   a. lumbar veins.
   b. right gonadal vein.
   c. left gonadal vein.
   d. renal veins.
   e. right adrenal vein.

8. What is the most effective adjunctive technique for radical nephrectomy and vena caval thrombectomy with an intra-atrial thrombus?
   a. Cardiopulmonary bypass
   b. Cardiopulmonary bypass with hypothermic circulatory arrest
   c. Caval-atrial shunt
   d. A Pringle maneuver
   e. Thoracic aortic arch occlusion

9. What is the maximum period of deep hypothermic circulatory arrest that can safely be maintained for most patients?
   a. 20 minutes
   b. 30 minutes
   c. 40 minutes
   d. 60 minutes
   e. 80 minutes

10. Adjunctive veno-venous bypass (caval-atrial shunt) is most helpful for removal of a vena caval thrombus in which setting?
    a. Tumor invasion of vena caval wall
    b. Intra-atrial vena caval thrombus
    c. Previous open heart surgery
    d. Subhepatic vena caval thrombus
    e. Intrahepatic vena caval thrombus

11. Acceptable criteria for performing partial nephrectomy with localized unilateral renal cell carcinoma and a normal opposite kidney include which of the following?
    a. Single tumor ≤6 cm, located in the upper or lower renal pole
    b. Single tumor ≤6 cm, any renal location
    c. Single tumor ≤4 cm, any renal location
    d. Up to two tumors ≤4 cm, any renal location
    e. Single tumor ≤4 cm, located in the upper or lower renal pole

12. The major disadvantage of partial nephrectomy compared with radical nephrectomy for localized low-stage renal cell carcinoma is the increased risk of which of the following?
    a. Perioperative renal failure
    b. Perioperative hemorrhage
    c. Postoperative distant metastasis
    d. Postoperative tumor recurrence in the remnant kidney
    e. Postoperative tumor recurrence in perirenal lymph nodes

13. What is the preferred surgical approach for performing partial nephrectomy for malignancy?
    a. Anterior subcostal transperitoneal
    b. Anterior subcostal extraperitoneal
    c. Flank extraperitoneal
    d. Posterior extraperitoneal
    e. Thoracoabdominal

14. What is the single most useful imaging study for surgical planning when performing partial nephrectomy for malignancy?
    a. Renal MRI with coronal and sagittal views
    b. Selective renal arteriography with oblique views
    c. Selective renal venography
    d. Intraoperative ultrasonography
    e. Three-dimensional renal CT

15. When a transverse partial resection of the upper half of the kidney is performed, particular care must be taken to avoid injury to which of the following renal arterial branches?
    a. Apical
    b. Anterior superior
    c. Posterior
    d. Anterior inferior
    e. Basilar

16. When partial nephrectomy for renal cell carcinoma is performed, what is the primary indication for surgical enucleation?
    a. Centrally located tumors
    b. von Hippel-Lindau disease
    c. Tuberous sclerosis
    d. Multiple sporadic tumors
    e. Papillary tumors

17. Which surgical technique is seldom necessary for performing partial nephrectomy for malignancy?
    a. Wedge resection of lateral tumor
    b. Transverse renal resection
    c. Segmental polar resection
    d. Wedge resection of central tumor
    e. Extracorporeal renal resection

18. What are the two most common complications following partial nephrectomy for renal malignancy?
    a. Hemorrhage and acute renal failure
    b. Hemorrhage and urinary fistula
    c. Urinary fistula and ureteral obstruction
    d. Urinary fistula and acute renal failure
    e. Ureteral obstruction and acute renal failure

19. Following partial nephrectomy for pT2N0M0 renal cell carcinoma, it is necessary to perform surveillance abdominal CT how frequently?
    a. Never
    b. Every 6 months
    c. Every year
    d. Every 2 years
    e. Every 4 years

20. Following partial nephrectomy in a solitary kidney, what is the most effective method of screening for hyperfiltration nephropathy?
    a. Urinary dipstick test for protein
    b. 24-hour urinary protein measurement
    c. Iothalamate glomerular filtration measurement
    d. Serum creatinine measurement
    e. Renal biopsy

21. Progressive renal artery obstruction with ischemic atrophy of the kidney is least likely to occur in which of the following?
    a. Atherosclerosis
    b. Medial fibroplasia

c. Perimedial fibroplasia
d. Intimal fibroplasia
e. Intramural dissection

22. Surgical treatment of a renal artery aneurysm is indicated when it is:

    a. calcified and larger than 2 cm.
    b. noncalcified and larger than 2 cm.
    c. associated with medial fibroplasia.
    d. noncalcified, of any size.
    e. associated with atherosclerosis.

23. What is the primary indication for endovascular stenting of the renal artery?

    a. Intimal fibroplasia
    b. Ostial atherosclerosis
    c. Medial fibroplasia
    d. Nonostial atherosclerosis
    e. Renal artery aneurysm

24. Revascularization to preserve renal function for atherosclerotic renal artery disease is primarily indicated in which situation?

    a. 80% right renal artery stenosis, normal left renal artery, serum creatinine level 4.0 mg/dl
    b. Bilateral 80% renal artery stenosis, serum creatinine level 2.1 mg/dl
    c. 50% right renal artery stenosis, 80% left renal artery stenosis, serum creatinine level 1.6 mg/dl
    d. Bilateral 50% renal artery stenosis, serum creatinine level 4.5 mg/dl
    e. 80% stenosis of the renal artery to a solitary kidney, serum creatinine level 4.5 mg/dl

25. What is the preferred technique for surgical revascularization of the right kidney in patients with severe atherosclerotic disease of both the abdominal aorta and the renal artery?

    a. Abdominal aortorenal bypass
    b. Thoracic aortorenal bypass
    c. Aortic endarterectomy
    d. Hepatorenal bypass
    e. Iliorenal bypass

26. What is the most common complication following direct end-to-end anastomosis of the right hepatic and renal arteries?

    a. Hepatic dysfunction
    b. Common bile duct obstruction
    c. Ischemic cholecystitis
    d. Renal artery thrombosis
    e. Portal vein injury

27. What is the preferred incision for performing thoracic aortorenal revascularization of the left kidney?

    a. Bilateral anterior subcostal transperitoneal
    b. Anterior midline transperitoneal
    c. Supracostal flank extraperitoneal
    d. Thoracoabdominal
    e. Anterior midline transperitoneal with median sternotomy

28. When aortorenal bypass is performed, what is the optimal bypass graft source for renal artery replacement?

    a. Polytetrafluoroethylene
    b. Gonadal vein
    c. Cephalic vein
    d. Saphenous vein
    e. Hypogastric artery

29. Operative mortality following surgical revascularization for atherosclerotic renal artery disease can be reduced by all of the following except which one?

    a. Preoperative screening for coronary disease
    b. Preoperative screening for cerebrovascular disease
    c. Avoidance of an operation on a diseased abdominal aorta
    d. Bilateral simultaneous renal revascularization
    e. Perioperative pulmonary wedge pressure monitoring

30. Surgical unroofing of renal cysts in autosomal dominant polycystic kidney disease is most likely to result in which of the following?

    a. Improvement of hypertension
    b. Improvement of renal function
    c. Extended stabilization of renal function
    d. Relief of associated pain
    e. Reduced frequency of urinary infections

31. What is the preferred surgical approach for performing surgery on a horseshoe kidney?

    a. Dorsal lumbotomy
    b. Flank extraperitoneal
    c. Anterior midline transperitoneal
    d. Anterior subcostal extraperitoneal
    e. Thoracoabdominal

Answers

1. **c. 30 minutes.** The extent of renal damage following normothermic arterial occlusion depends on the duration of the ischemic insult. Canine studies have shown that warm ischemic intervals of up to 30 minutes can be sustained with eventual full recovery of renal function. For periods of warm ischemia beyond 30 minutes, there is generally significant immediate functional loss, and late recovery of renal function is either incomplete or absent. [p 3574]

2. **d. Surface hypothermia.** Local hypothermia is the most efficacious and commonly employed method for protecting the kidney from ischemic damage. Lowering renal temperature reduces energy-dependent metabolic activity of the cortical cells, with a resultant decrease in both the consumption of oxygen and the breakdown of ATP. In situ renal hypothermia can be achieved with external surface cooling or perfusion of the kidney with a cold solution instilled into the renal artery. These two methods are equally effective; however, the latter is an invasive technique that requires direct entry into the renal artery. Surface cooling of the kidney is a simpler and more widely used method that has been accomplished by a variety of techniques such as surrounding the kidney in a cold solution. [pp 3574–3575]

3. **a. Proximal tubule.** Histologically, renal ischemia is most damaging to the proximal tubular cells, which may show varying degrees of necrosis and regeneration, whereas the glomeruli and blood vessels are generally spared. [p 3574]

4. **a. Leaving the kidney covered with ice slush for 10 minutes before beginning the renal operation.** Most urologists currently prefer ice slush cooling for surface renal hypother-

mia because of its relative ease and simplicity. The mobilized kidney is surrounded with a rubber sheet on which sterile ice slush is placed to completely immerse the kidney. An important caveat with this method is to keep the entire kidney covered with ice for 10 to 15 minutes immediately after occluding the renal artery and before commencing the renal operation. This amount of time is needed to obtain core renal cooling to a temperature (approximately 20°C) that optimizes in situ renal preservation. [p 3575]

5. **b. Large upper pole right renal tumor.** The thoracoabdominal approach is desirable for performing radical nephrectomy in patients with large tumors involving the upper portion of the kidney. It is particularly advantageous on the right side, where the liver and its venous drainage into the upper vena cava can limit exposure and impair vascular control as the tumor mass is being removed. [p 3583]

6. **d. Removal of the kidney outside Gerota's fascia.** Perhaps the most important aspect of radical nephrectomy is removal of the kidney outside Gerota's fascia because capsular invasion with perinephric fat involvement occurs in 25% of patients. [p 3589]

7. **c. Left gonadal vein.** During performance of radical nephrectomy, intraoperative hemorrhage can occur from the inferior vena cava or its tributaries. Lumbar veins enter the posterolateral aspect of the vena cava at each vertebral level, and undue traction on the cava can result in their avulsion with troublesome bleeding. A second predictable bleeding site is the entry of the right gonadal vein into the anterolateral surface of the vena cava. A third predictable site of bleeding lies at the level of the renal veins, where large lumbar veins will often course posteriorly from the left renal vein just lateral to the aorta, or from the posterior aspect of the vena cava close to the entry of the right renal vein. A fourth predictable site of bleeding is at the level of the right adrenal vein, which enters the inferior vena cava. [pp 3593–3594]

8. **b. Cardiopulmonary bypass with hypothermic circulatory arrest.** In patients with renal cell carcinoma and an intrahepatic or suprahepatic inferior vena cava thrombus, the difficulty of surgical excision is significantly increased. Several different surgical maneuvers have been used to provide adequate exposure, prevent severe bleeding, and achieve complete tumor removal in this setting. At The Cleveland Clinic, we have preferred to employ cardiopulmonary bypass with deep hypothermic circulatory arrest for most patients with complex supradiaphragmatic tumor thrombi and for all patients with right atrial tumor thrombi. We initially reported a favorable experience with this approach in 43 patients, and a subsequent study has shown excellent long-term cancer-free survival following its use in patients with right atrial thrombi. [pp 3596, 3598]

9. **c. 40 minutes.** When the patient is under deep hypothermic circulatory arrest, the entire interior lumen of the vena cava can be directly inspected to ensure that all fragments of thrombus are completely removed. Hypothermic circulatory arrest can be safely maintained for at least 40 minutes without incurring a cerebral ischemic event. [p 3600]

10. **e. Intrahepatic vena caval thrombus.** In patients with nonadherent supradiaphragmatic vena caval tumor thrombi that do not extend into the right atrium, veno-venous bypass in the form of a caval-atrial shunt is a useful technique. [p 3600]

11. **c. Single tumor ≤4 cm, any renal location.** Studies have clarified the role of partial nephrectomy in patients with localized unilateral renal cell carcinoma and a normal contralateral kidney. These data indicate that radical nephrectomy and partial nephrectomy provide equally effective curative treatment for such patients who present with a single, small (<4 cm), and clearly localized renal cell carcinoma. [p 3603]

12. **d. Postoperative tumor recurrence in the remnant kidney.** The major disadvantage of partial nephrectomy for renal cell carcinoma is the risk of postoperative local tumor recurrence in the operated kidney, which has been observed in 4% to 6% of patients. These local recurrences are most likely a manifestation of undetected microscopic multifocal renal cell carcinoma in the renal remnant. [p 3603]

13. **c. Flank extraperitoneal.** It is usually possible to perform partial nephrectomy for malignancy in situ by using an operative approach that optimizes exposure of the kidney and by combining meticulous surgical technique with an understanding of the renal vascular anatomy in relation to the tumor. We employ an extraperitoneal flank incision through the bed of the 11th or 12th rib for almost all of these operations; we occasionally use a thoracoabdominal incision for very large tumors involving the upper portion of the kidney. These incisions allow the surgeon to operate on the mobilized kidney almost at skin level and provide excellent exposure of the peripheral renal vessels. [pp 3603–3604]

14. **e. Three-dimensional renal CT.** Three-dimensional volume-rendered CT is a new noninvasive imaging modality that can accurately depict the renal parenchymal and vascular anatomy in a format familiar to urologic surgeons. The data integrate essential information from arteriography, venography, excretory urography, and conventional two-dimensional CT into a single imaging modality, and this method obviates the need for more invasive imaging. [p 3603]

15. **c. Posterior.** When a transverse resection of the upper part of the kidney is performed, care must be taken to avoid injury to the posterior segmental renal arterial branch, which may also occasionally supply the basilar renal segment. Preoperative selective renal arteriography with oblique views is integral to identifying and preserving the posterior segmental artery at surgery and to thereby avoid devascularizing a major portion of the healthy remnant kidney. [p 3605]

16. **b. von Hippel-Lindau disease.** The technique of enucleation is currently employed only in occasional patients with von Hippel-Lindau disease and multiple low-stage encapsulated tumors involving both kidneys. [p 3610]

17. **e. Extracorporeal renal resection.** Although some urologic surgeons have found that almost all patients undergoing partial nephrectomy for renal cell carcinoma can be managed satisfactorily in situ, others have continued to recommend an extracorporeal approach for selected patients. [p 3610]

18. **d. Urinary fistula and acute renal failure.** A study has detailed the incidence and clinical outcome of technical or renal-related complications occurring after 259 partial nephrectomies for renal tumors at The Cleveland Clinic. The most common complications were urinary fistula formation and acute renal failure. [p 3612]

19. **d. Every 2 years.** Surveillance for recurrent malignancy after nephron-sparing surgery for renal cell carcinoma can be tailored according to the initial pathologic tumor stage. Abdominal or retroperitoneal tumor recurrence is uncommon in pT2 patients, particularly early after nephron-sparing surgery, and these patients require only occasional follow-up abdominal CT; the author recommends that this be done every 2 years in this category. [p 3613]

20. **b. 24-hour urinary protein measurement.** Patients with more than 50% reduction in overall renal mass are at greatest risk for proteinuria, glomerulopathy, and progressive re-

nal failure. Structural or functional renal damage in such cases is usually antedated by the appearance of proteinuria. Therefore, the follow-up of patients after partial nephrectomy in a solitary kidney should include a 24-hour urinary protein determination in addition to the usual renal function and tumor surveillance studies. [p 3613]

21. **b. Medial fibroplasia.** For patients with renovascular hypertension caused by fibrous dysplasia, candidacy for surgical intervention is guided by the specific pathologic process, as determined by angiographic findings, and its associated natural history. Medical management of medial fibroplasia is the initial approach because loss of renal function from progressive obstruction is uncommon, and intervention is reserved for those patients with difficult-to-control hypertension. Renal artery disease caused by intimal or perimedial fibroplasia is often associated with progressive obstruction, which can result in ischemic renal atrophy. [p 3615]

22. **b. noncalcified and larger than 2 cm.** Renal artery aneurysms may require repair when they result in significant hypertension or for prevention of rupture when they are larger than 2 cm and noncalcified. [p 3615]

23. **b. Ostial atherosclerosis.** Whereas percutaneous transluminal angioplasty is associated with a successful blood pressure result for nonostial atherosclerosis, the long-term success rate with ostial lesions is poor owing to a higher incidence of restenosis. The results with endovascular stenting for ostial lesions are better than are those with percutaneous transluminal angioplasty. [pp 3615–3616]

24. **b. Bilateral 80% renal artery stenosis, serum creatinine level 2.1 mg/dl.** Knowledge of the natural history of atherosclerotic renal artery disease permits identification of patients at risk for ischemic nephropathy. Those at highest risk are patients with high-grade stenosis (>75%) involving the entire renal mass (bilateral disease or disease in a solitary kidney). Intervention in these patients is for the purpose of preservation of renal function. [p 3616]

25. **d. Hepatorenal bypass.** Hepatorenal bypass is the preferred vascular reconstructive technique for patients with a troublesome aorta who require right renal revascularization. [p 3622]

26. **c. Ischemic cholecystitis.** Despite the resulting total or segmental hepatic dearterialization in patients with direct end-to-end anastomosis of the right hepatic and renal arteries, postoperative liver function study results have remained normal. However, the gallbladder is more susceptible to ischemic damage and may undergo necrosis when its blood supply from the right hepatic artery is interrupted. [p 3623]

27. **d. Thoracoabdominal.** For left renal revascularization, a left thoracoabdominal incision is made below the 8th rib and extended medially across the midline. This incision provides excellent simultaneous exposure of the thoracic aorta and renal artery with no need for extensive abdominal visceral mobilization. [p 3624]

28. **e. Hypogastric artery.** Although a variety of surgical revascularization techniques are available for treating patients with renal artery disease, aortorenal bypass with a free graft of autogenous saphenous vein or hypogastric artery remains the preferred method in patients with a nondiseased abdominal aorta. An arterial autograft is theoretically advantageous. [p 3616]

29. **d. Bilateral simultaneous renal revascularization.** In recent years, several policies have been adopted to reduce operative mortality following surgical revascularization in patients with atherosclerotic renal artery disease. These include preliminary screening and correction of existing coronary or cerebrovascular occlusive disease, avoidance of bilateral simultaneous renal operations, and reliance on methods of revascularization that avoid operation on a badly diseased aorta. [p 3631]

30. **d. Relief of associated pain.** Multiple cyst punctures and unroofing of cysts (Rovsing's operation) do not appear to improve renal function or prevent further deterioration. However, this approach can provide long-term pain relief in symptomatic patients. [p 3638]

31. **d. Anterior subcostal extraperitoneal.** When surgery on a horseshoe kidney is performed, an anterior subcostal extraperitoneal approach is preferred. This provides good access to the isthmus as well as to the pelvis and ureter, which are rotated anteriorly. [p 3639]

Chapter 103

Laparoscopic Surgery of the Kidney

Jay T. Bishoff • Louis R. Kavoussi

Questions

1. Contraindications to laparoscopic kidney surgery include all of the following except which one?
   a. Severe cardiopulmonary disease
   b. Uncorrected coagulopathy
   c. Prior extensive abdominal surgery
   d. Dilated loops of bowel
   e. Untreated infection

2. Simple nephrectomy is indicated in the treatment of all of the following renal diseases except which one?
   a. Renovascular hypertension
   b. Symptomatic acquired renal cystic disease
   c. Nephrosclerosis
   d. Symptomatic autosomal dominant polycystic kidney disease
   e. Indeterminate enhancing renal mass

3. During the laparoscopic simple nephrectomy, dissection of the ureter:
   a. is performed after dissection of the upper pole and the renal hilum.
   b. should be avoided because the ureter is fragile and may tear.
   c. is performed early in the procedure and the ureter is divided soon after recognition.
   d. assists in the identification and dissection of the hilar blood vessels.
   e. is avoided to prevent bleeding from the gonadal vessels.

4. All of the following statements about laparoscopic donor nephrectomy are true except which one?
   a. Dual-phase spiral CT with three-dimensional reconstruction is adequate for detecting multiple renal arteries and veins.
   b. The presence of multiple renal vessels is a contraindication to laparoscopic donor nephrectomy.
   c. Laparoscopic donor nephrectomy has not been shown to have adverse effects on allograft survival or function.
   d. Pneumoperitoneum has been shown to decrease renal blood flow during the procedure.
   e. Patients who have had prior abdominal surgery near the intended operative field may be considered for laparoscopic donor nephrectomy.

5. Ureteral complications after laparoscopic donor nephrectomy can occur as a result of which of the following?
   a. Pneumoperitoneum, resulting in decreased blood flow to the kidney
   b. Aggressive dissection of the gonadal vein
   c. Division of the gonadal vein at the level of the iliac vessels
   d. Aggressive dissection of the periureteral tissue
   e. Lower pole elevation of the kidney during hilar dissection

6. What is the most compelling reason to perform a right-sided laparoscopic donor nephrectomy instead of left-sided nephrectomy?
   a. Renal function is decreased on the right compared with the left kidney in the donor.
   b. The right renal vein is longer than the left renal vein.
   c. The spleen obstructs the visualization and dissection of the renal hilum.
   d. Left-sided nephrectomy requires a muscle-splitting incision.
   e. The right renal artery is longer than the left renal artery.

7. Compared with open donor nephrectomy, the laparoscopic approach has been shown to significantly decrease all of the following except which one?
   a. Blood loss
   b. Readmission rates
   c. Length of hospital stay
   d. Recipient renal function
   e. Time for donor to return to unrestricted activities

8. Compared with open donor nephrectomy, laparoscopic donor nephrectomy results in which of the following?
   a. A higher serum creatinine value 12 months after transplantation
   b. A slight decrease in overall graft survival at 12 months
   c. Higher long-term complication rates in the recipient
   d. An increased incidence of acute rejection
   e. Equivalent graft survival 2 years after transplantation

9. Hand-assisted laparoscopic donor nephrectomy as an alternative to laparoscopy and open surgery has resulted in which of the following?
   a. Decreased warm ischemic times
   b. Shorter operative times
   c. Decreased donor complications
   d. Decreased hospital costs
   e. Decreased ureteral complication rate

10. Laparoscopic renal biopsy is not indicated in which of the following cases?
    a. Failed percutaneous biopsy
    b. Patients requiring anticoagulation
    c. Morbidly obese patients
    d. Patients with a solitary kidney
    e. Patients with uncontrolled hypertension

11. What is the most common complication seen after laparoscopic renal biopsy?
    a. Inadequate tissue sample for diagnosis
    b. Infection
    c. Pneumonia
    d. Hemorrhage
    e. Pneumothorax

12. Which of the following statements concerning the laparoscopic treatment and evaluation of symptomatic and indeterminate renal cysts is accurate?
    a. They are contraindicated because aspiration is effective and has a low complication rate.
    b. They allow rapid localization of intraparenchymal cysts.
    c. They are contraindicated in patients with autosomal dominant polycystic kidney disease.
    d. They allow biopsy and conversion to nephrectomy in case of malignancy.
    e. They are contraindicated because the collecting system may be entered during the procedure.

13. Symptomatic nephroptosis is a rare condition that:
    a. presents most commonly in middle-aged, obese females.
    b. can be diagnosed by renal ultrasonography.
    c. may be present when the kidney descends more than one vertebral body.
    d. is usually associated with irritable bowel or peptic ulcer disease.
    e. should be shown to cause obstruction of the kidney before repair.

14. Laparoscopic pyelolithotomy is indicated in all of the following cases except which one?
    a. Failed extracorporeal shock wave lithotripsy
    b. Pelvic or otherwise ectopic kidney
    c. Failed attempt to fragment a cystine stone
    d. Pregnancy with a symptomatic ureteropelvic junction stone
    e. Failed ureteroscopic stone extraction

15. In the treatment of urologic malignancy, port site seeding has been most frequently described in which condition?
    a. Renal cell carcinoma
    b. Prostate cancer
    c. Testicular cancer
    d. Transitional cell carcinoma
    e. Penile cancer

16. Which of the following statements concerning the preoperative clinical staging of renal cell carcinoma with CT is true?
    a. It is more likely to lead to overstaging than understaging of a renal mass.
    b. It allows accurate staging in 35% to 55% of patients.
    c. It is an inadequate study to allow morcellation of renal specimens.
    d. It should be correlated with renal angiography.
    e. It is inadequate for predicting lymph node involvement.

17. Laparoscopic radical nephrectomy is contraindicated in which of the following cases?

    a. History of ipsilateral renal surgery including extracorporeal shock wave lithotripsy
    b. Perinephric inflammation seen by CT
    c. Prior transabdominal surgery
    d. Tumors invading the adrenal gland or perinephric tissues (T3a)
    e. Tumors grossly extending into the renal vein or vena cava (T3b)

18. Which of the following statements concerning morcellation of a radical nephrectomy specimen is true?

    a. It should not be performed, because pathologic staging information is lost.
    b. It should be performed after placement of the kidney in an Endocatch retrieval device.
    c. It is associated with a high incidence of trocar site seeding.
    d. It should be monitored intra-abdominally with the laparoscope.
    e. It should not be performed after placement of the kidney in a LapSac.

19. What is the approximate actuarial 5-year disease-free survival rate for clinically localized renal cell carcinoma treated with laparoscopic radical nephrectomy?

    a. 95% to 100%
    b. 85% to 90%
    c. 75% to 80%
    d. 65% to 70%
    e. 55% to 60%

20. What is the reported approximate overall complication rate from laparoscopic radical nephrectomy?

    a. 40% to 45%
    b. 30% to 35%
    c. 20% to 25%
    d. 10% to 15%
    e. 0% to 5%

21. Laparoscopic partial nephrectomy mimics open partial nephrectomy in all of the following ways except which one?

    a. Tissue is removed under direct vision.
    b. Margin status is determined at the time of surgery.
    c. Inspection of the surface allows identification and treatment of multifocal disease.
    d. The collecting system can be resected with the specimen and closed.
    e. Arterial occlusion with hypothermia can be performed.

22. Laparoscopic partial nephrectomy is a recent advancement in the treatment of small T1 renal tumors. What is the reported 3-year disease-free survival rate?

    a. 100%
    b. 90%
    c. 80%
    d. 70%
    e. 60%

23. Laparoscopic cryosurgical ablation of renal tumors requires which of the following?

    a. Tumor tissue temperatures less than −20°C
    b. CT monitoring of the ice ball
    c. MRI of the ice ball
    d. Intraoperative ultrasonographic monitoring of the ice ball
    e. A double freeze cycle

24. Reported complications of laparoscopic cryosurgical ablation of renal tumors include all of the following except which one?

    a. Tumor recurrence
    b. Urinary fistula formation
    c. Hemorrhage
    d. Small bowel obstruction
    e. Skin necrosis

25. Which of the following statements concerning radiofrequency ablation of renal tumors is true?

    a. It can be reliably monitored by using ultrasonography and MRI.
    b. It requires tissue temperatures of higher than 45°C to induce tissue necrosis.
    c. It causes increased tissue temperatures indirectly through local ion vibration.
    d. It must be delivered with a temperature-based feedback system.
    e. It results in little temperature drop from the center of the probe to the periphery.

26. Common areas of postoperative bleeding after laparoscopic kidney surgery include all of the following except which one?

    a. Adrenal gland
    b. Large bowel mesentery
    c. Gonadal vessels
    d. Psoas muscle
    e. Ureteral stump

27. Which of the following statements concerning bowel injuries during laparoscopic surgery is true?

    a. They occur in 1 in 100 cases.
    b. They are usually the result of a Veress needle placement.
    c. They most commonly involve the large bowel.
    d. They are the result of electrocautery in half of the cases.
    e. They are usually recognized at the time of surgery.

28. The presentation of unrecognized bowel injury most commonly involves all of the following signs or symptoms except which one?

    a. Pain out of proportion at one trocar site
    b. Nausea
    c. Diarrhea
    d. Low-grade fever
    e. Elevated white blood cell count

29. As a surgeon learns to perform laparoscopic nephrectomy, complications may occur. Seventy percent of these complications have been reported to occur during the first how many cases?

    a. 5
    b. 10
    c. 20
    d. 30
    e. 40

30. Conversion from laparoscopic to open kidney surgery occurs most often during procedures performed for which indication?

    a. Malignancy.
    b. Stones.
    c. Obstruction.
    d. Infection.
    e. Renovascular hypertension.

31. What is the most common cause for conversion from laparoscopic to open surgery?

    a. Failure to progress
    b. Inability to visualize the renal hilum
    c. Perinephric adhesions
    d. Difficulty finding the ureter
    e. Bleeding

Answers

1. **c. Prior extensive abdominal surgery.** Prior abdominal surgery may alter the choice between transperitoneal or retroperitoneal approaches, patient positioning, and placement site of trocars, but it is not a contraindication to laparoscopic surgery. [p 3646]

2. **e. Indeterminate enhancing renal mass.** Indications include renovascular hypertension, symptomatic acquired renal cystic disease in dialysis patients, nephrosclerosis, symptomatic patients with autosomal dominant polycystic disease, chronic pyelonephritis, reflux/obstructive nephropathy, multicystic dysplastic kidney, and post–kidney transplant hypertension. [p 3648]

3. **d. Assists in the identification and dissection of the hilar blood vessels.** Once identified, the ureter is elevated and followed proximally to the lower pole and hilum of the kidney. The ureter is not divided at this time, as it can be used to help elevate the kidney. [p 3649]

4. **b. The presence of multiple renal vessels is a contraindication to laparoscopic donor nephrectomy.** The presence of multiple vessels is not a contraindication to laparoscopic donor nephrectomy, but preoperative identification allows the surgeon to anticipate their presence early in the operation. [p 3656]

5. **d. Aggressive dissection of the periureteral tissue.** Aggressive dissection of the periureteral tissue to expose the ureter can lead to ureteral strictures in the recipient. [p 3657]

6. **a. Renal function is decreased on the right compared with the left kidney in the donor.** Right-sided nephrectomies are performed when indicated by the relative renal function or vascular configuration. The right side is more technically difficult to approach because of the short renal vein and need for liver retraction to allow dissection of the upper pole. The application of the endovascular GIA stapler on the right renal vein can result in a loss of 1.0 cm of length. [p 3658]

7. **d. Recipient renal function.** Compared with open donor nephrectomy, the laparoscopic approach has been shown to significantly decrease blood loss, readmission rates, time to resume oral intake, analgesic requirements, length of hospital stay, time to full activity, and time to return to work. [p 3659]

8. **e. Equivalent graft survival 2 years after transplantation.** The long-term graft survival, at 1 and 2 years, is the same for both open and laparoscopic groups (98% and 97%, respectively). [p 3660]

9. **a. Decreased warm ischemic times.** The warm ischemic time and operative times have been shown to be improved over the laparoscopic approach, and there is no difference to the donor in terms of hospital stay and time to full recovery. [p 3661]

10. **e. Patients with uncontrolled hypertension.** Renal biopsy under direct vision is indicated in three primary categories of patients: failed percutaneous needle biopsy, anatomic variations, and high risk of bleeding complication. Factors that may make a patient unsuitable for percutaneous biopsy include morbid obesity, multiple bilateral cysts, a body habitus that makes localization impossible, and a solitary functioning kidney. [p 3661]

11. **d. Hemorrhage.** Hemorrhage is the most common major complication associated with laparoscopic renal biopsy. [p 3663]

12. **d. They allow biopsy and conversion to nephrectomy in case of malignancy.** The base of the cyst should be carefully inspected and biopsies performed using 5 mm laparoscopic biopsy forceps. If there is no evidence of malignancy, the parenchymal surface of the cyst wall can be fulgurated with electrocautery or the argon beam coagulator. Surgical cellulose (Surgicell, Johnson & Johnson, Arlington, TX) can be packed into the cyst base. If malignancy is noted, the patient should have a partial or radical nephrectomy, as indicated. Once the decortication is complete, careful inspection for hemostasis should be performed. [p 3666]

13. **e. Should be shown to cause obstruction of the kidney before repair.** Either erect and supine intravenous urograms or renal scans documenting obstruction are the best diagnostic studies for nephroptosis. Descent of the symptomatic kidney by two vertebral bodies and obstruction or diminished flow to the symptomatic side should be documented before surgical repair. [p 3668]

14. **d. Pregnancy with a symptomatic ureteropelvic junction stone.** Individuals to be considered for this approach include those in whom extracorporeal shock wave lithotripsy, percutaneous, or ureteroscopic procedures have failed; patients with unusual anatomy such as a pelvic kidney; and patients with stones resistant to fragmentation such as those of cystine composition. [p 3669]

15. **d. Transitional cell carcinoma.** In the laparoscopic staging and treatment of transitional cell carcinoma, there have been five reports of port site seeding. [p 3671]

16. **a. It is more likely to lead to overstaging than understaging of a renal mass.** One study concluded that clinical CT staging of low-stage renal tumors is reliable and tends to overstage rather than understage renal tumors. [p 3671]

17. **e. Tumors grossly extending into the renal vein or vena cava (T3b).** Contraindications to laparoscopic radical nephrectomy include tumors with renal vein or vena cava thrombi. [p 3671]

18. **d. It should be monitored intra-abdominally with the laparoscope.** If the specimen is to be morcellated, a LapSac (Cook Urological, Spencer, IN) fabricated from a double layer of plastic and nondistensible nylon, is used. This sac has been shown to be impermeable to bacteria and tumor cells even after use for morcellation. [p 3673]

19. **b. 85% to 90%.** The calculated disease-free rates for laparoscopic and open radical nephrectomy were 95% and 86% at 5 years, respectively, whereas the actuarial survival rates for laparoscopic and open radical nephrectomy were 86% and 75% at 5 years, respectively. [p 3676]

20. **d. 10% to 15%.** Complications occurred in 10 patients (15%) of the laparoscopic group and 8 (15%) in the open group. Six laparoscopic patients (8%) required blood transfusions compared with 11 in the open group. [p 3676]

21. **e. Arterial occlusion with hypothermia can be performed.** An extension of laparoscopy in the treatment of small renal lesions has been the partial nephrectomy, which mimics the fundamentals of open surgery. Tissue is removed under direct vision with margin status being assessed intraoperatively. Direct vision and laparoscopic ultrasonography permit the laparoscopist to identify multifocal tumors, determine an adequate surgical margin, and maintain orientation with respect to the collecting system and renal hilum. If necessary,

the collecting system can be resected with the surgical specimen to obtain adequate margins and then repaired. [p 3678]

22. **a. 100%.** A combined European series included 53 patients who underwent laparoscopic nephron-sparing surgery for renal mass less than 5 cm in size. Hemostasis was obtained at the time of wedge resection using bipolar coagulation and fibrin glue–coated cellulose. Thirty-five patients were found to have renal cell carcinoma. At a mean follow-up of 3 years, they reported a 100% disease-free survival rate. [p 3678]

23. **d. Intraoperative ultrasonographic monitoring of the ice ball.** Laparoscopy permits use of intraoperative laparoscopic ultrasound (IOLUS) monitoring of the progression of the ice ball. One study demonstrated that the ice ball visualized on IOLUS must extend at least 3.1 mm beyond the outer edge of the renal lesion of interest to ensure that a temperature of −20°C is reached in the tissues farthest from the cryoprobe. [p 3679]

24. **e. Skin necrosis.** Potential complications of cryosurgery include urinary fistula formation, post-treatment hemorrhage, and injury to adjacent structures to include the collecting system, bowel, and liver. Given that even momentary contact of the active cryoprobe can lead to necrosis and fibrosis, disastrous results could soon follow. One study in a porcine model noted severe adhesions between cryoablated kidney and overlying bowel in nonretroperitonealized kidneys. There was no evidence of bowel injury or fistulas. Another study reported the complication of small bowel obstruction when the cryoprobe inadvertently contacted a loop of small bowel during porcine laparoscopic renal cryoablation. Certain reports of short-term local tumor recurrences mandate further investigation to predict cryotherapy's ultimate role in the treatment of renal tumors. [p 3679]

25. **c. It causes increased tissue temperatures indirectly through local ion vibration.** The probe carries an alternating current of high-frequency radio waves that causes the local ions to vibrate, and the resistance in the tissue creates heat to the point of desiccation (thermal coagulation). [p 3679]

26. **d. Psoas muscle.** Common areas of postoperative intra-abdominal bleeding include the adrenal gland, mesentery, gonadal vessels, and ureteral stump. [p 3680]

27. **d. They are the result of electrocautery in half of the cases.** One of the most devastating complications occurring as a result of laparoscopic surgery is that of unrecognized bowel injury. Because only 10% of the laparoscopic instrument is in the visual field, these injuries can occur out of the surgeon's field of view. The combined incidence of bowel injury in the literature is 1.3 per 1000 cases. Most injuries (69%) are not recognized at the time of surgery. Small bowel segments account for 58% of injuries, followed by colon (32%) and stomach (7%). Fifty percent of bowel injuries are caused by electrocautery, and 32% occur during Veress needle or trocar insertion. [p 3680]

28. **e. Elevated white blood cell count.** Patients with unrecognized bowel injury after laparoscopy typically present with persistent and increased trocar site pain at the site closest to the bowel injury. Later signs and symptoms include nausea, diarrhea, anorexia, low-grade fever, persistent bowel sounds, and a low or normal white blood cell count. [p 3680]

29. **c. 20 cases.** In fact, 70% of the complications occurred during the first 20 cases at each institution. A learning curve of approximately 20 laparoscopic nephrectomy cases is also supported by other reports. [p 3681]

30. **d. Infection.** The majority of patients who had conversion to open surgery had infectious causes of renal pathology as the leading indication for kidney removal. [p 3681]

31. **e. Bleeding.** Bleeding was the most common cause of open conversion, followed by inability to visualize the renal hilum for dissection. [p 3681]

Chapter 104

Other Applications of Laparoscopic Surgery

Howard N. Winfield • Jeffrey A. Cadeddu

Questions

1. Laparoscopic pelvic lymph node dissection would be considered a valuable staging technique for cancer of the prostate in all of the following situations except which one?
   a. Gleason score of 4+4 on all biopsy specimens
   b. Clinical stage T3a prostate cancer
   c. Prostate-specific antigen (PSA) value of less than 10 ng/ml (Hybritech assay)
   d. PSA of greater than 20 ng/ml (Hybritech assay)
   e. A 52-year-old healthy man with clinical stage D0 tumor

2. All of the following anatomic statements related to laparoscopic pelvic lymph node dissection are correct except which one?
   a. For a transperitoneal approach, the initial incision through the posterior peritoneum should be medial to the medial (obliterated) umbilical ligament.
   b. For a transperitoneal approach, the initial incision through the posterior peritoneum should be lateral to the medial (obliterated) umbilical ligament.
   c. The obturator vein and artery are medial to the obturator nerve.
   d. The inferior apex of the obturator lymph node packet should be defined just before the tissue extending into the femoral canal.
   e. Dissection out to the genitofemoral nerve is normally not necessary for laparoscopic staging of prostate cancer.

3. Laparoscopic retroperitoneal lymphadenectomy is a good surgical procedure to consider in all of the following situations except which one?

   a. Clinical stage I nonseminomatous testis tumor
   b. Evidence of elevated testis tumor markers (β-human chorionic gonadotropin, α-fetoprotein)
   c. Slender patient with no previous abdominal surgery
   d. Patients who are less likely to be compliant with radiologic surveillance
   e. Testis histologic results showing the presence of embryonal carcinoma in the presence of negative radiologic and biochemical evaluation

4. Laparoscopic bladder diverticulectomy should be considered under which of the following conditions?

   a. If the diverticulum is located on the posteroinferior aspect of the bladder
   b. If the diverticulum is intimately involved with the ureter
   c. It the diverticulum is located on the anterolateral aspect of the bladder
   d. If the patient has had bladder tumor resection in the past year
   e. If the patient has an obstructing prostate measured as greater than 100 g by transrectal ultrasonographic study

5. Laparoscopic varicocele ligation includes all of the following maneuvers except which one?

   a. Incision of the posterior peritoneum lateral to spermatic vessels
   b. Complete mobilization of the spermatic vascular bundle
   c. Preservation of the vas deferens and associated vessels
   d. Division of the entire vascular bundle including veins and artery
   e. Careful identification of the gonadal artery

6. Laparoscopic seminal vesicle dissection includes all of the following maneuvers except which one?

   a. Puncture and drainage of a large seminal vesicle cyst to minimize risk of injury to adjacent organs
   b. Incision of the peritoneum overlying the rectovesical pouch
   c. Identification and mobilization of the ureter to prevent inadvertent injury
   d. Exposure of the surface of the seminal vesicles from a medial to a lateral direction
   e. Division of the seminal vesicle arteries between clips

7. As compared with radical retropubic prostatectomy, laparoscopic radical prostatectomy has a:

   a. lower blood transfusion rate.
   b. lower urinary continence rate.
   c. lower impotence rate.
   d. higher rectal injury rate.
   e. shorter hospital stay.

8. When planning and performing a laparoscopic lymphocele ablation, what should the surgeon do?

   a. Open a very small window in the lymphocele for fear of injuring adjacent structures
   b. Use laparoscopic ultrasonography to differentiate the lymphocele from the bladder or transplanted kidney
   c. Instill a sclerosing agent into any loculation within the lymphocele
   d. Anchor a loop of small bowel to the edge of the lymphocele window
   e. Obtain an MRI scan in every case to localize the lymphocele

9. Laparoscopic radical prostatectomy includes all of the following maneuvers except which one?

   a. Division of the urachus and development of the space of Retzius
   b. Late division of the dorsal vein complex
   c. Preplacement of sutures in the urethra for subsequent vesicourethral anastomosis
   d. Intact specimen extraction through a small incision
   e. Division of Denonvillier's fascia before incising the endopelvic fascia

Answers

1. **c. Prostate-specific antigen (PSA) value of less than 10 ng/ml (Hybritech assay).** Indications for this procedure include the following: (1) clinical stage T2b to T3a cancer, regardless of the follow-up treatment under consideration; (2) patients with a serum PSA value of greater than 20 ng/ml (Hybritech assay); (3) Gleason scores of 7 to 10; (4) positive seminal vesicle biopsies (T3c); and (5) biopsy-proven persistent adenocarcinoma of the prostate after a full course of radiotherapy in patients being considered for salvage prostatectomy. [p 3688]

2. **a. For a transperitoneal approach, the initial incision through the posterior peritoneum should be medial to the medial (obliterated) umbilical ligament.** To access the obturator-iliac nodal packets, an initial incision must be made through the posterior peritoneal membrane beginning just lateral to the medial (obliterated) umbilical ligament. [p 3689]

3. **b. Evidence of elevated testis tumor markers (β-human chorionic gonadotropin, α-fetoprotein).** Indications for this procedure include the following: (1) clinical stage I nonseminomatous testis tumor; (2) negative results for testis tumor markers; (3) candidate otherwise considered for surveillance; (4) no absolute contraindications to laparoscopic surgery; and (5) residual isolated abdominal or pelvic mass after chemotherapy in the presence of negative testis tumor markers. These cases must be individualized and approached very cautiously. [p 3692]

4. **c. If the diverticulum is located on the anterolateral aspect of the bladder.** Diverticula that involve the lateral, dome, or anterior regions of the bladder are easily accessible to dissection and repair by laparoscopic techniques. [p 3702]

5. **d. Division of the entire vascular bundle including veins and artery.** Once its location is confirmed, each vein is clipped (5 mm clip applier) or ligated and divided so that only the artery remains. [p 3696]

6. **c. Identification and mobilization of the ureter to prevent inadvertent injury.** Throughout the dissection, care must be taken to stay on the vas deferens and seminal vesicle to prevent injury to the rectum, the ureter posterior and lateral to the vas deferens, and the neurovascular bundles laterally. [pp 3697–3698]

7. **a. Lower blood transfusion rate.** Blood loss and transfu-

sion rates are lower with laparoscopic radical prostatectomy than with radical retropubic prostatectomy. [p 3700]

8. **b. Use laparoscopic ultrasonography to differentiate the lymphocele from the bladder or transplanted kidney.** If the location is unclear, real-time transabdominal and laparoscopic ultrasonographic studies allow differentiation from the bladder, as it is distended and drained, and from a transplanted kidney. [p 3701]

9. **c. Preplacement of sutures in the urethra for subsequent vesicourethral anastomosis.** Between the previously placed sutures, the dorsal vein is divided to expose the urethra. Additional hemostatic maneuvers are rarely needed. The urethral catheter is withdrawn and the urethra is divided completely. With a finger in the rectum for assistance, the surgeon then divides the rectourethralis muscle and remaining attachments in the midline to free the prostate completely. The specimen is placed in a laparoscopic bag and set aside to be removed after the vesicourethral anastomosis is completed. The vesicourethral anastomosis is the most difficult step in the procedure. If the bladder neck is deemed too large, a "tennis racquet" closure, with 2-0 polyglycolic acid suture, can be performed. The anastomosis is completed with 3-0 polyglycolic acid suture in either a running manner or with up to 12 interrupted simple sutures (see Fig. 104–17). A Foley catheter is placed and the anastomosis is tested for leakage. A single suction drain is positioned through one of the inferior lateral trocar sites, and the specimen is extracted through a small incision that incorporates a port site. [pp 3699–3700]

Chapter 105

Genitourinary Trauma

Jack W. McAninch • Richard A. Santucci

Questions

1. What is the most appropriate technique to evaluate microhematuria in a stable patient with a transthoracic gunshot wound?
    a. Abdominal sonography
    b. Intravenous pyelography (IVP)
    c. Immediate laparotomy (celiotomy) in the operating room, with intraoperative "one-shot" IVP
    d. Clinical observation on the hospital ward
    e. Immediate CT with use of intravenous contrast material

2. What method is used to perform one-shot intraoperative IVP in a 50 kg woman?
    a. Inject a 50 ml bolus of intravenous contrast agent followed by a full IVP series, including abdominal compression to evaluate the ureters.
    b. Inject a 100 ml bolus of intravenous contrast agent followed in exactly 10 minutes by a flat plate of the abdomen on the operating room table.
    c. Inject a 50 ml bolus of intravenous contrast agent followed in exactly 10 minutes by a flat plate of the abdomen on the operating room table.
    d. Determine the patient's scrum creatinine level before administration of intravenous contrast agent to make sure that the patient will not experience renal failure as a result of reaction to the contrast agent.
    e. Inject 100 ml of intravenous contrast and get a kidney, ureter, bladder scan (KUB) once the patient is safely out of surgery.

3. What is the first step in managing an intraoperatively discovered renal gunshot wound with large perirenal hematoma and intraoperative one-shot IVP showing urinary extravasation?
    a. Immediate nephrectomy
    b. Immediate renorrhaphy
    c. Expectant (nonoperative) management
    d. Isolation of the renal vein and artery with silicone loops
    e. Opening of Gerota's fascia and inspection of the kidney for injury

4. A patient is discovered to have a grade IV renal injury during open surgical exploration. What is the best way to evaluate associated injuries to the renal pelvis or ureter?
    a. Visual inspection of the renal pelvis and ureter, plus injection of 2 ml of methylene blue into the renal pelvis and inspection for extravasation of dye
    b. Occlusion of the distal ureter, allowing it to fill with urine to demonstrate a watertight proximal ureter and renal pelvis
    c. Retrograde pyelography
    d. Incision of the renal pelvis and inspection for injuries from within
    e. Ureteral stent placement

5. In the treatment of grade IV renal injury, the lowest complication rate and best preservation of renal function result from which of the following?
    a. Expectant (nonoperative) management
    b. Placement of a ureteral stent via a renal pelvis incision
    c. Renorrhaphy
    d. Nephrectomy
    e. Transcatheter embolization of the kidney

6. One-shot IVP shows nonvisualization of the right kidney and a normal left kidney. A rapidly enlarging retroperitoneal hematoma is present, and the patient is hemodynamically unstable, despite adequate intravenous blood and crystalloid administration. What are the most likely diagnosis and its recommended treatment?
    a. Right grade V injury (avulsion of the renal vessels); vessel isolation followed by nephrectomy
    b. Right grade V injury (avulsion of the renal vessels); immediate nephrectomy
    c. Right grade V injury (avulsion of the renal vessels); expectant (nonoperative) management

d. Right grade IV injury (deep parenchymal laceration involving the collecting system, or renal artery thrombosis, or partial renal vessel injury with contained hilar hematoma); vessel isolation followed by immediate nephrectomy
e. Right grade IV injury (deep parenchymal laceration involving the collecting system, or renal artery thrombosis, or partial renal vessel injury with contained hilar hematoma); transcatheter embolization

7. A patient has two shallow lacerations (<1 cm deep) in the renal parenchyma. What is the injury grade according to the American Association for the Surgery of Trauma Organ Injury Severity Scale?

    a. I
    b. II
    c. III
    d. IV
    e. V

8. The most important piece of clinical information to obtain in the follow-up of patients with significant renal injuries will be provided by which of the following?

    a. Serum creatinine value
    b. CT of the kidneys
    c. Renal ultrasonographic study
    d. Blood pressure measurement
    e. Serum potassium level

9. What is the best treatment for a multiply injured trauma patient with coagulopathy and hypotension who, at laparotomy, is found to have unilateral renal artery thrombosis and a normal contralateral kidney?

    a. Autotransplantation
    b. Open repair of renal artery thrombosis with hypogastric artery interposition graft
    c. Expectant (nonoperative) management
    d. Nephrectomy
    e. Splenorenal arterial bypass

10. What is the best option for repair of mid-ureteral transection after a stab wound?

    a. Ureteroureterostomy
    b. Transureteroureterostomy
    c. Boari flap
    d. Psoas hitch
    e. Stenting without repair

11. When ureteroureterostomy is performed, which of the following is required?

    a. Postoperative retroperitoneal suction drain
    b. Postoperative nephrostomy drain
    c. Spatulated, watertight repair
    d. Nonabsorbable sutures
    e. Intraperitonealization of the ureteral anastomosis

12. Which maneuver is cited as a cause of ureteral injury during stone basketing?

    a. Ureteroscopy without dilating the ureteral orifice first
    b. Ureteroscopy in nondilated systems
    c. Use of the holmium laser
    d. Pulsatile saline irrigation to assist visualization
    e. Persistence in stone basketing attempts in the face of a ureteral tear

13. Which of the following is a contraindication to transureteroureterostomy for repair of significant lower ureter injury?

    a. History of urolithiasis
    b. History of ureteral trauma
    c. Obesity
    d. Neurogenic bladder
    e. Spinal fracture

14. What is the treatment of choice for a ureteral contusion by a high-velocity bullet?

    a. Observation
    b. Ureteral stent placement
    c. Transureteroureterostomy
    d. Ureteroureterostomy
    e. Oversewing the contusion with healthy ureteral tissue

15. Which imaging technique is most useful for detecting ureteral injuries after trauma?

    a. CT without use of contrast material
    b. CT with use of contrast agent, obtained immediately after injection of the contrast agent
    c. CT with the use of contrast material, obtained 20 minutes after injection of the contrast agent
    d. Intravenous pyelography
    e. Furosemide (Lasix) renography

16. Which of the following statements is true about ureteral injuries during laparoscopy?

    a. The total number of injuries has stayed steady over the years.
    b. Surgery for endometriosis greatly increases the risk.
    c. Bipolar cautery use during tubal ligation eliminates risk.
    d. Most are recognized immediately.
    e. Use of indigo carmine dye eliminates the risk of injury.

17. Which of the following is neither a relative nor an absolute indication for open repair of bladder injury?

    a. Significant extraperitoneal bladder rupture in a patient scheduled to undergo laparotomy for associated intra-abdominal injuries by the general surgery team
    b. Significant extraperitoneal bladder rupture in a patient scheduled for open anterior repair of pelvic fracture by the orthopedic surgery team
    c. Significant extraperitoneal bladder rupture and a concern by the urology team that the complication rates of conservative treatments are unacceptably high
    d. Intraperitoneal bladder rupture
    e. "Pie in the sky" bladder

18. Which of the following is true about cystography for diagnosis of bladder injury?

    a. If the patient is already undergoing CT, a good method is antegrade filling of the bladder after intravenous administration of radiographic contrast material.
    b. The preferred method is retrograde filling of the bladder with at least 350 ml of contrast material.
    c. Contrast material should not be diluted if CT-cystography is performed.
    d. If plain film cystograms are obtained, postdrainage films are not necessary.
    e. If plain film cystograms are obtained, oblique films are always needed.

19. Which of the following is true about bladder injuries?

    a. They are present in 6% to 10% of patients with pelvic fracture.
    b. Physical findings of abdominal pain, tenderness, and bruising are pathognomonic.
    c. Delayed diagnosis is the rule.
    d. Bladder contusions commonly result in gross hematuria.
    e. They are associated with a 50% rate of urethral tear.

20. The risk of complications from nonoperative treatment of extraperitoneal bladder rupture is increased by associated:

a. ureteral injury.
b. renal injury.
c. rectal perforation.
d. pelvic fracture.
e. distal urethral injury.

21. In a blunt trauma patient with pelvic fracture in whom no urine is returned to catheter placement, what is the best method to evaluate urethral injury?

    a. Retrograde urethrography
    b. CT with intravenous contrast material and clamping of the urethral catheter
    c. Flexible cystoscopy in the operating room
    d. Percutaneous antegrade cystography
    e. Use of urethral sounds

22. What is a reasonable first step in treating a partial posterior urethral distraction injury found on retrograde urethrography?

    a. A single attempt at urethral catheterization by a urologist at the bedside
    b. Open placement of a large-bore (22 Fr) suprapubic tube in the operating room
    c. Percutaneous placement of a 12 Fr punch suprapubic catheter at the bedside
    d. Rigid bedside cystoscopy and placement of a urethral catheter
    e. Open surgical repair of the urethral distraction injury

23. In a patient with a posterior urethral distraction injury on retrograde urethrography who already has a urethral catheter in the bladder, what would the next step be to evaluate the lower urinary tract?

    a. Cystography, then open suprapubic tube placement and repair of bladder injuries, if present
    b. No further work-up
    c. Antegrade CT-cystography with clamping of the urethral catheter after intravenous injection of contrast material
    d. CT of the pelvis
    e. Cystoscopy

24. One statement will complete the following sentence correctly: Acute open suture repair of urethral distraction injuries:

    a. results in a high incidence of impotence and incontinence.
    b. carries a very low risk of subsequent urethral stricture.
    c. is simple and safe.
    d. is indicated in all cases of urethral distraction injury.
    e. is preferable to acute endoscopic realignment.

25. Three months after a urethral distraction injury, a patient develops a 2 cm posterior urethral obliterative stricture and wishes repair. Which of the following is true about the operation?

    a. Good results can be achieved with one-stage, open, perineal anastomotic urethroplasty.
    b. Two-stage (Johanson) urethroplasty will be required.
    c. "Cut-to-the-light" or core-through posterior urethrotomy is both safe and very effective.
    d. Use of the UroLume endoprosthesis is the best method.
    e. The patient will likely be incontinent after any open urethral stricture repair surgery.

26. Type II urethral distraction injuries, as described by Colapinto and McCallum, are the most common. They are characterized by which of the following?

    a. Urethral stretch injury
    b. Urethral disruption distal to the genitourinary diaphragm
    c. Urethral disruption proximal to the genitourinary diaphragm
    d. Distal urethral disruption
    e. Bulbar urethral disruption

27. The primary goal when evaluating a patient with genital gunshot wounds is to determine the presence or absence of which of the following?

    a. Major associated vascular injuries
    b. Associated urethral injury
    c. Testicular disruption
    d. Penile fracture
    e. Vas deferens injury

28. Which test should be performed before exploration of every penile gunshot wound?

    a. Femoral angiography
    b. CT of the abdomen
    c. Retrograde urethrography
    d. Nuclear medicine radionuclide scan of the scrotum
    e. Ultrasonography of the penis

29. An 80% transection of the anterior urethra is confirmed after penile gunshot wound with a 22-caliber pistol. What is the most appropriate therapy?

    a. Spatulated, stented, tensionless, watertight repair of the urethra with absorbable sutures
    b. Suprapubic tube and healing by secondary intention of the urethral injury
    c. Suprapubic tube and urethral catheter, and healing of the urethra by secondary intention
    d. Immediate onlay graft urethroplasty with buccal mucosa or penile skin
    e. Nonsurgical therapy

30. If a patient gets his penis caught in his zipper, what should the first step be?

    a. Local anesthetic block, lubrication, and a single attempt at opening the zipper
    b. Pulling the zipper apart with pliers
    c. General anesthetic and operating room exploration
    d. Coaching the patient through releasing the penis from the zipper
    e. Cutting apart the pants and removing the zipper in pieces

31. During exploration after scrotal gunshot wound, 40% of the left testicular capsule is found to be destroyed. What should the next approach be?

    a. Left orchidectomy
    b. Left testicular débridement and primary closure of the capsule of the testicle
    c. Watchful waiting
    d. Left orchidectomy and immediate testicular prosthesis
    e. Wet dressings and delayed testicular surgery

32. The blood in a hematocele is contained in which of the following?

    a. The tunica albuginea
    b. The tunica vaginalis
    c. Colles' fascia
    d. Scarpa's fascia
    e. Camper's fascia

33. What is the best option for coverage of acute penile skin loss?

    a. A foreskin flap for small distal lesions
    b. A scrotal rotation flap for distal lesions
    c. Avulsed skin retrieved from the scene
    d. An immediate skin graft after penile skin removal for Fournier's gangrene
    e. A meshed skin graft in a young child

Answers

1. **e. Immediate CT with use of intravenous contrast material.** The preferred imaging study for renal trauma is contrast-enhanced CT. [p 3710]

2. **b. Inject a 100 ml bolus of intravenous contrast agent followed in exactly 10 minutes by a flat plate of the abdomen on the operating room table.** Only a single film is taken 10 minutes after intravenous injection (IV push) of 2 ml/kg of contrast material. [p 3710]

3. **d. Isolation of the renal vein and artery with silicone loops.** The renal vessels are isolated before exploration to provide the immediate capability to occlude them if massive bleeding should ensue once Gerota's fascia is opened. [p 3711]

4. **a. Visual inspection of the renal pelvis and ureter, plus injection of 2 ml of methylene blue into the renal pelvis and inspection for extravasation of dye.** If a ureteral or renal pelvis injury is suspected intraoperatively, 1 to 2 ml of methylene blue dye can be injected into the renal pelvis with a 27-gauge needle. [p 3717]

5. **c. Renorrhaphy.** In our hands, renal repair in these injuries has been successful with minimal complications. [p 3712]

6. **a. Right grade V injury (avulsion of the renal vessels); vessel isolation followed by nephrectomy.** Grade V injury, according to the American Association for the Surgery of Trauma's Organ Injury Scaling Committee, includes laceration (completely shattered kidney) and vascular injury (avulsion of the renal hilum, devascularizing the kidney). In the unstable patient, one cannot risk an attempt at renal repair if a normal contralateral kidney is present, and nephrectomy is recommended. [pp 3708, 3713]

7. **b. II.** According to the scale, grade II laceration is 1 cm or less parenchymal depth of the renal cortex without urinary extravasation; grade III laceration is greater than 1 cm parenchymal depth of renal cortex without collecting system rupture or urinary extravasation; grade IV laceration is parenchymal laceration extending through renal cortex, medulla, and collecting system; and grade V laceration is a completely shattered kidney. [p 3708]

8. **d. Blood pressure measurement.** Hypertension is seldom noted in the early postinjury period, but postinjury blood pressure measurements are often not obtained consistently, as patients often do not return for follow-up evaluation. When hypertension is present, the basic mechanisms for arterial hypertension as a complication of trauma are (1) renal vascular injury, leading to stenosis or occlusion of the main renal artery or one of its branches; (2) compression of the renal parenchyma with extravasated blood or urine; and (3) post-trauma arteriovenous fistula. In these instances, the renin-angiotensin axis is stimulated by partial renal ischemia, resulting in hypertension. [pp 3713–3715]

9. **d. Nephrectomy.** Total nephrectomy would be indicated immediately in extensive renal injuries when the patient's life would be threatened by attempted renal repair. [p 3713]

10. **a. Ureteroureterostomy.** Ureteroureterostomy, so-called end-to-end repair in injuries to the upper two thirds of the ureter, is common (up to 32% of one large series) and has a reported success rate as high as 90%. [p 3718]

11. **c. Spatulated, watertight repair.** Repair ureters under magnification with spatulated, tension free, stented, watertight anastomosis, placing retroperitoneal drains afterward. [p 3718]

12. **e. Persistence in stone basketing attempts in the face of a ureteral tear.** One factor cited as a cause of injury was the persistence in stone basket attempts after recognition of a ureteral tear, and current recommendations are to stop and place a ureteral stent. [p 3716]

13. **a. History of urolithiasis.** Some authors believe that this operation is contraindicated in patients with a history of urothelial calculi. [p 3720]

14. **d. Ureteroureterostomy.** Ureteral contusions, although the most "minor" of ureteral injuries, often heal with stricture or break down later if microvascular injury results in ureteral necrosis. Severe or large areas of contusion should be treated with excision and ureteroureterostomy. [p 3718]

15. **c. CT with the use of contrast material, obtained 20 minutes after injection of the contrast agent.** Because modern helical CT scanners can obtain images before intravenous contrast dye is excreted in the urine, delayed images must be obtained (5 to 20 minutes after contrast material injection) to allow contrast material to extravasate from the injured collecting system, renal pelvis, or ureter. [p 3717]

16. **b. Surgery for endometriosis greatly increases the risk.** A large percentage of ureteral injuries after gynecologic laparoscopy occur during electrosurgical or laser-assisted lysis of endometriosis. [p 3716]

17. **e. "Pie in the sky" bladder.** In some cases, associated pelvic fractures will require open reduction and plating by the orthopedic service. If open plating of the symphysis pubis is planned, the urology team should be alerted and the bladder repaired at the same time. Several reasons support this. Intraperitoneal ruptures require open operative repair. [pp 3724, 3727]

18. **b. The preferred method is retrograde filling of the bladder with at least 350 ml of contrast material.** We infuse 350 ml of 30% contrast material (iohexol, Nycomed) by gravity into the urinary catheter (less is infused only if the patient complains of pain). [p 3722]

19. **a. They are present in 6% to 10% of patients with pelvic fracture.** Bladder injuries after blunt trauma are overwhelmingly associated with pelvic fracture, occurring in 6% to 10% of all cases. [p 3721]

20. **c. Rectal perforation.** Some authors have listed several contraindications to such conservative management: bone fragment projecting into the bladder (which is unlikely to heal), open pelvic fracture, and rectal perforation. [pp 3723–3724]

21. **a. Retrograde urethrography.** Because classic findings are seen in less than 50%, urethral disruption is discovered only when a urethral catheter cannot be placed by the emergency room trauma team or when it is misplaced into pelvic hematoma. When blood at the urethral meatus is discovered, it is our policy to obtain an immediate retrograde urethrogram to rule out urethral injury. [p 3725]

22. **a. A single attempt at urethral catheterization by a urologist at the bedside.** We make one gentle attempt to place a urethral catheter for suspected partial disruption. [p 3727]

23. **a. Cystography, then open suprapubic tube placement and repair of bladder injuries, if present.** If a urethral injury is demonstrated by urethrography, the patient is brought to the operating room for placement of a formal suprapubic urinary catheter, bladder exploration, and repair of bladder injuries if present. [pp 3725–3726]

24. **a. Results in a high incidence of impotence and incontinence.** We do not recommend open primary realignment for urethral distraction injuries, as it is reportedly associated with an unsatisfactory degree of impotence and incontinence. We favor the indirect method of primary realignment (the newer definition), in which the urethral gap is bridged acutely with a urethral catheter, when possible, to promote urethral healing, but open dissection of the injured area is minimized. [p 3727]

25. **a. Good results can be achieved with one-stage, open, perineal anastomotic urethroplasty.** Anastomotic urethroplasty is the procedure of choice for posterior or bulbar strictures resulting from trauma. [p 3731]

26. **c. Urethral disruption proximal to the genitourinary diaphragm.** The location of most posterior urethral distraction injuries is described by a three-part classification scheme in which type II is urethral disruption proximal to the genitourinary diaphragm. [p 3726]

27. **a. Major associated vascular injuries.** Potentially fatal injuries, such as intra-abdominal wounds or femoral vessel transection, must be aggressively sought and treated. [p 3733]

28. **c. Retrograde urethrography.** Urethrography is suggested for all patients with penetrating penile injury, as up to half will have urethral involvement. [p 3733]

29. **a. Spatulated, stented, tensionless, watertight repair of the urethra with absorbable sutures.** Associated anterior urethral injuries should be closed primarily with a watertight, spatulated, catheter-stented technique and absorbable suture. [p 3734]

30. **a. Local anesthetic block, lubrication, and a single attempt at opening the zipper.** These patients should be given a local anesthetic penile block. After lubrication of the zipper with mineral oil, a single attempt at opening it should be made. [p 3736]

31. **b. Left testicular débridement and primary closure of the capsule of the testicle.** Necrotic testicular tissue should be débrided and the capsule closed with running absorbable suture. In some cases, loss of capsule will require removal of intratesticular tissue to allow closure. [p 3736]

32. **b. The tunica vaginalis.** With more force, the tunica albuginea ruptures, resulting in scrotal blood collection that is contained by the tunica vaginalis (hematocele). [p 3736]

33. **a. A foreskin flap for small distal lesions.** In uncircumcised patients, some have advocated using foreskin to cover and allow primary closure of middle to distal penile skin loss, such as occurs with burns to the penile shaft. [p 3738]

Chapter 106

Use of Intestinal Segments and Urinary Diversion

W. Scott McDougal

Questions

1. When a portion of stomach is to be used for augmentation, it should:

   a. always be based on the right gastroepiploic artery.
   b. include only the antrum.
   c. never extend to the pylorus.
   d. include a significant portion of the lesser curve.

2. How does the ileum differ from the jejunum?

   a. It has a larger diameter.
   b. The mesentery is thinner.
   c. It has multiple arcades.
   d. The vessels in the mesentery are larger.

3. When stomach is used for urinary diversion, which electrolyte abnormality may occur?

   a. Hyperchloremic metabolic acidosis
   b. Hypochloremic metabolic alkalosis
   c. Hyperkalemic metabolic alkalosis
   d. Hypokalemic metabolic acidosis

4. Postoperative bowel obstruction is most common when which of the following segments is used for diversion?

   a. Colon
   b. Stomach
   c. Sigmoid
   d. Ileum

5. Mechanical bowel preparation results in:

   a. smaller bacterial counts per gram of enteric contents.
   b. a reduction in bacterial count in the jejunum.
   c. a reduction in total number of bacteria in the bowel.
   d. a reduction in the bacterial counts in the stomach.

6. When should systemic antibiotics in elective surgery be given?

   a. Before the patient is anesthetized
   b. Before the skin incision is made
   c. Intraoperatively before closure commences
   d. Any time as long as they are given in the perioperative period

7. What is the most common cause of a lethal bowel complication?

   a. Use of prior irradiated bowel
   b. Lack of mechanical bowel preparation
   c. Lack of antibiotic bowel preparation
   d. Placement of a drain adjacent to the anastomosis

8. What is the difference between stapled anastomoses and sutured anastomoses?

a. Fewer leaks
b. Less compatibility with urine
c. Reduced overall operative time
d. Less incidence of bowel obstruction

9. The use of a nasogastric tube in the postoperative period:

    a. hastens the return of intestinal motility.
    b. reduces the incidence of bowel leak.
    c. reduces postoperative vomiting.
    d. increases the risk of aspiration.

10. The abdominal stoma for a conduit should be:

    a. flush with the skin.
    b. placed through the belly of the rectus muscle.
    c. made as a loop to reduce parastomal hernia.
    d. made with colon for the lowest complication rate.

11. The loop end ileostomy is best used in what type of patient?

    a. The obese patient
    b. The thin patient
    c. The patient in whom a stoma is revised
    d. The female patient

12. Ureteral strictures occurring after an ileal conduit not associated with the ureteral intestinal anastomosis most frequently occur where?

    a. At the ureteropelvic junction
    b. In the right ureter several centimeters proximal to the ureteral intestinal anastomosis
    c. On the left side where the ureter crosses the aorta
    d. In the mid-ureter

13. Renal deterioration after a conduit diversion with normal kidneys occurs in what percentage of renal units?

    a. 20%
    b. 40%
    c. 60%
    d. 80%

14. What is the most common cause of death in patients with ureterosigmoidostomies over the long term?

    a. Cancer
    b. Renal failure
    c. Electrolyte abnormalities
    d. Their primary disease

15. What is the minimal glomerular filtration rate necessary for a continent diversion?

    a. 70 ml/minute
    b. 50 ml/minute
    c. 35 ml/minute
    d. 25 ml/minute

16. Which urinary diversion has the fewest number of intraoperative and immediately postoperative complications?

    a. Ileal conduit
    b. Colon conduit
    c. Kock pouch
    d. Indiana pouch

17. The jejunal conduit syndrome is manifested by which of the following?

    a. Hyperchloremic metabolic acidosis
    b. Hypochloremic metabolic alkalosis
    c. Hyperkalemic, hyponatremic metabolic acidosis
    d. Hypokalemic, hyponatremic metabolic alkalosis

18. What is the primary advantage of a transverse colon conduit?

    a. Its ease of construction
    b. The ability to use a nonrefluxing anastomosis
    c. That it is unlikely to be injured by radiation in those who have received pelvic radiation
    d. Its reduced electrolyte problems

19. Total body potassium depletion is most common in which of the following?

    a. Ureterosigmoidostomy
    b. Ileal conduit
    c. Colon conduit
    d. Sigmoid conduit

20. In urinary intestinal diversion, the serum creatinine level may not be an accurate reflection of renal function because:

    a. the intestine produces substances that interfere with its analysis.
    b. of secretion in the tubule.
    c. of reabsorption in the tubule.
    d. of reabsorption in the bowel.

21. Patients with urinary diversions who have a hyperchloremic metabolic acidosis over time:

    a. retain the ability to maintain the acidosis.
    b. lose the ability for electrolyte transport in the intestinal segments.
    c. compensate for the metabolic acidosis, thus eliminating risk.
    d. intermittently absorb ammonia when infection is present.

22. Which of the following statements is true concerning bone density abnormalities?

    a. They are unlikely to occur when the ileum is used.
    b. They are most likely to occur with colon.
    c. They are more common in patients who have a persistent hyperchloremic metabolic acidosis.
    d. They occur in patients with total body potassium depletion.

23. The effect of urinary intestinal diversion on growth:

    a. is unknown.
    b. is not a problem.
    c. has been shown to be adverse.
    d. accelerates growth.

24. Cancer occurring in urinary intestinal diversion is most likely to occur in which of the following?

    a. Augmentations
    b. Colon conduits
    c. Ileal conduits
    d. Ureterosigmoidostomies

25. Reconfiguring the bowel over the long term results in:

    a. decreased motor activity.
    b. increased volume.
    c. decreased metabolic complications.
    d. decreased absorption of lutes.

Answers

1. **c. Never extend to the pylorus.** When a wedge of fundus is employed, it should not include a significant portion of the antrum and should never extend to the pylorus or all the way to the lesser curve of the stomach. [p 3746]

2. **c. It has multiple arcades.** The ileum, being more distal in location, has a smaller diameter. It has multiple arterial arcades, and the vessels in the arcades are smaller than those in the jejunum. [p 3746]

3. **b. Hypochloremic metabolic alkalosis.** Complications specific to the use of stomach include the hematuria-dysuria syndrome and uncontrollable metabolic alkalosis in some patients with chronic renal failure. When stomach is used, a hypochloremic, hypokalemic metabolic alkalosis may ensue. [p 3748]

4. **d. Ileum.** The incidence of postoperative bowel obstruction is 4%, less than that occurring with ileum. [p 3749]

5. **c. A reduction in total number of bacteria in the bowel.** The mechanical preparation reduces the amount of feces, whereas the antibiotic preparation reduces the bacterial count. A mechanical bowel preparation reduces the total number of bacteria but not their concentration. [p 3749]

6. **a. Before the patient is anesthetized.** Systemic antibiotics must be given before the operative event if they are to be effective. [p 3751]

7. **a. Use of prior irradiated bowel.** In one study of urinary intestinal diversion, 75% of the lethal complications that occurred in the postoperative period were related to the bowel. Eighty percent of these patients had received radiation before the intestinal surgery. [p 3752]

8. **b. Less compatibility with urine.** In general, sutured anastomoses are preferable for intestinal segments that are exposed to urine. [p 3752]

9. **c. Reduces postoperative vomiting.** There was no significant difference in major intestinal complications between the two study groups; however, those who did not have gastric decompression showed a much greater incidence of abdominal distention, nausea, and vomiting. [p 3757]

10. **b. Placed through the belly of the rectus muscle.** All stomas should be placed through the belly of the rectus muscle and be located at the peak of the infraumbilical fat roll. [p 3760]

11. **a. The obese patient.** The loop end ileostomy obviates some of these problems and is usually easier to perform than the ileal end stoma in the patient who is obese. [p 3761]

12. **c. On the left side where the ureter crosses the aorta.** It is important to note that ureteral strictures also occur away from the ureterointestinal anastomosis. This stricture is most common in the left ureter and is usually found as the ureter crosses over the aorta beneath the inferior mesenteric artery. [p 3770]

13. **a. 20%.** Patients who are studied over the long term show a significant degree of renal deterioration. Indeed, 20% of renal units have shown significant anatomic deterioration. [p 3770]

14. **b. Renal failure.** The most common cause of death in patients who have had a ureterosigmoidostomy for more than 15 years is acquired renal disease (i.e., sepsis or renal failure). [p 3770]

15. **c. 35 ml/minute.** If the patient is able to achieve a urine pH of 5.8 or less after an ammonium chloride load, has a urine osmolality of 600 mOsm/kg or greater in response to water deprivation, has a glomerular filtration rate that exceeds 35 ml/minute, and has minimal protein in the urine, the patient may be considered for a retentive diversion. [p 3771]

16. **a. Ileal conduit.** It is the simplest type of conduit diversion to perform and is associated with the fewest number of intraoperative and immediately postoperative complications. [p 3771]

17. **c. Hyperkalemic, hyponatremic metabolic acidosis.** The early and long-term complications are similar to those listed for ileal conduit except that the electrolyte abnormality that occurs is hyperkalemic, hyponatremic metabolic acidosis instead of the hyperchloremic metabolic acidosis of ileal diversion. [p 3773]

18. **c. That it is unlikely to be injured by radiation in those who have received pelvic radiation.** The transverse colon is used when one wants to be sure that the segment of conduit employed has not been irradiated in individuals who have received extensive pelvic irradiation. [p 3773]

19. **a. Ureterosigmoidostomy.** Hypokalemia and total body depletion of potassium may occur in patients with urinary intestinal diversion. This is more common in patients with ureterosigmoidostomies than it is with patients who have other types of urinary intestinal diversion. [p 3779]

20. **d. Of reabsorption in the bowel.** Because urea and creatinine are reabsorbed by both the ileum and the colon, serum concentrations of urea and creatinine do not necessarily accurately reflect renal function. [p 3779]

21. **a. Retain the ability to maintain the acidosis.** The ability to establish a hyperchloremic metabolic acidosis, however, appears to be retained by most segments of ileum and colon over time. [p 3779]

22. **c. They are more common in patients who have a persistent hyperchloremic metabolic acidosis.** Osteomalacia in urinary intestinal diversion may be due to persistent acidosis, vitamin D resistance, and excessive calcium loss by the kidney. It appears that the degree to which each of these contributes to the syndrome may vary from patient to patient. [p 3780]

23. **c. Has been shown to be adverse.** There is considerable evidence to suggest that urinary intestinal diversion has a detrimental effect on growth and development. [p 3781]

24. **d. Ureterosigmoidostomies.** The highest incidence of cancer occurs when the transitional epithelium is juxtaposed to the colonic epithelium and both are bathed by feces. [p 3783]

25. **b. Increased volume.** Reconfiguring bowel usually increases the volume, but its effect on motor activity and wall tension over the long term is unclear at this time. [p 3784]

Chapter 107

Cutaneous Continent Urinary Diversion

Mitchell C. Benson • Carl A. Olsson

Questions

1. As a child, a 45-year-old man underwent ileal conduit diversion for bladder extrophy. He reports requesting continent diversion. The serum creatinine value is 2.0 mg/dl. A Loopogram shows bilaterally thin ureters with small kidneys. Which of the following is the best procedure?

   a. Ureterosigmoidostomy
   b. A T-pouch utilizing the ileal conduit
   c. Abandoning the idea of continent diversion
   d. A Penn pouch utilizing the ileal conduit

2. As a child, a 45-year-old man underwent ileal conduit urinary diversion for bladder extrophy. He reports requesting continent diversion. The serum creatinine value is 2.0 mg/dl. A Loopogram shows bilateral hydronephrosis and a pipe-stem conduit. What is the best course of action?

   a. Use of a Mainz II to avoid problems with his dilated ureters
   b. T-pouch and abandoning his diseased conduit
   c. Abandoning the idea of the continent diversion
   d. Draining the upper tracts and reassessing renal function

3. A patient undergoing cystectomy and attempted continent cutaneous diversion has positive ureteral margin biopsy results up to 2 cm above each iliac artery, at which point negative biopsy results are seen. What is the best course of action?

   a. Utilize the terminal ileum for ureteral implantation and a Mitrofanoff continence mechanism.
   b. Abandon the idea of continent diversion.
   c. Mobilize the kidneys and stretch the ureters to the reservoir.
   d. Use a T-pouch with a long chimney.

4. Preservation of the ileocecal valve can be maintained with which of the following catheterizable pouches?

   a. T-pouch or Kock pouch
   b. LeBag
   c. Indiana pouch
   d. Mainz I or II pouch

5. In which situation in a repair of a nipple valve would resection of additional bowel be required routinely?

   a. Stones on exposed staples
   b. Nipple valve slippage
   c. Nipple valve atrophy
   d. Pinhole leak

6. A 10-year-old child has undergone urinary diversion by ileal conduit for myelomeningocele. The conduit was replaced on two occasions for pipe-stem conduit development. The conduit is again affected by the same process. The patient's family desires a continent diversion. Which of the following is the best procedure?

   a. Ureterosigmoidostomy
   b. Revision of the conduit
   c. T-pouch utilizing the ileal conduit
   d. Penn pouch utilizing the ileal conduit

7. A patient with chronic active hepatitis and invasive bladder cancer associated with intravesical carcinoma in situ reports for treatment. The serum creatinine value is 1.0 mg/dl. Prostatic urethral biopsy shows mild atypia. What is the best approach?

   a. Cystoprostatectomy and a T-pouch
   b. Cystoprostatectomy and an ileal conduit
   c. Cystoprostatectomy and a right colon reservoir
   d. Cystoprostatectomy and a Mainz II pouch

8. The highest reoperation rate in patients with catheterizable pouches occurs with what type of sphincter:

   a. In situ appendix
   b. Imbricated terminal ileum
   c. Plicated terminal ileum
   d. Nipple valves

9. Which of the Mitrofanoff sphincter deficiencies can be corrected surgically?

   a. The length of the appendix
   b. Absence of the appendix
   c. Stenosis of the appendix
   d. All of the above

10. Hematuria and skin breakdown may occur with what type of pouch?

    a. T-pouch
    b. Gastric pouch
    c. Mainz pouch
    d. Right colon pouch

11. Preoperative colonoscopy is indicated in candidates for which of the following procedures?

    a. Small intestinal reservoir
    b. Gastric reservoir
    c. Rectal reservoirs
    d. All of the above

12. What condition may complicate absorbable stapled ileal pouches?

    a. Urine leaks
    b. Valve failure
    c. Hydronephrosis
    d. Ischemic pouch contraction

13. Anastomotic transitional cell carcinoma develops in a patient who has undergone cystectomy and continent cutaneous urinary diversion. What is the best treatment?

    a. Distal ureterectomy and reimplantation if feasible
    b. Conversion to an ileal conduit
    c. Ileal ureter interposition
    d. Nephroureterectomy

14. Drainage of mucus is hardest with which sphincteric mechanism?

    a. A Kock valve
    b. In situ appendix
    c. Imbricated ileum
    d. Plicated ileum

15. Which continent cutaneous diversion allows for a refluxing ureteroenteric anastomosis?

    a. A Mitrofanoff with implantation of the ureters into terminal ileum
    b. A Mitrofanoff with implantation of the ureters into the colon
    c. A T-pouch
    d. A Kock pouch

16. Three years after radical cystectomy and construction of a Kock pouch, a patient presents with right lower quadrant discomfort and associated spurts of urinary leakage. What is the most important diagnostic test?

    a. CT
    b. Intravenous pyelography
    c. Urine culture and sensitivity
    d. Pouch-o-Gram

17. Three years after cystectomy and use of a Kock pouch for bladder cancer, a patient presents with recurrent episodes of bilateral pyelonephritis. What is the most important diagnostic test?

    a. CT
    b. Intravenous pyelography
    c. Urine culture and sensitivity
    d. Pouch-o-Gram

18. What is the most important feature in preventing nipple valve slippage?

    a. Using absorbable staples
    b. The length of the intussusception
    c. Resecting adequate mesentery
    d. Attaching the nipple valve to the side wall of the reservoir

19. In a patient with pipe-stem conduit and bilateral hydronephrosis desiring continent diversion, nephrostomy drainage results in clearance values of 40 ml/min on the right and 10 ml/min on the left. The serum creatinine value is 1.8 mg/dl. What should the surgeon do?

    a. Mainz II pouch to avoid problems with dilated ureters
    b. T-pouch and abandon the idea of disease conduit
    c. Abandon the idea of continent diversion
    d. Ureterosigmoidostomy

20. A patient with squamous cell cancer of the bladder desires cystectomy and continent diversion. He has a 10 lb weight loss noted in the month before surgery. Which procedure is helpful in his management?

    a. Increase oral intake
    b. Preoperative hyperalimentation
    c. Postoperative hyperalimentation
    d. Proceed directly with surgery

21. Preoperative evaluation with an oatmeal enema is required in which of the following procedures?

    a. Right colon reservoir
    b. Mainz I pouch
    c. Mainz II procedure
    d. LeBag

22. Follow-up urinary cytology and colonoscopy should be employed in which type of continent diversion?

    a. Ureterosigmoidostomy
    b. Mainz II
    c. Right colon reservoir
    d. All of the above

23. Nocturnal emptying of the patient's reservoir is required in which type of diversion?

    a. Ureterosigmoidostomy
    b. T-pouch
    c. Right colon reservoir
    d. Penn pouch

24. The appendix is sacrificed in patients undergoing which of the following pouch constructions?

    a. Indiana pouch
    b. LeBag
    c. Mainz I
    d. All of the above

25. Pouch stone development occurs most commonly with which of the following operations?

    a. T-pouch
    b. A Kock pouch
    c. A Penn pouch
    d. Gastric-ileal composite pouch

26. Which of the following is a typical catheter used for appendiceal sphincters?

    a. 22 Fr straight tip catheter
    b. 22 Fr coudé tip catheter
    c. 14 Fr straight tip catheter
    d. 14 Fr coudé tip catheter

27. Urinary retention resulting from continent diversion occurs most commonly with what type of sphincter?

    a. Appendiceal stoma
    b. Benchekroun hydraulic valve
    c. Nipple valve sphincter
    d. Imbricated Indiana mechanism

28. Immediate postoperative initial pouch capacity is least in which of the following pouches?

    a. A T or Kock ileal pouch
    b. A right colon pouch
    c. A gastric pouch
    d. A Mainz I pouch

29. Elevated pouch pressures would potentially facilitate the continence mechanism seen with which of the following valves or sphincters?

    a. A Benchekroun ileal valve
    b. A Kock valve
    c. An appendiceal tunnel
    d. All of the above

30. The long-term failure rate of continence mechanisms is greatest with which of the following mechanisms?

    a. A T-pouch valve
    b. An appendiceal tunnel

c. A Benchekroun hydraulic valve
d. An imbricated terminal ileum

31. The use of absorbable staples in continent urinary diversion is best suited to what type of pouch?

   a. Ileal reservoir
   b. Right colon reservoir
   c. Gastric-ileal composite reservoir
   d. None of the above

32. When a large intestinal reservoir is created from absorbable staples, why is bowel eversion necessary?

   a. Staples should not be utilized in reservoir construction.
   b. To inspect the inside of the reservoir.
   c. To avoid injury to the mesenteric blood supply.
   d. To allow application of the second row of staples.

33. Which of the following groups of patients may not be suitable candidates for continent urinary diversion?

   a. Patients with multiple sclerosis
   b. Quadriplegic individuals
   c. The very frail or mentally impaired
   d. All of the above

34. Which of the following sutures should not be used in the construction of a reservoir?

   a. Chromic catgut
   b. Plain catgut
   c. Silk
   d. Polyglycolic acid (Dexon)

35. Which of the following diversions is at risk for the development of a late malignancy?

   a. A ureterosigmoidostomy
   b. A T-pouch
   c. A Mainz II
   d. All of the above

36. Which of the following diversions is at greatest risk for the development of a late malignancy?

   a. A ureterosigmoidostomy
   b. A T-pouch
   c. A Mainz II pouch
   d. An Indiana reservoir

37. Continent urinary diversion has which of the following effects?

   a. It results in a psychotic depression.
   b. It results in an improved psychosocial adjustment.
   c. It has been associated with violent behavior.
   d. None of the above.

38. Which of the following is NOT true of continent urinary diversion?

   a. It is the "gold standard" of urinary diversion.
   b. It is a safe and reliable urinary diversion.
   c. It is associated with an increased complication rate.
   d. It is appropriate for selected individuals.

39. Which of the following circumstances would contraindicate a rectal bladder?

   a. Prior pelvic irradiation
   b. Dilated ureters
   c. Lax anal sphincter tone
   d. All of the above

40. During the construction of a continent cutaneous urinary diversion, what should the surgeon do?

   a. Not be concerned about the continence mechanism because the mechanism will mold to the catheter
   b. Test the continence mechanism for ease of catheterization
   c. Not be concerned about pouch integrity, because the pouch will seal itself
   d. None of the above

41. If the urine in a continent cutaneous reservoir is found to be infected, what should be done?

   a. Nothing need be done in the absence of symptoms.
   b. The urine should always be sterilized with appropriate antibiotics.
   c. The patient should have the infection eradicated and then be given prophylactic antibiotics.
   d. The patient should undergo intravenous pyelography to check for upper tract damage.

42. What is the most appropriate and conservative care for pouch rupture?

   a. Broad-spectrum antibiotic therapy
   b. Careful radiologic imaging and antibiotic therapy
   c. Surgical exploration for repair of the rupture and broad-spectrum antibiotic therapy
   d. Pouch drainage and broad-spectrum antibiotic therapy

43. Which was the first pouch to employ the Mitrofanoff principle?

   a. Mainz I pouch
   b. Penn pouch
   c. Kock pouch
   d. Indiana pouch

44. Which of the following represents an advantage of the gastric pouch?

   a. Electrolyte reabsorption is reduced.
   b. It does not result in absorptive malabsorption.
   c. Acid urine may reduce the risk of infection.
   d. All of the above.

45. When converting from an ileal conduit to a continent diversion, what should be done with the conduit?

   a. It should be discarded because it is older and subject to more complications.
   b. It should always be preserved for the ureteroileal anastomosis.
   c. It should be incorporated into the continent diversion when possible.
   d. None of the above.

46. Which of the following is true of absorbable staples?

   a. Their use has been shown to shorten operative time.
   b. They are safe and reliable.
   c. Unlike nonabsorbable staples, they must not be overlapped.
   d. All of the above.

Answers

1. **c. Abandoning the idea of continent diversion.** The reabsorption and recirculation of urinary constituents and other metabolites require that serum creatinine levels are in the normal range or certainly below the level of 1.8 mg/dl. [p 3790]

2. **d. Draining the upper tracts and reassessing renal function.** In patients with bilateral hydronephrosis, where renal functional improvement might be anticipated upon relief of the ureteral obstruction, the urologist may veer from the serum creatinine and creatinine clearance standards. The authors' prejudice in such cases is to drain the upper tract (by percutaneous nephrostomies, if needed) with re-evaluation of renal function thereafter, before opting for a continent diversion. [p 3790]

3. **a. Utilize the terminal ileum for ureteral implantation and a Mitrofanoff continence mechanism.** The appendix with a detubularized right colon reservoir and refluxing ureters implanted end-to-side into terminal ileum are used. This procedure is uniquely capable of affording continent cutaneous diversion to the patient with short ureters because the terminal ileum can be left long enough to reach high into the retroperitoneum. The appendix or other pseudo-appendiceal (Mitrofanoff) mechanisms can be used for continence. [p 3824]

4. **a. T-pouch or Kock pouch.** This procedure and the similarly constructed T-pouch are the only catheterizable continent diversions that preserve the ileocecal valve. All other pouches are of right colon, so that the ileocecal valve is sacrificed. [p 3807]

5. **c. Nipple valve atrophy.** In addition to slippage, nipple valves are subject to ischemic atrophy. When this occurs, a new nipple valve must be fashioned from a new bowel segment. [p 3805]

6. **b. Revision of the conduit.** The best procedure is to revise the conduit. It should be noted that some patients have developed rather striking diarrhea or steatorrhea following the loss of the ileocecal valve. This may be particularly true in the pediatric patient when there is neurogenic bowel dysfunction (myelomeningocele patient). [pp 3794, 3805]

7. **b. Cystoprostatectomy and an ileal conduit.** The best approach is cystoprostatectomy and a conduit. The reabsorption and recirculation of urinary constituents and other metabolites require that liver function be normal and that serum creatinine levels be in the normal range or certainly below the level of 1.8 mg/dl. [p 3790]

8. **d. Nipple valves.** The creation of nipple valves is by far the most technologically demanding of all the continence mechanisms and is associated with the highest complication and reoperation rate. [p 3805]

9. **d. All of the above.** The caliber of Mitrofanoff mechanisms, the length of the appendix, stenosis, and even absence of the appendix can be resolved by surgical variations. It is the authors' opinion that these criticisms are more theoretical than real and the appendiceal or pseudo-appendiceal continence mechanism remains a very attractive and reliable continence mechanism. [p 3804]

10. **b. Gastric pouch.** Peristomal skin irritation from acid secretion with use of a gastric pouch occurred in two patients but was not considered severe. This is a more frequent complication in other reports and has resulted in skin breakdown in some instances. [p 3826]

11. **c. Rectal reservoirs.** Procedures that require the use of a large intestinal segment should always be preceded by a radiologic or colonoscopic assessment of the entire large intestine. Sigmoidoscopy only for a sigmoid colon procedure is insufficient because more proximal disease may leave the patient with a short colon syndrome. [p 3790]

12. **d. Ischemic pouch contraction.** Urodynamic evaluation at 6 months of patients in whom absorbable staplers were used to create W-stapled ileal neobladders, however, documented a small-capacity reservoir requiring augmentation enterocystoplasty in 3 of 25 patients (12%). The author attributed this complication to either the size of the staples or reservoir fibrosis secondary to foreign body reaction. [p 3831]

13. **a. Distal ureterectomy and reimplantation if feasible.** For an isolated anastomotic recurrence, distal ureterectomy and reimplantation are appropriate. An additional segment of ileum can serve as a proximal limb to the reservoir. If nephrectomy is necessary, careful attention must be paid to the residual renal function. [p 3792]

14. **b. In situ appendix.** The large amount of mucus produced by an intestinal reservoir is more easily emptied or irrigated by using a catheter of 20 to 22 French size rather than the typical catheter that would be admitted through an appendiceal stump (14 to 16 Fr). [p 3804]

15. **a. A Mitrofanoff with implantation of the ureters into terminal ileum.** We have utilized the in situ appendix with a detubularized right colon reservoir and the native ileocecal valve as an antireflux mechanism (refluxing ureters implanted end-to-side into terminal ileum). [p 3824]

16. **c. Urine culture and sensitivity.** A condition has been described that is manifested by pain in the region of the pouch along with increased pouch contractility (pouchitis). It should be mentioned that this condition, although infrequent, may result in temporary failure of the continence mechanism because of the hypercontractility of the bowel segment employed for construction of the pouch. The patient typically presents with a history of sudden explosive discharge of urine through the continence mechanism (rather than dribbling incontinence) along with discomfort in the region of the pouch. The most important diagnostic test is urine culture. [p 3806]

17. **d. Pouch-o-Gram.** Episodes of recurrent pyelonephritis should be evaluated by a Pouch-o-Gram searching for a failure of the antireflux mechanism or appearance of upper tract stones. [p 3806]

18. **d. Attaching the nipple valve to the side wall of the reservoir.** The second major advance has been the attachment of the nipple valve to the reservoir wall itself. This has been achieved by two or three different stapling techniques as well as by a suturing technique. Nevertheless, nipple valve failure can be anticipated in 10% to 15% of cases even in the hands of the very best and experienced surgeons. Attaching the nipple valve to the sidewall of the pouch results in a relative lengthening of the valve rather than a foreshortening of the valve with pouch filling. [p 3805]

19. **c. Abandon the idea of continent diversion.** In cases in which renal function is borderline, creatinine clearance should be measured. A minimal level of creatinine clearance of 60 ml/min should be documented before deeming the patient an appropriate candidate for continent diversion. Continent diversion should be abandoned and simple replacement of the conduit considered. [p 3790]

20. **b. Preoperative hyperalimentation.** If the patient is nutritionally depleted to begin with, hyperalimentation has been suggested to be of value if initiated during the preoperative interval. [pp 3792, 3802]

21. **c. Mainz II procedure.** Any procedure that relies on the intact anal sphincter for continence, such as the Mainz II pouch, requires an assessment of the sphincter before carrying out the operation. Our preference has been to utilize 400 to 500 ml of a thin mixture of oatmeal and water that the patient is asked to retain for 1 hour in the upright position. [p 3794]

22. **d. All of the above.** Urinary cytology should be performed in all patients undergoing a continent urinary diversion starting no later than 10 years after the procedure, whether or not the diversion was performed secondary to a malignancy. When the ureters are directed into the fecal stream, routine colonoscopy should also be performed. Because of an increased risk of malignancy even in the absence of admixture of urine and stool, all large intestinal pouches should be subjected to annual investigation by pouchoscopy as well as cytology. [p 3792]

23. **a. Ureterosigmoidostomy.** Routine nightly insertion of a rectal tube is advocated in the long-term care of the patient. However, many patients will reject this practice as uncomfortable and unappealing. Nighttime urinary drainage must be mandated, on the other hand, in any patient who cannot maintain electrolyte homeostasis with oral medication (e.g., patients with ureterosigmoidostomy owing to the additional risk of metabolic acidosis). [pp 3798–3799]

24. **d. All of the above.** In all instances, unless the appendix is being utilized as a continence mechanism, appendectomy must be performed because the in situ appendix would serve as a nidus for infection and abscess formation. [pp 3814–3815]

25. **b. A Kock pouch.** A final feature of stapled nipple valves is the potential for stone formation on exposed staples. Pouch stone development occurs most commonly with the Kock pouch. [p 3805]

26. **d. 14 Fr coudé tip catheter.** The appropriate angle of entry can be taught to the patient until the patient is comfortable with the use of the new catheter. In fact, the authors' preference is to routinely utilize coudé catheters with non-nipple valve pouches. The best catheter for draining an appendiceal sphincter pouch would be a 14 Fr coudé tip tube. [p 3806]

27. **c. Nipple valve sphincter.** Urinary retention is an infrequent but serious occurrence in catheterizable pouches. It is most commonly seen with pouches whose continence mechanism consists of a nipple valve. If the chimney of the nipple valve is not near the surface of the abdomen, the catheter can be misdirected into folds of bowel rather than through the nipple valve. [p 3806]

28. **a. A T or Kock ileal pouch.** In the case of ileal pouches, pouch capacity will initially be low (150 ml). Small bowel pouches have initial capacities that are much lower than right colon pouches. [p 3806]

29. **a. A Benchekroun ileal valve.** The premise of Benchekroun was that as the reservoir filled, the pressure within the valve would also increase, thereby creating continence. [p 3824]

30. **c. A Benchekroun hydraulic valve.** Concerns regarding the long-term durability of the Benchekroun hydraulic ileal valve mechanism have resulted in this procedure being largely abandoned. [pp 3805, 3824]

31. **b. Right colon reservoir.** In our experience, colonic pouches appear better suited for construction with the absorbable stapler because of their relatively larger lumen. With large bowel pouches, there is no problem with staple lines causing subsequent bowel ischemia. [p 3831]

32. **d. To allow application of the second row of staples.** It is necessary to evert the bowel to continue subsequent staple applications. The bowel is everted, a cut is made beyond the end of the staple line, and the next line of staples is applied. [p 3828]

33. **d. All of the above.** Patients with multiple sclerosis, quadriplegic individuals, and the very frail or mentally impaired patient will at some point in their lives require the care of members of the family or visiting nurse, and we view such patients as poor candidates for any form of continent diversion. [pp 3789–3790]

34. **c. Silk.** All sutures utilized in the urinary tract should be absorbable. [p 3791]

35. **d. All of the above.** Late malignancy has been reported in all bowel segments exposed to the urinary stream, whether or not there is a commingling with feces. [p 3792]

36. **a. A ureterosigmoidostomy.** Although late malignancy has been reported in all bowel segments exposed to the urinary stream, whether or not there is a commingling with feces, the mixture of urothelium, urine, and feces poses the greatest risk. [p 3792]

37. **b. It results in an improved psychosocial adjustment.** Many studies from throughout the world have suggested an improved psychosocial adjustment of the patient undergoing continent urinary and fecal diversion compared with those patients with diversions requiring collecting appliances. [p 3793]

38. **a. It is the "gold standard" of urinary diversion.** The process of patient counseling that the authors employ always refers to ileal conduit urinary diversion as the gold standard against which the newer operations must be compared. [p 3793]

39. **d. All of the above.** If the urologist selects one of these procedures, the preoperative evaluation should include all of the caveats of ureterosigmoidostomy. Dilated ureters are not acceptable. The patient with extensive pelvic irradiation is not a candidate. Existing renal insufficiency disqualifies a patient from candidacy. Anal sphincteric tone must be judged competent before electing these operations, and, finally colonoscopy must be carried out before the procedure to ensure against preexisting colorectal disease as well as after the procedure to guard against the potential development of colonic cancer after surgery. [p 3793]

40. **b. Test the continence mechanism for ease of catheterization.** The continence mechanism is catheterized to ensure ease of catheter passage. This is an extremely important and crucial maneuver because the inability to catheterize is a serious complication that will often result in the need for reoperation. [p 3805]

41. **a. Nothing need be done in the absence of symptoms.** Because all patients with catheterized pouches will have chronic bacteriuria, the problem of antibiotic management should be discussed. Most authors would suggest that bacteriuria in the absence of symptoms does not warrant antibiotic treatment. [p 3806]

42. **c. Surgical exploration for repair of the rupture and broad-spectrum antibiotic therapy.** In general, these patients require immediate pouch decompression and radiologic pouch studies. For patients with large defects, surgical exploration and pouch repair are required. If the amount of

urinary extravasation is small, and the patient does not have a surgical abdomen, catheter drainage and antibiotic administration may suffice in treating intraperitoneal rupture of a pouch. Patients managed with this conservative approach require careful monitoring. [pp 3806–3807]

43. **b. Penn pouch.** The Penn pouch was the first continent diversion employing the Mitrofanoff principle wherein the appendix served as the continence mechanism. [p 3823]

44. **d. All of the above.** First, electrolyte reabsorption would be greatly diminished by utilizing this bowel segment in the reservoir. This would potentially make the stomach the selected reservoir for individuals with preexisting metabolic acidosis or renal insufficiency. Hyperchloremic acidosis would not be an anticipated problem; in fact, in addition to presenting a barrier against the absorption of chloride and ammonium, the gastric mucosa secretes chloride ions. Furthermore, in patients in whom shortening of the bowel may be expected to lead to degrees of malabsorption, the use of stomach is an attractive alternative. The acid pH of the urine may also reduce the risk of bacterial colonization. Finally, when the entire lower bowel has been irradiated, the stomach may provide healthy nonirradiated tissue to use in performing continent diversion. [p 3825]

45. **c. It should be incorporated into the continent diversion when possible.** It is the authors' preference to utilize the conduit in some form whenever possible. The use of an existing bowel segment has the potential to diminish metabolic sequelae and may result in a lower complication rate. [pp 3827–3828]

46. **d. All of the above.** The use of absorbable staplers has substantially reduced the time required to fashion bowel reservoirs and has demonstrated short-term and long-term reliability with respect to reservoir integrity and volume. However, it is very important to note that the absorbable poly-GIA staples must not overlap, because this will result in the failure of the staples to lock together. This is in direct contrast to metal staples, which are meant to overlap to create anastomotic integrity. [p 3828]

Chapter 108

Orthotopic Urinary Diversion

John P. Stein • Donald G. Skinner

Questions

1. Before 1950, what was the most common form of urinary diversion performed?

   a. Colon conduit
   b. Orthotopic neobladder
   c. Ileal conduit
   d. Ureterosigmoidostomy

2. What long-term complication is not commonly associated with ureterosigmoidostomy urinary diversion?

   a. Renal deterioration
   b. Hyperchloremic metabolic acidosis
   c. Hypercalcemia
   d. Secondary malignancy

3. What is the most common long-term complication associated with the ileal conduit?

   a. Ureteroileal stenosis
   b. Pyelonephritis
   c. Stomal stenosis
   d. Nephrolithiasis

4. With regard to orthotopic urinary diversion, all the following statements are true except which one?

   a. Voiding is accomplished by a Valsalva maneuver and relaxation of the external sphincter.
   b. Most patients are continent.
   c. The rhabdosphincter complex is responsible for the continent mechanism.
   d. Most patients require intermittent catheterization to empty their neobladder.

5. With regard to renal function before continent urinary diversion, which of the following statements is true?

   a. A minimum creatinine clearance of 60 ml/minute should be documented.
   b. A serum creatinine value of 2.0 mg/dl or less should be documented.
   c. Patients with ureteral obstruction should first undergo decompression to determine the true baseline level.
   d. All of the above.

6. Patients with borderline renal function may be best served with what form of orthotopic diversion?

   a. Gastric neobladder
   b. Ileal neobladder
   c. Colonic neobladder
   d. Ileal colonic neobladder

7. Regarding patient age and orthotopic diversion, which of the following statements is true?

   a. Orthotopic diversion should not be performed in patients older than 80 years of age.
   b. Orthotopic diversion should not be performed in patients younger than 30 years of age.
   c. Differentiation between physiologic and chronologic age should be made.
   d. Advanced age is an absolute contraindication to orthotopic diversion.

8. Which of the following is an absolute contraindication to an orthotopic bladder substitute?

   a. An obese patient
   b. Patients with lymph node–positive bladder cancer after cystectomy
   c. A female with bladder neck tumor involvement with an uninvolved urethra

d. A male with an intraoperative positive distal surgical margin at the proximal urethra

9. Which orthotopic bladder substitute shape will accommodate the largest volume with the lowest pressures?

   a. Tube structure
   b. Cylindrical structure
   c. Spherical structure
   d. U-shaped structure

10. Innervation of the striated rhabdosphincter complex, which is crucial in the continence mechanism in patients undergoing orthotopic diversion, is from which of the following?

    a. The parasympathetic fibers from the sacral segments
    b. The sympathetic fibers from the superior hypogastric plexus
    c. A combination of both the parasympathetic and sympathetic fibers
    d. The pudendal innervation

11. To best preserve the pudendal innervation and the continence mechanism in patients undergoing cystectomy and orthotopic diversion, one should:

    a. perform minimal dissection along the pelvic floor.
    b. perform minimal dissection along the lateral aspect of the rectum.
    c. perform a nerve-sparing cystectomy.
    d. perform minimal dissection along the lateral aspect of the vagina in women.

12. The ultimate decision to perform an orthotopic bladder substitution after cystectomy for bladder cancer can be made:

    a. preoperatively at the time of consultation with the patient.
    b. only if there is not gross evidence of extravesical tumor extension.
    c. if the urethra is palpably normal.
    d. if the intraoperative frozen section analysis of the distal surgical margin (urethra) is normal.

13. In women who have a penetrating posterior bladder wall tumor, it is best to:

    a. never perform an orthotopic bladder substitution.
    b. remove the anterior vaginal wall en bloc with the bladder.
    c. remove the entire vagina en bloc with the bladder.
    d. strip the bladder off the anterior bladder wall.

14. Options for vaginal reconstruction in women at the time of anterior exenteration for bladder cancer include which of the following?

    a. Myocutaneous flap
    b. Detubularized bowel
    c. Omental flap
    d. All of the above

15. With regard to urethral recurrence after cystectomy for transitional cell carcinoma of the bladder, which of the following statements is true?

    a. The overall risk for men of a urethral recurrence after cystectomy is approximately 10%.
    b. Urethral recurrence is not thought to represent a failure of definitive treatment of the primary tumor but rather a manifestation of the multicentric defect of transitional cell carcinoma.
    c. Prostatic tumor involvement with the primary tumor is a risk factor for a urethra recurrence in the retained urethra after cystectomy.
    d. All of the above.

16. What is the greatest risk factor for a urethral tumor recurrence after cystectomy for bladder cancer?

    a. Lymph node tumor involvement
    b. Presence of carcinoma in situ
    c. Tumor multifocality
    d. Prostatic stroma involvement

17. Which of the following statements is correct in patients undergoing cystectomy with the intent for orthotopic reconstruction for bladder cancer?

    a. Preoperative prostate biopsies are mandatory in all patients considering orthotopic diversion to exclude prostatic tumor involvement.
    b. Intraoperative frozen section analysis of the urethra (distal surgical margin) is mandatory in all patients considering orthotopic diversion.
    c. Patients with a history of prostatic mucosa tumor involvement must be excluded from orthotopic diversion.
    d. Intraoperative frozen section analysis of the urethra is an unreliable method to evaluate for tumor involvement.

18. Which of the following statements is correct regarding urethral tumor involvement in women with bladder cancer?

    a. Bladder neck tumor involvement is the most significant risk factor for urethral tumor involvement.
    b. The urethra is the most common site of tumor involvement in women.
    c. Women with bladder neck tumors will always have concomitant urethral tumor involvement.
    d. Women with urethral tumors will always have lymph node–positive disease.

19. Which of the following statements is true regarding a woman with a history of transitional cell carcinoma of the bladder and with bladder neck tumor involvement?

    a. There is approximately an 80% chance of having tumor in the urethra.
    b. There is approximately a 50% chance of having tumor in the urethra.
    c. There is approximately a 20% chance of having tumor in the urethra
    d. There is an extremely low (<5%) chance of having tumor in the urethra.

20. Which of the following statements is true regarding urethral tumor involvement in women with bladder cancer?

    a. Women with urethral tumor will almost always have bladder neck tumor involvement.
    b. Approximately 50% of women with bladder neck or anterior vaginal wall involvement will have concomitant urethral tumor involvement.
    c. Anterior vaginal wall tumor involvement is a significant risk factor for urethral tumor involvement.
    d. All of the above.

21. Intraoperative frozen section analysis of the proximal urethra in women (considering orthotopic diversion) who are undergoing cystectomy for bladder cancer:

    a. is an unreliable means of evaluating the proximal urethra.
    b. should not be performed in women with bladder neck tumor involvement.
    c. is mandatory to exclude tumor in all women considering an orthotopic bladder substitution.
    d. is necessary only in women with a history of multifocal carcinoma in situ.

22. Which of the following statements is true regarding intraoperative frozen section analysis of the proximal urethra in patients considering orthotopic diversion?

a. It is mandatory in all women.
b. It is mandatory in all men.
c. It is a reliable method for evaluating the urethra.
d. All of the above.

23. Which of the following statements is true regarding local pelvic recurrence after radical cystectomy for bladder cancer?
    a. Local recurrence after cystectomy occurs in less than 10% of all patients.
    b. A local recurrence rate of approximately 50% is seen in patients with lymph node–positive disease.
    c. A local recurrence rate of approximately 30% is seen in patients with extravesical, lymph node–negative disease.
    d. Local recurrence rates do not relate to the pathologic stage.

24. Patients who develop a local pelvic tumor recurrence after radical cystectomy and orthotopic diversion should in general:
    a. expect involvement with the neobladder.
    b. undergo a conversion to a cutaneous form of diversion.
    c. expect normal neobladder function.
    d. have bilateral percutaneous nephrostomy tubes placed.

25. Orthotopic urinary diversion after definitive radiation therapy:
    a. is an absolute contraindication.
    b. may be performed in properly selected individuals.
    c. is associated with a significantly higher incidence of urinary retention rate.
    d. may require intermittent catheterization in most patients.

26. Male patients undergoing orthotopic diversion after definitive radiation therapy should be counseled that:
    a. they may require placement of an artificial urinary sphincter.
    b. there is a significantly high incidence of urinary retention rate.
    c. they may require intermittent catheterization in most cases.
    d. all of the above.

27. Which of the following statements concerning reflux prevention is true?
    a. It is controversial only in those undergoing a continent cutaneous form of urinary diversion.
    b. It is not controversial in those undergoing an orthotopic form of urinary diversion.
    c. It has been clearly shown in randomized studies not to be a crucial issue in patients undergoing an orthotopic form of urinary diversion.
    d. None of the above.

28. Which of the following statements concerning patients undergoing an orthotopic bladder substitution is true?
    a. They may have infected urinary constituents.
    b. They will likely require intermittent catheterization to empty the neobladder.
    c. They should have an antireflux mechanism incorporated regardless of the incidence of obstruction with the antireflux technique.
    d. All of the above.

29. Which of the following statements is correct regarding renal deterioration in patients undergoing an ileal conduit?
    a. It may occur even in the face of normal radiographic studies.
    b. It may take 20 years to occur.
    c. It is thought to be related to the combination of obstruction and reflux of infected urinary constituents.
    d. All of the above.

30. Complications associated with the antireflux intussuscepted nipple valve of the Kock ileal reservoir occur in:
    a. 10% of patients.
    b. 30% of patients.
    c. 80% of patients.
    d. only those with a continent cutaneous Kock ileal reservoir.

31. What is the most common complication associated with the antireflux intussuscepted nipple valve of the Kock ileal reservoir?
    a. Afferent nipple stenosis
    b. Prolapse of the afferent nipple (extussusception)
    c. Stones
    d. None of the above

32. Which of the following statements is true regarding the "serous-lined tunnel" technique to create an antireflux mechanism?
    a. This is a flap-valve technique.
    b. This requires an isoperistaltic afferent limb.
    c. This requires the use of staples to create.
    d. Only ileum can be used to construct this antireflux mechanism.

33. Which of the following statements is true regarding the T-mechanism as described by Stein and Skinner?
    a. This is a flap-valve technique.
    b. It can be incorporated into an antireflux (afferent) and a continent catheterizable (efferent) limb.
    c. This technique can be applied in cases in which there are dilated and or shortened ureters.
    d. All of the above.

34. Which of the following statements is true regarding the orthotopic T-pouch ileal neobladder?
    a. This reservoir maintains the same geometric configuration as the Kock ileal neobladder.
    b. Vascular arcades are preserved to the afferent limb to maintain the blood supply.
    c. No staples are required in the construction of this neobladder.
    d. All of the above.

35. The etiology of Kock pouch stones in the orthotopic ileal neobladder is thought to be related primarily to which of the following?
    a. Infected urine
    b. Retained mucus
    c. Exposed metallic staples
    d. Prolapse of the intussuscepted nipple

36. Which of the following statements is NOT true when comparing an orthotopic neobladder to an ileal conduit?
    a. There is definitely an increased complication rate with an orthotopic form of diversion over an ileal conduit.
    b. The orthotopic reservoir may provide an improved cosmetic result compared with an ileal conduit.
    c. The operative time required to create an orthotopic neobladder is similar to that for an ileal conduit.
    d. The hospitalization required for those receiving an orthotopic neobladder is similar to those receiving an ileal conduit.

37. Which of the following statements is NOT true regarding

the application of absorbable stapling techniques to orthotopic diversions?

    a. The application should decrease operative time.
    b. Detubularization and folding of the bowel are still required.
    c. The staple line usually does not provide a watertight seal.
    d. Recent advancements have decreased the bulk of the stapler and facilitated the application of this technique.

38. Which of the following statements is true regarding quality of life assessment after cystectomy and urinary diversion?

    a. Quality of life issues are becoming more important in the evaluation of patients undergoing urinary diversion.
    b. A well-validated measure of assessing quality of life is important in this evaluation.
    c. Most early studies evaluating quality of life had methodologic problems that limited their conclusions.
    d. All of the above.

39. Which of the following statements is true regarding an orthotopic bladder substitute?

    a. Most patients are continent and volitionally void per urethra.
    b. There does not appear to be an increased complication rate compared with other forms of diversion.
    c. Quality of life studies are favorable for this diversion.
    d. All of the above.

Answers

1. **d. Ureterosigmoidostomy.** Ureterosigmoidostomy remained the diversion of choice until the late 1950s. [p 3836]

2. **c. Hypercalcemia.** Electrolyte imbalances, renal problems, and secondary malignancies arising at the ureteral implantation site were described. [p 3836]

3. **b. Pyelonephritis.** Problems with stomal stenosis, pyelonephritis, calculus formation, ureteral obstruction, and renal deterioration became more apparent with longer follow-up times (see Table 108–1). [p 3836]

4. **d. Most patients require intermittent catheterization to empty their neobladder.** This form of lower urinary tract reconstruction relies on the intact rhabdosphincter continence mechanism, eliminating the need for intermittent catheterization. Voiding is accomplished by concomitantly increasing intra-abdominal pressure (the Valsalva maneuver), with relaxation of the pelvic floor. The majority of patients undergoing orthotopic reconstruction are continent. [p 3837]

5. **d. All of the above.** Permanently compromised renal function (serum creatinine level greater than 2.0 mg/dl) should be considered a contraindication to continent urinary diversion. A minimum creatinine clearance of 60 ml/minute should be documented before orthotopic diversion. Patients with an elevated serum creatinine value secondary to ureteral obstruction should undergo upper urinary tract decompression (via percutaneous nephrostomy) allowing recovery, and redetermination of the true baseline renal function before the decision to perform the particular urinary diversion. [p 3838]

6. **a. Gastric neobladder.** Patients with borderline renal function, who otherwise would be candidates for lower urinary tract reconstruction, may be more appropriate candidates for a gastric form of neobladder. [p 3838]

7. **c. Differentiation between physiologic and chronologic age should be made.** Although controversial, the patient's age alone should not necessarily be a contraindication to orthotopic diversion. Therefore, a differentiation between physiologic and chronologic age should be made. [p 3838]

8. **d. A male with an intraoperative positive distal surgical margin at the proximal urethra.** A contraindication to orthotopic diversion in male and female patients includes those patients demonstrating carcinoma in situ or overt carcinoma of the urethral margin detected on intraoperative frozen section analysis. [p 3847]

9. **c. Spherical structure.** The increase of volume capacity achieved in the intestinal segment depends on its shape; volume is almost double in a U-shaped pouch and is still greater in an S-shaped, a W-shaped, or a Kock pouch, closely resembling that of a sphere. [p 3839]

10. **d. The pudendal innervation.** Most interested investigators agree that the rhabdosphincter is probably supplied by the branches of the pudendal nerve. [p 3840]

11. **a. Perform minimal dissection along the pelvic floor.** In any pelvic surgery that involves maintaining the rhabdosphincter innervation and ultimate function, excessive dissection along the pelvic floor should be avoided, where the branches of the pudendal nerve course to the sphincteric complex. Therefore, minimal dissection should be performed, during any pelvic surgery, along the pelvic floor levator musculature to avoid injury to the rhabdosphincter innervation. [pp 3840–3841]

12. **d. If the intraoperative frozen section analysis of the distal surgical margin (urethra) is normal.** Regardless of the technique, frozen section analysis of the distal urethral margin (prostatic apex) on the cystectomy specimen is performed to exclude tumor involvement. The decision to perform an orthotopic bladder substitution is ultimately made at this time. [p 3842]

13. **b. Remove the anterior vaginal wall en bloc with the bladder.** Alternatively, in the case of a deeply invasive posterior bladder tumor, with concern for an adequate surgical margin, the anterior vaginal wall may be removed en bloc with the cystectomy specimen. [p 3842]

14. **d. All of the above.** Vaginal reconstruction by a clam-shell (horizontal) or side-to-side (vertical) technique is required. Other means of vaginal reconstruction may include a rectus myocutaneous flap, a detubularized cylinder of ileum, a peritoneal flap, and an omental flap. [p 3843]

15. **d. All of the above.** It is generally believed that urethral tumors in patients with a history of bladder cancer represent a second manifestation of the multicentric defect of the primary transitional cell mucosa that led to the original bladder tumor. The overall risk of a urethral recurrence for transitional cell carcinoma after cystectomy is approximately 10%. There is a growing body of data to suggest that, by far, the most ominous criterion for a urethral tumor recurrence is prostatic urethral involvement. [p 3843]

16. **d. Prostatic stroma involvement.** Collectively, these studies suggest that prostatic stromal invasion is the strongest single predictor for subsequent recurrence in the anterior urethra after cystectomy for bladder cancer. [p 3844]

17. **b. Intraoperative frozen section analysis of the urethra (distal surgical margin) is mandatory in all patients considering orthotopic diversion.** Data are emerging to suggest that it may be reasonable to abandon the preoperative prostatic biopsies and perform frozen section analysis on the prostatic urethral apex at the time of surgery to determine appropriate patients for orthotopic urinary diversion in men. [p 3845]

18. **a. Bladder neck tumor involvement is the most significant risk factor for urethral tumor involvement.** The authors emphasized that the only consistent risk factor found for urethral tumor involvement was concurrent tumor at the bladder neck. [pp 3845–3846]

19. **b. There is approximately a 50% chance of having tumor in the urethra.** All patients with an uninvolved bladder neck also had an uninvolved urethra, whereas approximately 50% of patients with a bladder neck tumor had concomitant urethral tumor involvement. [p 3846]

20. **d. All of the above.** Patients with urethral involvement also had concomitant bladder neck involvement regardless of the presence or absence of carcinoma in situ. In addition to bladder neck involvement, one study identified anterior vaginal wall tumor involvement (P4) as a major risk factor for simultaneous urethral tumor, and 50% of these patients also demonstrated urethral tumors. [p 3846]

21. **c. Is mandatory to exclude tumor in all women considering an orthotopic bladder substitution.** These data suggest that intraoperative frozen section analysis of the distal surgical margin may provide an accurate and reliable means of evaluating the proximal urethra and should determine which female patients would be appropriate candidates to undergo orthotopic diversion. [p 3846]

22. **d. All of the above.** Intraoperative frozen section analysis of the distal surgical margin in both men (apical prostatic urethra) and women (proximal urethra) provides an accurate assessment of the urethra and may appropriately determine candidacy for orthotopic diversion. [p 3847]

23. **a. Local recurrence after cystectomy occurs in less than 10% of all patients.** In this large series, an overall local pelvic recurrence rate of 7% was observed for the entire group of patients. [p 3847]

24. **c. Expect normal neobladder function.** One study concluded that most patients may anticipate normal neobladder function even in the presence of recurrent disease or until death. Local recurrence rates following cystectomy are low even in high-risk patients and seldom affect the function of the neobladder or the ability to deliver therapy. [pp 3847–3848]

25. **b. May be performed in properly selected individuals.** It is becoming more clear that in carefully selected patients, orthotopic lower urinary tract reconstruction can be performed after definitive, full-dose pelvic irradiation. [p 3849]

26. **a. They may require placement of an artificial urinary sphincter.** All patients should be informed that incontinence rates after salvage cystectomy and orthotopic diversion are significant and in nearly 25% of subjects may require the need for an artificial urinary sphincter placement. [p 3849]

27. **d. None of the above.** Controversy exists regarding the need to incorporate an antireflux mechanism in patients undergoing an orthotopic form of urinary diversion. First, it must be emphasized that it will be only after well-designed, prospective, randomized studies with appropriate patient numbers and with long-term follow-up that a convincing answer can be obtained. To date, this study has not been performed. [p 3849]

28. **a. They may have infected urinary constituents.** These data suggest that a significant number of patients with an orthotopic bladder substitute will have chronically infected urinary constituents. [p 3850]

29. **d. All of the above.** Upper tract urinary deterioration may not become clinically apparent until as long as 10 to 20 years after urinary diversion. In addition, deterioration of renal function may occur even in the face of normal radiographic findings. The development of renal insufficiency was thought to be related to or a combination of high pressures, obstruction, and chronically infected urine. [pp 3849–3850]

30. **a. 10% of patients.** An overall complication rate of 10% was observed with the intussuscepted antireflux nipple in more than 800 patients (undergoing either a continent cutaneous or an orthotopic Kock ileal reservoir) with long-term follow-up (median, 6 years). [p 3850]

31. **c. Stones.** The three most common complications related to the intussuscepted afferent nipple included the formation of calculi (usually on exposed staples that secure the afferent nipple valve) in 5%, afferent nipple stenosis (thought to be caused by ischemic changes resulting from the mesenteric stripping required to maintain the intussuscepted limb) in 4%, and extussusception (prolapse of the afferent limb) in 1% of patients. [p 3850]

32. **a. This is a flap-valve technique.** If a tubular structure (ureter, appendix, or intestine) is laid in this trough, the incised intestinal mucosa on either side can be sutured together (covering the tubular structure) and transform the trough into a serous-lined tunnel—an effective flap-valve technique. [p 3851]

33. **d. All of the above.** Stein and Skinner subsequently developed and described a modification of this technique, which has been called the T-mechanism. This flap-valve T-mechanism is a versatile technique that can easily be applied as an antireflux mechanism, as well as a continent cutaneous mechanism. Advantages of this technique include application even in the face of grossly dilated ureters and/or in the presence of concomitant pathology of the distal ureters that may result in shortened ureteral length. [p 3851]

34. **d. All of the above.** The orthotopic T-pouch ileal neobladder maintains exactly the same geometric configuration as the Kock ileal neobladder, the only difference being the antireflux technique. The unique aspect of the T-pouch is maintaining the vascular arcades by opening the windows of Deaver, which then allows permanent fixation of a segment of ileum within a serous-lined ileal trough to create an effective flap-valve technique. [p 3854]

35. **c. Exposed metallic staples.** Because no exposed staples exist within the reservoir, pouch stones typically associated with exposed metallic staples used to maintain the intussuscepted nipple should not develop. [p 3854]

36. **a. There is definitely an increased complication rate with an orthotopic form of diversion over an ileal conduit.** There was no significant difference in the perioperative mortality and complication rates when comparing these different forms (conduit versus continent) of urinary diversion. These findings were similar to those from a previous study that found no difference in hospitalization stay, complication rate, and reoperation rate when comparing patients undergoing an ileal conduit and various forms of orthotopic diversion. [pp 3860–3861]

37. **c. The staple line usually does not provide a watertight seal.** To reduce the operative time, the use of absorbable staples has been applied in the construction of the urinary

reservoir. The initial application of this technology was hampered by the fact that the stapler was bulky and difficult to manipulate. Improvements in the staples and the applicators (absorbable staplers) have now facilitated the application to continent diversion. This technique allows for a secure, watertight staple line. [p 3862]

38. **d. All of the above.** Quality of life issues are becoming increasingly important in the selection of the type of urinary diversion and are likely to play a larger role in future management of patients undergoing lower urinary tract reconstruction following cystectomy. Most of the aforementioned studies, evaluating and comparing quality of life issues in patients undergoing various forms of urinary diversion, have been criticized for the methodologic problems that may limit their conclusions. In the future, large, well-designed, randomized, prospective studies will be required to better understand and evaluate quality of life issues in patients undergoing various forms of urinary diversion. Furthermore, these studies must incorporate well-validated measures or surveys to evaluate patients. [pp 3862–3863]

39. **d. All of the above.** Overall, most patients undergoing orthotopic diversion are continent, have the luxury of voiding every 4 to 6 hours with excellent voided volumes, retain a more routine micturition pattern, avoid the need for a cutaneous stoma or external urostomy appliance, and live a more normal life with an improved self-image. [p 3864]

Chapter 109

Surgery of the Seminal Vesicles

Jay I. Sandlow • Richard D. Williams

Questions

1. What is the embryologic origin of the seminal vesicles?
    a. Müllerian duct
    b. Ectodermal ridge
    c. Distal mesonephric duct
    d. A swelling off of the distal paramesonephric duct
    e. Neural crest cells

2. What percentage of the seminal plasma volume is made up of seminal vesicle secretions?
    a. 5%
    b. 25%
    c. 60%
    d. 90%
    e. 0% (the seminal vesicle does not contribute to the seminal plasma volume)

3. What is the major blood supply to the seminal vesicle?
    a. Hypogastric artery
    b. Vesiculodeferential artery
    c. Inferior vesicle artery
    d. Internal iliac artery
    e. Deep dorsal penile artery

4. Decreased T1 signal intensity on MRI, along with increased T2 intensity of seminal vesicles, is indicative of which process?
    a. Inflammation of the seminal vesicles
    b. Hemorrhage within the seminal vesicles
    c. Seminal vesicle tumors
    d. Seminal vesicle cysts
    e. Normal seminal vesicles

5. Agenesis of the seminal vesicle is associated with significant ipsilateral renal anomalies. What is the embryologic reason for this?
    a. A genetic defect that links seminal vesicle agenesis to renal agenesis.
    b. A mutation of the cystic fibrosis transmembrane regulator gene.
    c. An insult to the mesonephric duct at approximately 12 weeks of gestation.
    d. An embryologic insult to the mesonephric duct earlier than 7 weeks of gestation.
    e. None (there is no association between agenesis of the seminal vesicle and ipsilateral renal anomalies).

6. What disorder is frequently associated with bilateral agenesis of the seminal vesicles?
    a. Cystic fibrosis
    b. Kartagener's syndrome
    c. Young's syndrome
    d. Kallmann's syndrome
    e. Klinefelter's syndrome

7. What causes the majority of seminal vesicle cysts?
    a. Genetic abnormality
    b. Obstruction of the ejaculatory duct
    c. Inflammation
    d. Renal agenesis
    e. Genetic abnormalities

8. What is the most common type of malignant neoplasm found in seminal vesicles?
    a. Primary adenocarcinoma
    b. Sarcoma
    c. Cystosarcoma phyllodes
    d. Metastatic tumors
    e. Amyloidosis

9. What is the best first test for a suspected seminal vesicle abnormality?
    a. CT
    b. Transrectal ultrasonography
    c. MRI
    d. Fine-needle biopsy
    e. Vasography

10. Vasography is useful for providing information regarding all of the following conditions except which one?

a. The presence of a seminal vesicle
b. The level of obstruction of the seminal vesicle and/or ejaculatory duct
c. Pathology of the seminal vesicle
d. Epididymal or vasal obstruction
e. None of the above

11. What is the best method for differentiating a benign from a malignant seminal vesicle mass?

a. Biopsy of the lesion
b. Contrast-enhanced CT
c. Gadolinium-enhanced MRI
d. Transrectal ultrasonography
e. Rectal examination

12. What is the best surgical approach to a congenital lesion of the seminal vesicle?

a. The perineal route, as this results in a quicker recovery
b. The transcoccygeal route, as these lesions are usually large
c. The abdominal route, so that the ipsilateral kidney can be dealt with concomitantly
d. The paravesical route, as this has a lower incidence of postoperative erectile dysfunction
e. The transvesical route, as rectal injury is much less likely

13. What is the best indication for the transcoccygeal approach to the seminal vesicle?

a. Need for exploration of the ipsilateral kidney
b. Individuals who have had previous suprapubic and/or perineal surgery
c. Patients wishing to maintain potency
d. Patients with bilateral large seminal vesicle lesions
e. None of the above

14. In a patient with a seminal vesicle abscess, what is the treatment of choice?

a. Laparoscopic unroofing
b. Transvesical excision of the seminal vesicle
c. Aspiration and antibiotic instillation
d. Endoscopic unroofing via deep transurethral resection
e. Use of a retropubic approach to unroof the abscess

Answers

1. **c. Distal mesonephric duct.** Separate symmetrical buds extend from the distal mesonephric duct just proximal to the ejaculatory duct at approximately 12 weeks to form the seminal vesicles (see Fig. 109–1 C). [p 3870]

2. **c. 60%.** The secretions from the seminal vesicle contribute approximately 50% to 80% of the ejaculate volume, with an average volume of 2.5 ml and a pH in the neutral to alkaline range. [p 3870]

3. **b. Vesiculodeferential artery.** The blood supply to the seminal vesicle is from the vesiculodeferential artery, a branch of the umbilical artery. [p 3871]

4. **a. Inflammation of the seminal vesicles.** In the normal situation, the anatomic relationships of the seminal vesicles shown by MRI are similar to those shown by CT except that on T1-weighted images, seminal vesicles are of low signal intensity that increases substantially on T2-weighted images (see Fig. 109–5 A and B). In contrast to the normal hypointense T1-weighted image, inflammation results in a less intense image. The normally hyperintense signal found on a T2-weighted image is increased further with inflammation. [pp 3873, 3876]

5. **d. An embryologic insult to the mesonephric duct earlier than 7 weeks of gestation.** It may be associated with unilateral absence of the vas deferens, as well as ipsilateral renal anomalies (see Fig. 109–7). This is thought to result from an embryologic insult before the separation of the ureteral bud from the mesonephric duct, which typically occurs at 7 weeks of gestation. [pp 3874, 3875]

6. **a. Cystic fibrosis.** Bilateral absence of the seminal vesicles is frequently found in association with congenital bilateral absence of the vas deferens. This is commonly associated with a mutation of the cystic fibrosis transmembrane receptor. Seventy percent to 80% of men with bilateral absence of the vas and/or seminal vesicles are carriers for the genetic mutation associated with cystic fibrosis. Conversely, 80% to 95% of men with cystic fibrosis have bilateral absence of the vas deferens or seminal vesicles. [pp 3874–3875]

7. **b. Obstruction of the ejaculatory duct.** Cysts of the seminal vesicles may be either congenital or acquired and are thought to be due to obstruction of the ejaculatory duct. [p 3876]

8. **d. Metastatic tumors.** The main difficulty encountered with seminal vesicle neoplasms is determining that they are in fact primary within the seminal vesicles. Indeed, it is more common for carcinoma of the bladder, adenocarcinoma of the prostate, lymphoma, or rectal carcinoma to secondarily involve the seminal vesicle. [p 3877]

9. **b. Transrectal ultrasonography.** Ultrasonography, by either the transabdominal or the transrectal (preferred) route, has become one of the most accurate methods of evaluating the seminal vesicle. Patients with a suspected seminal vesicle abnormality or mass felt on a rectal examination should first undergo transrectal ultrasonography. [pp 3871, 3874]

10. **c. Pathology of the seminal vesicle.** Vasography does not provide accurate demonstration of the pathology of the seminal vesicles in patients with vesiculitis, cysts, or tumors. [p 3874]

11. **a. Biopsy of the lesion.** Ultrasonographically guided transrectal or perineal aspiration cytologic studies or core biopsies can be useful to diagnose a seminal vesicle neoplasm. [p 3872]

12. **c. The abdominal route, so that the ipsilateral kidney can be dealt with concomitantly.** For the most part, congenital lesions require an abdominal approach so that the ipsilateral kidney can be dealt with concomitantly, if necessary. [p 3878]

13. **b. Individuals who have had previous suprapubic and/or perineal surgery.** In individuals in whom the perineal or supine position may be difficult to maintain, or who have had multiple suprapubic or perineal surgeries, the transcoccygeal approach may be very useful. [p 3881]

14. **d. Endoscopic unroofing via deep transurethral resection.** If the cyst or abscess is adjacent to the prostate (not in the middle or distal end of the seminal vesicle), it may be possible to unroof the cavity with a deep transurethral resection into the prostatic substance just distal to the bladder neck at the 5- or 7-o'clock position. [p 3881]

Chapter 110

Surgery of the Penis and Urethra

Gerald H. Jordan • Steven M. Schlossberg

Questions

1. In reference to tissue transfer terms with the skin as a model, which of the following statements is true?

   a. The superficial layer is the adventitial dermis.
   b. The deep layer is termed the lamina.
   c. The dermal layer has two sublayers.
   d. The reticular dermis lies immediately superficial to the lamina.

2. With regard to the physical characteristics of tissue, which of the following statements is true?

   a. They are a function of the collagen-elastin architecture as it is suspended in a mucopolysaccharide matrix.
   b. Only select tissues have inherent tissue tension.
   c. Extensibility can be used synonymously with compliance.
   d. The vesicoelastic property of tissue relaxation is also termed creep.

3. In tissue transfer terms, which of the following statements concerning grafts is true?

   a. The process of take occurs over 48 hours.
   b. A graft is tissue that is excised from a donor site and then re-establishes its blood supply by revascularization.
   c. During inosculation, the first phase of take, the graft exists at below core body temperature.
   d. The process of take is a reflection of only the host bed conditions.

4. With regard to the microanatomy of the grafts discussed, which of the following statements is true?

   a. Anatomically, the intradermal plexus is at the interface of the superficial dermis and the deep dermis.
   b. The subdermal plexus is carried at the juncture of the deep dermis and the underlying tissue.
   c. The lymphatics are most richly distributed in the adventitial dermis.
   d. The adventitial dermis, because of its collagen content, accounts for the majority of the physical characteristics.

5. Grafts of all kinds can be termed split thickness or full thickness. Choose the best answer below with regard to these.

   a. A split-thickness skin graft exposes the vessels of the subdermal plexus.
   b. Exposing the subdermal plexus conveys less fastidious vascular characteristics.
   c. Mesh grafts are created by cutting slits in the epidermis or epithelium.
   d. A full-thickness skin graft is fastidious because of the nature of the subdermal plexus, among other variables.

6. With regard to the grafts used most commonly in genitourinary reconstructive surgery, which of the following statements is true?

   a. Thin full-thickness skin is an optional replacement for the tunica albuginea of the corpora cavernosa.
   b. Bladder epithelial graft is fastidious because of the nature of the superficial lamina.
   c. Buccal mucosa graft is thought to have a panlaminar plexus.
   d. According to the vascular literature, the vein graft does not take via the process of revascularization.

7. In tissue transfer terms, which of the following statements regarding flaps is most accurate?

   a. The terms *pedicle graft* and *flap* are synonymous.
   b. Flaps take because of vascular anastomosis.
   c. A flap with a defined cuticular vascular territory is termed a paddle.
   d. A flap without a defined cuticular vascular territory is termed a random flap.

8. If a flap is classified according to elevation technique, which of the following statements is true?

   a. All peninsula flaps would by definition be a random flap.
   b. An island flap would by definition be an axial flap.
   c. A true island flap could also be called a paddle.
   d. The microvascular free transfer flap relies on the principle of flap delay.

9. With regard to the anatomy of the penile shaft, which of the following statements is true?

   a. Throughout most of the length of the penis, the septum is a true competent septum.
   b. The erectile tissues of the normal corpora cavernosa are separated from the tunica by the space of Smith.
   c. The dorsal arteries of the penis are carried in envelope fashion in the dartos fascia.
   d. Buck's fascia is loosely areolar and lies immediately beneath the skin.

10. The urethra can be subdivided into five entities. Which of the following statements is most accurate?

    a. The fossa navicularis is that portion of the urethra that is most dorsally displaced with regard to the surrounding spongy erectile tissue.
    b. The bulbous urethral portion is invested by the thickest portion of the corpus spongiosum.
    c. The bulbous urethra at its proximal extent is part of the posterior urethra.
    d. The membranous urethra is invested by the most proximal aspect of the corpus spongiosum.

11. Which of the following statements is true regarding the blood supply to the superficial structures of the penis?

    a. It is a continuation of the deep external pudendal artery.
    b. It eventually arborizes into Buck's fascia.

c. It allows for elevation of the skin on its random blood supply while carrying skin islands on the fascia.
d. For venous drainage, it depends on the intermediate venous system.

12. With regard to the venous drainage of the penis, which of the following statements is true?

    a. The deep system includes the deep dorsal vein.
    b. The intermediate system runs within the dartos fascia.
    c. The deep system begins distally as the subcoronal plexus.
    d. The deep system, which includes the crural and cavernosal veins, drains to the periprostatic plexus and to the femoral/iliac veins.

13. Which of the following statements regarding the arterial system to the deep structures of the penis is true?

    a. It is derived from the superficial external pudendal vessel.
    b. It consists of the common penile artery and its distal branches.
    c. It consists of the dorsal artery, which travels along the dorsum in the dartos fascia.
    d. It consists of the arteries to the glans, which represent the dominant blood supply to the corpora cavernosa.

14. With regard to the innervation to the penis, which of the following statements is true?

    a. The cavernosal nerves are purely parasympathetic and are the extensions of the nervi erigentes.
    b. The pudendal nerves accompany the vessels as they run through the obturator foramen.
    c. The dorsal nerve arises in Alcock's canal as a branch of the nerve there.
    d. The dorsal nerves throughout their course are prominent, large nerve bundles.

15. With regard to Colles' fascia, which of the following statements is true?

    a. Colles' fascia is the perineal component of Camper's fascia.
    b. Colles' fascia attaches at its posterior margin to the midline fusion of the ischial cavernosus muscle.
    c. Colles' fascia joins with the dartos fascia (tunica dartos) of the scrotum.
    d. Colles' fascia becomes contiguous with Buck's fascia in the posterior triangle of the perineum.

16. With regard to the anterior triangle of the perineum, which of the following statements is true?

    a. The ischiocavernosus muscles laterally attach to the inner surface of the ischium and insert in the midline into Buck's fascia.
    b. The bulbous spongiosum muscles (midline fusion of the ischial cavernosus muscles) insert posteriorly to the central tendon of the perineum.
    c. The perineal body represents a confluence of fascial structures.
    d. The perineal body has a prominent neurovascular pedicle within it that provides autonomic innervation to the pelvic diaphragm.

17. Which of the following statements concerning urethral hemangioma is true?

    a. When one encounters the endoscopic findings consistent with urethral hemangioma, one must be alert to exclude the diagnosis of urethral carcinoma.
    b. Laser therapy has been very successfully employed for the management of large urethral hemangiomas.
    c. Reiter's syndrome includes the triad of stomatitis, arthritis, and urethritis.
    d. In Reiter's syndrome, the urethritis is usually mild and self-limiting.

18. With regard to balanitis xerotica obliterans (BXO), which of the following statements is true?

    a. BXO is the genital manifestation of psoriasis.
    b. BXO is one, if not the most frequent, cause of meatal stenosis.
    c. BXO is a disease of middle-aged adults and is virtually never seen in younger adults or adolescents.
    d. Because BXO has been linked to the presence of gram-negative cocci, long-term treatment with fluoroquinolones has been suggested.

19. With regard to fistulas complicating urethral reconstruction, which of the following statements is true?

    a. Fistulas are an early complication that present inevitably within the first 3 weeks after surgery.
    b. Fistulas often recur, not because of a problem at the fistula site but because of stenosis or obstruction distal to the fistula site.
    c. In acute fistulas, one should consider resuturing and reinstitution of diversion.
    d. Fistula closure, in the majority of cases, requires tissue transfer.

20. Which of the following statements concerning urethral fistulas is true?

    a. Urethral fistula, not associated with a history of urethral reconstruction, can be the initial presenting symptom of urethral carcinoma.
    b. Fistulas associated with inflammatory strictures usually resolve with aggressive antibiotic therapy.
    c. Congenital diverticula in the prostatic urethra associated with the verumontanum are usually vestiges of the wolffian duct.
    d. Congenital diverticula of the bulbous urethra are vestiges of the müllerian duct.

21. With regard to urethral meatal stenosis in childhood, which of the following statements is true?

    a. Meatal stenosis is a frequent complication of phimosis.
    b. Meatal stenosis of childhood is frequently associated with upper tract changes, and all patients should be evaluated with ultrasonography and voiding cystourethrography.
    c. When ammoniacal meatitis is noted, often a short course of meatal dilatation and steroid cream application will resolve the problem.
    d. When meatal stenosis is present, usually a dorsally based Y-V advancement flap repair is preferred.

22. With regard to failure of previously performed reconstruction for hypospadias, which of the following statements is true?

    a. Most cases can be significantly improved with technically straightforward minimal procedures.
    b. Not uncommonly, patients who had their initial operations in the 1960s or 1970s will still have significant dorsal hooded skin, which can be useful for subsequent repairs.
    c. Residual chordee after previously performed reconstruction for hypospadias is rarely encountered.
    d. In older patients, the only reliable assessment for residual chordee is a challenge of intercavernosal vasoactive agents in the office to demonstrate the deformity.

23. With regard to secondary operations for exstrophy, which of the following statements is true?

    a. Residual chordee is inevitably the result of incompletely excised dysgenetic tissues.

b. Division of the tethering urethra is almost always required to correct residual chordee.
c. If urethral transposition of the epispadiac urethra is being considered, care must be taken in dissecting proximally to avoid injury to the corpus spongiosum.
d. Reconstruction of the abdominal wall is seldom required, as most problems have to do with dyssymmetric distribution of the penile skin.

24. When one is confronted with a patient with penile amputation, which of the following statements is true?

    a. Replantation is not a consideration in self-inflicted injury, as most patients are chronically psychotic and will eventually try to amputate the penis again.
    b. If the distal part of the penis is not available, even if the amputation involves mostly skin with much of the shaft preserved, it is recommended that the remaining shaft be buried in the scrotum.
    c. The classic technique for replantation involves coaptation of the dorsal nerves, the deep dorsal vein, and the cavernosal arteries.
    d. The McRoberts technique of macro-replantation is not the preferred method of management for these patients, but when the situation warrants it, it is very successful.

25. With regard to the management of external trauma, which of the following statements is accurate?

    a. Because of the nature of the genital tissues, aggressive initial débridement must be undertaken.
    b. The eventual effect of a genital burn may be to unacceptably tether and/or incarcerate the penis.
    c. The gracilis flap is ideally suited for coverage of large perineal or groin wounds.
    d. Complications of direct irradiation to the penis can usually be reconstructed with split-thickness grafts (STSGs).

26. Concerning genital lymphedema, which of the following statements is true?

    a. Reconstruction for lymphedema that is the consequence of the indirect effects of radiation is best accomplished with excision of the tissues and coverage with STSGs.
    b. In reconstruction for lymphedema, it is essential to maintain the parietal tunica vaginalis of the testicles intact with grafting over that location.
    c. When considering reconstruction for lymphedema, full-thickness skin grafts (FTSGs) are preferable because of the distribution of the lymphatics in the superficial (adventitial) dermis.
    d. Local skin flaps are often useful and desirable because of superior cosmetic results obtained.

27. Which of the following statements concerning urethral stricture is true?

    a. It causes limitation of the urethral lumen because of the bulk of the scar.
    b. It most often is limited to the urethral epithelium.
    c. It implies a scarring process, usually involving both the epithelium and the underlying spongy erectile tissue of the corpora cavernosa.
    d. It causes limitation of the urethral lumen because of contraction and noncompliance of the scar.

28. Which of the following statements concerning posterior urethral stricture is true?

    a. It involves the tissues of the epithelium as well as the underlying erectile tissue of the corpora cavernosa.
    b. It involves the tissues of the epithelium as well as the underlying erectile tissue of the corpus spongiosum.
    c. It is not a true stricture but rather fibrosis that results from distraction of the urethra.
    d. The stricture process can often be occult because of the unpredictable involvement of the urethral tissues.

29. Most anterior urethral strictures currently result from which of the following?

    a. Catheter-induced urethritis
    b. Inflammation associated with BXO
    c. Delay in diagnosis and treatment of infectious urethritis
    d. Crushing trauma to the bulbous urethra

30. Which of the following statements regarding strictures resulting from BXO is true?

    a. They are usually associated with scarring extending deeply into the corpus spongiosum.
    b. They usually begin as meatal stenosis associated with ammoniacal balanitis.
    c. They often resolve with the use of antibiotics.
    d. They are probably the result of inflammation of the urethral epithelium caused by *Borrelia burgdorferi*.

31. When the urologist is confronted with a patient in retention or a case of difficult catheter placement, which of the following statements is true?

    a. Endoscopy nicely defines the nature of the difficulty.
    b. The patient can usually be effectively treated with filiform follower dilatation.
    c. Optimal management may mean placement of a suprapubic catheter.
    d. Imaging results are usually uninformative.

32. In determining the anatomy of the stricture, all of the following provide useful information except which one?

    a. MRI
    b. High-resolution ultrasonography
    c. Contrast studies
    d. Urethroscopy

33. With regard to the modalities for evaluation of the urethra, which of the following statements is true?

    a. Extravasation of contrast material during retrograde urethrography inevitably implies poor technique.
    b. Distention of the urethra during ultrasonographic study often confuses findings.
    c. Contrast material suitable for intravenous injection should be used for all retrograde urethral studies.
    d. Thickened contrast layers better define the stricture length.

34. With regard to planning of reconstruction for urethral stricture, which of the following statements is true?

    a. Even if a patient does not have retention, placement of a suprapubic tube may help define strictured areas.
    b. Tightly stenotic areas should be dilated to pass endoscopes proximally.
    c. The effects of hydrodilatation are manifested most immediately distal to the area of narrowest stenosis.
    d. Calibration of strictured areas to 16 Fr or greater reliably predicts the potential for segments to contract.

35. With regard to direct visual internal urethrotomy, which of the following statements is true?

    a. Strictures are best incised at the 12-o'clock position because of the efficiency of most urethrotomes when used in this orientation.
    b. It can be associated with the creation of erectile dysfunction.

c. It has been estimated and reported to have long-term success rates of approximately 50%.
d. It would be the first procedure considered for a stricture of the pendulous urethra.

36. Concerning permanently implanted urethral stents, which of the following statements is true?

    a. Available data show that these stents are best employed for short bulbous urethral strictures associated with minimal spongiofibrosis.
    b. When properly employed, they have success rates of almost 95%.
    c. They are rarely complicated by persistent perineal pain.
    d. They are useful for short strictures of the pendulous urethra.

37. All of the following are either absolute or strong relative contraindications to the use of the Urolume stent except which one?

    a. Distraction injuries of the membranous urethra
    b. Patients who have failed prior substitution urethral reconstruction
    c. Patients with short strictures of the bulbous urethra that are not associated with significant spongiofibrosis
    d. Patients who are younger than 50 years old who are reasonable candidates for urethral reconstruction

38. With regard to the use of laser urethrotomy, which of the following statements is most accurate?

    a. Several lasers have been used for urethrostomy with results superior to those of cold knife urethrotomy.
    b. The neodymium:yttrium-aluminum-garnet (Nd:YAG) laser in theory would be a better laser for urethrotomy than the holmium:YAG laser.
    c. The KTP laser is not useful because it is not fiber deliverable.
    d. The holmium:YAG laser has significant vaporizing as well as cutting properties with little forward scatter.

39. Concerning anterior urethral reconstruction, which of the following statements is true?

    a. Excision and primary anastomosis treatment is severely limited and useful only for very proximal strictures 1 to 2 cm in length.
    b. Performance of the excision and primary anastomosis technique is facilitated by dissection of the corpus spongiosum to the level of the glans penis.
    c. Success requires total excision of the fibrosis with a widely spatulated anastomosis.
    d. Reconstruction is facilitated by development of the intracrural space with infrapubectomy.

40. With regard to techniques of urethral reconstruction, which of the following statements is true?

    a. The Monseur technique employed the use of mesh split-thickness skin.
    b. The excision with strip anastomosis technique can be used with graft onlay techniques.
    c. The Barbagli operation combines the use of excision with staged augmented anastomosis.
    d. The use of the spongioplasty maneuver requires the total excision of all spongiofibrosis.

41. With regard to genital skin flap operations for anterior urethral reconstruction, which of the following statements is true?

    a. Flap operations are best applied as individual techniques and require the surgeon to become intimately familiar with the individual steps of all techniques.
    b. The operations can conceptually become one operation with multidimensional application.
    c. The operations are all based on mobilization of the extended Buck fascia.
    d. The operations require a comfortable understanding of the extended circumflex iliac superficial vascular pattern.

42. With regard to flap procedures for anterior urethral reconstruction, which of the following statements is true?

    a. The scrotal skin island is a problematic flap and should be avoided at all cost.
    b. Circular skin islands, mechanically, are facilitated by dividing the dartos fascial flaps ventrally.
    c. "Tubed flaps" in general are optimal for cases of short to moderate length strictures.
    d. The length of tubed segments can be limited by the aggressive mobilization of the corpus spongiosum.

43. With regard to strictures associated with BXO, which of the following statements is true?

    a. Urolume has proved to be an excellent option.
    b. Staged skin graft procedures have yielded excellent durable results.
    c. Because BXO is a generalized skin condition, buccal mucosa has been considered for reconstruction with initial encouraging results.
    d. Flap techniques have provided excellent long-term success rates.

44. Which of the following statements concerning urethral distraction injuries is true?

    a. They are usually associated with full-thickness spongiofibrosis.
    b. Although they can involve any part of the membranous urethra, they most frequently occur at the juncture of the membranous urethra with the bulbous urethra.
    c. They can be partial, and this difference is easily defined by contrast-enhanced studies.
    d. They are best managed with an aligning catheter placed to traction.

45. Membranous urethral distraction injuries are:

    a. best first evaluated with contrast-enhanced studies.
    b. often evaluated with an endoscope in the anterior urethra and a cystogram with the patient straining to void.
    c. virtually always defined with simultaneous cystogram and retrograde urethrogram.
    d. virtually always complicated by postoperative incontinence when contrast material is seen in the posterior urethra.

46. Which of the following statements regarding reconstruction for posterior urethral distraction is true?

    a. It often requires the use of flaps or grafts to span the distraction defect.
    b. It usually is accomplished within weeks of the acute trauma.
    c. It can often be done distal to the external sphincter.
    d. It often requires total pubectomy to facilitate exposure.

47. With regard to continence after reconstruction for membranous urethral distraction, which of the following statements is true?

    a. Location of the injury along the course of the membranous urethra is not associated with continence postoperatively.

b. Continence can be accurately predicted by contrast-enhanced studies.
c. Continence is best predicted by the appearance of the bladder neck on endoscopy.
d. Continence is best addressed after a procedure to re-establish urethral continuity is performed.

48. A maneuver that allows for reconstruction of posterior distraction injuries without creating chordee or foreshortening of the penis is:

    a. development of the intracavernosal (intracrural) space.
    b. infrapubectomy.
    c. mobilization of the proximal corpus spongiosum.
    d. all of the above.

49. With regard to follow-up after urethral reconstruction, choose the single most accurate modality.

    a. Flow study
    b. Flexible endoscopy
    c. Voiding cystourethrography
    d. Retrograde ureterography

50. With regard to failures of reconstruction of posterior urethral distraction primary anastomotic technique, which of the following statements is true?

    a. Most failures are due to technical anastomotic procedures.
    b. Long-segment failures are readily amenable to direct-vision internal urethrotomy with Urolume placement.
    c. Patients with one intact pudendal artery are at risk for ischemic stenosis of the corpus spongiosum.
    d. Patients with reconstitution of an injured pudendal vessel, even if reconstitution was a unilateral phenomenon, are excellent candidates for posterior urethral reconstruction.

51. In the authors' opinion:

    a. Cut for light procedures in virtually all cases rarely open the urethra; patency must be maintained with chronic catheter dilation.
    b. Cut for light procedures in inexperienced hands can be a dangerous undertaking.
    c. No cut for light series compares with open surgical series from large centers, and thus cut for light procedures should be reserved for patients who are not open surgical candidates.
    d. All of the above.

52. With regard to the Devine-Horton classification of congenital curvatures, which of the following statements is true?

    a. Type IV is merely a forme fruste of hypospadias.
    b. Type V is the most commonly encountered type.
    c. The term *congenital curvature of the penis* is reserved for cases in which there is solitary, relative asymmetric compliance of the tunica albuginea of the corpus spongiosum.
    d. Types I, II, and III are all forms of acquired curvature.

53. In dealing with the entity of chordee without hypospadias, which of the following statements is true?

    a. Correction of curvature is often achieved with mobilization of the corpus spongiosum alone.
    b. It can often be corrected with maneuvers that lengthen the foreshortened ventral skin.
    c. There is a stepwise progression of ventral dissection of dysgenetic tissues, correction of skin tethering, elevation of mobilization of the corpus spongiosum, midline ventral septotomy, and often dorsal plication.
    d. When it is found, division of the urethra is virtually always indicated.

54. With regard to congenital curvature of the penis, which of the following statements is true?

    a. If length is an issue, the patient probably is more correctly characterized as having chordee without hypospadias.
    b. It is optimally managed with incision and grafting to avoid foreshortening of the penis.
    c. In most cases, despite dissection and incision of tissues that appear inelastic, most patients require incision with grafting.
    d. Correction is facilitated by tourniquet occlusion during artificial erection.

55. With regard to acquired curvatures of the penis that are not Peyronie's disease, which of the following statements is true?

    a. Most are characterized by prominent dorsal scars.
    b. In most cases, global cavernosal veno-occlusive dysfunction (CVOD) is not a complicating factor.
    c. They are virtually never associated with "minimal" buckling trauma.
    d. Patients often have significant complaints of penile foreshortening.

Answers

1. **c. The dermal layer has two sublayers.** In the case of the skin as a model, the superficial layer of the skin is termed the *epidermis* (thickness 0.8 to 1.0 mm). The deep layer of the skin is termed the *dermis*. The dermis has two layers: a superficial layer, or the adventitial dermis (also called the papillary or periadnexal dermis, depending on the anatomy), and the deep layer, or the reticular dermis. [p 3887]

2. **a. They are a function of the collagen-elastin architecture as it is suspended in a mucopolysaccharide matrix.** All tissue has inherent physical characteristics, and those are extensibility, inherent tissue tension, and vesicoelastic properties of stress relaxation and creep. The physical characteristics of a transferred unit are primarily a function of the helical arrangement of collagen along with the elastin cross-linkages. The collagen-elastin architecture is suspended in a mucopolysaccharide matrix that influences the vesicoelastic properties. [p 3887]

3. **b. A graft is tissue that is excised from a donor site and then re-establishes its blood supply by revascularization.** Tissue can be transferred as a graft (see Fig. 110–1). The term *graft* implies that tissue has been excised and transferred to a graft host bed, where a new blood supply develops via a process that has been termed *take*. Take requires approximately 96 hours and occurs in two phases. The initial phase, termed *imbibition*, takes about 48 hours, and during that phase the graft survives by drinking nutrients from the adjacent graft host bed. During that phase, the graft temperature is less than body temperature. The second phase, termed *inosculation*, also requires about 48 hours and is the phase during which true microcirculation is re-established in

the graft. During that phase, the temperature of the graft rises to core body temperature. The process of take is influenced both by the nature of the grafted tissue and by the conditions of the graft host bed. Processes that interfere with the vascularity of the graft host bed thus interfere with graft take. [pp 3887–3888]

4. **b. The subdermal plexus is carried at the juncture of the deep dermis and the underlying tissue.** At approximately that interface is the superficial plexus. In the case of skin as a model, the plexus is the intradermal plexus. There are some lymphatics in the superficial dermal or tunica layer. In the deep dermal layer or deep lamina, the deep plexus is carried. In the case of skin, this is the subdermal plexus. In that layer are most of the lymphatics, and the collagen content of that layer is much greater than in the superficial dermal layer. The reticular dermis is generally thought to account for the physical characteristics of the tissue. [p 3888]

5. **d. A full-thickness skin graft is fastidious because of the nature of the subdermal plexus, among other variables.** If a graft is carried as a full-thickness unit (FTG), it carries the covering. It carries the superficial dermis or lamina with all of the characteristics attributable to that layer. In most cases, the plexus (subdermal plexus) is composed of larger vessels that are more sparsely distributed. The graft is thus fastidious in its vascular characteristics. [p 3888]

6. **c. Buccal mucosa graft is thought to have a panlaminar plexus.** In the case of the buccal mucosal graft, there is a panlaminar plexus. In the case of the bladder epithelial graft (see Fig. 110–1 *B*), there is a superficial and a deep plexus; however, the plexuses are connected by many more perforators. The dermal graft for years has been used to augment the tunica albuginea. Mature vein grafts show evidence of take to the vasa vasorum. [pp 3887–3889]

7. **d. A flap without a defined cuticular vascular territory is termed a random flap.** The term *flap* implies that the tissue is excised and transferred with the blood supply either preserved or surgically re-established at the recipient site. When one refers to terms of tissue transfer, the term *graft* implies a specific unit of transfer, and thus terms such as *pedicle graft* or *free graft* are confusing. It is best to avoid these terms when discussing tissue transfer. A random flap is a flap without a defined cuticular vascular territory. [p 3889]

8. **b. An island flap would by definition be an axial flap.** A peninsula flap is a flap in which the vascular and the cutaneous continuity of the flap base are left intact. An island flap (see Fig. 110–3 *B*) is a flap in which the vascular continuity is maintained; however, the cuticular continuity is divided. The microvascular free transfer flap (free flap) (see Fig. 110–3 *C*) has both the vascular continuity and the cuticular continuity interrupted. The vascular continuity is then re-established at the recipient site. A true island flap would be elevated on dangling vessels. [pp 3889–3890]

9. **b. The erectile tissues of the normal corpora cavernosa are separated from the tunica by the space of Smith.** The corpora cavernosa are not separate structures but constitute a single space with free communication through an incompetent midline septum, composed of multiple strands of elastic tissue similar to that making up the tunica albuginea. The erectile tissue is separated from the tunica albuginea by a thin layer of areolar connective tissue that was described by Smith. [p 3890]

10. **b. The bulbous urethral portion is invested by the thickest portion of the corpus spongiosum.** The fossa navicularis is contained within the spongy erectile tissue of the glans penis and terminates at the junction of the urethral epithelium with the skin of the glans. The bulbous urethra is covered by the midline fusion of the ischiocavernosus musculature and is invested by the bulbospongiosum and corpus spongiosum. It becomes larger and lies closer to the dorsal aspect of the corpus spongiosum, exiting from its dorsal surface prior to the posterior attachment of the bulbospongiosum to the perineal body. The membranous urethra is the portion that traverses the perineal pouch and is surrounded by the external urethral sphincter. This segment of the urethra is unattached to fixed structures, has the distinction of being the only portion of the male urethra that is not invested by another structure, and is lined with a delicate transitional epithelium. [pp 3891–3892]

11. **c. It allows for elevation of the skin on its random blood supply while carrying skin islands on the fascia.** Blood is supplied to the skin of the penis by the left and right superficial external pudendal vessels. A flap of skin may be elevated, and the fascia containing its blood supply can be mobilized, to create a subcutaneous pedicle allowing distal islands of preputial or penile skin to be transferred to virtually any part of the urethra. [pp 3892–3893]

12. **d. The deep system, which includes the crural and cavernosal veins, drains to the periprostatic plexus and to the femoral/iliac veins.** The superficial veins are contained in the dartos fascia on the dorsolateral aspects of the penis. The intermediate system contains the deep dorsal and circumflex veins, lying within and beneath Buck's fascia. The deep dorsal vein is formed by five to eight small veins emerging from the glans penis to form the retrocoronal plexus. The deep drainage system consists of the crural and cavernosal veins. The crural veins arise in the midline, in the space between the crura. Normally, they are small and almost indiscernible, joining the deep dorsal vein or the periprostatic plexus. Three or four small cavernosal veins emerge from the dorsolateral surface of each crus and course laterally between the bulbospongiosum and the crus of the penis for 2 to 3 cm, before draining into the internal pudendal veins. [pp 3893–3894]

13. **b. It consists of the common penile artery and its distal branches.** The blood supply to the deep structures of the penis is derived from the common penile artery, which is a continuation of the internal pudendal artery after it gives off its perineal branch. [p 3894]

14. **c. The dorsal nerve arises in Alcock's canal as a branch of the nerve there.** The cavernosal nerves are a combination of the parasympathetic and visceral afferent fibers that constitute the autonomic nerves of the penis. These provide the nerve supply to the erectile apparatus. The pudendal nerves enter the perineum with the internal pudendal vessels through the lesser sciatic notch at the posterior border of the ischiorectal fossa. They run in the fibrofascial pudendal canal of Alcock to the edge of the urogenital diaphragm (see Fig. 110–10 *A*). Each dorsal nerve of the penis arises in Alcock's canal as the first branch of the pudendal nerve. On the shaft, their fascicles fan out to supply proprioceptive and sensory nerve terminals in the tunica of the corpora cavernosa and sensory terminals in the skin. [pp 3895, 3896]

15. **c. Colles' fascia joins with the dartos fascia (tunica dartos) of the scrotum.** Colles' fascia joins with the dartos fascia (tunica dartos) of the scrotum, and a fold of this fascia projects backward beneath the fibers of the bulbospongiosus muscle. Anteriorly, Colles' fascia fuses and becomes continuous with the membranous layer of the subcutaneous con-

nective tissue of the anterior abdominal wall (Scarpa's fascia). [p 3898]

16. **a. The ischiocavernosus muscles laterally attach to the inner surface of the ischium and insert in the midline into Buck's fascia.** The ischiocavernosus muscles cover the crura of the corpora cavernosa. They attach to the inner surfaces of the ischium and ischial tuberosities on each side and insert at the midline into Buck's fascia, surrounding the crura at their junction below the arcuate ligament of the penis. The bulbospongiosus muscles are located in the midline of the perineum. They are attached to the perineal body posteriorly, and to each other in the midline, as they encompass the bulbospongiosum and crura of the corpora cavernosa at the base of the penis. These muscles are confluent with the ischiocavernosus muscles laterally, and at their insertion into Buck's fascia. [p 3898]

17. **d. In Reiter's syndrome, the urethritis is usually mild and self-limiting.** Because all reported cases of urethral hemangioma have been benign, management is dependent on the size and location of the lesion. For smaller lesions, laser treatment has been successful and produces less scarring. The preferred treatment for larger lesions is open excision and urethral reconstruction. Reiter's syndrome is characterized by a classic triad of arthritis, conjunctivitis, and urethritis. Urethral involvement is usually mild, self-limiting, and a minor portion of the disease. [p 3900]

18. **b. BXO is one, if not the most frequent, cause of meatal stenosis.** BXO is the term used to describe genital lichen sclerosus et atrophicus in the male. The most common cause of meatal stenosis, BXO appears as a whitish plaque that may involve the prepuce, glans penis, urethral meatus, and fossa navicularis. Several reports have suggested the association with chronic infection by a spirochetal infection, *Borrelia burgdorferi*. Although previously thought to be rare, BXO is commonly found at the time of circumcisions performed beyond the neonatal period. Long-term antibiotic therapy may also be helpful to improve the inflammation because secondary infection of the inflamed tissue may occur. We have typically used tetracycline, but a trial of long-term penicillin (or advanced-generation erythromycin) may be warranted. [p 3900]

19. **b. Fistulas often recur, not because of a problem at the fistula site but because of stenosis or obstruction distal to the fistula site.** Treatment of a urethral fistula must be directed not only toward the defect but also the underlying process leading to its development. In cases of urethral reconstruction, especially reconstruction for hypospadias, fistula often occurs or recurs because of distal obstruction and high-pressure voiding. After urethral surgery, fistulas can develop immediately or as delayed complications. Repair of the fistula may be delayed at a minimum of 6 months to allow for complete resolution of the inflammation. [p 3901]

20. **a. Urethral fistula, not associated with a history of urethral reconstruction, can be the initial presenting symptom of urethral carcinoma.** Fistulas associated with inflammatory strictures occur as periurethral tracts and develop secondary to high-pressure voiding of infected urine. Repair requires suprapubic drainage, and treatment of the infection requires incision and drainage of any abscesses present. One must be very cautious in treating the patient with urethral fistulas but without a chronic history of obstructive voiding symptoms. In many cases, fistula or periurethral abscess may be the hallmark symptom of urethral carcinoma. In males, a congenital urethral diverticulum may result from incomplete development of the urethra, with a defect in only the ventral wall and subsequent distention. A congenital diverticulum in the prostatic urethra may be a large remnant of the müllerian duct associated with defects of diminished virilization. [pp 3902–3903]

21. **c. When ammoniacal meatitis is noted, often a short course of meatal dilatation and steroid cream application will resolve the problem.** Meatal stenosis in the male child appears to be a consequence of circumcision, which allows for ammoniacal meatitis. In children seen with ammoniacal meatitis, we usually start them with meatal dilatation using steroid cream. Within a week, the process seems to settle down. Anecdotally, the fusion of the ventral meatal skin, which causes meatal stenosis, seems to be avoided. [p 3904]

22. **b. Not uncommonly, patients who had their initial operations in the 1960s or 1970s will still have significant dorsal hooded skin, which can be useful for subsequent repairs.** Many of these patients will have persistent chordee and a subcoronal meatus. In an older patient, a reliable preoperative assessment of residual chordee can be made on the basis of history and photographs taken at home. Patients who were initially operated on before the late 1970s likely underwent either a graft or some form of repair using almost exclusively ventral tissue. Some of these patients will still have the remnants of a dorsal hood or enough dorsal skin to perform a dorsal transverse penile skin island type of reconstruction. We believe that surgical correction of complex cases requires an aggressive approach by the surgeon. [p 3907]

23. **c. If urethral transposition of the epispadiac urethra is being considered, care must be taken in dissecting proximally to avoid injury to the corpus spongiosum.** Relative shortening, dorsal chordee, and sometimes torsion of the penis may be caused by one or more of the following factors: (1) inelastic fibrous bands of scar tissue that attach the penis to the bone or fascia in the anterior part of the ring of the pelvis; (2) shortness of a dorsally placed native urethra or shortness and possible scarring of a previously constructed neourethra; (3) inelasticity of abnormal attachments of the deeper dartos and Buck's fascial layers; (4) dysgenetic development or inelasticity of the dorsal aspect of the tunica albuginea of the paired corpora cavernosa. When making the decision to divide an adequate urethra, albeit tethering, a number of factors must be considered, including how to reconstruct the resultant urethral defect, realizing that tubed repairs are always less than optimal. In addition, one must realize that tubed graft repairs are always less adequate and fraught with short-term and late complications compared with tubed flap procedures. This tissue of the proximal corpus spongiosum lies deep to the urethra in the midline, between the divergent proximal ends of the corporal bodies. Bleeding from the thin-walled venous spaces of the corpus spongiosum may be troublesome if entered and, if transposing the urethra is contemplated, could adversely affect vascularity. [p 3909]

24. **d. The McRoberts technique of macro-replantation is not the preferred method of management for these patients, but when the situation warrants it, it is very successful.** Often, the amputation is self-inflicted, usually during an acute psychotic break. This should not preclude reimplantation unless the patient adamantly refuses such treatment. Even then, with court order and/or the agreement of two or more surgeons, replantation may be undertaken. If so, replantation by the technique described by McRoberts should be carried out. His series and other series show that a high degree of success can be expected after replantation without microvascular reanastomosis. If the patient presents with the distal part having been disposed of or otherwise unavailable, the wound should be closed. Often the penis will have been

stretched out during the amputation, and an excess of skin will have been removed, leaving a length of intact but denuded shaft structures proximal to the amputation wound. We close the corporal bodies with 4-0 or 5-0 polydioxanone suture, spatulate the urethral meatus to the tunica, and immediately cover the penile shaft with a split-thickness skin graft (STSG). If the testicles are avulsed as part of the injury, replantation is not usually an option because of stretch injury to the spermatic vessels. [p 3912]

25. **b. The eventual effect of a genital burn may be to unacceptably tether and/or incarcerate the penis.** The physiologic functions of genital tissues cannot be accurately duplicated. The unique vascularity of genital tissue allows for less aggressive rather than more aggressive débridement. In many patients, the penis will have become incarcerated in contracted scar tissue after healing of the acute injury. Successful transposition of a gracilis musculocutaneous flap introduces compliant vascular tissue and skin into the area, allowing release of the penile shaft. For coverage of large perineal or groin defects, the posterior thigh flap offers excellent bulky, sensate tissues. Therapeutic radiation can produce chronic suppurative gangrene. These lesions are not amenable to reconstruction. [pp 3913–3914]

26. **a. Reconstruction for lymphedema that is the consequence of the indirect effects of radiation is best accomplished with excision of the tissues and coverage with STSGs.** Patients with lymphedema can readily undergo reconstruction. When the lymphedematous tissue has been excised, the testicles will be free and, as in a degloving injury, they must be fixed in the midline in an anatomically correct position. The shaft of the penis should be covered with a STSG. If the scrotum cannot be closed, a meshed STSG is utilized to cover the testicles, as described. Not uncommonly, these patients have hydroceles, the parietal tunica vaginalis must be excised, and grafting can be done directly onto the visceral tunica vaginalis of the testicles. Unlike the FTSG, split-thickness skin carries little of the reticular dermis and hence few of the lymphatic channels. Reaccumulation of lymphedema will occur within a FTSG and can recur in a thick split-thickness graft. Local skin flaps should be avoided, as they seldom give good cosmetic results. [pp 3914–3915]

27. **d. It causes limitation of the urethral lumen because of contraction and noncompliance of the scar.** The term *urethral stricture* generally refers to anterior urethral disease, or a scarring process involving the spongy erectile tissue of the corpus spongiosum. In some cases, the scarring process extends through the tissues of the corpus spongiosum and into adjacent tissues. Contraction of this scar reduces the urethral lumen. [p 3915]

28. **c. It is not a true stricture but rather fibrosis that results from distraction of the urethra.** Posterior urethral "strictures" are not included in the common definition of urethral stricture. Posterior urethral stricture is an obliterative process of the posterior urethra that has resulted in fibrosis and is generally the effect of distraction in that area. Although the distraction defect can be lengthy in some cases, the actual process involving the tissues of the urethra is usually confined. [p 3915]

29. **d. Crushing trauma to the bulbous urethra.** Any process that injures the urethral epithelium and/or the underlying corpus spongiosum to the point that healing results in a scar can cause anterior urethral stricture. Today, most urethral strictures are the result of trauma (usually straddle trauma). We are, however, seeing an increase in strictures associated with BXO, and those strictures clearly behave much more like inflammatory strictures than traumatically induced isolated scars. Inflammatory strictures associated with gonorrhea were most commonly seen in the past. The place of chlamydia and *Ureaplasma urealyticum* in the development of anterior urethral strictures is not clear. [p 3916]

30. **a. They are usually associated with scarring extending deeply into the corpus spongiosum.** Some evidence suggests that the progression of the stricture to eventually involve the entire anterior urethra may be due to high-pressure voiding that causes intravasation of urine into the glands of Littre, inflammation of these glands, and, perhaps, microabscesses and deep spongiofibrosis. Whether the urethral changes and eventual fibrosis are also related to bacterial injury, to our knowledge, has not been well defined. Literature does not show resolution of the stricture process with the use of antibiotics. [p 3916]

31. **c. Optimal management may mean placement of a suprapubic catheter.** When a patient cannot void, an attempt is made to pass a urethral catheter. If the catheter does not pass, the nature of the obstruction is determined via dynamic retrograde urethrography. Thus, most cases are managed with acute dilatation, and clearly there are many instances in which this is not the best course for the patient. When there is doubt, we determine the nature of the stricture when possible, and not uncommonly we place a suprapubic cystostomy catheter to treat the acute situation and allow time for a more appropriate treatment plan to be devised. Although detailed imaging is not always available, flexible endoscopy is almost universally available. [p 3917]

32. **a. MRI.** To devise an appropriate treatment plan, it is important to determine the location, length, depth, and density of the stricture (spongiofibrosis). The length and location of the stricture can be determined using radiographs, urethroscopy, and ultrasonography. The depth and density of the scar in the spongy tissue can be deduced from the physical examination, the appearance of the urethra in contrast studies, the amount of elasticity noted on urethroscopy, and the depth and density of fibrosis as evidenced by ultrasonographic evaluation of the urethra, although the absolute length of spongiofibrosis may not be evident on ultrasonographic evaluation. [p 3917]

33. **c. Contrast material suitable for intravenous injection should be used for all retrograde urethral studies.** Extravasation during retrograde urethrography is possible in patients in whom the urethra is markedly inflamed. For this reason, contrast studies should be carried out with contrast material that is suitable for intravenous injection. Contrast materials that have been thickened with lubricating jelly can be a source of problems and offer little benefit. Real-time ultrasonographic evaluation of the urethra after it has been filled with a lubricating jelly or saline has been described by McAninch. If the patient is not in a steep lateral oblique position for the retrograde urethrogram, the length of stricture will be underestimated. [p 3918]

34. **a. Even if a patient does not have retention, placement of a suprapubic tube may help define strictured areas.** In selected patients, we have found it useful to place a suprapubic tube to defunctionalize the urethra. After 6 to 8 weeks, if there is going to be constriction of an area that was hydrodilated with voiding, the tendency for that constriction to occur should become apparent. It is imperative, however, to completely evaluate the urethra proximal and distal to the stricture with endoscopy and bougienage during surgery, to ensure that all of the involved urethra is included in the reconstruction. Whereas hydraulic pressure generated by voiding may keep segments proximal to the stricture patent, unless these segments are included in the repair, they

are at risk for contraction after obstruction of the narrow caliber segment is relieved with reconstruction. For this reason, any abnormal areas of the urethra that are proximal to a narrow caliber segment of the stricture must be treated with suspicion. If the lumen does not appear to demonstrate evidence of diminished compliance, then we presume that area to be uninvolved in active stricture disease. However, coning down of the urethra suggests its involvement in the scar. [pp 3918–3919]

35. **b. It can be associated with the creation of erectile dysfunction.** Many surgeons have learned to perform internal urethrotomy by making a single incision at the 12-o'clock position. This location might be questioned, however, based on the location of the urethra within the corpus spongiosum. Distally, although the anterior aspect of the corpus spongiosum is thicker, a deep incision in the more distal aspects of the anterior urethra will certainly enter the corpora cavernosa, and these incisions have been associated with the creation of erectile dysfunction. The most common complication of internal urethrotomy is recurrence of stricture. Less commonly noted complications of internal urethrotomy include bleeding and extravasation of irrigation fluid into the perispongiosal tissues. One report using actuarial techniques showed the curative success rate of internal urethrotomy to be approximately 20%. Other evaluations showed the curative success rate of direct visual internal urethrotomy to be approximately 30% to 35%. The data showed that strictures at the bulbous urethra that are less than 1.5 cm in length and not associated with dense, deep spongiofibrosis (i.e., straddle injuries) can be managed with internal urethrotomy with a 74% moderately long-term success rate. Pansadora's study did not have any long-term successes for treated strictures outside the bulbous urethra. [pp 3919–3920]

36. **a. Available data show that these stents are best employed for short bulbous urethral strictures associated with minimal spongiofibrosis.** Removable urethral stents are designed to prevent the process of epithelialization from incorporating the stent into the urethral wall and are left in place for as long as 6 months to a year before they are removed. The greatest experience with these removable stents comes from Israel, and centers there report good success in small series. The majority of experience with permanently implantable stents comes from Europe and the United Kingdom. One study reported a success rate of 84% at 4.5 years using the permanently implantable Urolume. Available data show that the stent is best employed for relatively short strictures of the bulbous urethra associated with minimal spongiofibrosis. Some patients (particularly young patients) complain of perineal pain, often with vigorous activity, even following implantation of the stent in the deep bulbous urethra. [p 3920]

37. **c. Patients with short strictures of the bulbous urethra that are not associated with significant spongiofibrosis.** There are also specific contraindications to the use of the Urolume. Patients who have undergone prior substitution urethral reconstruction, particularly when skin has been incorporated into the urethra, have been shown to be poor candidates for implantation with the Urolume stent. Patients who fall into this category are those who have had urethral distraction injuries and straddle injuries associated with deep fibrosis. The product insert clearly contraindicates the use of the Urolume in patients with posterior urethral distraction defects. Some centers in Europe are now advocating the use of the Urolume only in patients who are older than 50 years of age and/or who have other significant medical problems that make the option of lengthy open urethral reconstruction less appealing. [pp 3920–3921]

38. **d. The holmium:YAG laser has significant vaporizing as well as cutting properties with little forward scatter.** For both the argon and Nd:YAG lasers, the predominant mode of action is thermal necrosis, which leads to a significant potential for peripheral tissue injury rather than vaporization. The Nd:YAG laser has also been used with a bare fiber in the contact mode. A bare fiber carries with it a risk of forward scatter. Advocates of the use of a contact laser suggest that it obliterates the scar via vaporization; however, results of using these fibers are no better than those using direct cold knife visual internal urethrotomy. A KTP laser is essentially a Nd:YAG laser that has passed through a KTP crystal, resulting in a reduced depth of penetration. The holmium:YAG laser has similar properties to the KTP laser, and like the KTP laser, provides both direct contact cutting and vaporization with minimal forward scatter. Experience is accumulating with the use of the holmium:YAG laser, and anecdotally, it may have a place in the management of some strictures, in particular strictures that are relatively isolated and short. The excimer laser is a true vaporizing laser that has little forward scatter or peripheral tissue necrosis associated with it. There has been little experience reported with the use of this laser. [pp 3922–3923]

39. **c. Success requires total excision of the fibrosis with a widely spatulated anastomosis.** It has now been demonstrated with certainty that the most dependable technique of anterior urethral reconstruction is the complete excision of the area of fibrosis, with a primary reanastomosis of the normal ends of the anterior urethra. The best results are achieved when the following technical points are observed: (1) the area of fibrosis is totally excised; (2) the urethral anastomosis is widely spatulated, creating a large ovoid anastomosis; and (3) the anastomosis is tension-free. With vigorous mobilization, development of the intercrural space, and detachment of the bulbospongiosum from the perineal body, significant lengths of stricture can be excised and reanastomosed. For very proximal short bulbous strictures, tension-free anastomosis can be facilitated by the dissection of the membranous urethra. As a rule, the closer the stricture is to the membranous urethra, the longer it can be and still be reconstructed via anastomotic techniques. [pp 3923–3924]

40. **b. The excision with strip anastomosis technique can be used with graft onlay techniques.** Four grafts that have been used for urethral reconstruction are the FTSG, the STSG, the bladder epithelial graft, and the buccal mucosal graft. The use of the spongioplasty procedure requires that the corpus spongiosum adjacent to the area of the stricture be relatively normal and free of fibrosis. We prefer the use of a lateral urethrostomy or dorsal graft onlay. In that modification, the urethrostomy is through the stricture on the dorsal wall. A graft is then applied, spread fixed, in the area of the urethrostomy to the triangular ligament and/or corpora cavernosa. In turn, the edges of the stricture are then sutured to the edges of the graft as well as the adjacent structures. The dorsal graft onlay technique can be utilized with stricture excision and strip anastomosis (augmented anastomotic procedure). [pp 3924–3926]

41. **b. The operations can conceptually become one operation with multidimensional application.** A number of applications of genital skin islands, mobilized on either the dartos fascia of the penis or the tunica dartos of the scrotum, have been proposed for repair of urethral stricture disease. In the past, these flap operations were considered to be separate procedures. We suggest that all of these procedures are really different applications of a single concept, proposed by the microinjection studies of Quartey. Skin islands, as mentioned, can be viewed as passengers on fascial flaps, and the

design of flaps for urethral reconstruction can be paralleled to the design of flaps for reconstruction in general. These procedures utilizing skin islands oriented on the penile dartos fascia have been also useful for reconstruction of the fossa navicularis. There are three important considerations for the use of flaps in urethral reconstruction: (1) the nature of the flap tissue; (2) the vasculature of the flap; and (3) the mechanics of flap transfer. The skin must be nonhirsute for urethral reconstruction. In addition, for donor site consideration, it is most convenient to use the areas of redundant nonhirsute genital skin. [p 3926]

42. **d. The length of tubed segments can be limited by the aggressive mobilization of the corpus spongiosum.** The literature has made it clear that onlay procedures (graft or flap) are attended with a higher success rate than are tubularized grafts or tubularized skin islands. Tubularized grafts and skin islands should therefore be avoided, if possible. When tubularized segments cannot be avoided, the length of these segments can be limited by combining aggressive mobilization and excision. Tubularized flaps, without question, provide better results than tubularized grafts. [p 3929]

43. **c. Because BXO is a generalized skin condition, buccal mucosa has been considered for reconstruction with initial encouraging results.** Special mention must be made regarding reconstruction for strictures associated with BXO. With the advent of flap techniques, many centers embraced these techniques for these strictures. However, analysis of results of these patients from several large centers has shown a very high recurrence rate. Because of that, these centers adjusted by applying staged graft techniques. Interestingly, staged graft techniques using skin grafts again had a very high recurrence rate on a number of analyses. It is theorized that because BXO is a skin condition, the use of skin as a flap, a single-stage graft, or a staged graft does not preclude involvement of the skin with the BXO inflammatory process. At the time of this writing, this center has completed a cursory assessment of our series of patients with BXO-associated strictures who underwent reconstruction with flap-skin island techniques and skin graft. Preliminary results at our center are not as dismal as from other centers, but the success rate is clearly less (approximately 60%) than for non-BXO-associated strictures. At present, a number of centers now believe that, for reconstruction of strictures associated with BXO, staged buccal graft techniques should be employed. Short follow-up suggests better success with this approach. [p 3930]

44. **b. Although they can involve any part of the membranous urethra, most frequently occur at the juncture of the membranous urethra with the bulbous urethra.** Urethral distraction injuries are the result of blunt pelvic trauma and accompany about 10% of pelvic fracture injuries. Although it is possible to totally disrupt the urethra with a straddle injury, these injuries most commonly involve only the bulbous urethra. Distraction injuries of the membranous urethra have been compared to plucking an apple (prostate) off its stem (the membranous urethra). This analogy implies that the injury most frequently occurs at the apex of the prostate. Experience shows that this is not the case, however, and the most frequent point of distraction is at the departure of the membranous urethra from the bulbospongiosum. In the postpubescent male, the injury seldom involves the prostatic urethra. In the prepubescent male, in whom the prostatic urethra is more fragile, the injury can extend into that area. Many injuries appear not to totally distract the entire circumference of the urethra. Instead, a strip of epithelium is left intact. In these patients, the placement of an aligning catheter may allow the urethra to heal virtually unscarred or with an easily managed stricture. Because of flexible endoscopy equipment, placement of an aligning catheter is relatively straightforward. Because of the ready availability of flexible cystoscopes, some centers are now evaluating acutely these injuries only with endoscopy. Aligning catheters are just what the name implies, a guide, not a mechanism, for placing traction on the bladder and prostate. [p 3930]

45. **a. Best first evaluated with contrast-enhanced studies.** Although location of the distraction injury has been demonstrated to be an important factor in continence after reconstruction, this information should be a factor only in patient counseling before the reconstruction and not in the treatment approach. The length of the defect is an important consideration and must be determined as precisely as possible. Lack of contrast material in the posterior urethra gives some information, albeit inconclusive, about the integrity of the bladder neck. When the patient is successfully relaxing to void and the cystogram outlines the posterior urethra, a simultaneous retrograde urethrogram nicely outlines the length of the distraction defect. However, this situation is the exception rather than the rule, and retrograde urethrograms are most useful for determining whether the anterior urethra is normal. If the anterior urethra is normal, it has been our experience as well as others' that a successful anastomotic repair is ensured. In fact, a primary anastomosis has been shown to be possible even with some involvement of the anterior urethra. Thus, primary anastomosis is unquestionably the goal in all of these patients until it is proved impossible to do. When the proximal urethra is not visualized on simultaneous cystogram with urethrogram, endoscopy through the suprapubic tract in combination with retrograde urethrogram can be used to outline the defect. [p 3931]

46. **c. It can often be done distal to the external sphincter.** The timetable for reconstruction of distraction defects is determined by the type and extent of associated injuries. In the majority of cases, distraction injuries are not long, and the resultant obliteration is amenable to a technically straightforward mobilization of the corpus spongiosum with a primary anastomotic technique. The classic reconstruction consists of a spatulated anastomosis of the proximal anterior urethra to the apical prostatic urethra. Experience has demonstrated, however, that anastomosis of the proximal anterior urethra to any segment of the posterior urethra can be successfully accomplished using a widely spatulated anastomosis in which optimal epithelial apposition is achieved. Use of a transpubic or an abdominal perineal approach is not necessary for the reconstruction of distraction injuries. Also, the use of pubectomy can be associated with long-term sequelae, which include shortening of the penis, destabilization of erection, and destabilization of the pelvis, resulting in a chronic pain syndrome with exercise. [pp 3931–3933]

47. **d. Continence is best addressed after a procedure to re-establish urethral continuity is performed.** We have found, and others have reported, that the competence of the bladder neck is difficult to accurately assess before the re-establishment of urethral continuity. Even in cases in which an obvious scar is noted to involve the bladder neck, follow-up of these patients after the urethral reconstruction establishes continuity of the urethra has found many patients with more than adequate continence. Still other patients are believed to have incontinence due to scar incarceration of the bladder neck. In our experience, however, this is an infrequent occurrence, and the appearance of the bladder neck by any modality available is not predictive of continence. It is currently our practice to re-establish the continuity of the urethra, and in cases in which there are concerns about conti-

nence, forewarn the patient before the urethral reconstruction. [p 3933]

48. **d. All of the above.** Development of the intracrural space, mobilization of the corpus spongiosum, infrapubectomy, and, if needed, rerouting of the corpus spongiosum all shorten the course that the corpus spongiosum must traverse and allow for reconstruction without attendant chordee. [pp 3935–3936]

49. **b. Flexible endoscopy.** At approximately 6 months, and again at 1 year, postoperatively, the patients are evaluated with a flexible endoscope. At that time we consider the reconstruction to be mature, and it should be widely patent. In the absence of the reappearance of symptoms, no further routine follow-up is done. We have almost completely replaced postoperative retrograde studies with the use of flexible endoscopy. We have not found flow studies to be valuable in following these patients and have found in many cases (anterior urethral reconstruction) that retrograde urethrography was more confusing than helpful. [p 3937]

50. **d. Patients with reconstitution of an injured pudendal vessel, even if reconstitution was a unilateral phenomenon, are excellent candidates for posterior urethral reconstruction.** With the techniques discussed, or similar techniques, curative rates for reconstruction of posterior urethral distraction injuries are in the high 90% range. Failures are not, in large centers, due to technical problems (i.e., anastomotic restenosis). In general, failures are indicative of ischemia of the proximal corpus spongiosum with ensuing stenosis of the mobilized corpus spongiosum. We found that many patients had evidence of either unilateral or bilateral pudendal artery lesions but that most had evidence of vascular reconstitution. We found that patients with an intact pudendal artery on one side often were potent and were reliably cured with reconstruction. We found that patients with only reconstituted vessels, either unilateral or bilateral, never were potent but were reliably reconstructed. [pp 3937–3938]

51. **d. All of the above.** Using the maneuvers outlined above, we have found that virtually all distraction injuries can be reconstructed via a perineal approach using an anastomotic technique. We have therefore abandoned a transpubic approach as applied to posterior urethral distraction injuries. We have found that the endoscopic management of urethral distraction defects is not a simple procedure and must be undertaken by a skilled and experienced surgeon. Many of these procedures can be categorized as a "cut for light" procedure. Although there are surgeons who report success, the majority of these procedures are not done with sufficient precision to allow for adequate realignment of the urethra. We have seen many disasters that have resulted from these procedures, and in most cases we condemn the use of these modalities. In addition, no cut for light series compares favorably, with regard to long-term success rates, with series from large centers that use primary anastomotic techniques. Patients whose medical condition, age, or concomitant orthopedic injury prevents them from being placed in the exaggerated lithotomy position and/or undergoing reconstruction via a transpubic approach may be managed with this technique. [p 3940]

52. **c. The term *congenital curvature of the penis*** is reserved for cases in which there is solitary, relative asymmetric compliance of the tunica albuginea of the corpus spongiosum. In some patients, there is an intimate association between congenital curvature and the hypospadias anomaly. There is a spectrum of penetrance, and the hypospadias anomaly can represent a spectrum from a perineal location of the meatus, with total malfusion of the ventral tissues involving the scrotum and the shaft of the penis, to a normally located urethral meatus, fused preputial skin, and apparently properly fused ventral penile skin, but persistent abnormalities of the fascial layers or corpus spongiosum. In type I congenital curvature, the urethral meatus is at the tip of the glans. None of the surrounding layers are normally formed, however, and the epithelial urethra is associated with malfusion of the corpus spongiosum and all of the tissues superficial to the urethra. Skin coverage of the epithelial tube is present. In type II, a dysgenetic band of fibrous tissue thought to be derived from the mesenchyma, which would have produced Buck's fascia and the dartos fascia, lies beneath and lateral to the urethra. However, the urethra is contained within a normally developed and fused corpus spongiosum. In type III, the urethra, corpus spongiosum, and Buck's fascia are all normally developed and ventrally fused. However, there is a short area of inelastic tissue in the dartos layer of the penis that causes a relatively sharp bend. In type IV, although the urethra, corpus spongiosum, and fascial layers are normally developed, there is relative shortness or inelasticity of one aspect of the tunica albuginea of the corpora cavernosa. Experience has shown that most patients whose congenital curvature is type IV seem to actually demonstrate evidence of a hypercompliance of the tunica albuginea. Type V congenital curvature is also known as the congenital short urethra. If type V congenital curvature exists at all, it occurs so rarely that when it is encountered one should doubt the findings. The congenital curvatures types I, II, and III all represent forms of the hypospadias anomaly, and we prefer to refer them collectively under the term chordee without hypospadias. We prefer to refer to the type IV anomaly as congenital curvature of the penis. Although, as mentioned, the type V anomaly is so rarely encountered that it deserves its own diagnosis, we believe its correction is best discussed with types I, II, and III, under the category of chordee without hypospadias. [pp 3942–3943]

53. **c. There is a stepwise progression of ventral dissection of dysgenetic tissues, correction of skin tethering, elevation of mobilization of the corpus spongiosum, midline ventral septotomy, and often dorsal plication.** Patients with chordee without hypospadias usually present with either ventral curvature or ventral curvature associated with torsion. In many cases, there are abnormalities of the ventral penile skin. In patients who have chordee without hypospadias, the photograph will reveal an erect penis commensurate with the size of the detumesced penis, whereas in the congenital curvature patient, the erect penis will be noticeably large. Many of our patients are also evaluated preoperatively by our sex therapy colleague. Because of their congenital anomaly, these patients often become relatively reclusive and have poor self and genital images. Even in patients with obvious abnormalities of the corpus spongiosum (i.e., poor ventral fusion or frank bifid corpus spongiosum), wide mobilization usually reveals that it is not the corpus spongiosum that remains as the ventral limiting factor. In most patients, the penis will remain curved due to the inelasticity of the ventral aspect of the corpora cavernosa themselves. If the epithelial tube has served as an adequate urethra (i.e., it is not stenotic), the morbidity of urethral division and subsequent need for urethral reconstruction must be considered before undertaking such a procedure. In children, after mobilization and excision of the dysgenetic tissues, the residual chordee can usually be corrected by making a longitudinal incision with a sharp blade. If this maneuver is not sufficient, the dorsal neurovascular structures can be mobilized in concert with Buck's fascia, and a small ellipse or ellipses of dorsal tunica albuginea excised and closed with watertight plicating sutures. [pp 3943–3945]

54. **a. If length is an issue, the patient probably is more correctly characterized as having chordee without hypospadias.** Patients with congenital curvature of the penis can have ventral, lateral (which is most often to the left), and/or unusually dorsal curvature. Patients usually present as otherwise healthy young men between the ages of 18 and 30. Many of these patients will have noticed curvature before puberty but will have presumed it to be normal. With puberty, however, they discover that the curvature is not normal. We do not routinely recommend a tourniquet device because constricting devices can conceal the proximal limits of the curvature. This is of most significance in cases of ventral curvatures that frequently extend proximal. In patients with ventral curvature, there may be some illusion of thickening of the dartos fascia and Buck's fascia, and in those patients, the fibrous tissue is mobilized and completely excised. After these tissues are excised, the artificial erection is repeated, and an occasional patient will have a completely straightened curvature. Most patients, however, suffer from a differential elasticity between the dorsal and ventral aspects of the corporal bodies, and although the curvature may have been lessened, it will persist, unless further procedures are done to straighten the penis. Because the size of the erect penis is usually not a problem in these cases of congenital curvature, we have chosen the second option. If the patient falls into the category of chordee without hypospadias, if shortness of the penis is an issue, we do not hesitate to use incisions with grafts to correct the curvature. [p 3945]

55. **b. In most cases, global cavernosal veno-occlusive dysfunction (CVOD) is not a complicating factor.** When a young man presents with an acquired curvature of the penis, one must always allow the possibility of Peyronie's disease. Occasionally, however, a patient or his initial care physician will ignore the stigmata of the trauma (often described as "minimal" by patients), and the patient will present with a noticeable lateral scar that causes both indentation of the lateral aspect of the penis and, in some cases, curvature. Patients who had preexisting lateral curvature may actually notice that their penis has been straightened by the trauma, but they are disturbed by the concavity caused by the scar. The pathology of a subclinical fracture of the penis is believed to be due to the disruption of the outer longitudinal layer of the tunica albuginea during the buckling trauma. These patients usually have normal erectile function, and there is no association with concomitant global CVOD. However, the association of CVOD and trauma of the penis continues to be seen, and some patients after fracture-type injuries of the penis will have significant problems with erectile dysfunction. These injuries are not associated with shortening of the penis. It is the lack of erectile dysfunction and penile shortening that help distinguish these patients from those with Peyronie's disease. Although foreshortening of the penis is not a characteristic of either the injury itself or the resulting scar in either of these injuries, these patients are not thought to be best treated by approaching the opposite aspect of the scar and excising an ellipse of the tunica. This would result in bilateral scars, which will cause bilateral indentations of the penis, and although the penis will have been straightened by the correction, most patients are upset by the cosmetic and functional result of a near-circumferential indentation of the penis. [pp 3946–3947]